ANNALS OF THE NEW YORK ACADEMY OF SCIENCES

Volume 872

EDITORIAL STAFF

Executive Editor
BILL M. BOLAND

Managing Editor
JUSTINE CULLINAN

Associate Editor
COOK KIMBALL

The New York Academy of Sciences
2 East 63rd Street
New York, New York 10021

HEMATOPOIETIC STEM CELLS
BIOLOGY AND TRANSPLANTATION

ANNALS OF THE NEW YORK ACADEMY OF SCIENCES
Volume 872

HEMATOPOIETIC STEM CELLS
BIOLOGY AND TRANSPLANTATION

Edited by Donald Orlic, Thomas A. Bock, and Lothar Kanz

The New York Academy of Sciences
New York, New York
1999

Cover: Neues Schloss, Meersburg, Germany, site of the conference.

Library of Congress Cataloging-in-Publication Data

Hematopoietic stem cells : biology and transplantation / edited by
Donald Orlic, Thomas A. Bock, and Lother Kanz.
      p.   cm. — (Annals of the New York Academy of Sciences, ISSN
0077-8923 ; v. 872)
      Includes bibliographical references and index.
      ISBN 1-57331-188-X (alk. paper). — ISBN 1-57331-189-8 (pbk. :
alk. paper)
      1. Hematopoietic stem cells Congresses.   2. Hematopoietic stem
cells—Transplantation Congresses.   I. Orlic, Donald.   II. Bock,
Thomas A.   III. Kanz, Lothar.   IV. New York Academy of Sciences.
V. Series.
      [DNLM: 1. Hematopoietic Stem Cells —physiology Congresses.
2. Hematopoietic Stem Cell Transplantation Congresses.   WH 380
H4875 1999 / W1 AN626YL v.872 1999]
Q11.N5 vol. 872
[QP92]
500 s—dc21
[612.4'1]
DNLM/DLC
for Library of Congress   99-26840
                                                                      CIP

GYAT / PCP
Printed in the United States of America
ISBN 1-57331-188-X (cloth)
ISBN 1-57331-189-8 (paper)
ISSN 0077-8923

ANNALS OF THE NEW YORK ACADEMY OF SCIENCES
Volume 872
April 30, 1999

HEMATOPOIETIC STEM CELLS
BIOLOGY AND TRANSPLANTATION[a]

Editors and Conference Chairs
DONALD ORLIC, THOMAS A. BOCK, AND LOTHAR KANZ

CONTENTS

[a]This volume contains the papers from a conference entitled *Hematopoietic Stem Cells II: International Symposium and Workshop*, which was hosted by the University of Tübingen in Meersburg, Germany on July 1–4, 1998.

Financial assistance was received from:
- AMGEN, GERMANY
- AMGEN, EUROPE
- KIRIN, JAPAN

Preface

This second International Symposium and Workshop on "Hematopoietic Stem Cells" was held on July 1–4, 1998 at the Neues Schloss, Meersburg, Germany. The conference was hosted by the University of Tübingen. A group of thirty-five basic and clinical scientists presented their latest *in vitro* and *in vivo* studies on hematopoietic stem cell (HSC) biology. These included new data on: 1) molecular controls, 2) microenvironment, 3) gene therapy, 4) animal models of hematopoiesis, and 5) clinical applications.

The concept that HSCs are immortal and possess multiple developmental capabilities has always intrigued researchers in this field. Data presented at this conference demonstrate that major insights into these fundamental characteristics of HSCs may soon be achieved. For example, the recently discovered suppressor of cytokine signaling (SOCS) proteins were shown to suppress differentiation of a blood cell line in response to cytokines. Molecular pathways such as this represent model systems that can be used for studies of HSC self-renewal and differentiation. Greater control of the molecular pathways that regulate self-renewal and commitment will enhance our ability to mobilize, expand and direct HSC differentiation and will ultimately result in improved therapy for malignancies. Advances in our capacity to induce HSC cycling will also improve prospects for gene therapy as a protocol for treating inherited blood cell disorders such as severe combined immunodeficiency and thalassemia.

Major advances were reported from investigations on the origin of hematopoietic cells from embryonic stem cells and from cells located in the yolk sac and aorta-gonad-mesonephros region of the developing embryo. It is likely that these studies will lead to a better understanding of how colonization of hematopoietic organs occurs in the developing fetus and how homing occurs in bone marrow transplant recipients. The egress of blood cells from bone marrow to the peripheral circulation is also under intense scrutiny and appears to result largely from an interaction between blood cells and factors secreted by stromal cells.

Progress in the early years of HSC biology was essentially directed towards the identification of a single, uniform population of cells. The heterogeneity within the HSC population did not become clear until cell sorting by flow cytometry was used to fractionate subpopulations of HSCs on the basis of surface markers. Although controversial, data presented at this conference demonstrated that in addition to the well characterized $CD34^+$ HSCs a subpopulation of $CD34^-$ HSCs can also be isolated from mouse and human bone marrow. Both mouse and human $CD34^-$ HSCs were able to repopulate the hematopoietic system when injected into adult mice and fetal sheep, respectively. Clarification of whether $CD34^+$ or $CD34^-$ HSCs are the more primitive subpopulation may require further analysis of their molecular behavior.

Continued development of analytical techniques such as single cell reverse transcription polymerase chain reaction (RT-PCR), as reported at this conference, may resolve some of the remaining ambiguities of HSC identity by analysis of gene expression in single HSCs.

Finally, there now exist nonobese diabetic severe combined immunodeficient (NOD/SCID) mouse and fetal sheep xenotransplant models for the study of human

HSC behavior. These animal models provide an opportunity to observe the developmental patterns of human hematopoiesis. Based in part on these findings, clinical protocols were initiated to study the limitations of genetic histocompatibility barriers in the transplant setting. Transplantation of megadoses of highly purified, cytokine-mobilized peripheral blood CD34$^+$ cells into patients reduced the expected adverse effects commonly seen with a 1–3 human leukocyte antigen (HLA) mismatch. A similar favorable outcome was achieved when 1–3 HLA mismatched cord blood cells were transplanted.

We thank the New York Academy of Sciences for agreeing to communicate the conference proceedings via the *Annals* series, and particularly, for doing so in a very timely manner. We are especially grateful to Dr. Saul J. Sharkis and Dr. Wolfram Brugger for their contribution to the organization of the scientific program. Roxanne Fischer, Peggy McKoy, and Lisa Hoffman were responsible for the transcription of all of the discussions. Our special thanks to Amgen, Germany; Amgen, Europe; and Kirin, Japan for their generous support, which made this conference possible.

Donald Orlic
Thomas A. Bock
Lothar Kanz

Introduction to Stem Cell Biology *in Vitro*

Threshold to the Future

C. EAVES,[a,d] C. MILLER,[a] E. CONNEALLY,[a] J. AUDET,[b] R. OOSTENDORP,[a] J. CASHMAN,[a] P. ZANDSTRA,[b] S. ROSE-JOHN,[c] J. PIRET,[b] AND A. EAVES[a]

[a]*Terry Fox Laboratory, British Columbia Cancer Agency, Vancouver, British Columbia, V5Z 1L3, Canada*
[b]*Biotechnology Laboratory, University of British Columbia, Vancouver, British Columbia, Canada*
[c]*Mainz University, Mainz, Germany*

ABSTRACT: Transplantable hematopoietic cells with multilineage reconstituting ability can be quantitated in suspensions of human or murine cells using similar assay procedures. The incorporation into these assays of stringently defined functional endpoints ensures a high degree of specificity for the cells detected. Application of these assays to stem cell-containing suspensions after they have been stimulated for several days with defined cytokines *in vitro*, or by a mixture of defined and/or undefined factors *in vivo*, has shown that net amplifications in these populations can be obtained under both circumstances. Such studies have allowed cytokine conditions that support stem cell self-renewal divisions to be identified and have also provided evidence that stem cell regeneration can be manipulated both *in vitro* and *in vivo* by altering the molecular milieu of the responding cells. These observations pave the way to future delineation of mechanisms that control the normal behavior, pathology and future clinical exploitation of hematopoietic stem cell populations.

INTRODUCTION

In medicine, the significance of hematopoietic stem cells is well established, and even their industrial potential is now widely recognized. At the same time, from both a biological and a developmental perspective, the continuing mysteries of what makes these cells unique and how their activities are regulated command undiminished fascination. FIGURE 1 illustrates diagrammatically the players and specific processes of interest to the present discussion. The latter include the regulation of stem cell viability, proliferation and differentiation (vs. death, quiescence and self-maintenance, respectively).

Identification of the molecular events that mediate and/or control these cellular changes requires a working definition of what a hematopoietic stem cell is (and of what it is not) that can be used to quantitate stem cells independent of their frequency in a given tissue or cell suspension. Much controversy has arisen from the diversity of interests that drive investigations of hematopoietic stem cell biology and, hence,

[d]Address for correspondence, Dr. C. Eaves, Terry Fox Laboratory, 601 West 10th Avenue, Vancouver, BC, V5Z 1L3, Canada. Phone, 604/877-6070; fax, 604/877-0712; e-mail, connie@terryfox.ubc.ca

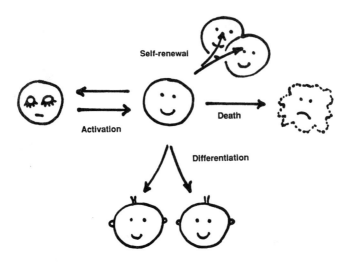

FIGURE 1. Targets for regulation of primitive hematopoietic cells. Schematic diagram of biological "functions" of hematopoietic stem cells whose alteration may be reversible or irreversible, and which may involve both shared and unique intracellular pathways, but in each case provide a distinct mechanism for changing the size of the stem cell compartment.

the particular defining properties considered relevant. However, such arguments have also stimulated a greater appreciation of the array of pathways that stem cells may follow, and have enlarged our concept of developmental programs that include ontologically distinct regulatory mechanisms.

The cellular properties that our group has focused on for a number of years as defining activities of hematopoietic stem cells are those that allow engraftment of intravenously transplanted recipients coupled to a sustained output (at the single cell level) of large numbers of lymphoid and myeloid progeny. The assay we developed to allow such cells to be not only detected in variously manipulated populations, but also quantitated and distinguished from either developmentally earlier or later cell types, is shown in FIGURE 2. The cells thus identified are referred to operationally as competitive repopulating units (CRUs).[1] Note that in this assay, the competitive characteristic is an independently variable qualitative property that can be discriminated by the number and type(s) of cells used to ensure the viability of the recipient mice independent of the test cells. The frequency of CRUs in the test cell suspension is then determined by varying the number of test cells injected into groups of recipients and assessing the proportion of "negative" mice in each group, where a negative mouse is one that fails to meet all of the endpoint criteria adopted. If the frequency of negative mice is determined solely by the input cell of interest, then its frequency can be calculated using Poisson statistics.

Specificity of this assay for transplantable cells with long-term multilineage hematopoietic repopulating activity is achieved by restricting the definition of positive mice to those that contain both lymphoid and myeloid cells of test cell origin with the requirement that these are predominant in groups of mice injected with limited numbers of transplantable test cells. To date assessment of recipients 4 months post-

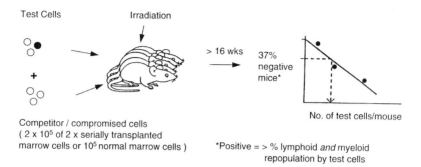

FIGURE 2. Schematic diagram illustrating the key features of the CRU assay for quantitating transplantable hematopoietic "stem" cells with longterm *in vivo* lympho-myeloid reconstituting activity, as described by Szilvassy *et al.* (1990) and subsequently modified and simplified with retention of the same specificity and sensitivity.[3,4] The use of sublethally irradiated, highly immunocompromised NOD/SCID mice as recipients allows human CRUs to be detected and quantitated by the same procedure.[5,34]

transplant has ensured the detection of murine CRUs with engrafting activity that consistently extends for $\geq$ one year.[2,3] Maximal sensitivity is achieved by pretreatment of the recipients with a myeloablative dose of irradiation and then cotransplantation of the test cells with a second population containing no more than ~10 other CRUs of adult marrow origin.[1,4] Recently, we have found that an equivalent sensitivity of murine CRU detection can be achieved using W^{41}/W^{41} recipients given a sublethal dose of irradiation (400 cGy).[3] This eliminates the need for the preparation and injection of a second source of stem cells and thus simplifies the practicalities of performing the assay. Since W^{41}/W^{41} mice are also fertile, their use requires only that the test cells be from a congenic (C57Bl/6) background.

The principles of the murine CRU assay can also be applied to the detection and quantitation of human stem cells with transplantable lympho-myeloid repopulating properties using sublethally irradiated (350 cGy) nonobese diabetic/severe combined immunodeficient (NOD/SCID) mice as recipients.[5,6] However, the sensitivity of human CRU detection under these conditions appears to require some additional human cells to be coinjected[7] and, even then, may significantly underestimate the frequency of cells with the biological properties of murine CRUs assessed in a syngeneic model.[8]

CRU AMPLIFICATION

A variety of marking studies have allowed the self-replicative ability of transplantable totipotent hematopoietic stem cells to be demonstrated.[9–12] On the other hand, the well-known decline in yield of progeny stem cells after serial transplantation[13–15] has raised doubts about the sustainability of transplantable hematopoietic stem cell self-renewal activity. One possibility is that this ability is restricted to a minor subset of cells, which prevents a net expansion of any input CRU population. Alternatively, it is possible that the self-renewal activity of CRUs can be

TABLE 1. Expansion of the CRU population *in vivo*

I. During ontogeny		
Day 14 fetal liver[31]	$\longrightarrow$	Adult BM (10× one femur)[1]
1,000		20,000
		Expansion = 20×

II. Post-transplant — fetal liver[32]		
No. injected/mouse	$\longrightarrow$	Number after 8–12 months
10–1,000		1,500–6,200
		Expansion = 6–150×

III.Post-transplant — BM[3] or day-4 FU BM[32,33]		
No. injected/mouse	$\longrightarrow$	Number after 4–12 months
1–1,000		30–1,800
		Expansion = 2–30×

modulated by the nature and timing of the exogenous stimulation that they receive. The historical failure to identify *in vitro* conditions that allow CRU numbers to be amplified, in spite of evidence that some may undergo extensive self-renewal when cultured on stromal feeder layers[16] has reinforced concern that large-scale CRU production *ex vivo* might not be feasible. On the other hand, determination of the number of CRUs present in mice at different stages of ontogeny, or after hematologic recovery posttransplant, indicates that CRU numbers can be expanded in both of these situations *in vivo* (TABLE 1).

Recently, we showed that, even *in vitro*, a modest but significant net expansion of adult mouse marrow CRUs can be achieved when Sca-1⁺lin⁻ cells are incubated in the absence of stroma, but in the presence of three factors normally produced by stroma; i.e., flt3-ligand (FL), steel factor (SF) and interleukin-11 (IL-11).[3] Moreover, this amplification of the CRU population *in vitro*, although accompanied by a rapid accumulation of more differentiated cells, is not associated with a loss of *in vivo* CRU regenerating activity, as the latter remains quantitatively (and qualitatively) indistinguishable from that of the starting Sca-1⁺lin⁻ marrow cells (FIG. 3). Evidence that IL-11 signals exclusively through gp 130[17,18] suggested that other molecules that similarly activate gp 130 might elicit the same response. Experiments using a hybrid cytokine consisting of IL-6 fused to the soluble IL-6 receptor via a flexible linker[19] in place of IL-11 have now shown this to be the case.[20] Similarly, use of a fluorescent dye tracking strategy that allows sequential cell generations to be separately isolated[21] has provided independent evidence of the ability of murine CRU to execute self-renewal divisions in suspension cultures of lin⁻ adult mouse marrow cells.[22]

Expansion of human CRU numbers in liquid suspensions of primitive subsets of human cord blood cells has been recently reported by Bhatia *et al.*[23] as well as our own group[5] In this case, the factors able to stimulate this result were FL, SF, IL-3, IL-6 and granulocyte colony-stimulating factor (G-CSF), again suggesting that the

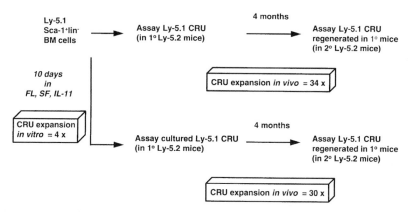

FIGURE 3. CRUs amplified *in vitro* subsequently expand normally *in vivo*. Outline of the experimental procedure used to demonstrate the CRU expansion that occurs in 10-day suspension cultures of Sca-1+lin- marrow cells containing FL, SF and IL-11 and their subsequent undiminished CRU regenerative activity determined by evaluation in secondary recipients of the CRU content of primary recipients of freshly isolated vs. cultured marrow cells. (Adapted from Miller *et al.*[3])

combined signaling of Flt3, c-kit and gp 130 may be important for the maintenance of stem cell functions upon their mitogenic stimulation.

IN VIVO MANIPULATION OF STEM CELL DECISIONS

A number of lines of evidence suggest the existence of genes whose products may alter the rapidity or type of reprogramming that forces or prevents the differentiation of primitive hematopoietic cells. Whether or not these intrinsic regulators of cellular differentiation, or their functional status, can be altered by changing the nature or frequency of interactions between cells and their environment remains more controversial. For example, even if an altered behavior can be demonstrated at the population level (e.g., reproducible and significant differences in CRU numbers obtained after exposing equal aliquots of the same original cell suspension to two different conditions for the same period of time), a selective rather than a deterministic mechanism may be invoked. To rule out the latter requires evidence that different outcomes can be associated with the same original target population. This, in turn, typically depends on the use of single cell analyses.

Although still tedious to perform, experiments of this type are now at least feasible owing to the progress that has been made in methodologies and equipment for obtaining highly enriched populations of very primitive hematopoietic cells at reasonable yields. Two examples of single cell studies that we have reported[24] involved monitoring the retention or loss of properties that allow human cells to be detectable as long-term culture-initiating cells (LTC-IC), as defined by a 6-week version of the original assay.[25] The modified assay[26] allows the additional detection of even more primitive hematopoietic cells so that their numbers remain correlated with CRU fre-

TABLE 2. Clone formation and progenitor expansion after 10 days in single cell serum-free suspension cultures of CD34[+]CD38[−] cells[a]

Cytokine concentration (ng/ml)		% of cells forming clones	Progenitor Expansion[b]	
FL/SF	IL-3/IL-6/ G-CSF		LTC-IC	CFC
300	60	52 ± 7	57 ± 18	570 ± 50
30	6	61 ± 9	1.2 ± 0.5	430 ± 90

[a]Data from Zandstra et al.[24]
[b]Fold-increase on day 10 of culture under the cytokine conditions shown relative to day 0 values.

quencies even after being cultured for a few days.[27] In the studies alluded to above[24] it could be shown that CD34[+]CD38[−] cells isolated from normal adult human marrow can be stimulated to produce the same number of clones when exposed to different cytokine cocktails, in spite of marked differences in the numbers of daughter cells within these clones that still possess LTC-IC activity (TABLE 2).

More recently, we have documented a 10-fold enhancement in the number of human CRUs regenerated in NOD/SCID mice given various human cytokines after transplantation of human cord blood cells.[8] Interestingly, this enhancement is selective for this very primitive population and is not, as noted previously,[28,29] shared by any other regenerated human cell type monitored. In this case, the mechanisms involved will be more difficult to establish. However, it has been reported that some of the same murine cytokines can have a similar effect when administered to previously myeloablated mice after completion of their hematologic recovery from a syngeneic transplant.[30] In addition, it was noted that the effects seen were not accompanied by a discernible increase in the proliferative activity of the regenerated CRU population, suggesting that the cytokine-induced increase in CRU numbers might reflect a change in the self-renewal activity of the stimulated cells. These and other possibilities will obviously dictate the design of future experiments to clarify the role that exogenously administered cytokines may play in regulating CRU numbers *in vivo*.

ACKNOWLEDGMENTS

The work described in this review was made possible by grants from the National Cancer Institute of Canada (NCIC) with funds from the Terry Fox Run, Novartis Canada, the NHLBI of the NIH (PO1 55435) and the Science Council of British Columbia (BC). C. Eaves is a Terry Fox Cancer Research Scientist of the NCIC. E. Conneally held an NCIC Terry Fox Physician–Scientist Fellowship. J. Audet and P. Zandstra both held studentships from the Natural Sciences and Engineering Research Council of Canada and scholarships from the Science Council of BC. We also thank B. Fox for assistance in preparing the manuscript.

REFERENCES

1. SZILVASSY, S.J. *et al.* 1990. Quantitative assay for totipotent reconstituting hematopoietic stem cells by a competitive repopulation strategy. Proc. Natl. Acad. Sci. USA **87:** 8736–8740.

2. JORDAN, C.T. *et al.* 1990. Clonal and systemic analysis of long-term hematopoiesis in the mouse. Genes Dev. **4:** 220–232.
3. MILLER, C.L. *et al.* 1997. Expansion *in vitro* of adult murine hematopoietic stem cells with transplantable lympho-myeloid reconstituting ability. Proc. Natl. Acad. Sci. USA **94:** 13648–13653.
4. REBEL, V.I. *et al.* 1994. Amplification of Sca-1$^+$ Lin$^-$ WGA$^+$ cells in serum-free cultures containing steel factor, interleukin-6, and erythropoietin with maintenance of cells with long-term *in vivo* reconstituting potential. Blood **83:** 128–136.
5. CONNEALLY, E. *et al.* 1997. Expansion in vitro of transplantable human cord blood stem cells demonstrated using a quantitative assay of their lympho-myeloid repopulating activity in nonobese diabetic-*scid/scid* mice. Proc. Natl. Acad. Sci. USA **94:** 9836–9841.
6. BHATIA, M. *et al.* 1997. Purification of primitive human hematopoietic cells capable of repopulating immune-deficient mice. Proc. Natl. Acad. Sci. USA. **94:** 5320–5325.
7. VERSTEGEN, M.M.A. *et al.* 1998. Transplantation of human umbilical cord blood cells in macrophage-depleted SCID mice: Evidence for accessory cell involvement in expansion of immature CD34$^+$CD38$^-$ cells. Blood **91:** 1966–1976.
8. CASHMAN, J.D. *et al.* 1999. Human growth factor-enhanced regeneration of transplantable human hematopoietic stem cells in NOD/SCID mice. Blood **93:** 481–487.
9. WU, A.M. *et al.* 1968. Cytological evidence for a relationship between normal hematopoietic colony-forming cells and cells of the lymphoid system. J. Exp. Med. **127:** 455–464.
10. DICK, J.E. *et al.* 1985. Introduction of a selectable gene into primitive stem cells capable of long-term reconstitution of the hemopoietic system of W/Wv mice. Cell **42:** 71–79.
11. LEMISCHKA, I.R. *et al.* 1986. Developmental potential and dynamic behavior of hematopoietic stem cells. Cell **45:** 917–927.
12. KELLER, G, *et al.* 1990. Life span of multipotential hematopoietic stem cells *in vivo*. J. Exp. Med. **171:** 1407–1418.
13. SIMINOVITCH, L. *et al.* 1964. Decline in colony forming ability of marrow cells subjected to serial transplantation into irradiated mice. J. Cell. Comp. Physiol. **64:** 23–32.
14. MAUCH, P. *et al.* 1989. Loss of hematopoietic stem cell self-renewal after bone marrow transplantation. Blood **74:** 872–875.
15. HARRISON, D.E. *et al.* 1982. Loss of stem cell repopulating ability upon transplantation. Effects of donor age, cell number, and transplantation procedure. J. Exp. Med. **156:** 1767–1779.
16. FRASER, C.C. *et al.* 1992. Proliferation of totipotent hematopoietic stem cells *in vitro* with retention of long-term competitive *in vivo* reconstituting ability. Proc. Natl. Acad. Sci. USA **89:** 1968–1972.
17. NANDURKAR, H.H. *et al.* 1996. The human IL-11 receptor requires gp130 for signalling: demonstration by molecular cloning of the receptor. Oncogene **32:** 585–593.
18. KAROW, J. *et al.* 1996. Mediation of interleukin-11 dependent biological responses by a soluble form of the interleukin-11 receptor. Biochemistry **318:** 489–495.
19. FISCHER, M. *et al.* 1997. A bioactive designer cytokine for human hematopoietic progenitor cell expansion. Nat. Biotechnol. **15:** 142–145.
20. AUDET, J. *et al.* 1998. *In vitro* expansion of *in vivo* repopulating hematopoietic stem cells from adult mouse bone marrow using hyperIL-6, an engineered hybrid cytokine of human interleukin-6 and its soluble receptor [abstract]. Exp. Hematol. **26:** 700.
21. NORDON, R.E. *et al.* 1997. High resolution cell division tracking demonstrates the Flt3-ligand-dependence of human marrow CD34$^+$CD38$^-$ cell production *in vitro*. Br. J. Haematol. **98:** 528–539.
22. Oostendorp, R. *et al.* 1998. High resolution tracking of cell divisions demonstrates similar cell cycle entry kinetics of hematopoietic stem cells stimulated in vitro and *in vivo* [abstract]. Exp. Hematol. **26:** 814.
23. BHATIA, M. *et al.* 1997. Quantitative analysis reveals expansion of human hematopoietic repopulating cells after short-term *ex vivo* culture. J. Exp. Med. **186:** 619–624.

24. ZANDSTRA, P.W. *et al.* 1997. Cytokine manipulation of primitive human hematopoietic cell self-renewal. Proc. Natl. Acad. Sci. USA **94:** 4698–4703.
25. SUTHERLAND, H.J. *et al.* 1990. Functional characterization of individual human hematopoietic stem cells cultured at limiting dilution on supportive marrow stromal layers. Proc. Nat. Acad. Sci. USA **87:** 3584–3588.
26. HOGGE, D.E. *et al.* 1996. Enhanced detection, maintenance and differentiation of primitive human hematopoietic cells in cultures containing murine fibroblasts engineered to produce human steel factor, interleukin-3 and granulocyte colony-stimulating factor. Blood **88:** 3765–3773.
27. CONNEALLY, E. *et al.* 1998. Efficient retroviral-mediated gene transfer to human cord blood stem cells with *in vivo* repopulating potential. Blood **91:** 3487–3493.
28. VORMOOR, J. *et al.* 1994. Immature human cord blood progenitors engraft and proliferate to high levels in severe combined immunodeficient mice. Blood **83:** 2489–2497.
29. CASHMAN, J. *et al.* 1997. Sustained proliferation, multi-lineage differentiation and maintenance of primitive human haematopoietic cells in NOD/SCID mice transplanted with human cord blood. Br. J. Haematol. **98:** 1026–1036.
30. ISCOVE, N.N. *et al.* 1997. Hematopoietic stem cells expand during serial transplantation *in vivo* without apparent exhaustion. Curr. Biol. **7:** 805–808.
31. MILLER, C.L. *et al.* 1997. Impaired steel factor responsiveness differentially affects the detection and long-term maintenance of fetal liver hematopoietic stem cells *in vivo*. Blood **89:** 1214–1223.
32. PAWLIUK, R. *et al.* 1996. Evidence of both ontogeny and transplant dose-regulated expansion of hematopoietic stem cells *in vivo*. Blood **88:** 2852–2858.
33. SAUVAGEAU, G. *et al.* 1995. Overexpression of HOXB4 in hematopoietic cells causes the selective expansion of more primitive populations *in vitro* and *in vivo*. Genes Dev. **9:** 1753–1765.
34. WANG, J.C.Y. *et al.* 1997. Primitive human hematopoietic cells are enriched in cord blood compared with adult bone marrow or mobilized peripheral blood as measured by the quantitative *in vivo* SCID-repopulating cell assay. Blood **89:** 3919–3924.

DISCUSSION

L. KANZ (*Eberhard Karls University*): Do you have any data on the effect of thrombopoietin on this kind of experiment?

EAVES: The Piacabello combo (that is, FL plus TPO only) is not very good in the type of short-term cultures we have studied with cord blood. We have not done long-term suspension cultures and Dr. Piacabello never documented big increases in the short-term either.

Hematopoietic Commitment during Embryogenesis

SCOTT ROBERTSON,[a] MARION KENNEDY,[a] AND GORDON KELLER, [a,b,c]

[a]National Jewish Medical and Research Center, 1400 Jackson Street, Denver, Colorado 80206, USA

[b]The Department of Immunology, University of Colorado Health Sciences Center, Denver, Colorado 80262, USA

ABSTRACT: Hematopoiesis develops initially as discrete blood islands in the extraembryonic yolk sac of the embryo. These blood islands consist of clusters of primitive erythrocytes surrounded by developing angioblasts that ultimately form the yolk sac vasculature. The close developmental association of these early hematopoietic and endothelial cells has led to the hypothesis that they develop from a common precursor, a cell known as the hemangioblast. Using a developmental model system based on the *in vitro* differentiation capacity of embryonic stem (ES) cells, we have identified a precursor with the capacity to generate endothelial as well as primitive and definitive hematopoietic progeny. The developmental potential of this precursor population suggests that it represents the *in vitro* equivalent of the hemangioblast.

INTRODUCTION

The hematopoietic system undergoes dramatic changes throughout ontogeny both with respect to the site of activity as well as to the lineages produced.[1] Most of our understanding of lineage relationships and regulation of growth and differentiation within the hematopoietic system has come from studies on adult bone marrow and fetal liver. While there are some notable differences between fetal and adult hematopoiesis, in general they share many similarities including the simultaneous development of multiple lineages that derive from a common precursor known as the multipotential stem cell.[2–4] Stem cells of both fetal and adult origin are able to provide long-term hematopoietic repopulation following transplantation into adult recipient animals, a characteristic that distinguishes them from all other cells in the hematopoietic system. Prior to the development of the fetal liver, hematopoietic activity is found in the extraembryonic yolk sac, the first site of hematopoietic commitment.[1,5] In contrast to the fetal and adult systems, yolk sac hematopoiesis shows unique developmental patterns which suggest the presence of novel precursor populations.[1,5]

[c]Address for correspondence: Gordon Keller, Ph.D., National Jewish Medical and Research Center, 1400 Jackson Street, Denver, Colorado 80206-2761. Phone, 303/398-1813; fax, 303/398-1396; e-mail, kellerg@njc.org

YOLK SAC HEMATOPOIESIS

The embryonic hematopoietic system initiates as discrete blood islands in the early yolk sac at approximately day 7.5 of gestation.[1,5] The potential of the first stage of the embryonic program is distinct from that of fetal liver and adult marrow hematopoiesis in that it appears to be restricted to the generation of two lineages: embryonic erythrocytes, which represent the major hematopoietic component of the blood islands, and macrophages that are dispersed throughout the yolk sac.[1,5] These early erythroid cells, known as primitive erythrocytes, are large, remain nucleated and produce the embryonic forms of globlin.[5–7] Given this potential, this stage of yolk sac development is known as primitive hematopoiesis. Cells of the endothelial lineage represent the second component of the blood islands and are first detected as a layer of developing angioblasts which surround the inner clusters of primitive erythrocytes. The observation that the hematopoietic and endothelial lineages develop simultaneously in close proximity in the blood islands provided the basis for the hypothesis that they share a common precursor, a cell called the hemangioblast (reviewed in Refs. 8 and 9). Although experimental evidence supporting this notion has accumulated since the original hypothesis was put forward almost 100 years ago, a cell with these characteristics has not yet been isolated from the developing mouse embryo.

While the initial stages of yolk sac hematopoiesis appear to be restricted, precursors for other hematopoietic lineages, including definitive erythroid, myeloid, and mast cells can be detected within 12–48 hours following the development of the blood islands.[10–12] These cells, which are collectively referred to as definitive hematopoietic precursors, appear in the yolk sac prior to the establishment of intraembryonic hematopoiesis, suggesting that they are produced at this site. However, in contrast to the primitive erythroid and macrophage precursors that mature in the yolk sac, these precursors do not undergo significant differentiation in this environment. Although these precursors can be detected in the yolk sac by 8.0 to 9.0 days of gestation, transplantable stem cells capable of providing long-term repopulation in adult recipients are not easily detected until day 10.5 to 11.[13] Interestingly, these cells are found within the embryo proper slightly earlier than in the yolk sac, leading to the suggestion that they develop at some site within the embryo and then migrate to the yolk sac. Reports of lymphoid precursors within the yolk sac are somewhat variable with respect to stage of development and have been detected between 8.5 and 9.5 days of gestation.[14–16] One of the most recent studies demonstrated that lymphoid potential is present in both the yolk sac and embryo proper as early as day 8.5.[17] However, these precursors appear to develop from multipotential rather than from lymphoid committed cells and therefore the actual stage at which lymphoid-restricted precursors develop may be later than originally reported.

The embryonic developmental sequence in which primitive erythroid cells appear before definitive erythroid/myeloid precursors and long-term repopulating stem cells (LTRSC) is reverse to that predicted by most models of fetal or adult hematopoiesis. These models typically position the LTRSC as the most immature cell within the system. There are at least several explanations for these unusual observations. First, it is possible that yolk sac hematopoiesis is established by an embryonic multipotential precursor that initially produces primitive erythroid progeny, then definitive hematopoietic cells, and finally LTRSC and lymphoid precursors. These consecutive waves of differentiation including the late development of the repopulating stem cell would simply reflect maturation of the system. This putative multipotential cell could be considered as the primordial hematopoietic precursor, the pre-LTRSC. A second possibility is that the yolk sac hematopoietic program is distinct from that of intraembryonic hematopoiesis and restricted to the development of primitive erythroid, definitive erythroid and myeloid precursors.

Yolk sac hematopoietic activity declines dramatically between days 10 and 12 of gestation, concomitant with the initiation of intraembryonic hematopoiesis in the developing fetal liver.[1,12] The transition from yolk sac to fetal liver defines the switch from primitive to definitive hematopoiesis and the replacement of the primitive erythroid program by multilineage hematopoiesis including definitive erythropoiesis, myelopoiesis, and lymphopoiesis.[1,12] Definitive erythroid cells generated in the fetal liver differ from primitive erythrocytes in the yolk sac in that they are small and that they enucleate and produce adult globins.[6,7]

HEMATOPOIETIC DEVELOPMENT OF ES CELLS IN CULTURE RECAPITULATES YOLK SAC HEMATOPOIESIS

To define the developmental events involved in the establishment of the hematopoietic and endothelial lineages, it is important to focus on the early yolk sac at a stage prior to the appearance of the blood islands. Most attempts to study these early differentiation steps have been severely hampered by the inaccessibility of the embryo at this stage of development as well as by the limited numbers of cells available. To overcome these problems a number of groups have utilized the ES *in vitro* differentiation system as a model for early hematopoietic and endothelial development. Under appropriate conditions, ES cells will differentiate and form colonies known as embryoid bodies (EBs), which contain developing precursor populations from multiple lineages, including those of the hematopoietic and vascular systems.[18] During the past 8 years cell culture systems and techniques have advanced significantly such that it is now possible to routinely generate both the primitive and definitive erythroid lineages, most myeloid lineages, and endothelial cells in a predictable pattern from developing EBs.[18–25]

One concern with this model system is whether or not it reflects the developmental program in the normal embryo. While this is difficult to determine in all aspects, several findings do indicate that at least the early events in hematopoietic and endothelial commitment in the EBs are similar to those found *in utero*. First, precursor analysis of the EBs clearly demonstrated that the primitive erythroid and macrophage lineages are the first to develop, followed by those of the definitive erythroid and other myeloid lineages, a pattern reminiscent of that of the early yolk sac.[21] Moreover, as observed in the yolk sac, the primitive erythroid lineage within the EB appears to be transient, generated between days 4 and 10 of differentiation. Second, kinetic analysis of gene expression within the developing EBs indicates that markers expressed in mesoderm appear earlier than those expressed in hematopoietic and endothelial precursors, which in turn precede those that define specific hematopoietic lineages.[21] These gene expression patterns are consistent with the well-established biological data that demonstrate that the hematopoietic and endothelial lineages develop from mesoderm. Together, these findings suggest that, at least for the early events, hematopoietic commitment in the ES/EB system is comparable to that of the early embryo.

THE PRIMITIVE AND DEFINITIVE HEMATOPOIETIC LINEAGES DEVELOP FROM A COMMON PRECURSOR IN EBs

As indicated earlier, one model for the unusual pattern of lineage development in the yolk sac could be the development of a multipotential cell with the potential to generate both primitive and definitive hematopoietic progeny. The initial production of the primitive erythroid lineage followed by the development of definitive precursors would reflect maturation of the system resulting from molecular changes within this precursor population and/or changes in the microenvironment. To determine whether a multipotential cell with both primitive and definitive hematopoietic potential does exist, we analyzed EBs prior to the establishment of the primitive erythroid lineage, specifically before day 4 of differentiation. Using this approach, we identified a transient vascular endothelial growth factor (VEGF)-responsive precursor that developed in EBs within 2.5 days of differentiation and persisted for approximately 24 hours.[26] In methylcellulose cultures containing VEGF and conditioned medium from an embryonic endothelial cell line (D4T), these precursors generate colonies consisting of undifferentiated blast cells. Replating studies demonstrated that these blast cell colonies contain both primitive and definitive hematopoietic precursors and, as such, documented for the first time that these lineages can develop from a common precursor, the blast colony-forming cell (BL-CFC).[26] To further characterize the developmental status of the blast cell colonies, individual colonies were analyzed via RT–PCR for the expression of genes representing mesodermal, endothelial, and early and late hematopoietic precursors. This analysis included Brachyury,[27] flk-1,[28,29] SCL,[30–32] CD34,[33,34] GATA-1,[35] and βH1 and β major globins. None of the blast colonies analyzed expressed Brachyury, indicating that they represent a stage of development more advanced than mesoderm. All of the colonies analyzed did, however, express flk-1, SCL/TAL-1, CD34 and GATA-1, suggesting that they contain hematopoietic precursors representing various stages of development, a finding consistent with their replating potential. Many of the blast colonies also expressed βH1 and β major globin, a finding that further supports the notion that they have both primitive and definitive hematopoietic potential.

THE VEGF-RESPONSIVE BL-CFC HAS BOTH HEMATOPOIETIC AND ENDOTHELIAL POTENTIAL

The finding that the BL-CFC responded to VEGF and that the blast colonies expressed flk-1 suggested that these colonies may have endothelial in addition to hematopoietic potential. To determine whether this was true, individual blast colonies were cultured in liquid in microtiter wells in the presence of cytokines that support the development of both the hematopoietic and endothelial lineages. Approximately 30–40% of blast colonies from day-3.25 EBs were able to generate both hematopoietic and adherent cells under these conditions. The remainder gave rise to only hematopoietic progeny. Analysis of the adherent population indicated that these cells expressed markers characteristic of endothelial cells, including PECAM-1, flk-1, tie-2, and flt-1. In addition, they displayed the capacity to take up acetylated low-density lipoprotein (LDL), also a characteristic of endothelial cells. The observation that blast colonies contained both hematopoietic and endothelial precursors strongly suggests that the BL-CFC they derive from has the properties of a hemangioblast.[36] As indicated above, not all blast colonies displayed endothelial potential. Kinetic analysis revealed that the proportion with endothelial potential was highest (approximately 75%) in blast colonies generated from day-2.5 EBs. The proportion of bi-lineage blast colonies dropped dramatically as the age of the EBs from which they were generated increased. Fewer than 25% of the blast colonies from day-3.5 EBs showed both hematopoietic and endothelial potential. These findings suggest that the bi-potential BL-CFC represented a transient population that persists in EBs for approximately 24 hours between day 2.5 and 3.5 of differentiation. Analysis of the hematopoietic potential of the blast colonies with endothelial potential indicated that most contain precursors for multiple lineages. However, a small number of these colonies appeared to be more restricted and generated only primitive erythroid and adherent cell progeny. These findings suggest that populations of hemangioblasts with different potentials may exist.

CONCLUSIONS

The identification of the VEGF-responsive BL-CFC provides the first demonstration that the primitive and definitive hematopoietic and endothelial lineages can develop from a common precursor. That fact that these blast colonies develop in response to VEGF indicates that this precursor expresses Flk-1, and that this interaction is required for the development of these early populations. This interpretation is consistent with *in vivo* gene-targeting studies which demonstrated that a functional Flk-1 receptor is required for the development of these lineages in the embryo.[37] Taken together, the characteristics of the BL-CFC are consistent with the interpretation that it represents the *in vitro* equivalent of the hemangioblast and suggests that a comparable precursor should be present in the developing embryo. Current experiments are aimed at identifying the BL-CFC in early embryos. Utilizing the ES/EB system we have also been able to identify and characterize a novel colony that spans mesodem to hemangioblast commitment and as such likely develops from a precursor earlier than the BL-CFC. The majority of these colonies express Brachyury, flk-1 and SCL, indicating the presence of mesodermal and hemangioblastic cells. In addition a subpopulation of these colonies also express GATA-1, βmajor and βH1, demonstrating further commitment to the hematopoietic lineages. Access to these unique colonies will allow for a molecular analysis of the specification of mesoderm to earliest stages of enothelial and hematopoietic development.

REFERENCES

1. METCALF, D. & M. MOORE. 1971. Haemopoietic Cells. Frontiers in Biology, Vol. 24. A. Neuberger and E.L. Tatum, Eds. North-Holland Publishing Co. London.
2. KELLER, G. 1992. Hematopoietic stem cells. Curr. Opin. Immunol. **4:** 133–139.
3. UCHIDA, N., W. FLEMING, E. ALPERN & I. WEISSMAN. 1993. Heterogeneity of hematopoietic stem cells. Curr. Opin. Immunol. **5:** 177–184.
4. MORRISON, S.J., N. UCHIDA & I.L. WEISSMAN. 1995. The biology of hematopoietic stem cells. Annu. Rev. Cell. Dev. Biol. **11:** 35–71.
5. RUSSEL, E. 1979. Hereditary anemias of the mouse: a review for geneticists. Adv. Genet. **20:** 357–459.
6. BARKER, J. 1968. Development of the mouse hematopoietic system. I. Types of hemoglobin produced in embryonic yolk sac and liver. Dev. Biol. **18:** 14-29.
7. BROTHERTON, T., D. CHUI, J. GAULDIE & M. PATTERSON. 1979. Hemoglobin ontogeny during normal mouse fetal development. Proc. Natl. Acad. Sci. USA **76:** 2853–2857.
8. WAGNER, R.C. 1980. Endothelial cell embryology and growth. Adv. Microcirc. **9:** 45–75.
9. RISAU, W. & I. FLAMME. 1995. Vasculogenesis. Annu. Rev. Cell. Dev. Biol. **11:** 73–91.
10. WONG, P., S. CHUNG, D. CHUI & C. EAVES. 1986. Properties of the earliest clonogenic hemopoietic precursor to appear in the developing murine yolk sac. Proc. Natl. Acad. Sci. USA **83:** 3851–3854.
11. SONODA, T., C. HAYASHI & Y. KITAMURA. 1983. Presence of mast cell precursors in the yolk sac of mice. Dev. Biol. **97:** 89–94.
12. JOHNSON, G. & D. BARKER. 1985. Erythroid progenitor cells and stimulating factors during murine embryonic and fetal development. Exp. Hematol. **13:** 200–208.
13. MULLER, A.M., A. MEDVINSKY, J. STROUBOULIS, F. GROSVELD & E. DZIERZAK. 1994. Development of hematopoietic stem cell activity in the mouse embryo. Immunity **1:** 291–301.
14. LIU, C. & R. AUERBACH. 1991. *In vitro* development of murine T cells from prethymic and preliver embryonic yolk sac hematopoietic stem cells. Development **113:** 1315–1323.
15. CUMANO, A., C. FURLONGER & C. PAIGE. 1993. Differentiation and characterization of B cell precursor detected in the yolk sac and embryo body of embryos beginning at the 10- to 12-somite stage. Proc. Natl. Acad. Sci. USA **90:** 6429–6433.
16. HUANG, H., L. ZETTERGREN & R. AUERBACH. 1994. *In vitro* differentiation of B cells and myeloid cells from the early mouse embryo and its extraembryonic yolk sac. Exp. Hematol. **22:** 19–25.
17. GODIN, I., F. DIETERLEN-LIEVRE & A. CUMANO. 1995. Emergence of multipotent hemopoietic cells in the yolk sac and para-aortic splanchnopleura in mouse embryos, beginning at 8.5 days postcoitus. Proc. Natl. Acad. Sci. USA **92:** 773–777.
18. KELLER, G. 1995. *In vitro* differentiation of embryonic stem cells. Curr. Opin. Cell Biol. **7:** 862–869.
19. SCHMITT, R., E. BRUYNS & H. SNODGRASS. 1991. Hematopoietic development of embryonic stem cells *in vitro*: cytokine and receptor gene expression. Genes Dev. **5:** 728–740.
20. BÜRKERT, U., T. VON RÜDEN & E. WAGNER. 1991. Early fetal hematopoietic development from *in vitro* differentiated embryonic stem cells. New Biol. **13:** 698–708.
21. KELLER, G., M. KENNEDY, T. PAPAYANNOPOULOU & M.V. WILES. 1993. Hematopoietic commitment during embryonic stem cell differentiation in culture. Mol. Cell. Biol. **13:** 473–486.
22. NAKANO, T., H. KODAMA & T. HONJO. 1994. Generation of lymphohematopoietic cells from embryonic stem cells in culture. Science **265:** 1098–1101.

23. RISAU, W., H. SARIOLA, H.G. ZERWES, J. SASSE, P. EKBLOM, R. KEMLER & T. DOET-
    SCHMAN. 1988. Vasculogenesis and angiogenesis in embryonic-stem-cell-derived
    embryoid bodies. Development **102:** 471–478.
24. WANG, R., R. CLARK & V.L. BAUTCH. 1992. Embryonic stem cell-derived cystic
    embryoid bodies form vascular channels: an *in vitro* model of blood vessel devel-
    opment. Development **114:** 303–316.
25. VITTET, D., M.H. PRANDINI, R. BERTHIER, A. SCHWEITZER, H. MARTIN-SISTERON, G.
    UZAN & E. DEJANA. 1996. Embryonic stem cells differentiate *in vitro* to endothe-
    lial cells through successive maturation steps. Blood **88:** 3424–3431.
26. KENNEDY, M., M. FIRPO, K. CHOI, C. WALL, S. ROBERTSON, N. KABRUN & G.
    KELLER. 1997. A common precursor for primitive erythropoiesis and definitive
    haematopoiesis. Nature **386:** 488–493.
27. HERRMANN, B.G., S. LABEIT, A. POUSTKA, T.R. KING & H. LEHRACH. 1990. Cloning
    of the T gene required in mesoderm formation in the mouse. Nature **343:** 617–622.
28. YAMAGUCHI, T.P., D.J. DUMONT, R.A. CONLON, M.L. BREITMAN & J. ROSSANT. 1993.
    flk-1, an flt-related receptor tyrosine kinase is an early marker for endothelial cell
    precursors. Development **118:** 489–498.
29. MILLAUER, B., S. WIZIGMANN-VOOS, H. SCHNURCH, R. MARTINEZ, N.P. MOLLER, W.
    RISAU & A. ULLRICH. 1993. High affinity VEGF binding and developmental
    expression suggest Flk-1 as a major regulator of vasculogenesis and angiogenesis.
    Cell **72:** 835–846.
30. BEGLEY, C.G., P.D. APLAN, S. DENNING, B.F. HAYNES, T.A. WALDMANN & S.S. KIR-
    SCH. 1989. The gene SCL is expressed during early hematopoiesis and encodes a
    differentiation-related DNA-binding motif. Proc. Natl. Acad. Sci. USA **86:** 10128–
    10132.
31. ROBB, L., I. LYONS, R. LI, L. HARTLEY, F. KONTGEN, R.P. HARVEY, D. METCALF &
    C.G. BEGLEY. 1995. Absence of yolk sac hematopoiesis from mice with a targeted
    disruption of the scl gene. Proc. Natl. Acad. Sci. USA **92:** 7075–7079.
32. SHIVDASANI, R., E. MAYER & S.H. ORKIN. 1995. Absence of blood formation in mice
    lacking the T-cell leukemia oncoprotein tal-1/SCL. Nature **373:** 432–434.
33. CIVIN, C.I., L.C. STRAUSS, C. BROVALL, M.J. FACKLER, J.F. SCHWARTZ & J.H.
    SHAPER. 1984. Antigenic analysis of hematopoiesis. III. A hematopoietic progeni-
    tor cell surface antigen defined by a monoclonal antibody raised against KG-1a
    cells. J. Immunol **133:** 157–165.
34. KATZ, F.E., R. TINDLE, D.R. SUTHERLAND & M.F. GREAVES. 1985. Identification of a
    membrane glycoprotein associated with haemopoietic progenitor cells. Leukemia
    Res. **9:** 191–198.
35. ORKIN, S. 1992. GATA-binding transcription factors in hematopoietic cells. Blood
    80: 575–581.
36. CHOI, K., M. KENNEDY, A. KAZAROV, J.C. PAPADIMITRIOU & G. KELLER. 1998. A
    common precursor for hematopoietic and endothelial cells. Development **125:**
    725–732.
37. SHALABY, F., J. ROSSANT, T.P. YAMAGUCHI, M. GERTSENSTEIN, X.F. WU, M.L.
    BREITMAN & A.C. SCHUH. 1995. Failure of blood-island formation and vasculogen-
    esis in Flk-1-deficient mice. Nature **376:** 62–66.

DISCUSSION

S.J. SHARKIS *(Johns Hopkins Oncology Center)*: I know that this is an *in vitro* session, but have you taken any of these transitional colonies and transplanted them into on-the-hoof mice?

KELLER: We are starting to look at that. We have decided to follow the model developed by Merv Yoder and transplant conditioned newborn pups with both the blast colonies and the transitional colonies. The other approach is to expand the blast colonies and the transitional colonies in different combinations of cytokines or on different stromal cell lines prior to transplantation. I think we also have to entertain the possibility that we are looking at a developmental program that may never give rise to long-term repopulating stem cells.

R. MÖHLE *(Eberhard Karls University)*: There are some data from partial Flk-1 knockouts that there is a common mesodermal precursor which populates both yolk sac and AGM (aorta-gonad-mesonehros) region. Migration of this cell depends on Flk-1. Is this cell identical with your blast colony cell?

KELLER: I would hope it is a comparable cell. We have not done much sorting from normal embryos. We have started to grow blast cell colonies from mid-streak stage embryos. Our preliminary studies indicate that the normal embryo does contain blast colony-forming cells. We are trying to determine whether they can generate both hematopoietic and endothelial progeny.

D.A. WILLIAMS *(Riley Hospital for Children)*: Two questions, both probably trivial. When you talk about myeloid precursors in the yolk sac are those primitive or definitive myeloid precursors?

KELLER: I don't know.

WILLIAMS: The second question has to do with your genomics; based on whatever criteria you are going to use, what percentage of the 1,500 sequences fall into the category that you are going to want to analyze in detail? In other words, how formidable a task is it going to be to run these?

KELLER: It is not as bad as it sounds. Of the 1,500 sequences, we have eliminated the known genes and are now in the process of determining what proportion are differentially expressed between the driver and tracer. Using the slot blots with nine different samples, we can probably analyze 700–800 clones in several months.

Humoral Regulation of Hematopoietic Stem Cells[a]

MAKIO OGAWA,[b] AND TAKUYA MATSUNAGA

Department of Veterans Affairs Medical Center and the Department of Medicine, Medical University of South Carolina, Charleston, South Carolina, USA, and The Fourth Department of Internal Medicine, Sapporo Medical University, Sapporo, Japan

ABSTRACT: During the last two decades, studies using primarily cell culture methods disclosed that a number of hematopoietic cytokines possess stimulatory effects on primitive hematopoietic progenitors. More recently, investigators in a number of laboratories, including ours, used murine transplantation models to characterize the cytokines regulating the hematopoietic stem cells. The results are in general agreement with the cytokine interactions defined in culture. The positive cytokines may be separated into two groups: one consisting of steel factor and flt3/flt2 ligand and the other consisting of interleukin (IL)-6, IL-11, IL-12, leukemia inhibitory factor, granulocyte colony-stimulating factor (G-CSF) and thrombopoietin. Interactions of two cytokines belonging to different groups appear necessary to positively regulate the kinetics of stem cells. Surprisingly, IL-3 and IL-1 proved to have profound negative effects on hematopoietic stem cells. Studies of human hematopoietic stem cells are now necessary.

INTRODUCTION

It is generally accepted that, in the steady-state bone marrow, primitive hematopoietic progenitors and stem cells are cell-cycle dormant, while maturer progenitors are active. During the last two decades a number of cytokines have been discovered that regulate the cycling state of the primitive hematopoietic progenitors. As summarized in an earlier review,[1] the list includes interleukin (IL)-3, granulocyte/macrophage colony-stimulating factor (GM-CSF), IL-4, IL-6, granulocyte-CSF (G-CSF), IL-11, leukemia inhibitory factor (LIF), IL-12 and steel factor (SF, c-kit ligand). More recently flt3/flk-2 ligand (FL)[2] and thrombopoietin (TPO, mpl ligand)[3] were added to the list of the early-acting cytokines. The evidences for the effects of these cytokines on the primitive progenitors were obtained primarily in studies utilizing cell cultures. First, serial observations (mapping) of the development of blast cell colonies identified a number of cytokine combinations that regulate the cell cycle kinetics of primitive progenitors.[4–6] Because the progenitors for the blast cell colonies are dormant in the cell cycle,[7] the cytokines that stimulates the

[a]This work was supported by the Office of Research and Development, Medical Research Service, Department of Veterans Affairs, NIH grants RO1 DK32294 and RO1 DKHL 48714 and a grant from the Japan Society for the Promotion of Science (JSPS-RFTF97100201).

[b]Address correspondence to: Makio Ogawa, MD, PhD, Department of Veterans Affairs Medical Center, 109 Bee Street, Charleston, SC 29401-5799. Phone, 843/577-5011, ext. 6712; fax, 843/953-6433; e-mail: ogawam@musc.edu

cycling of the progenitors hasten the development of blast cell colonies. The second line of evidence was provided by studies of colony formation from cell populations that are highly enriched for cell-cycle dormant, primitive progenitors. For example, colony formation from CD34[+] human leukocyte antigen (HLA-DR[-]) human marrow cells required combinations of the early-acting cytokines listed above.[8] The third line of evidence was provided by the observation of cytokine combinations that support the proliferation of lymphohematopoietic progenitors in culture. For a long time after the development of clonal cell culture technology, the clonal assays were limited to progenitors that are committed to myeloid and erythroid differentiation. Several years ago we developed a two-stage methylcellulose culture assay for lymphohematopoietic progenitors that are capable of myeloid and B-lymphoid differentiation.[9] Subsequently, we demonstrated that the progenitors assayable in this system have T-cell[10] and natural killer (NK) cell[11] potentials as well. While the original assay was dependent on the media conditioned by pokeweed mitogen-stimulated spleen cells (PWM-SCM), we later identified the cytokine combinations that support the bilineage differentiation. Again, the effective cytokine combinations proved to be very similar to those supportive of the cell-cycle dormant progenitors. Based on these cell culture studies, a model was proposed in which the cytokines were divided into three groups. The first group consists of IL-3, IL-4 and GM-CSF, which individually can support proliferation of multipotential progenitors. The second group consists of IL-6, IL-11, G-CSF, LIF, IL-12 and TPO. Cytokines in this group, as a single agent, are unable to support formation of multilineage colonies. In addition, IL-6, IL-11, IL-12 and LIF appear to be structurally related to each other or through receptor structure, namely, gp 130. The third group consists of SF and FL, which are ligands for receptors with tyrosine kinase activity. Cytokine interactions are important because, for the effective stimulation of the proliferation of dormant progenitors, combinations of at least two cytokines are required, each belonging to different groups.[1]

EFFECTS OF CYTOKINES ON STEM CELLS

Demonstration that these cytokines do regulate the cell kinetics of hematopoietic stem cells was made in transplantation studies using syngeneic mice. A typical experimental approach was to incubate bone marrow cells that are enriched for stem cells in suspension culture for 1 to 2 weeks, transplant the cells into lethally irradiated recipients together with 'compromised' marrow cells and analyze the ability of the transplanted cells to provided long-term hematopoietic reconstitution. The cells incubated in culture in the presence of combinations of early-acting cytokines were capable of providing long-term reconstitution.[12,13]

Negative Regulations of Stem Cells

During our studies of the effects of recombinant cytokines supporting the proliferation of lymphohematopoietic progenitors, we discovered that the IL-3 or IL-1 can negatively regulate the B-lymphoid potentials of the progenitors.[14] When IL-3 or IL-1 was added to permissive combinations of two cytokines, such as SF and IL-6, SF and IL-11 or FL and IL-11, IL-3 or IL-1 independently abolished the B-lymphoid potentials of the primary colonies. Subsequently, we observed that both the T-cell potential[10] and the NK cell potential[11] of the lymphohematopoietic progenitors were also abolished by IL-3 or IL-1. These observations then raised a question whether or not IL-3 or IL-1 can negatively regulate the earlier process of hematopoiesis, namely, self-renewal of stem cells. Therefore, in the next series of experiments we tested the capabilities of the early-acting cytokines to expand the population of cells capable of long-term reconstitution. Similar to the effects on the lymphoid potentials of the primary colonies, both IL-3 and IL-1 severely compromised the abilities of cultured cells to provide a long-term reconstitution in irradiated recipient mice.[12,13] There are known differences in the structures of mouse and human IL-3 receptors. While there are 2 signal-transducing β proteins (βc and βIL-3) for the mouse IL-3 receptor, the human IL-3 receptor has only βc.[15] We tested the role of βc and βIL-3 in the transduction of the negative signals of IL-3 on mouse stem cells by studying βc-null and βIL-3-null mice. Both βc and βIL-3 transduced the negative signals of IL-3.[16] While the physiological significance of these observations is not clear, this raises a serious question about the use of IL-3 for *in vitro* expansion of human stem cells. Because βc protein is the signal-producing protein of the GM-CSF receptor, we also examined GM-CSF. It had no effects on either lymphohematopoietic progenitors or stem cells.[16] This observation is consistent with the report of McKinstry *et al.*[17] that GM-CSF receptor a protein is not expressed by mouse Rhodamine-123[low] lineage-negative (Lin⁻) Ly-6A/E (Sca-1)⁺ c-kit⁺ cells. FIGURE 1 depicts the interactions of cytokines that positively regulate stem cells.

Mechanisms of the Effects of the Cytokines on Stem Cells

While these studies convincingly demonstrated the direct effects of the early-acting cytokines on stem cells, their mechanisms need to be elucidated. One of the questions we addressed was whether or not these cytokines supported mere survival of stem cells or actively stimulated cell proliferation and self-renewal of the stem cells. In order to answer this question, we examined three cytokines, IL-6, FL, and

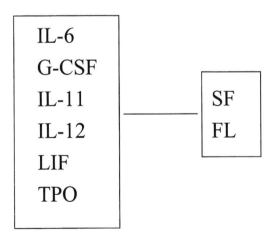

FIGURE 1. A model of interactions of cytokines regulating stem cells.

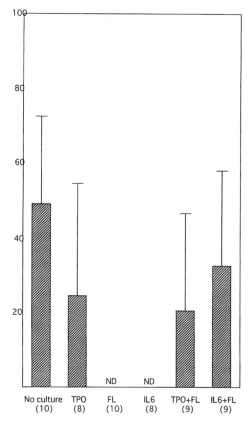

FIGURE 2. Long-term reconstituting abilities of freshly sorted bone marrow cells and cultured cells at 5 months posttransplantation. Data represent mean ± SD of donor cells in the peripheral blood mononuclear cells of the recipient mice. The numbers in parentheses indicate the number of recipient mice.

TPO in suspension culture. In the first experiment, we tested the abilities of the cytokines, as single agents and in combinations, to maintain the cell and progenitor numbers during 1-week suspension culture. Lin⁻ Ly6A/E⁺, c-kit⁺ marrow cells from 5-fluorouracil (5-FU)-treated mice were cultured in suspension for 1 week in the presence and absence of cytokines and tested for total cells and colony-forming units in culture (CFU-C). The results are presented in TABLE 1. While both cells and CFU-C declined in number in the presence of single cytokines, they increased during incubation in the presence of IL-6 and either FL or TPO. These results are consistent with the cytokine interactions defined in culture and described above. We then tested the reconstituting abilities of the cultured cells in transplantation experiments. We used the Ly-5 markers for identification of donor cells and the general transplantation plans described earlier.[12,13] The level of engraftment at 5 months after transplantation is presented in FIGURE 2. As a single agent only TPO was able to maintain

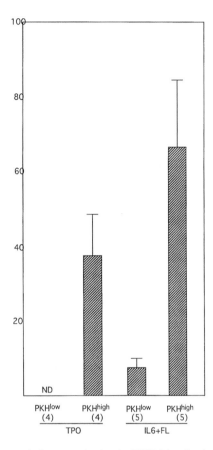

FIGURE 3. Hematopoietic reconstitution by PKH-26-stained cells. The four cell populations were prepared by sorting, and their in vivo reconstituting abilities were analyzed at 5 months posttransplantation. Data represent mean ± SD of donor cells in the peripheral blood mononuclear cells of the recipient mice. The numbers in parentheses indicate the number of recipient mice.

the survival of stem cells. In agreement with the results of cells and CFU-C in TABLE 1, the combination of FL and IL-6 was capable of maintaining the survival of stem cells. Since the maintenance of stem cells by the combination of FL and IL-6 was associated with cell and progenitors proliferation, we wished to test the hypothesis that it reflects cell divisions and self-renewal of the stem cells rather than mere survival of the stem cells. We used a lipid-soluble dye, PKH-26 (PKH), which binds irreversibly to the lipid components of the cell membrane. Using this dye we could study the divisional history of the stem cells. The enriched post-5-FU marrow cells were stained with PKH, and incubated in suspension culture in the presence of either TPO alone or a combination of FL and IL-6 for 1 week. The cells were then separated into PKH^{low} and PKH^{high} cells by fluorescence-activated cell sorter (FACS), and

TABLE 1. Relative change of total cells and progenitors in suspension culture

Cytokines	Cells	Total CFU-C
None	0 ± 0	0 ± 0
FL	0.2 ± 0.1	0 ± 0
TPO	0.4 ± 0.2	0.5 ± 0.2
IL-6	0.2 ± 0.1	0.1 ± 0.1
FL, TPO	0.6 ± 0.1	0.6 ± 0.2
FL, IL-6	4.3 ± 0.8	4.5 ± 0.9
TPO, IL-6	4.2 ± 1.2	2.5 ± 1.0

NOTE: One thousand Lin-Sca-1^+ c-kit$^+$ cells prepared from the marrow of 5-FU-treated mice were cultured in the presence of designated cytokine(s). On day 7 of culture, cells were counted and analyzed for CFU-C in methylcellulose culture. Data represent mean $\pm$ SD of 3 experiments. Day 0 numbers were given a relative value of 1.

each population was analyzed for stem cells by transplantation into lethally irradiated recipients. PKH^{low} cells represented cells that had undergone a number of cell divisions, while PKH^{high} cells represented the cells that remained dormant during incubation. The result of the analyses of the engraftment levels at 5 months post-transplantation is shown in FIGURE 3. Of the cells cultured with TPO alone, only PKH^{high} cells revealed long-term reconstitution. Of the cells cultured in the presence of FL and IL-6, the majority of the reconstitution was from PKH^{high} cells; however, 7.5% of the stem cells with divisional histories (PKH^{low} cells) was also capable of long-term engraftment. These results indicated that some degree of self-renewal of stem cells takes place but that the majority of stem cells remain dormant in culture with cytokines. It is possible that hitherto unknown cytokines are necessary for stimulation of all stem cells. The results, however, clearly demonstrated that expansion of total cells and progenitors cannot be taken as a sign of expansion of stem cells.

REFERENCES

1. OGAWA, M. 1993. Differentiation and proliferation of hematopoietic stem cells. Blood **81:** 2844–2853.
2. HIRAYAMA, F., S.D. LYMAN, S.C. CLARK & M. OGAWA. 1995. The FLT3 ligand supports proliferation of lymphohemopoietic progenitors and early B-lymphoid progenitors. Blood **85:** 1762–1768.
3. KU, H., Y. YONEMURA, K. KAUSHANSKY & M. OGAWA. 1996. Thrombopoietin, the ligand for the Mpl receptor, synergises with steel factor and other early-acting cytokines in supporting proliferation of primitive hematopoietic progenitors of mice. Blood **87:** 4544–4551.
4. IKEBUCHI, K., G.G. WON., S.C. CLARK, J.N. IHLE, Y. HIRAI & M. OGAWA. 1987. Interleukin 6 enhancement of interleukin 3 dependent proliferation of multipotential hemopoietic progenitors. Proc. Natl. Acad. Sci. USA **84:** 9035–9039.
5. IKEBUCHI, K., S.C. CLARK, J.N. IHLE, L.M. SOUZA & M. OGAWA. 1988. Granulocyte colony-stimulating factor enhances interleukin 3-dependent proliferation of multipotential hemopoietic progenitors. Proc. Natl. Acad. Sci. USA **85:** 3445–3449.
6. MUSASHI, M., Y-C YANG, S.R. PAUL, S.C. CLARK, T. SUDO & M. OGAWA. 1991. Direct and synergistic effects of interleukin 11 on murine hemopoiesis in culture. Proc. Natl. Acad. Sci. USA **88:** 765–769.
7. NAKAHATA, T. & M. OGAWA. 1982. Identification in culture of a new class of hemopoietic colony-forming units with extensive capability to self renew and generate multipotential hemopoietic colonies. Proc. Natl. Acad. Sci. USA **79:** 3843–3847.

8. LEARY, A.G., H-Q. ZENG, S.C. CLARK & M. OGAWA. 1992. Growth factor requirements for survival in G0 and entry into the cell cycle of primitive human hemopoietic progenitors. Proc. Natl. Acad. Sci. USA **89:** 4013–4017.

9. HIRAYAMA, F., J-P. SHIH, A. AWGULEWITSCH, G.W. WARR, S.C. CLARK & M. OGAWA. 1992. Clonal proliferation of murine lymphohemopoietic progenitors in culture. Proc. Natl. Acad. Sci. USA **89:** 5907–5911.

10. HIRAYAMA, F. & M. OGAWA. 1995. Negative regulation of early T-lymphopoiesis by interleukin-3 and interleukin-1a. Blood **86:** 4527-4531.

11. AIBA, Y. & M. OGAWA. 1997. Development of natural killer (NK) cells, B lymphocytes, macrophages and mast cells from single hematopoietic progenitors in culture of murine fetal liver cells. Blood **90:** 3923–3930.

12. YONEMURA, Y., H. KU, F. HIRAYAMA, L.M. SOUZA & M. OGAWA. 1996. Interleukin-3 or interleukin-1 abrogates the reconstituting ability of hematopoietic stem cells. Proc. Natl. Acad. Sci. USA **93:** 4040–4044.

13. YONEMURA, Y., H. KU, S.D. LYMAN & M. OGAWA. 1997. In vitro expansion of hematopoietic progenitors and maintenance of stem cells: Comparison between FLT3/FLK2 ligand and KIT ligand. Blood **89:** 1915–1921.

14. HIRAYAMA F., S.C. CLARK & M. OGAWA. 1994. Negative regulation of early B-lymphopoiesis by interleukin-3 and interleukin-1a. Proc. Natl. Acad. Sci. USA **91:** 469–473.

15. HARA, T. & A. MIYAJIMA. 1992. Two distinct functional high affirmity receptors for mouse interleukin-3 (IL-3). EMBO J. **11:** 1875–1884.

16. MATSUNAGA, T., F. HIRAYAMA, Y. YONEMURA, R. MURRAY & M. OGAWA. Negative regulation by interleukin-3 of mouse early B-cell progenitors and stem cells in culture: Transduction of the negative signals by bc and bIL-3 proteins of interleukin-3 receptor and absence of negative regulation by GM-CSF. Blood. In press.

17. MCKINSTRY, W.J., C-L. LI, J.E.J. RASKO, N.A. NICOLA, G.R. JOHNSON & D. METCALF. 1997. Cytokine receptor expression of hematopoietic stem and progenitor cells. Blood **89:** 65.

DISCUSSION

G.J. SPANGRUDE (*University of Utah Medical Center*): I am interested in the IL-3 effect on mouse stem cells. We heard from Connie Eaves that there was a dose sensitive effect and I saw in your data you tried a high and low dose and saw your effect. I have always been intrigued by the possibility that this is predominantly a post 5-FU phenomenon. Tell me whether you see this effect in normal bone marrow studies or whether you have only seen it in post 5-FU studies?

OGAWA: We see it with cells from normal mice. Also the human cells are not post 5-FU cells.

S.J. SHARKIS (*Johns Hopkins Oncology Center*): If I read your data correctly, there is a little controversy as to whether or not cells are in cycle. Connie told us that it was the cells in cycle after *in vitro* culture that had reconstituting capacity, but if I am correct, you are telling us in fact that it was only the cells that remained PKH-bright that had the capacity to reconstitute.

OGAWA: We cannot be too dogmatic. We do not have the sophisticated technique that Connie has. Therefore, I said that the cells are relatively dormant in cycling. I cannot exclude the possibility that the cells divided a couple of times.

C.J. EAVES (*Terry Fox Laboratory*): I noticed that the data you showed was for TPO alone or Flt-3 ligand + IL-6. In our hands we also do not see amplification of stem cells with either of those conditions. Therefore, I think our findings and yours are quite consistent. I think you need additional factors to get a significant amplification.

G. KELLER (*Howard Hughes Medical Institute*): This is a question for Connie. Have you seen any repopulation with CD34⁻ cells in the NOD-SCID model?

EAVES: We have not yet really looked properly. We did try a couple of years ago but did not try high enough numbers of cells given what we know from other people's data. We certainly are working with CD34⁻ cells and can isolate subpopulations which have progenitor activity especially after being cultured in the presence of growth factors so I am persuaded that there are definitely very interesting cells in that population However, we do not have NOD-SCID data to talk about, but John Dick does.

Expression of Novel Surface Antigens on Early Hematopoietic Cells[a]

HANS-JÖRG BÜHRING,[b,d] MARTINA SEIFFERT,[b] THOMAS A. BOCK,[b] STEFAN SCHEDING,[b] ANDREAS THIEL,[c] ALEXANDER SCHEFFOLD,[c] LOTHAR KANZ,[b] AND WOLFRAM BRUGGER[b]

[b]Department of Hematology and Oncology, University of Tübingen, Tübingen, Germany
[c]Department of Immunology, German Rheuma Research Center, Berlin, Germany

ABSTRACT: The purpose of this report is to demonstrate the expression of very recently identified surface antigens on CD34[+] and AC133[+] bone marrow (BM) cells. Coexpression analysis of AC133 and defined antigens on CD34[+] BM cells revealed that the majority of the CD164[+], CD135[+], CD117[+], CD38[low], CD33[+], and CD71[low] cells resides in the AC133[+] population. In contrast, most of the CD10[+] and CD19[+] B cell progenitors and a fraction of the CD71[high] population are AC133[-], indicating that CD34[+]AC133[+] cells are enriched in primitive and myeloid progenitor cells, whereas CD34[+]AC133[-] cells mainly consist of B cell and late erythroid progenitors. This corresponds to the highly reduced percentage of CD10[+] B cells and the absence of CD71[high] erythroid progenitors on AC133[+] selected BM cells. A portion of 0.2–0.7% of the AC133[+] selected cells do not coexpress CD34. These cells are very small and define a uniform CD71[-], CD117[-], CD10[-], CD38[low], CD135[+], HLA-DR[high], CD45[+] population with unknown delineation. Four color analysis on CD34[+]CD38[-] BM cells revealed that virtually all of these primitive cells express AC133. Using an improved liposome-enhanced labeling technique for the staining of weakly expressed antigens, subsets of this population could be identified which express the angiopoietin receptors TIE (67.6%) and TEK (36.8%), the vascular endothelial growth factor receptors FLT1 (7%), FLT4 (3.2%), and KDR (10.4%), or the receptor tyrosine kinases HER-2 (15.4%) and FLT3 (CD135; 77.6%). Our results suggest that the CD34[+]CD38[-] population is heterogeneous with respect to the expression of the analyzed receptor tyrosine kinases.

INTRODUCTION

In an attempt to define the surface marker profile of hematopoietic stem cells, monoclonal antibodies against cell surface antigens were developed which either selectively recognize immature hematopoietic cells or further dissect populations within the stem cell compartment. Based on the establishment of such antibodies most of the hematopoietic stem cells can now be defined by the

[a]These studies were supported by the Deutsche Forschungsgemeinschaft (SFB 510, project A1), by a grant from the Research Program of the University Clinic of Tübingen (fortüne; project 433), and by a grant from the Federal Ministry of Education and Research and the Interdisciplinary Clinical Research Center (project IIA1).

[d]Correspondence to: Hans-Jörg Bühring, Ph.D., Department of Hematology and Oncology, University of Tübingen, FACS-Laboratory, Otfried-Müller-Str.10, 72076 Tübingen, Germany. Phone, +49-7071-298 2730; fax, +49-7071-29 2730; e-mail, hjbuehri@med.uni-tuebingen.de

CD34[high]CD90[+]CD38[-] phenotype.[1-4] Recently, a primitive CD34-negative stem cell population was described which is negative for most of the cell surface markers that are generally attributed to primitive hematopoietic cells.[5-7] Very recently, a pentaspan molecule defined by the antibody AC133[8,9] with homolgy to mouse prominin[10,11] and C. elegans protein F08B12.1[12] was identified, which appears to be exclusively expressed on a subpopulation of hematopoietic CD34[+] cells.[8] In this report we describe the expression of AC133 on CD34[+] and CD34[+]CD38[-] human bone marrow cells as well as the coexpression patterns of the angiopoietin receptors TIE and TEK, and the vascular endothelial growth factor (VEGF) receptors FLT1, FLT4, and KDR. Since these receptors are only expressed at very low copy numbers on the cell surface, we applied a novel magnetofluorescent liposome staining technique to increase the sensitivity of immunofluorescence.[13]

MATERIALS AND METHODS

Source of Human Cells

Bone marrow (BM) cells from healthy donors were obtained after informed consent according to the guidelines of our local ethics committee. Mononuclear cells were separated on a Ficoll-Hypaque (Biochrome, Berlin, Germany) density gradient (1.077 g/ml).

Immunomagnetic Separation

AC133[+] or CD34[+] BM cells were purified on magnetic activated cell sorting (MACS) columns using microbead-conjugated AC133 or anti-CD34 antibodies (Miltenyi Biotech, Bergisch Gladbach, Germany). Separation on MiniMACS devices was performed according to the manufacturer's recommendations (Miltenyi Biotech).

Antibodies

The following antibody conjugates were used for immunofluorescence staining: anti-CD10-FITC, CD38-FITC, CD71-FITC, HLA-DR-FITC, CD34-PerCP, and CD38-APC were obtained from Becton Dickinson, Heidelberg, Germany; anti-CD33-FITC were purchased from Immunotech, Hamburg, Germany, and anti-CD117 from Hoelzel, Cologne, Germany. Biotinylated anti-FLT1 antiserum was obtained from R&D, Wiesbaden, Germany. AC133-PE was a kind gift from Dr. D. Buck, Sunnyvale, California, and 4G8-FITC, BV10-biotin (both anti-CD135), and 24D2-biotin (anti-HER-2) were produced and conjugated in our own facilities.[14-17] Biotinylated antibodies with specificities for TIE and FLT4 were a kind gift from Dr. K. Alitalo, Helsinki, Finland. Biotinylated anti-TEK was kindly provided by Dr. T. Suda, Kumamoto, Japan, and biotinylated anti-KDR by Dr. P. Reusch, Freiburg, Germany.

Preparation of Reagents for Staining with Liposome Conjugates

Streptavidin (Pierce, Rockford, USA) was coupled to digoxigenin (DIG) (Boehringer Mannheim, Mannheim, Germany) according to the manufacturer's instructions (Boehringer Mannheim). The preparation of magnetofluorescent liposomes and coupling with $F(ab)_2'$ fragments of anti-DIG antibodies (Boehringer Mannheim) was described previously.[13]

Immunofluorescence Staining and Flow Cytometric Analysis

Three-color staining

MACS-selected AC133[+] or CD34[+] BM cells were stained with the following antibodies for 30 minutes on ice: Anti-CD34-PerCP, AC133-PE, and FITC-conjugates of the indicated antibodies. After washing twice in staining buffer (PBS, 1% BSA, 0.1% NaN_3) cells were analyzed on a FACSCalibur flow cytometer (Becton Dickinson, Heidelberg, Germany).

Four-color staining

Mononuclear BM cells were stained with the following antibodies for 30 minutes on ice: Anti-CD34-PerCP, anti-CD38-APC, AC133-PE, and biotin-conjugates of the indicated antibodies. After two washing steps cells were incubated with streptavidin-digoxigenin (SA-DIG) for 30 minutes on ice and washed twice. In the final step cells were incubated with anti-DIG conjugated magnetofluorescent liposomes for 30 minutes at room temperature. Tubes were vigorously shaken during incubation to keep liposomes and cells in suspension. After washing twice in staining buffer (PBS, 1% BSA, 0.1% NaN3), cells were analyzed on a FACSCalibur flow cytometer (Becton Dickinson, Heidelberg, Germany).

Flow cytometric analysis

Analyses of cells were performed on a FACSCalibur flow cytometer (Becton Dickinson, Heidelberg, Germany) equipped with an argon laser to excite FITC-; PE-; and PerCP fluorochromes, and an helium-neon laser to excite allophycocyanine (APC) fluorochromes. The time delay for the second laser was adjusted according to the manufacturer's recommendations. 10,000–20,000 CD34[+] or AC133[+] selected BM cells or 100,000 mononuclear cells were analyzed using the CellQuest software program (Becton Dickinson, Heidelberg, Germany).

FIGURE 1. Coexpression of AC133 and CD surface antigens on MACS-selected BM CD34[+] cells. Selected cells were labeled with anti-CD34-PerCP, AC133-PE, and FITC-conjugates of the indicated antibodies. Cells were analyzed on a FACSCalibur flow cytometer using the CellQuest software program. Plots show displays of AC133 versus CD antigens of cells gated on the CD34[+] population.

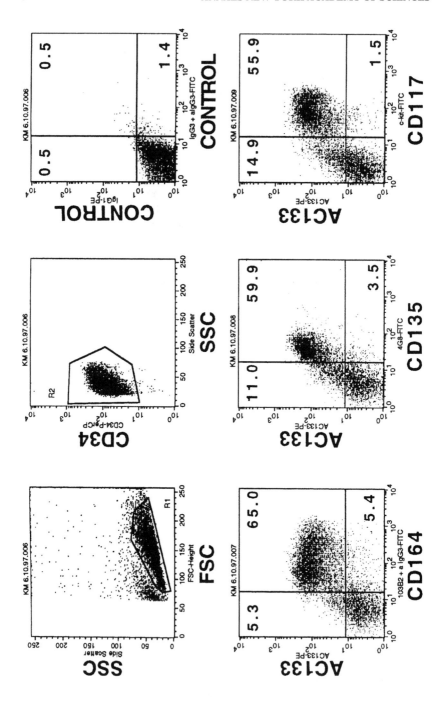

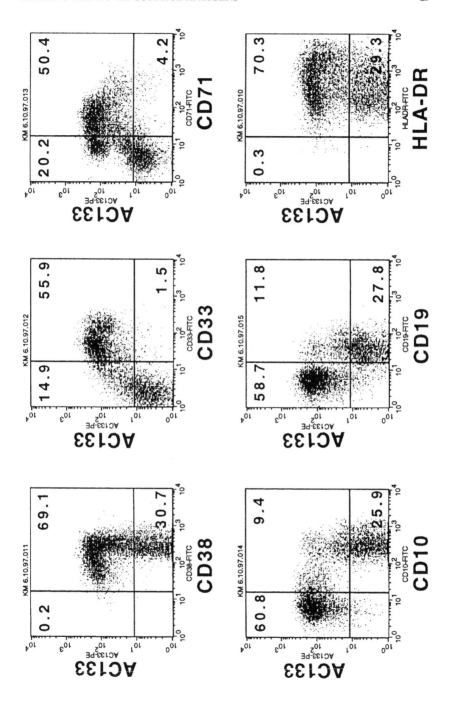

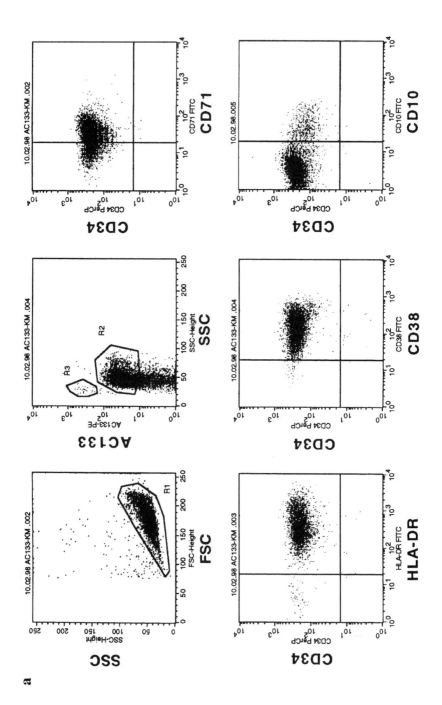

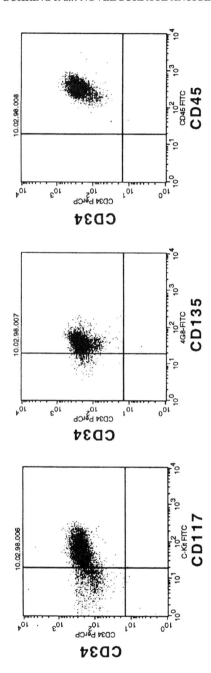

FIGURE 2. Coexpression of CD34 and CD antigens on MACS-selected BM AC133+ cells. Selected cells were labeled with anti-CD34-PerCP, AC133-PE, and FITC-conjugates of the indicated antibodies. Cells were analyzed on a FACSCalibur flow cytometer using the CellQuest software program. Plots show displays of CD34 versus CD antigens of cells gated on the AC133+ population. (**a**) Analysis of cells gated on the AC133low population as defined in the side scatter versus AC133 plot.

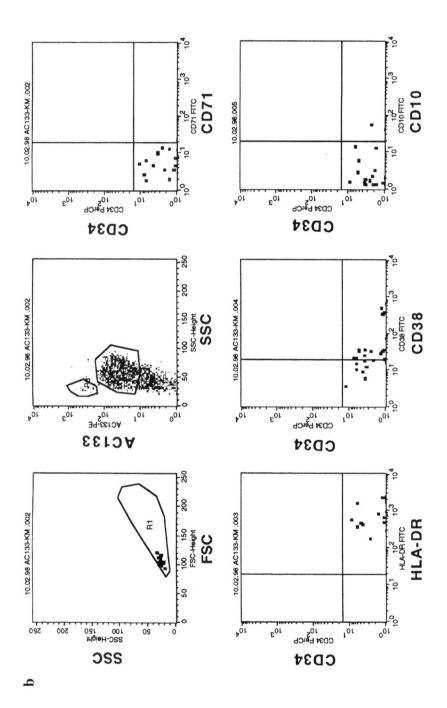

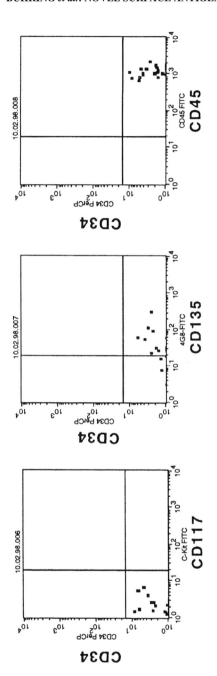

FIGURE 2. (b) Analysis of cells gated on the AC133^{high} population as defined in the side scatter versus AC133 plot. The cells in the dual scatter plot represent cells gated on the AC133^{high} population.

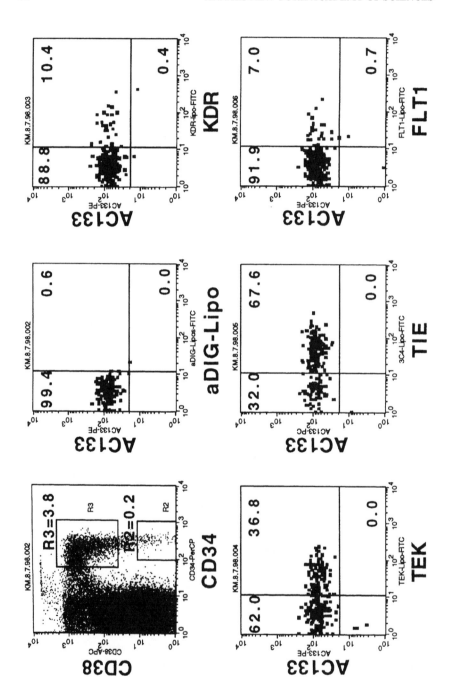

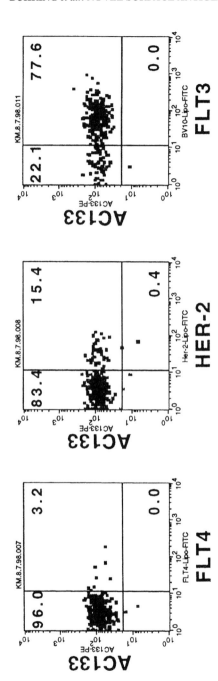

FIGURE 3. Coexpression of AC133 and receptor tyrosine kinases on CD34+CD38− BM cells. Cells were labeled with anti-CD38-APC, anti-CD34-PerCP, AC133-PE, and biotinylated conjugates of antibodies with the indicated specificities. The biotinylated antibodies were labeled with streptavidin-digoxigenin (SA-DIG) in the next step and with anti-DIG-liposomes[13] in the final step. Cells were analyzed on a FACSCalibur flow cytometer using the CellQuest software program. Plots show displays of AC133 versus receptor tyrosine kinase expression of cells gated on the CD34+CD38− population.

RESULTS AND DISCUSSION

Analysis of AC133 Expression on CD34+ BM Cells

In the first set of experiments the coexpression of AC133 and CD antigens was analyzed on CD34-selected BM cells. The plots in FIGURE 1 show that almost all the CD164+, CD135+, CD117+, CD33+, and CD71^{low} cells coexpress AC133, whereas most of the CD10+ and CD19+ cells are AC133-. In addition, CD34+ cells expressing the highest levels of CD71 are also negative for AC133. These results suggest that CD34+AC133+ cells are enriched in primitive hematopoietic cells and myeloid progenitors/precursors, whereas the CD34+AC133- fraction contains cells mainly committed to the B cell and erythroid lineages.

Analysis of CD34 Expression on AC133+ BM Cells

In the next experiments the coexpression of CD34 and CD antigens on AC133-selected BM cells was analyzed. FIGURE 2 shows two distinct AC133+ populations, a major population with a lower density of AC133 expression and a minor AC133^{high} population consisting of 0.1–0.7% of the AC133+ cells. Gating on the AC133^{low} cells revealed that, compared to CD34-selected cells, these CD34+ cells are enriched for CD71$^{low/-}$, CD38^{low}, CD117+, and CD135+, and almost depleted for CD10+ cells (FIG. 2a). These results are in line with the observation that CD34+AC133- cells mainly consist of CD10+ B cells and CD71^{high} erythroid cells.

FIGURE 2b shows the plots of cells gated on the AC133^{high} population. These cells are very small as demonstrated by backgating into the dual scatter plot, and define a uniform CD71-, CD117-, CD10-, CD38^{low}, CD135+, HLA-DRhigh, CD45+ population with unknown delineation. Since the phenotype of this population is very similar to the recently reported phenotype of CD34- stem cells,[6] we were interested whether AC133 is expressed on these cells. However, preliminary characterization of CD34- 'side population (SP)' cells in a dual-wavelength flow cytometry-defined analysis of cells stained with the Hoechst 33342 dye,[5] revealed that AC133+CD34- do not represent SP cells but rather rare B cells.

Coexpression of AC133 and Receptor Tyrosine Kinases on CD34+CD38- BM Cells

To further characterize the distribution of antigens which are expressed only at very low copy numbers on the cell surface of early hematopoietic cells, magnetofluorescent liposomes were used to increase the sensitivity of staining.[13] BM CD34+CD38- cells were analyzed by four-color analysis for their coexpression of AC133 and the angiopoietin receptors TIE and TEK, the vascular endothelial growth factor receptors FLT1, FLT4, and KDR, and the receptor tyrosine kinases (RTK) HER-2 and FLT3 (CD135). FIGURE 3 demonstrates that all receptors are expressed on CD34+CD38- subpopulations. The FLT3 receptor (76%+) and the angiopoietin receptors TIE (67%+) and TEK (36%+) showed the most prominent expression on these primitive cells, whereas expression of the VEGF receptors KDR (10%+), FLT1 (7%+), and FLT4 (3%+) and the class I RTK HER-2 (15%+) was found only on minor populations.

Our data demonstrate for the first time the surface expression of these RTK on primitive $CD34^+CD38^-$ BM cells. Additional studies are required to evaluate which fractions contain cells with the capacity to reconstitute long-term multilineage hematopoiesis in non obese severe combined immunodeficiency (NOD-SCID) mice[18] or in the human/sheep xenograft model.[19] The results would then provide significant information about the RTK-phenotype on pluripotent hematopoietic stem cells.[20] Using the novel liposome conjugates for improved resolution of antigen-negative cells and cells expressing only low copy numbers of surface antigens, it is now possible to reevaluate the findings of previous reports in which cobblestone area forming cells (CAFC) were found in either the $FLT3^+$ and $FLT3^-$ or the TIE^+ and TIE^- populations, respectively.[15,21]

ACKNOWLEDGMENTS

We thank H. Letzkus and A. Marxer for excellent technical assistance.

REFERENCES

1. BAUM, C.M., I.L. WEISSMAN, A.S. TSUKAMOTO *et al.* 1992. Isolation of a candidate human hematopoietic stem cell population. Proc. Natl. Acad. Sci. USA **89:** 2804–2808.
2. CRAIG, W., R. KAY, R.L. CUTLER *et al.* 1993. Expression of Thy-1 on human hematopoietic progenitor cells. J. Exp. Med. **177:** 1331–1342.
3. TERSTAPPEN, L.W.M., S. HUANG, M. SAFFORD *et al.* 1991. Sequential generations of hematopoietic colonies derived from single nonlineage-committed $CD34^+CD38^-$ progenitor cells. Blood **77:** 1218–1227.
4. DIGIUSTO, D., S. CHEN, J. COMBS *et al.* 1994. Human fetal bone marrow early progenitors for T, B, and myeloid cells are found exclusively in the population expressing high levels of CD34. Blood **84:** 421–432.
5. GOODELL, M.A., K. BROSE, G. PARADIS *et al.* 1996. Isolation and functional properties of murine hematopoietic stem cells that are replicating in vivo. J. Exp. Med. **183:** 1797–1806.
6. GOODELL, M.A., M. ROSENZWEIG, H. KIM *et al.* 1997. Dye efflux studies suggest that hematopoietic stem cells expressing low or undetectable levels of CD34 antigen exist in multiple species. Nat. Med. **3:** 1337–1345.
7. SHARKIS, S.J., M.I. COLLECTOR, J.P. BARBER *et al.* 1997. Phenotypic and functional characterization of the hematopoietic stem cell. Stem Cells **15** (Suppl. 1)**:** 41–45.
8. YIN, A.H., S. MIRAGLIA, E.D. ZANJANI *et al.* 1997. AC133, a novel marker for human hematopoietic stem and progenitor cells. Blood **90:** 5002–5012.
9. MIRAGLIA, S., W. GODFREY, A.H. YIN *et al.* 1997. A novel five-transmembrane hematopoietic stem cell antigen: Isolation, characterization, and molecular cloning. Blood **90:** 5013–5021.
10. CORBEIL, D., K. ROPER, A. WEIGMANN *et al.* 1998. AC133 hematopoietic stem cell antigen: Human homologue of mouse kidney prominin or distinct member of a novel protein family? Blood **91:** 2625–2626.
11. WEIGMANN, A., D. CORBEIL, A. HELLWIG *et al.* 1997. Prominin, a novel microvilli-specific polytopic membrane protein of the apical surface of epithelial cells, is targeted to plasmalemmal protrusions of non-epithelial cells. Proc. Natl. Acad. Sci. USA **94:** 12425–12430.
12. WILSON, R., R. AINSCOUGH, K. ANDERSON *et al.* 1994. 2.2 Mb of contiguous nucleotide sequence from chromosome III of C. elegans. Nature **368:** 32–38.

13. SCHEFFOLD, A., S. MILTENYI, A. RADBRUCH et al. 1995. Magnetofluorescent lipo-
    somes for increased sensitivity of immunofluorescence. Immunotechnology **1:**
    127–137.
14. ROSNET, O., H.-J. BÜHRING, S. MARCHETTO et al. 1996. The human FLT3/FLK2
    hematopoietic receptor tyrosine kinase is expressed on the surface of normal and
    malignant hematopoietic cells. Leukemia **10:** 238–248.
15. RAPPOLD, I., B.L. ZIEGLER, I. KOHLER et al. 1997. Functional and phenotypic charac-
    terization of cord blood and bone marrow subsets expressing FLT3 receptor
    tyrosine kinase. Blood **90:** 111–125.
16. BÜHRING, H.-J., D. BIRNBAUM, K. BRASEL et al. 1998. CD135 workshop panel report.
    In Leucocyte Typing VI. T. Kishimoto et al., Eds.: 875–879. Garland Publishing,
    Inc. New York.
17. BÜHRING, H.-J., I. SURES, B. JALLAL et al. 1995. The receptor tyrosine kinase
    p185HER2 is expressed on a subset of B-lymphoid blasts from patients with acute
    lymphoblastic leukemia and chronic myelogenous leukemia. Blood **86:** 1916–
    1923.
18. BOCK, T.A., D. ORLIC, C.E. DUNBAR et al. 1995. Improved engraftment of human
    hematopoietic cells in severe combined immunodeficient (SCID) mice carrying
    human cytokine transgenes. J. Exp. Med. **182:** 2037–2043.
19. ZANJANI, E.D., G. ALMEIDA-PORADA & A.W. FLAKE. 1996. The human/sheep
    xenograft model: A large animal model of human hematopoiesis. Int. J. Hematol.
    63: 1051–1055.
20. BOCK, T.A. 1997. Assay systems for hematopoietic stem and progenitor cells. Stem
    Cells **15**(Suppl. 1)**:** 185–195.
21. KUKK, E., U. WARTIOVAARA, Y. GUNJI et al. 1997. Analysis of TIE receptor tyrosine
    kinase in haematopoietic progenitor and leukaemia cells. Br. J. Haematol. **98:** 195–
    203.

DISCUSSION

J.D. GRIFFIN (*Dana Farber Cancer Insitute*): A standard FACS can probably detect about 500–1000 antigens per cell. Do you have any sense about how much more
sensitive this liposome technique is?

BÜHRING: I asked the group that produced the liposomes and they could not give
me a definite answer, but if I compare it with conventional staining methods, it definitely resolves antigens which I cannot resolve with the other method. Of course
you can estimate the sensitvity increase using standard reference beads, but we did
not perform this experiment.

C.J. EAVES (*Terry Fox Laboratory*): Our experience with anti-AC133 antibody
has been to get nice staining of cord blood cells and fetal liver but lousy staining of
bone marrow. Your bone marrow staining looked pretty nice and equivalent to cord
blood. Do you think that this is just a different preparation that we may have? Have
you encountered this finding?

BÜHRING: We always get nice staining of our bone marrow cells. Of course there
is one problem if you have AC133 selected cells and restain them — and at the moment you can only restain them with same antibody as used for selection — then you
get a reduced signal. But we get equivalent signals also in bone marrow cells. One
of the most important questions to me, and I would like to address this also to the
audience, is whether anyone already knows whether CD34⁻ stem cells do express the

AC133 antigen. At the moment we are trying to find this out using the Goodell method for detection of CD34$^-$ stem cells which reside in the Hoechst red-low Hoechst-blue-intermediate population. I would be very interested to know if anyone in the audience has data whether the AC133 antibody detects CD34$^+$ stem cells. If this were the case, the AC133 antibody would be superior to CD34 antibodies for stem cell selection.

L. KANZ (*Eberhard Karls University*): The expression of HER-2 somehow is frightening. There are many groups trying to use vaccination strategies with HER-2 related peptides and for dendritic cells fused with those peptides for specific immuno-therapy in breast or ovarian cancer. Could you comment on a possible induction of bone marrow aplasia in those patients?

BÜHRING: By conventional staining techniques you find low to absent HER-2 expression on normal CD34$^+$ stem cells, which is in contrast to the expression on some leukemic ALL blasts. Most probably HER-2 targeting strategies, which are efficient in ovarian and breast cancer, will not affect hematopoietic stem cells, because they express very low copy numbers of HER-2 on the cell surface. However, treating stem cells with anti-HER-2 peptides or HER-2-specific dendritic cells will answer your question.

Lymphohematopoietic Stem Cell Engraftment[a]

PETER J. QUESENBERRY,[b] F. MARC STEWART, SUJU ZHONG,
HOURI HABIBIAN, CHRISTINA MCAULIFFE, JUDY REILLY, JANE CARLSON,
MARK DOONER, SUSIE NILSSON, STEFAN PETERS, GARY STEIN,
JANET STEIN, ROB EMMONS, BRIAN BENOIT, IVAN BERTONCELLO, AND
PAMELA BECKER

University of Massachusetts Medical Center and University of Massachusetts Cancer Center, Worcester, Massachusetts 01605, USA

ABSTRACT: Traditional dogma has stated that space needs to be opened by cytoxic myeloablative therapy in order for marrow stem cells to engraft. Recent work in murine transplant models, however, indicates that engraftment is determined by the ratio of donor to host stem cells, i.e., stem cell competition. One hundred centigray whole body irradiation is stem cell toxic and nonmyelotoxic, thus allowing for higher donor chimerism in a murine syngeneic transplant setting. This nontoxic stem cell transplantation can be applied to allogeneic transplant with the addition of a tolerizing step; in this case presensitization with donor spleen cells and administration of CD40 ligand antibody to block costimulation.

The stem cells that engraft in the nonmyeloablated are in G_0, but are rapidly induced (by 12 hours) to enter the S phase after *in vivo* engraftment. Exposure of murine marrow to cytokines (IL-3, IL-6, IL-11 and steel factor) expands progenitor clones, induces stem cells into cell cycle, and causes a fluctuating engraftment phenotype tied to phase of cell cycle. These data indicate that the concepts of stem cell competition and fluctuation of stem cell phenotype with cell cycle transit should underlie any new stem cell engraftment strategy.

Traditionally, it has been considered that space needs to be opened by myeloablative therapy in order for there to be adequate lymphohematopoietic stem cell engraftment. However, previous studies by Micklem, Saxe, Brecher and others have indicated that marrow cells would engraft in nonablated animals.[1-5] Stewart *et. al.*[6] extended these observations showing high levels of long-term multilineage engraftment in nonmyeloablated BALB/c mice. A series of studies utilizing a male/female transplantation model in nonmyeloablated BALB/c hosts has shown that engraftment is essentially quantitative and appears to be determined by competition between infused marrow cells and host cells.[7-10] These studies show that high levels of engraftment were obtained in marrow, spleen and thymus, that the level of en-

[a]This work was supported in part by National Institutes of Health grants No: RO1 DK27424-14, Hematopoietic Cellular Interaction and Lithium, R01 DK49650-04, Repetitive Marrow Transplantation into Normal Mice, P01 DK50222-01A1, Stem Cell Biology and P01 HL56920-02, Hematopoietic Stem Cell Growth and Engraftment.

[b]Correspondence and requests for materials to: Peter J. Quesenberry, M.D., Director, Cancer Center, University of Massachusetts Medical Center and University of Massachusetts Cancer Center, Two BioTech, Suite 202, 373 Plantation Street, Worcester, MA 01605. Phone, 508/856-6956; fax, 508/856-1310; e-mail, Peter.Quesenberry@banyan.ummed.edu

TABLE 1. Engraftment into nonmyeloablated hosts

High levels of chimerism seen in marrow, spleen and thymus.
Chimerism persistent out to two years.
Chimerism multilineage.
Engraftment at stem cell level appears quantitative.

graftment was cell dose related and that high numbers of cells given in one injection gave equal levels of engraftment to the same number of cells divided over multiple injections, although the addition of heparin could enhance engraftment at very high levels of infused cells. Experiments were carried out where 40 million cells were infused on 20 separate occasions into the same mouse over time. This very high level of infusion led to very high levels of marrow engraftment but not to total replacement of marrow. These data are summarized in TABLE 1.

Further studies in this model has shown that highly purified lineage-negative, rhodamine-low, Hoescht-low murine stem cells also engraft well and give high levels of marrow chimerism in nonmyeloablated BALB/c mice.[11] Homing studies revealed a probable maximal window of 19 hours for marrow engraftment with fairly rapid clearance of stem cells from blood and lung.[12] No early homing was seen in thymus and very low levels in the spleen. Mapping of male cells in female nonmyeloablated hosts utilizing the fluorescence *in situ* hybridization (FISH) technique on fixed marrow sections revealed that by six weeks postengraftment virtually all of the engrafted male cells were adjacent to the endosteal surface.[11] In addition, it was clear that these cells had given rise to bone osteocytes which persisted out to six months post-marrow infusion.[12]

The above observations suggested that engraftment was dependent upon the ratio of host and donor stem cells, not upon any actions in 'opening space.' If this was in fact the case, treatments which could diminish host stem cells without toxicity, should be able to markedly increase the percent of donor chimerism by increasing the competitive advantage of transfused stem cells. This could provide a nontoxic way of augmenting the percentage of donor cells, while minimizing the severe nuetropenia and thrombocytopenia associated with conventional myeloablative conditioning regimines. Accordingly, we assessed the capacity of low doses of irradiation 1) to ablate engrafting stem cells in the host and 2) to enhance donor engraftment.[13] Exposure of BALB/c mice to a 100 cGy whole body irradiation markedly decreased the capacity of marrow stem cells to engraft long-term to a level of about 10% of normal. This left enough residual hematopoietic stem/progenitor cells to avoid any significant myeloablation. There were transient and moderate decreases in the white count and platelet count. Mice exposed to 100 cGy and infused with 40 million marrow cells showed high levels of persistent chimerism at 2, 5 and 8 months postinfusion. The chimerism was multilineage and was evidenced in marrow, spleen and thymus. Hosts exposed to 100 cGy whole body irradiation also showed relatively high levels of chimerism when infused with 10 million marrow cells, levels estimated to be those potentially obtainable in a clinical transplant setting. These results indicated that a 100-cGy whole body irradiation was very stem cell toxic, but nonmyelotoxic and allowed for very high levels of long-term donor cell chimerism.

TABLE 2. Murine allochimerism

B6 to BALB/c	Mismatch at h2 locus
Low level host treatment	100 cGy
High levels of infused stem cells	40×10^6 B6 marrow cells
Costimulator blockade	CD-40 ligand antibody — multiple injections

ALLOCHIMERISM

The combination of relatively high levels of infused stem cells and low-level ir-radiation offers an attractive approach for the nontoxic creation of chimerism. In or-der for these approaches to be useful for treatment of marrow disorders they must be applicable in an allogenesic stem cell transplantation setting. This introduces the problems of graft-versus-host disease (GVHD) and graft rejection. The keys to es-tablishing long-term stable allochimerism for the treatment of intrinsic marrow dis-eases, autoimmune disorders or cancer relates to avoiding GVHD and rejection and establishing long-term tolerance. Theoretically low-level host treatment avoids the 'cytokine storm' and its purported adverse effects on GVHD. The utilization of high levels of stem cells may also help overcome rejection and GVHD problems.

A powerful approach to tolerization has been costimulator blockade of CD40-CD40 ligand or B7-CD28 interactions. Accordingly, we have evaluated the combined use of high levels of stem cells, low-level host irradiation and costimulator blockade as an approach to the nontoxic creation of stable allochimerism (TABLE 2). Thus we evaluated our capacity to establish allochimerism in a completely H_2 mis-matched murine marrow transplantation model.

In one experiment 40×10^6 B6 cells were infused into 100 cGy-treated BALB/c hosts, and engraftment was quantitated utilizing monoclonal antibody marking and

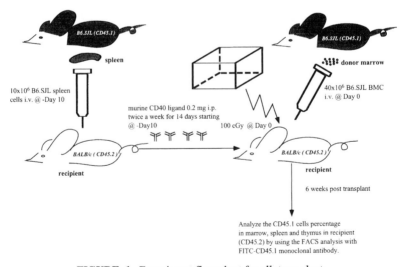

FIGURE 1. Experiment flow chart for allotransplant.

TABLE 3. B6.SJL: BALB/c allochimerism[a]

Group	Treatment	Average Marrow Engraftment Determined by FITC-CD45.1[d]
I	40×10^6 BMC + 100 cGy[b]	$18 + 7$
II	40×10^6 BMC + 100 cGy + 10×10^6 spleen cells[c]	$8 + 6$
III	40×10^6 BMC + 100 cGy + 10×10^6 spleen cells[c] + CD40 ligand antibody	$39 + 4$

[a]B6.SJL as donor is H-2K[s], CD45.1, BALB/c as recipient is H-2K[d], CD45.2
[b]All BALB/c host mice were treated with 100 cGy at transplant day.
[c]Group II & III received 10×10^6 B6.SJL spleen cell i.v. 10 days prior to transplant. Group III received CD40 ligand as outlined in FIGURE 1.
[d]Engraftment was determined 6 weeks after transplant, using FITC-CD45.1 monoclonal antibody to mark donor cells with analysis by FACS.

fluorescent activated cell sorting at 8 weeks post-marrow infusion (TABLE 3). When 100-cGy exposed BALB/c mice were infused with 40×10^6 marrow cells from B6.SJL mice, engraftment occurred with donor chimerism of $18 \pm 7\%$. If B6.SJL spleen cells (10^6) were injected intraperitoneally 10 days prior to infusion of 40×10^6 B6.SJL marrow cells to 100-cGy exposed BALB/c hosts, 4 of 5 mice rejected the graft. When CD40-ligand antibody was repetitively administered with and after the spleen cell injection and through the transplant, all mice showed high level chimerism at 8 weeks. The experimental details are outlined in FIGURE 1. Mice in these experiments appeared healthy at the time of sacrifice, with no gross evidence of GVHD. The combination of B6 spleen cell sensitization and CD40-ligand antibody blockade with infusion of B6 marrow into 100-cGy treated BALB/c hosts led to mean donor chimerism levels of $39 \pm 4\%$ donor. These data indicate that the nontoxic creation of allochimerism may be a feasible approach to a number of genetic marrow diseases such as thalassemia and sickle cell anemia, autoimmune diseases and cancer.

PHENOTYPE OF ENGRAFTING STEM CELL

The stem cell which engrafts *in vivo* in either irradiated or normal hosts is quiescent as determined by either *in vitro* tritiated thymidine or *in vivo* hydroxyurea suicide experiments. However, when these quiescent stem cells are infused into normal nonirradiated hosts, the majority rapidly enter active cell cycle, with approximately 50% being in S phase by 12 hours postinfusion as determined by *in vivo* hydroxyurea suicide.[14] This is consistent with previous results, utilizing different approaches, by Hendrikx *et al.*[15] *In vitro* cytokine stimulation of marrow cells results in maintenance or expansion of progenitors with stimulation of cell cycle transit. When BALB/c male marrow cells were exposed to interleukin-3 (IL-3), interleukin-6 (IL-6), interleukin-11 (IL-11) and steel factor in liquid culture for 48 hours progenitors (colony-forming cells (CFC) and high proliferative potential colony-forming cells (HPP-CFC)) were maintained or expanded, and cell cycle progression was stimulated.[16,17] However, at 48 hours of cytokine culture, engraftability into either normal or irradiated hosts was markedly impaired.[16,17] Lineage-negative,

TABLE 4. Critical concepts in stem cell engraftment strategies

Engraftment is determined by the ratio of host to donor stem cells.
Therapies which nontoxically reduce host stem cells will increase donor chimerism.
Stem cells giving long-term chimerism show marked fluctuation with cell cycle transit.
Donor cell priming and costimulator blockade facilitate tolerance and stable allochimerism.

rhodamine-low, Hoechst-low stem cells were purified from whole BALB/c marrow and incubated in liquid culture with IL-3, IL-6, IL-11 and steel factor, and their cell cycle transit was determined using tritium labeling and cell doublings.[18] The first cell cycle showed a 16–20-hour time interval from dormancy to S phase, and the first population doubling occurred at 36–40 hours; subsequent population doublings occurred every 12 hours indicating a markedly shortened G_1 phase. When engraftability at 2 or 6 months post-marrow infusion was determined for BALB/c male cells at varying times out to 80 hours in liquid culture, it was found that the capacity to engraft showed a fluctuating phenotype, with marked changes in engraftment being observed over 2–4-hour intervals.[19] There was an initial loss of long-term engraftment at an average of 33 hours in cytokine culture corresponding with late S, and early G_2 (as previously determined); a recovery of engraftment levels to that seen with input marrow was then seen at 40 hours of culture. These data suggest that bone marrow stem cells show a plastic reversible phenotype apparently linked to cell cycle transit.

In toto, these data indicate that certain critical concepts (TABLE 4) should form the intellectual base for stem cell transplant approaches in either the autologous or allogeneic setting.

REFERENCES

1. MICKLEM, H.S., C.M. CLARKE, E.P. EVANS & C.E. FORD. 1968. Fate of chromosome-marked mouse bone marrow cells transfused into normal syngeneic recipients. Transplantation **6**: 299.
2. TAKADA, A., Y. TAKADA & J.L. AMBRUS. 1970. Proliferation of donor spleen and marrow cells in the spleens and bone marrows of unirradiated and irradiated adult mice. Proc. Soc. Exp. Biol. Med. **136**: 222.
3. TAKADA, Y. & A. TAKADA. 1971. Proliferation of donor hematopietic cells in irradiated and unirradiated host mice. Transplantation **12**: 334.
4. BRECHER, G., J.D. ANSELL, H.S. MICKLEM, J.H. TJIO & E.P. CRONKITE. 1982. Special proliferative sites are not needed for seeding and proliferation of transfused bone marrow cells in normal syngeneic mice. Proc. Natl.Acad. Sci. USA **79**: 5085.
5. SAXE, D.F., S.S. BOGGS & D.R. BOGGS. 1984. Transplantation of chromosomally marked syngeneic marrow cells into mice not subjected to hematopoietic stem cell depletion. Exp. Hematol. **12**: 277.
6. STEWART, F.M., R. CRITTENDEN, P.A. LOWRY, S. PEARSON-WHITE & P.J. QUESENBERRY. 1993. Long-term engraftment of normal and post-5-fluorouracil murine marrow into normal nonmyeloablated mice. Blood **81**: 2566-2571.
7. RAMSHAW, H.S., S.S. RAO, R.B. CRITTENDEN, S.O. PETERS, H.U. WEIER & P.J. QUESENBERRY. 1995. Engraftment of bone marrow cells into normal unprepared hosts: effects of 5-fluorouracil and cell cycle status. Blood **86**(3): 924–929.
8. RAMSHAW, H., R.B. CRITTENDEN, M. DOONER, S.O. PETERS, S.S. RAO & P.J. QUESENBERRY. 1995. High levels of engraftment with a single infusion of bone marrow cells into normal unprepared mice. Biol. Blood Marrow Trans. **1**: 74-80.

9. RAO, S.S., S.O. PETERS, R.B. CRITTENDEN, F.M. STEWART, H.S. RAMSHAW & P.J. QUESENBERRY. 1997. Stem cell transplantation in the normal nonmyeloablated host: relationship between cell dose, schedule and engraftment. Exp. Hematol. **25:** 114–121.

10. BLOMBERG, M.E., S.S. RAO, J.L. REILLY, C.Y. TIARKS, S.O. PETERS, E.L.W. KITTLER & P.J. QUESENBERRY. 1998. Repetitive bone marrow transplantation in nonmyeloablated recipients. Exp. Hematol. **26:** 320–324.

11. NILSSON, S., M. DOONER, C. TIARKS, W. HEINZ-ULRICH & P.J. QUESENBERRY. 1997. Potential and distribution of transplanted hematopoietic stem cells in a nonablated mouse model. Blood **89:** 4013–4020.

12. NILSSON, S., M.S. DOONER & P.J. QUESENBERRY. Unpublished observations.

13. STEWART, F.M., S. ZHONG, J. WUU, C.C. HSIEH, S.K. NILSSON & P.J. QUESENBERRY. 1998. Lymphohematopoietic engraftment in minimally myeloablated hosts. Blood **91:** 3681–3687.

14. NILSSON, S.K., M.S. DOONER & P.J. QUESENBERRY. 1997. Synchronized cell-cycle induction of engrafting long-term repopulating stem cells. Blood **90:** 4646–4650.

15. HENDRIKX, P.J., A.C.M. MARTENS, A. HAGENBEEK, J.F. KEIJ & J.W.M. VISSER. 1996. Homing of fluorescently labeled hemopoietic stem cells. Exp. Hemato.l **24:** 129.

16. PETERS, S.O., E.L. KITTLER, H.S. RAMSHAW & P.J. QUESENBERRY. 1995. Murine marrow cells expanded in culture with IL-3, IL-6, IL-11, and SCF acquire an engraftment defect in normal hosts. Exp. Hematol. **23:** 461–469.

17. PETERS, S.O., E.L.W. KITTLER, H.S. RAMSHAW & P.J. QUESENBERRY. 1996. *Ex vivo* expansion of murine marrow cells with interleukin-3, interleukin-6, interleukin-11, and stem cell factor leads to impaired engraftment in irradiated hosts. Blood **87:** 30–37.

18. REDDY, G.P.V., C.Y. TIARKS, L. PANG & P.J. QUESENBERRY. 1997. Synchronization and cell cycle analysis of pluripotent hematopoietic progenitor stem cells. Blood **90:** 2293–2299.

19. HABIBIAN, H.K., S.O. PETERS, C.C. HSIEH, J. WUU, K. VERGILIS, C.I. GRIMALDI, J. REILLY, J.E. CARLSON, A.E. FRIMBERGER, F.M. STEWART & P.J. QUESENBERRY. 1998. The fluctuating phenotype of the lymphohematopoietic stem cell with cell cycle transit. J. Exp. Med. **188:** 393–398.

DISCUSSION

H.E. BROXMEYER (*Indiana University*): Could tell us a little more about your anti-CD40 ligand studies? Why did you chose that ligand? Did you look at anti-CD40? Did you look at anti-41BB or antibodies to any other members of the tumor necrosis factor (TNF) receptor family?

P.J. QUESENBERRY (*University of Massachusetts Medical Center*): We are doing B7 experiments with CD40 ligand antibody. We picked it based on work in our diabetes group at the University of Massachusetts. They have been doing extensive studies on skin grafting. They found that they can go to a mismatched combination with spleen priming and CD40 ligand antibody and obtain prolonged takes of skin grafts. We are very excited about this data. However, I found out in San Diego that we have been scooped, because Megan Sikes has very similar data. This area is moving very fast. We shall hear more later in this meeting about potential clinical application.

R. HOFFMAN (*University of Illinois College of Medicine*): We have been trying to do similar type experiments in larger animals, basically in baboons. The degree of allochimerism has been disturbingly low with what one would call minimal radiation doses or no radiation doses at all. I am perplexed by the discrepancies between the data in the mouse and those in larger animals. Is there some intrinsic difference between the baboon system and the murine system that would explain this? The experience in clinical human allogeneic transplantation would suggest, however, that some sort of preparative regimen is required for engraftment. So how would you explain this?

QUESENBERRY: As we look more and more it appears that the preparative regimen alters host-donor stem cell ratios rather than creating space. You can obtain high rates of donor chimerism with minimal to no treatment if you infuse enough stem cells. So I do not agree. I do not think you need much in the way of preparative regimens. It depends on the number of stem cells, and again I think we shall hear about that later. If you use very low numbers of stem cells (most previous experiments used low levels of stem cells), then you need aggressive preparative regimens. If you have high levels of stem cells, you need less aggressive to no preparative treatment. I shall give a disturbing trivial explanation why primate or any other animal system might be very different, and that is colony infections. We just had experience with a parvovirus infection effecting engraftment. One would have to look carefully at other factors within any animal system for engraftment. I have been very impressed with how different infections can totally wipe you out, so that may be a potential factor in the primate model.

HOFFMAN: No, that is not a factor, because with myeloablative doses of radiation we get engraftment.

QUESENBERRY: That is not convincing, because with myeloablative doses you may get engraftment with parvovirus, too. So, depending on your system, a current infection may or may not have a major effect on the result.

Y. REISNER (*Weizmann Institute of Science*): A comment on the stem cell dose effect. As you know we have been using it for many years in allogeneic transplants. One of the confusing issues when you look into allogeneic as opposed to the autologous setting, is that these CD34 cells can also tolerize and interfere with the rejection mediated by host T cells. Later, at the end of this meeting I shall show data about this. In early studies we found indications, based on the superiority of myeloablative agents vs immunosuppressive drugs, in enhancing T cell-depleted bone marrow allografts, that there is a competition between stem cells that play a role in engraftment. But also there is a major factor here of tolerizing the immune system. Altogether, in our primate experiments we find it more difficult to achieve engraftment with megadoses of stem cells. For example, in mice exposed to 650 rads we were able to achieve very nice donor type chimerism with 40 million T cell-depleted allogeneic bone marrow cells, whereas in monkeys we are currently using 700 rads and are still failing to achieve donor chimerism. We believe this difference is quantitative and not qualitative. We may have to find new approaches to deal with the more vigorous immune systems that are likely to be found in the outbred primate and in man. Perhaps your suggestion to use anti-CD40 ligand may be useful in combination with radiation, but you might find that 100 rads in the monkey is still not enough. You might have to use 700 rads plus anti-CD40 ligand to get where you want to be.

QUESENBERRY: I agree with that. And that may be a double blockade, the addition of a B7 block to CD40 blockade. Your other comment is very appropriate. I think the data in kidney transplant in animal models are impressive. Marrow chimerism may be able to get around a lot of the rejection problems with the kidney and also suggests very interesting strategies for bone marrow itself.

C. J. EAVES (*Terry Fox Laboratory*): Have you actually tried the bromodeoxyuridine (BrdU) experiment posttransplant to ask whether the rate of turnover is any different in a posttransplant scenario from what it is normally. We know the change in accumulation of stem cells is different, but is this explained either partly or wholly by a change in turnover?

QUESENBERRY: Actually we are doing those studies, but I do not have data. I would say from the hydroxyurea experiments we have done, and also from Visser's experiments, that when you infuse dormant marrow cells most of them go through cycle within a couple of days. Their kinetics would be very different from other people's studies with chronic BrdU. But the experiments to directly test that are appropriate and are going to be very interesting.

B. TOROK-STORB (*Fred Hutchinson Cancer Research Center*): I do not know how the monkey studies are being done, what the preparative regimen is, or how the cells are prepared. However, in our transplant program in Seattle we have cloned 6 human leukocyte antigen (HLA)-identical transplants with peripheral blood stem cells with only 200 cGy of irradiation and 35 days total of immunosuppression and have established stable chimerism in all these patients. We believe as you do that we are not making marrow space with the total body irradiation (TBI), but that we are establishing tolerance.

QUESENBERRY: We have done one patient at 100 cGy, and we are just measuring chimerism; but we have one tumor regression in that setting. It is a very exciting area.

TOROK-STORB: These 6 transplants have been done on an outpatient basis. The people were never hospitalized, and the one who is out 7 months is all donor now.

Homing of Long-Term and Short-Term Engrafting Cells *In Vivo*[a]

SOPHIE M. LANZKRON, MICHAEL I. COLLECTOR, AND SAUL J. SHARKIS[b]

Johns Hopkins Oncology Center, Baltimore, Maryland 21287-8967, USA

ABSTRACT: Long-term repopulating hematopoietic stem cells can be separated from cells which provided radioprotection (short-term repopulating cells) on the basis of size. This might be a result of the quiescent nature of long-term repopulating cells. To define the activity of these populations we utilized a dye, PKH26, which incorporates into the membrane of cells and is equally distributed to daughter cells when they divide. We were able to retrieve PKH26+-labeled cells posttransplant in the hematopoietic tissues of the recipients. We could also assess their cell cycle status and their ability, short-and long-term, to reconstitute secondary lethally irradiated hosts in limiting dilution. The results suggest that long-term repopulating cells remain quiescent in the bone marrow shortly after engraftment, whereas cells which radioprotect are more rapidly dividing. We could not detect labeled cells in the peripheral blood posttransplant, and even though cells homed to both the spleen and bone marrow the cells in the bone marrow were significantly more competent at reconstituting lethally irradiated secondary hosts.

INTRODUCTION

Stem cell homing is not well understood. We have established that short-term and long-term hematopoietic reconstituting cells exist.[1] Thirty-day survival (radioprotection) is due to cells which are larger in size than long-term reconstituting cells. Thus, small-sized cells obtained by counter flow-elutriation (flow rate 25, FR25) will long term reconstitute irradiated mice, but large cells (rotor off, R/O) only radioprotect but do not long-term repopulate. We have demonstrated that by limited dilution FR25 cells which are further purified by removal of lineage-positive cells (Lin⁻) can reconstitute the mouse for its lifetime.[2] Since only very few cells might be injected (as low as 1 cell per recipient), the mechanisms of stem cell homing must be exquisitely sensitive. Homing may be mediated by contact of stem cells with cells of the microenvironment through specific receptors.[3] The rarity of the stem cell has made it difficult to track these progenitors in vivo. PKH26 is a fluorescent marker that stains the cell membrane; the intensity of the stain within the cell decreases with each cell division. PKH26 has been utilized in the human,[4] to enrich for early progenitors. Hendrikx *et al.*[5] have used PKH26 dye to follow spleen colony-forming unit (CFU$_s$) localization in mice. We present data that utilize this dye to track and

[a]Supported in part by National Institutes of Health Grant Nos. HL54330, CA70970, and DK53812.

[b]Please address correspondence and reprint requests to: Saul J. Sharkis, Ph.D., Johns Hopkins Oncology Center, Room 2-127, 600 North Wolfe Street, Baltimore, MD 21287-8967. Phone, 410/955-2813; fax, 410/614-7279; e-mail, ssharkis@welchlink.welch.jhu.edu

more importantly to recover short- and long-term repopulating cells which have homed to the bone marrow of recipient mice.

MATERIALS AND METHODS

Animals

Male and female C57 BL/6Jx DBA/2 F1 (B6D2F1) mice (National Cancer Institute, Frederick, MD) 6 to 12 weeks of age, were used for all studies. Mice were housed in sterile microisolator cages. They were fed acidified water and sterilized lab chow *ad libitum*.

Isolating and Staining HSC

For each isolation experiment 20 male mice were killed by cervical dislocation and the hind legs removed. Bone marrow (BM) was flushed with medium from the medullary cavities of the femurs and tibias using a 25-gauge needle. Single-cell suspensions were produced by repeated passage through the needle. Approximately 30 million whole bone marrow (WBM) cells were set aside prior to counterflow centrifugal elutriation (CCE). These served as control cells for cell cycle analysis (see below). The cells were elutriated as previously described.[1] Cells were collected at a flow rate of 25 ml/min (FR25) and from the R/O fraction. The FR25 cells were then lineage depleted by placing 10^7 cells on Petri dishes absorbed with a cocktail of 60µg each rat-antimouse AA4.1, B220, CD5, GR-1, MAC-1 and TER119. After incubating at 4°C for 90 minutes the nonadherent cells (Lin⁻) were removed by gentle rocking and aspiration.

PKH26 Staining

The cells from each group (FR25Lin⁻, R/O) were washed in alpha-MEM without BSA or serum. Samples were then resuspended in PKH diluent and added to the PKH26 dye at 10-µM concentration. The cells were incubated at room temperature for 2–5 minutes with gentle agitation. To stop the reaction 2 ml of 100% serum was added and the cells incubated for one minute at room temperature with gentle agitation. Four milliliters of alpha-MEM with 10% FCS was added. The samples were centrifuged and washed twice with 10 ml alpha-MEM with 10% FCS. Male PKH26 stained cells from each group were then injected into female mice at a dose of 2.5 million cells per animal. A small number of cells were kept from each group to use as a control for staining efficiency. A single mouse was injected with 2.5 million stained WBM as a control.

Tracking of PKH+ Cells

At 48 hours posttransplant primary recipient mice were sacrificed. For the initial studies peripheral blood was obtained by retroorbital bleed prior to sacrificing recipient animals, but as the yield of PKH26⁺ cells from these samples was very low, the remainder of experiments was limited to spleen and BM. The spleen was harvested and ground over wire mesh into media. The spleen samples were then layered over Ficoll Hypaque and centrifuged at 1200 rpm for 45 minutes. The upper layer was extracted and washed. BM samples were harvested as described above. Bone marrow cells for transplant were treated with ammonium chloride and then layered over a fetal calf serum gradient to remove excess red blood cells. PKH26 fluorescence intensity was then measured on an Epics 740 flow cytometer (Counter Electronics, Hialeah, FL).

Cell Cycle Analysis

BM and spleen samples (PKH26$^+$ cells) collected by cell sorting were washed with PBS containing 0.2% BSA and then resuspended in citrate/sucrose buffer. They were treated with tryspin and incubated for 10 minutes. They were then incubated with *tryspin inhibitor* for 10 minutes, stained with propidium iodide and analyzed by flow cytometry.

Short-Term and Long-Term Reconstitution Assays

Mice that had been injected with PKH26 stained FR25Lin$^-$ or R/O cells as described above were sacrificed at 48 hours. The collected BM cells were then treated as above, and PKH26$^+$ cells were collected by flow cytometry. The male PKH$^+$ spleen and BM cells from each group were injected at a dose of 10^1, 10^2, 10^3, 10^4 cells along with 2×10^4 fresh female unstained R/O cells into female mice. Mice were observed for 30-day survival (short-term reconstitution, radioprotection). In addition, at 6, 12, and 24 weeks, mice receiving 10^2 PKH$^+$ cells underwent retroorbital bleeds for donor engraftment. Fluorescence in situ hybridization (FISH) for the Y chromosome was done as previously described[6] to evaluate over time long-term donor reconstitution.

RESULTS

At time 0, staining FR25Lin$^-$ bone marrow with PKH26 results in $92 \pm 5\%$ PKH$^+$ labeled cells. At 48 hours posttransplant, into female lethally irradiated recipients, we can recover $0.51 \pm 0.03\%$ labeled cells from the donor in the bone marrow of the recipient and $0.27 \pm 0.2\%$ in the spleen ($p < 0.01$). If we label R/O bone marrow cells with PKH26 we can identify less PKH bright cells in the bone marrow than the spleen($0.05 \pm 0.02\%$ versus $0.65 \pm 0.19\%$, $p < 0.01$). These results imply that long-term repopulating cells traffic differently than later precursors. The number of cells recovered were sufficient to allow cell cycle analysis and short- and long-term reconstitution assays. Examination of WBM for cell cycle at time 0 demonstrates 17.0% of cells are in S phase. Cell cycle analysis of elutriated populations (FR25, Lin$^-$ and R/O) reveal that at time 0 FR25Lin$^-$ cells are mostly in G_1/G_0 with less than 6% of cells in S phase, but R/O cells are distributed throughout the cell cycle (TABLE 1). At 48 hours posttransplant only a small increase in S phase cells are observed from FR25Lin- cells recovered both in bone marrow (8.5%) and spleen (3.0%) of primary recipients. On the other hand, recovered PKH$^+$ labeled R/O cells appear to have reduced cell cycle activity compared with their activity at time zero.

In a second set of experiments the PKH26$^+$ cells from the primary recipients' spleen and bone marrow were obtained by cell sorting. These male PKH26 bright cells were injected into secondary female recipients along with 2×10^4 unlabeled female R/O cells (in preliminary experiments PKH26 bright cells recovered from the FR25Lin$^-$ cell inoculum given alone failed to radioprotect secondary recipients after

TABLE 1. Cell cycle analysis of PKH26$^+$ cells^a

	Percent		
		G$_1$	S
FR25Lin$^-$ BM (preinjection)	87.0	6.0	7.0
FR25Lin$^-$ BM (48 hours)	85.0	9.0	5.0
FR25Lin$^-$ Spleen (48 hours)	92.0	3.7	4.0
R/O (preinjection)	60.0	29.0	11
R/O BM (48 hours)	77.0	14.0	6.0
R/O spleen (48 hours)	85.0	12.0	2.7
Whole bone marrow (preinjection)	78.0	17.0	4.8

^{a}PKH26 bright cells were labeled with propidium iodide and analyzed for % of cells in each phase of the cell cycle. FR25Lin$^-$ cells were less than 6% in DNA synthesis prior to transplant and only increased insignificantly ($p > 0.05$). R/O cells, on the other hand, remain from 12–29% in DNA synthesis pre- and posttransplant. A minimum of four separate experiments were performed, and the data shown are the mean values for all four experiments.

48 hours in the primary recipient; data not shown). We observed that FR25Lin-PKH26 bright cells which are harvested from the bone marrow have the ability to allow greater than 60-day survival of secondary recipients at doses from 10^1 to 10^3 cells (TABLE 2). Interestingly, if the FR25Lin- PKH26 bright cells are harvested from the spleen of primary recipients the cells fail to radioprotect most of the secondary recipients at concentrations as high as 10^4 cells per recipient (TABLE 2). The percent of male cells present at periods from three weeks to six months are shown (FIGURE 1) following injection of only 10^2 of these PKH26 bright cells from the bone marrow. Animals that received either 10^2 or 10^3 male R/O PKH26$^+$ cells that had been in the primary recipients for 48 hours only contributed in a limited fashion

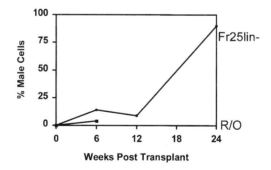

FIGURE 1. Engraftment of FR25Lin$^-$ or R/O cells into secondary recipients of PKH$^+$ cells. One hundred PKH bright cells recovered 48 hours posttransplant from male FR25Lin-donors •—• or male R/O donors ■—■ were injected into secondary female hosts. Peripheral blood was obtained from these recipients at 6, 12, and 24 weeks posttransplant and analyzed for the presence of male cells. Values represent the mean % male cells for 4–6 recipients. The standard error of the mean was less than 4% at six months. Secondary recipients receiving R/O PKH$^+$ cells did not survive to six months.

TABLE 2. Short-term reconstitution of secondary recipients of FR25Lin⁻ cells

Number & Type of Cells Injected[a]	% 30-Day Survival	Median Survival (Days)[b]
1,000 FR25Lin⁻ BM	100.0	>60 (4/4)
100 FR25Lin⁻ BM	78.5	>60 (11/14)
10 FR25Lin⁻ BM	20.0	19.0 (3/15)
10,000 FR25Lin⁻ spleen	12.5	18.0 (1/8)
1,000 FR25Lin⁻ spleen	0.0	16.0 (0/20)
100 FR25Lin⁻ spleen	0.0	17.0 (0/20)

[a]Animals received the number of FR25Lin⁻ cells indicated plus 20,000 female R/O cells.
[b]Numbers in parenthesis represent number alive/number injected. Animals receiving 20,000 female R/O cells alone died at 17–19 days.

to survival and not to long-term reconstitution of secondary recipients when given along with 2×10^4 female R/O cells (FIGURE 1).

DISCUSSION

Early after transplantation, cells enriched for both short-term radioprotection (R/O) and long-term engraftment (FR25Lin⁻) home to the hematopoietic organs of lethally irradiated recipient mice. We do not recover PKH26 labeled cells in the peripheral blood 48 hours following transplant but find these cells in the bone marrow and spleen of primary recipients. Thus, these cells rapidly home to hematopoietic tissues. Hendrikx *et al.* when examining CFU_s showed that this precursor rapidly undergoes proliferation *in vivo*.[5] The R/O population, enriched for later precursors, also are in cell cycle after transplant. We, however, further show that long-term repopulating cells (FR25Lin⁻) at 48 hours remain relatively quiescent. Nilsson *et al.*[7] recently showed that stem cells can be killed by 5-fluorouracil (5-FU) very shortly posttransplant, suggesting a rapid entering of these cells into cell cycle. However, their study did not directly measure the cell cycle activity shortly after transplant but relied on engraftment post-drug treatment six weeks later (at a time indicative of radioprotection). We believe our assay more directly studies the donor cells by direct harvest of PKH26 bright cells 48 hours posttransplant. At 48 hours FR25Lin⁻ cells can still engraft secondary recipients at low numbers (100 cells), whereas later progenitors (R/O cells) fail to do so. PKH26 has been utilized to select for human cells in vitro which are quiescent. Recent elegant studies[8,9] have shown by *in vitro* assay that human CD34-positive cells residing in G_0 are more primitive than those in G_1, and their responsiveness to cytokines may be different than cells in cycle. Our observation *in vivo* that our primitive population remains relatively quiescent at two days is consistent with the ability of these cells to continue to long-term repopulate a lethally irradiated host at small numbers. The cells which home to the spleen shortly after transplant (FR25Lin⁻ PKH26 bright cells) also fail to radioprotect secondary recipients. It is possible that the spleen microenvironment which does maintain the donor cells in a quiescent state (only 3% in S phase of the cell cycle, TABLE 1) is not inductive for stem cell proliferation reflected by a failure of the donor cells to radioprotect or to long-term engraft secondary recipients. Alternatively, but less likely, our stem cell population (FR25Lin⁻ cells) could be contaminated with lymphoid cells, not depleted by our panning step, take up PKH26 and are preferentially homing to the spleen. It is clear that cells from the same experiment which home to the bone marrow of primary recipients did have both radioprotection and long-term engraftment potential. We favor the hypothesis that stem cells early after transplant seek out microenvironments which aid in their proliferation and differentiation.

Future potential applications for this assay include its use in further defining the biology of stem cell homing. Papayannopoulou *et al.*[10] have demonstrated that cell surface antigens (i.e., very late antigen VLA-4) act as homing receptors for progenitors like CFU_S. Using an antibody to VLA-4, they have shown that lodgement of CFU_S within the bone marrow can be blocked, and that same group has shown that long-term reconstituting cells can be mobilized to the peripheral blood.[11] Given that our assay allows identification of quiescent cells shortly after injection, it could be used along with antibodies to cell surface adhesion molecules to investigate more closely the interaction of long-term engrafting cells with the microenvironment. We have described an assay of stem cell homing which allows us to further study the biology of stem cell growth in vivo and to identify and isolate cells that provide long-term engraftment.

ACKNOWLEDGMENT

We thank Marie C. Moineau for her assistance with manuscript preparation.

REFERENCES

1. JONES, R.J., J.E. WAGNER, P. CELANO, M.S. ZICHA & S.J. SHARKIS. 1990. Separation of pluripotent hematopoietic stem cells from multipotent progenitors (CFU-S). Nature **347:** 188–189.
2. JONES, R.J., M.I. COLLECTOR, J.P. BARBER, M.S. VALA, M.J. FACKLER, W.S. MAY, C.A. GRIFFIN, A.L. HAWKINS, B.A. ZEHNBAUER, J. HILTON, O.M. COLVIN & S.J. SHARKIS. 1996. Characterization of mouse lymphohematopoietic stem cells lacking spleen colony-forming activity. Blood **88:** 487–491.
3. AIZAWA, S. & M. TAVASSOLI. 1987. *In vitro* homing of hemopoietic stem cells is mediated by a recognition system with galactosyl and mannosyl specificities. Proc. Natl. Acad. Sci. USA **84:** 4485–4489.
4. BERARDI, A.C., A. WANG, J.D. LEVINE, P. LOPEZ & D.T. SCADDEN. 1995. Functional isolation and characterization of human hematopoietic stem cells. Science **267:** 104–108.
5. HENDRIKX, P.J., A.C.M. MARTENS, A. HAGENBEEK, J.F. KEIJ & J.W.M. VISSER. 1996. Homing of fluorescently labeled murine hematopoietic stem cells. Exp. Hematol. **24:** 129–140.
6. HAWKINS, A.L., R.J. JONES, B.A. ZEHNBAUER, M.S. ZICHA, M.I. COLLECTOR, S.J. SHARKIS & C.A. GRIFFIN. 1992. Fluorescence *in situ* hybridization to determine engraftment status after murine bone marrow transplant. Cancer Genet. Cytogenet. **64:** 145–148.
7. NILSSON, S.K., M.S. DOONER & P.J. QUESENBERRY. 1997. Synchronized cell-cycle induction of engrafting long-term repopulating stem cells. Blood **90:** 4646–4650.
8. LADD, A.C., R. PYATT, A. GOTHOT, S. RICE, J. MCMAHEL, C.M. TRAYCOFF & E.F. SROUR. 1997. Orderly process of sequential cytokine stimulation is required for acti-

vation and maximal proliferation of primitive human bone marrow CD34$^+$ hemato-poietic progenitor cells residing in G_0. Blood **90:** 658–668.

9. GOTHOT, A., R. PYATT, J. MCMAHEL, S. RICE & E. SROUR. 1997. Functional heteroge-neity of human CD34$^+$ cells isolated in subcompartments of the G_0/G_1 phase of the cell cycle. Blood **90:** 4384–4393.

10. PAPAYANNOPOULOU, T., C. CRADDOCK, B. NAKAMOTO, G.V. PRIESTLEY & N.S. WOLF. 1995. The VLA4/VCAM-1 adhesion pathway defines contrasting mechanisms of lodgement of transplanted murine hemopoietic progenitors between bone marrow and spleen. Proc. Natl. Acad. Sci. USA **92:** 9647–9651.

11. CRADDOCK, C.F., B. NAKAMOTO, R.G. ANDREWS, G.V. PRIESTLEY & T. PAPAYANNOP-OULOU. 1997. Antibodies to VLA4 integrin mobilize long-term repopulating cells and augment cytokine-induced mobilization in primates and mice. Blood **90:** 4779–4788.

DISCUSSION

P.J. QUESENBERRY (*University of Massachusetts Medical Center*): Are you mea-suring the cycle status by PKH or by Hoechst?

S.J. SHARKIS (*Johns Hopkins Oncology Center*): Neither. This is a propidium io-dide assay. We sort the cells on the basis of PKH but measure the cell cycle at 48 hours using propidium iodide.

QUESENBERRY: That would be consistent with our results. If you look at the kill at 20 hours, there is no kill with hydroxyurea. So there was a synchronous induction of cycle. Now you look at them later on, and they are out of cycle. Would that be consistent with what you are saying?

SHARKIS: We have not looked early, because we do not get enough cells. The dif-ference between the data that a number of people are presenting regarding the pos-sibility that these cells rapidly go into cycle versus our data is that we are looking at different stem cells. We select cells on the basis of quiescence using elutriation. These are different cells than those selected by the technology that has been de-scribed otherwise.

QUESENBERRY: We did the same experiment, and I think we have the same re-sults. At 12 hours they are all in cycle, and at 20 hours they are not in cycle.

G.J. SPANGRUDE (*University of Utah Medical Center*): You reisolated 100 PKH positive cells after 48 hours, and I assume you transplanted those with fresh rotor off cells to mediate radiation protection. Then you see 100% male cells in those recipi-ents six months later.

SHARKIS: The rotor off cells are female cells.

SPANGRUDE: However, you also showed that if you did the same experiment from spleen, then you did not see survival in that case.

SHARKIS: That is correct.

Spangrude: Your data are arguing that there are two kinds of cells within this frac-tion 25, or else there is a differential effect of the spleen microenvironment when they land in that environment.

SHARKIS: We favor the second of those two hypotheses.

SPANGRUDE: Do you find it remarkable that there is 100% male engraftment with 100 cells transplanted? This to me is pretty amazing.

SHARKIS: We have done it before with 10 cells. The PKH can be a positive selector for stem cells, but that is a bias on my part. I agree that a very small percentage of these cells filter into the bone marrow. However, if you can collect them, you have a population that can engraft.

SPANGRUDE: One of the difficulties I have with the male and female system is that it is difficult to phenotype those cells each time when you look with fluorescence *in situ* hybridization (FISH) analysis to find donor cells. Unless you go to more extensive efforts, you cannot easily tell whether they are lymphoid lineage or myeloid lineage. You have probably done that in a representative number of cases, but can you say you see both lineages in every case?

SHARKIS: We do not kill the animal until very late. We try to keep the animals alive for at least 9 months before we look in bone marrow and thymus and spleen. In every case where we do that, we do see both lymphoid and myeloid engraftment. The suggestion is that it is a multipotential progenitor that provides this engraftment.

D. METCALF (*P. O. Royal Melbourne Hospital*): For enlightenment, the percentage of cells in S phase was established from fluorescence-activated cell sorter (FACS) analysis.

SHARKIS: Yes.

METCALF: Am I correct in believing that the answer is only accurate if the length of the cell cycle is not changed?

SHARKIS: That is a correct assumption.

METCALF: Ninety-nine percent of current papers fall into this same error, because this is the thing that everyone uses whether you look at BCL2 or whatever.

SHARKIS: You and I are the only people old enough to remember that the very early data said that cell cycle in vivo only becomes rapid after 96 hours after transplant. Then it becomes much more rapid. It goes from 18 hours to 12 hours. Based upon those data, not the data that I am showing you, I would suggest that the length of the time of the cell cycle at 48 hours is likely to be the same as at time zero.

T. PAPAYANNOPOULOU (*University of Washington*): Some clarification. You said you recover about 0.48% of the cells injected in the marrow in 48 hours. How much do you recover in the spleen at the same time?

SHARKIS: They are similar amounts, and that is a representative experiment. We have done five or six experiments, and now 0.7% is the mean for bone marrow and spleen. The number of cells recovered in both organs is the same.

PAPAYANNOPOULOU: Is this the total bone marrow or the femur?

SHARKIS: This is just femur.

SPANGRUDE: I am confused. Are you looking at a percentage of injected cells rather than a percent of the organ?

SHARKIS: Yes, the former.

SPANGRUDE: What is the percent of the organ? Are you sorting for 1% of the total marrow? Is it an easily sortable number?

SHARKIS: We have not calculated that. We are happy to get a total of about 25,000 PKH bright cells for bioassay per mouse. I cannot tell you per organ at this point.

QUESENBERRY: We have been using PKH, and we assume that it is nontoxic. However, one of our colleagues studying diabetes has been using it in other cell systems, and it is not neutral.

SHARKIS: The proof is in the pudding. We got a 100 cell reconstitution in six months.

SPANGRUDE: To address Dr. Quesenberry's comment about the neutrality of PKH, I think there is some selection. When I became interested in these homing issues, we did a direct comparison between lymph node homing using PKH labeling of lymph node lymphocytes compared to a radioactive or cell surface antigen allelic marker. We found that PKH-labeled lymphocytes were 100-fold less able to home to lymph nodes than cells labeled by the other two methods. This is not a neutral technique, at least for lymph node homing by lymphocytes. I suspect there is some selection going on.

D.M. BODINE (*National Human Genome Research Institute/NIH*): This is a follow-up question on what Dr. Metcalf was saying. Have you looked at the PKH intermediate cells that you collect? These are the ones that are apt to have divided. What is the cell cycle status of those cells?

SHARKIS: We have not looked at these. We focused on the questions asked here. I think that this is the greatest assay in the world. This will help us with phenotyping and cell cycle questions. If we can recover enough cells from the fractions of PKH bright, dull, or whatever, we will have a tremendous amount of information about the biology of the stem cell after it has been in the appropriate microenvironment for varying periods of time.

QUESENBERRY: You have heard about the greatest assay in hemopoiesis, and we shall move on.

Further Characterization of CD34-Low/Negative Mouse Hematopoietic Stem Cells

HIROMITSU NAKAUCHI,[a] HINA TAKANO, HIDEO EMA, AND MASATAKE OSAWA[b]

Department of Immunology, Institute of Basic Medical Sciences and Center for TARA, University of Tsukuba, and CREST (JST), 1-1-1 Tennodai, Tsukuba Science-City, Ibaraki 305-8575, Japan

ABSTRACT: We have previously reported that in adult mouse bone marrow, $CD34^{low/-}$ c-kit$^+$ Sca-1$^+$ lineage markers negative (Lin$^-$) (CD34$^-$KSL) cells represent hematopoietic stem cells with long-term marrow repopulating ability whereas CD34$^+$ c-kit$^+$ Sca-1$^+$ Lin$^-$ (CD34$^+$KSL) cells are progenitors with short-term reconstitution capacity. To further characterize cells in those two populations, relative expression of various genes were examined by reverse transcriptase polymerase chain reaction (RT-PCR). In CD34$^-$KSL cells, none of the genes studied was found to be expressed with the exception of GATA-2, IL-1Rα, IL-2Rγ, AIC-2B, c-kit, EPO-R, and c-mpl. In contrast, expression of GATA-1 and all cytokine receptor genes examined except IL-2Rβ, IL-7Rα and IL-9Rα were found in CD34$^+$KSL.

The difference between these two populations was also shown in single cell culture analysis of these cells. When cells were clone-sorted and cultured in the presence of SCF, IL-3 and EPO, CD34$^-$KSL cells required much more time to undergo the first cell division than CD34$^+$KSL cells. Dormancy and random fashion of cell division by CD34$^-$KSL cells were also evident by the analysis of the second cell division, which was found to be delayed and unsynchronous compared with CD34$^+$KSL cells. Clonal culture analysis showed that CD34$^-$KSL cells were more potent in proliferation and multilineage differentiation capacities than CD34$^+$KSL cells. In a paired-daughter cell experiment, 75% of CD34$^-$KSL and 50% of CD34$^+$KSL paired-daughter-derived colonies were nonidentical with wide variety of lineage combinations. Taken together, these data support our previous notion that CD34$^-$KSL cells are at higher rank in hematopoietic hierarchy than CD34$^+$KSL cells. In addition, our results using highly enriched stem cell population directly obtained from mouse bone marrow support the proposed stochastic nature of lineage commitment.

INTRODUCTION

Hematopoietic stem cells (HSCs) supply all blood cells throughout life by making use of their self-renewal and multilineage differentiation capabilities. Despite the

[a]Corresponding author: Hiromitsu Nakauchi, Department of Immunology, Institute of Basic Medical Sciences, University of Tsukuba, Tsukuba-City, Ibaraki 305-8575, Japan. Phone, +81-298-53-3462; fax, +81-298-53-6966; e-mail, nakauchi@md.tsukuba.ac.jp
[b]Present address: KIRIN Pharmaceutical Research Laboratory, Gunma 370-1295, Japan.

crucial role of HSCs in normal hematopoiesis as well as in clinical bone marrow (BM) transplantation, our knowledge of their physical characteristics and the mechanisms that control their proliferation and differentiation remain elusive. Although isolation of HSCs is essential for further quantitative and molecular biological analyses of differentiation and self-renewal capabilities, it has been difficult because of their paucity in the BM.

However, recent progress in cell separation techniques and the development of monoclonal antibodies have enabled the isolation of HSC from mammalian bone marrow cells.[1] For example, a monoclonal antibody to c-kit clearly showed that this receptor tyrosine kinase is expressed on hematopoietic progenitor cells and can be used as a marker for HSC enrichment.[2,3] Three-color fluorescence-activated cell sorter (FACS) analysis and cell sorting experiments revealed that long-term marrow repopulating ability (LMRA) is exclusively enriched in c-kit$^+$Sca-1$^+$ fraction among mouse bone marrow lineage marker negative (Lin$^-$) cells.[4] However, a minimum of 30 c-kit$^+$Sca-1$^+$Lin$^-$ cells were still required to radioprotect lethally irradiated mice. We therefore needed another monoclonal antibody that could subdivide c-kit$^+$Sca-1$^+$Lin$^-$ cells for further enrichment.

CD34 is a cell surface sialomucin-like adhesion molecule that is expressed on 1–3% of BM cells. CD34 has been known as a marker of human HSCs, since all colony-forming activity is found in the CD34-positive fraction. Clinical transplantation as well as primate studies that used enriched CD34$^+$ BM cells also indicated the presence of HSCs with LMRA within this fraction.[5] After isolation of human CD34 gene,[6,7] the mouse homologue (mCD34) was isolated by cross hybridization.[8,9] With the expectation that mCD34 is expressed in mouse HSCs, a rat monoclonal antibody was raised against recombinant mCD34. This antibody (clone 49E8) reacted with $2.5 \pm 0.5\%$ of adult mouse BM cells that were mostly c-kit$^+$ and Lin$^-$, suggesting its expression in primitive hematopoietic cells. Using this mCD34 monoclonal antibody, we were indeed able to further subdivide c-kit$^+$Sca-1$^+$Lin$^-$ (KSL) cells. Day-12 spleen colony-forming units (CFU-Ss) and colony-forming units in culture (CFU-Cs) were found mainly in the CD34$^+$KSL fraction. However, contrary to our expectation, those cells in the CD34-positive fraction did not show LMRA. In adult mouse BM, HSCs with LMRA have a phenotype of CD34$^{low/-}$ c-kit$^+$Sca-1$^+$Lin$^-$ (CD34$^-$KSL) subpopulation, whereas CD34$^+$KSL fraction contains hematopoietic progenitors with short-term reconstitution ability.[10] In this report, we summarize the results of our more recent study on these highly enriched stem cell and progenitor subpopulations.

NEITHER CD34$^-$KSL NOR CD34$^+$KSL SUBPOPULATION ALONE CAN RADIOPROTECT LETHALLY IRRADIATED MICE

To study their radioprotective ability, c-kit$^+$Sca-1$^+$Lin$^-$ cells were fractionated into CD34-negative, CD34^{low} and CD34$^+$ subpopulations according to their mCD34 expression by FACS. As shown in FIGURE 1, although injection of 100 c-kit$^+$Sca-1$^+$Lin$^-$ cells was shown to radioprotect a lethally irradiated mouse,[3] injection of 300 cells from either CD34$^-$ or CD34$^+$ subpopulation alone showed poor radioprotection. When cells of both fractions were cotransplanted, rescue of lethally

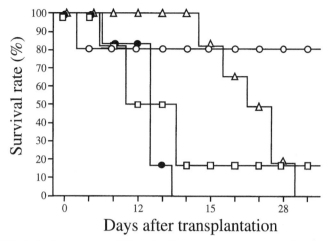

Days after transplantation

FIGURE 1. Radioprotective ability of c-kit⁺Sca-1⁺Lin⁻ bone marrow subpopulations. **(A)** Bone marrow c-kit⁺Sca-1⁺Lin⁻ were subdivided into three fractions according to the expression of mCD34. **(B)** Survival rate of recipient mice after transfer of cells. Groups of 30 mice from 4 separate experiments were lethally irradiated (9.5 Gy) and injected intravenously with either three hundred CD34⁻KSL cells (Fr. 1; *open squares*), CD34⁺KSL cells (Fr. 3; *open triangles*), or CD34 KSL cells plus CD34⁺KSL cells (*open circles*). *Closed circles* indicate negative control (without injection).

irradiated mice was observed. These results indicate that when limited number of HSCs are used for transplantation, both of committed progenitor cells that provide initial engraftment and HSCs responsible for delayed but durable engraftment are necessary for successful long-term reconstitution.

EXPRESSION OF VARIOUS GENES IN THE PURIFIED MOUSE HSCs

In order to examine expression of various genes in highly enriched hematopoietic stem cell subpopulations, mRNAs were obtained from sorted cells and reverse transcriptase polymerase chain reaction (RT-PCR) analysis was performed. Because these cells are rare in bone marrow, we sorted 2000 cells from each subpopulation. After first strand synthesis, polyA tailing reaction was performed by terminal deoxynucleotidyl transferase (TdT, Gibco-BRL). Then PCR amplification was performed with 1 mM (A/C/G)-dT18-R1-R0 primer as described by Brady *et al.*[11]

By using these amplified cDNAs, PCR reactions were performed with primers specific for various genes. FIGURE 2a confirms uniform amplification of cDNAs obtained from CD34⁻, CD34⁺ and Lin⁻ cells by using primers specific for house keeping genes. Then relative expression of various genes was examined by PCR. FIGURE 2b demonstrates that expression of GATA-1 began at the CD34⁺KSL cell stage, while that of GATA-2 began earlier at the CD34⁻KSL cell stage and diminished as they differentiated. Lin⁻ cells do not contain mature blood cells but include a number of lineage-committed progenitor cells. Thus, all cytokine receptors tested were

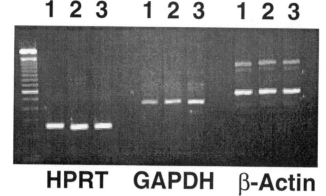

HPRT GAPDH β-Actin

FIGURE 2a. Expression of hypoxanthine guanine phosphoribosyl transferase (HPRT), glyceraldehyde-3-phosphate dehydrogenase (GAPDH) and β-actin genes in CD34⁻KSL (*lane 1*), CD34⁺KSL (*lane 2*) and Lin⁻ cells (*lane 3*).

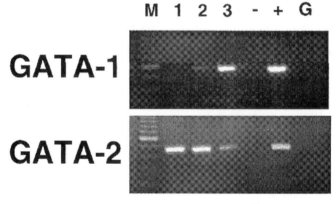

FIGURE 2b. Expression of GATA-1, GATA-2 in CD34⁻KSL (*lane 1*), CD34⁺KSL (*lane 2*) and Lin⁻ cells (*lane 3*). M, size marker; −, negative control; +, positive control; and G, genomic DNA.

found to be expressed in Lin⁻ cells. CD34⁺ progenitor cells express all but interleukin-2Rβ (IL-2Rβ), IL-7R and IL-9R. We can assume that CD34⁺ progenitor fraction are more primitive than Lin⁻ cell population that contains committed progenitor cells expressing IL-2Rβ, IL-7R or IL-9R. Most intriguing was the finding that, although supposedly being most primitive and multipotent, CD34-negative HSCs did not express most cytokine receptors including IL-3R. IL-6R and granulocyte/macrophage colony-stimulating factor receptor (GM-CSFR). These data are in accord with our previous observation that CD34⁻KSL cells do not form colonies in the presence of IL-3 alone, but CD34⁺KSL cells do.

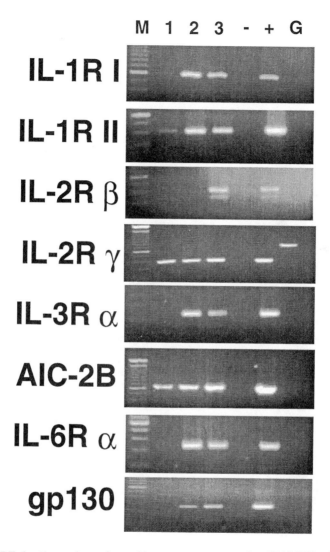

FIGURE 2c. Expression of cytokine receptor genes in CD34⁻KSL (*lane 1*), CD34⁺KSL (*lane 2*) and Lin⁻ cells (*lane 3*). M, size marker; −, negative control; +, positive control; and G, genomic DNA.

The fact that CD34-negative HSCs do not respond to single cytokines and require the presence of SCF and one other cytokine to form colonies may indicate that SCF mediates signals somehow act to induce expression of other cytokine receptors. By demonstrating expression of multiple cytokine receptors in the hematopoietic progenitor cells, Hu *et al.* proposed a promiscuous model in which unilineage commitment is prefaced by a phase of multilineage locus activation.[12] From our results,

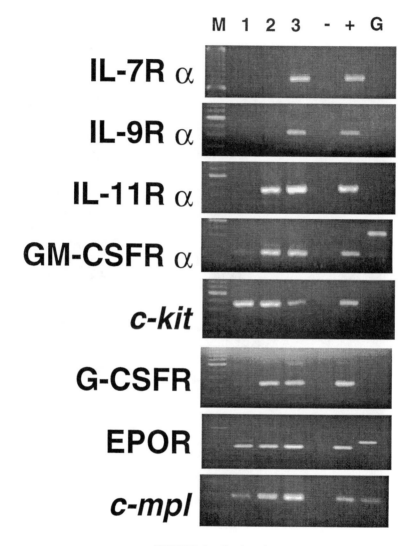

FIGURE 2c. Continued

however, this multilineage locus activation takes place not at the HSC level, but most probably at the CD34$^+$ progenitor cell stage.

Although most cytokine receptor α-chains were not expressed, mRNA for common signal transducing molecules such as IL-2R γ-chain and AIC-2B were detectable. As far as we examined, all known IL-2R γ-chain associated α- or β-chains were not expressed. There may be as yet unknown α-chain expressed in HSCs. It has been reported, however, that IL-2R γ-chain knockout mice showed minimum hematopoietic abnormalities.[13]

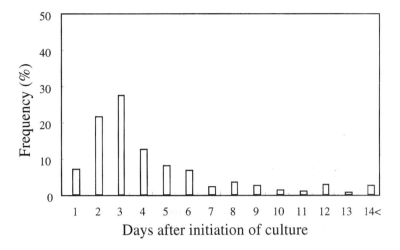

Days after initiation of culture

FIGURE 3. The time required to undergo first cell division after initiation of singe cell liquid culture. CD34⁻KSL cells were clone-sorted into wells of a 96-well culture plate by FACS and cultured in the presence of SCF, IL-3 and EPO. Cells were observed periodically under the microscope until the first cell division.

IN VITRO DIFFERENTIATION POTENTIAL OF THE CD34⁻KSL AND CD34⁺KSL CELLS

Individual CD34⁻KSL and CD34⁺KSL cells of the murine bone marrow were clone-sorted into a culture well and cultured in liquid medium with SCF, IL-3 and EPO. When cells were observed periodically under the microscope until the first cell division, half the CD34⁺KSL cells made the first cell division within 24 hours, and all the rest by day 4 of culture. On the other hand, CD34⁻KSL cells took more time with a lot of variation to undergo the first cell division. While many CD34⁻KSL cells divided within the first 3 days, 34% of them required 4 to 19 days (FIG. 3). More than 80% of the CD34⁺KSL cells made the second cell division within 24 hours. The second cell division for CD34⁻KSL cells also occurred somewhat earlier, but only 33% of them divided within 24 hours, and the rest divided unsynchronously over 14 days. Thus, compared with CD34⁺KSL cells, CD34⁻KSL cells are more dormant and have unique cell cycle status.

In this series of experiments, colonies were found in approximately 50% of the wells in both subpopulations. Large colonies containing more than 10^4 cells were more frequently formed by CD34⁻KSL cells (59%) than by CD34⁺KSL (30.6%), indicating higher proliferation potential of CD34⁻KSL over CD34⁺KSL (FIG. 4a). We then examined cells in each colony under the microscope after cytospin preparation and May-Giemsa staining. As shown in FIGURE 4b, CD34⁻KSL cell-derived colonies included a higher number of lineages per colony than those of CD34⁺KSL cells. Nearly 40% of colonies derived from CD34⁺KSL were single lineage (mostly macrophage) colonies, whereas over 40% of the colonies derived from CD34⁻KSL were

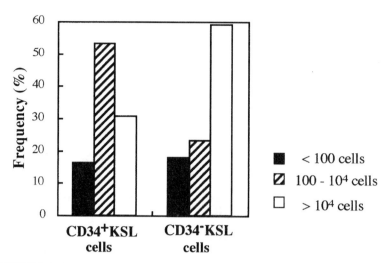

FIGURE 4a. Proliferation capacity of CD34⁻KSL and CD34⁺KSL cells. CD34⁻KSL or CD34⁺KSL cells were clone-sorted into well of a 96-well culture plate and cultured in the presence of SCF, IL-3 and EPO for 14 days. Then the number of cells in each well was estimated under the microscope.

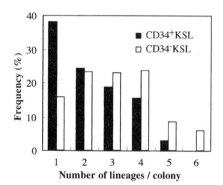

FIGURE 4b. Differentiation potential of CD34⁻KSL and CD34⁺KSL cells. CD34⁻KSL or CD34⁺KSL cells were clone-sorted into well of a 96-well culture plate and cultured in the presence of SCF, IL-3 and EPO for 14 days. Then the cells in each well were collected for cytologic examination. The number of lineage in a colony was determined by morphological examination of cytospin preparation after May-Giemsa staining.

four or more lineage colonies. These data indicate that CD34⁻KSL have higher multilineage differentiation and proliferation potential than CD34⁺KSL.

LINEAGE COMMITMENT OF THE CD34⁻KSL AND CD34⁺KSL CELLS

In early 1980s, Makio Ogawa and his colleagues performed a series of elegant experiments to study differentiation potential of isolated progenitors by use of micro-

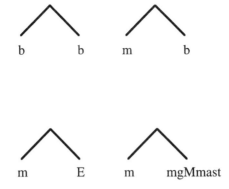

FIGURE 5. Examples of lineage combination in paired-daughter colonies. b, blast cells; m, macrophages; E, erythroblasts; g, granulocytes; M, megakaryocytes; and mast, mast cells.

manipulation techniques.[14] Analysis of colonies formed by two daughter cells derived from a single parent cell showed dissimilar combinations of lineages and sizes, consistent with the concept that stem cell commitment is a stochastic process.[15,16] In those experiments, IL-3-induced blast cells were used as parent cells. We attempted to reproduce this paired-daughter cell experiment using freshly isolated HSCs by FACS. Paired-daughter cells derived from single CD34⁻KSL or CD34⁺KSL cells were separated by micromanipulation technique and cultured in the presence of IL-3, SCF and EPO. Colonies formed by these paired-daughter cells were examined after cytospin preparation was made. Differential analysis of cells revealed that colonies derived from CD34⁻KSL cells showed significantly higher incidence (75%) of nonidentical lineage combinations between paired-daughter cells than those (50%) derived from CD34⁺KSL.

Furthermore, paired-daughter colonies derived from CD34⁻KSL showed wider variety of lineage combinations than those by CD34⁺KSL cells. For example, as in FIGURE 5, there was a combination in which one of the paired-daughter cells formed a macrophage colony while the other formed a colony that included macrophages, granulocytes, megakaryocytes, and mast cells. In other cases, differentiation into macrophage and erythroid colonies or macrophage to blast cells was observed. Thus, lineage commitment can widely split even in paired-daughter cells derived from a single parent cell cultured in the same environment.

Characterization of isolated CD34⁻KSL cells and CD34⁺KSL cells revealed significant difference in dormancy, proliferation and differentiation potentials *in vitro*. In addition, expression levels of various cytokine genes were strikingly different between the two populations. All these *in vitro* results, on top of previously reported *in vivo* data, point out that CD34⁻KSL cells are more primitive than CD34⁺KSL cells. In addition, our results of a paired-daughter cell experiment using highly enriched stem cell fraction directly isolated from BM support the previously proposed stochastic model of stem cell differentiation.

REFERENCES

1. VISSER, J.W. & B.D. VAN. 1990. Purification of pluripotent hemopoietic stem cells: past and present. Exp. Hematol. **18:** 248–256.
2. OGAWA, M., S. NISHIKAWA, K. YOSHINAGA, S. HAYASHI, T. KUNISADA, J. NAKAO, T. KINA, T. SUDO, H. KODAMA, AND S. NISHIKAWA. 1993. Expression and function of c-kit in fetal hemopoietic progenitor cells: transition from the early c-kit independent to the late c-kit-dependent wave of hemopoiesis in the murine embryo. Development **117:** 1089–1098.
3. OKADA, S., H. NAKAUCHI, K. NAGAYOSHI, S. NISHIKAWA, Y. MIURA & T. SUDA. 1992. *In vivo* and *in vitro* stem cell function of c-kit⁻ and Sca-1-positive murine hematopoietic cells. Blood **80:** 3044–3050.
4. OSAWA, M., K. NAKAMURA, N. NISHI, N. TAKAHASI, Y. TOKUOMOTO, H. INOUE & H. NAKAUCHI. 1996. *In vivo* self-renewal of c-kit$^+$ Sca-1$^+$ Lin(low/-) hemopoietic stem cells. J.Immunol. **156:** 32073214.
5. KRAUSE, D.S., M. J. FACKLER, C.I. CIVIN & W.S. MAY. 1996. CD34: structure, biology & clinical utility. Blood **87:** 1–13.
6. SIMMONS, D.L., A.B. SATTERTHWAITE, D.G. TENEN & B. SEED. 1992. Molecular cloning of a cDNA encoding CD34, a sialomucin of human hematopoietic stem cells. J. Immunol. **148:** 267–271.
7. NAKAMURA, Y., H. KOMANO & H. NAKAUCHI. 1993. Two alternative forms of cDNA encoding CD34. Exp. Hematol. **21:** 236–242.
8. BROWN, J., M.F. GREAVES & H.V. MOLGAARD. 1991. The gene encoding the stem cell antigen, CD34, is conserved in mouse and expressed in haemopoietic progenitor cell lines, brain, and embryonic fibroblasts. Int. Immunol. **3:** 175–184.
9. SUDA, J., T. SUDO, M. ITO, N. OHNO, Y. YAMAGUCHI & T. SUDA. 1992. Two types of murine CD34 mRNA generated by alternative splicing. Blood **79:** 2288–2295.
10. OSAWA, M., K. HANADA, H. HAMADA & H. NAKAUCHI. 1996. Long-term lymphohematopoietic reconstitution by a single CD34-low/negative hematopoietic stem cell. Science **273:** 242–245.
11. BRADY, G. & N.N. ISCOVE. 1993. Construction of cDNA libraries from single cells. Methods Enzymol. **225:** 611–623.
12. HU, M., D. KRAUSE, M. GREAVES, S. SHARKIS, M. DEXTER, C. HEYWORTH & T. ENVER. 1997. Multilineage gene expression precedes commitment in the hemopoietic system. Genes Dev. **11:** 774–785.
13. CHENG, J., S. BAUMHUETER, G. CACALANO, M.K. CARVER, H. THIBODEAUX, R. THOMAS, H.E. BROXMEYER, S. COOPER, N. HAGUE, M. MOORE & L.A. LASKY. 1996. Hematopoietic defects in mice lacking the sialomucin CD34. Blood **87:** 479–490.
14. OGAWA, M. 1993. Differentiation and proliferation of hematopoietic stem cells. Blood **81:** 2844–2853.
15. SUDA, J., T. SUDA & M. OGAWA. 1984. Analysis of differentiation of mouse hemopoietic stem cells in culture by sequential replating of paired progenitors. Blood **64:** 393–399.
16. SUDA, T., J. SUDA & M. OGAWA. 1984. Disparate differentiation in mouse hemopoietic colonies derived from paired progenitors. Proc. Natl. Acad. Sci. USA **81:** 2520–2524.

DISCUSSION

H.E. BROXMEYER (*Indiana University*): When you looked at the different lineages, you separated the cells and left them in the same dish. Do you think it would have made a difference if you had separated them and taken one of the cells out and put it into another dish? I wonder about the potential for cross-feeding even though there are only two cells in the dish.

NAKAUCHI: That is a formal possibility. The next time we do the experiments we should separate daughter cells into different wells. On the other hand, we would like to keep them in the same condition as much as possible.

D. ORLIC (*National Human Genome Research Institute/NIH*): Your model seems like one that could be interesting to use to look at the very earliest events that are involved in stem cell differentiation/self-renewal. Have you made any attempt to correlate your single cell gene expression studies with your cell division studies? In those cells that begin to divide at 18 days, have you looked to see if any of the genes that were not expressed in the CD34-negative population prior to division are now being expressed? Newly expressed genes might give insight into factors involved in releasing these cells from the block to cell division?

NAKAUCHI: That is a very difficult experiment to do.

B.P. SORRENTINO (*St. Jude Children's Research Hospital*): In your CD34⁻ purified stem cells, have you looked to determine if the cells express P-glycoprotein (P-gp) or have you looked at any surrogate assays for P-gp expression like rhodamine exclusion, given that a number of groups have identified this as a gene product expressed in primitive cells? In my paper I show that P-gp is functionally significant in terms of regulating stem cell maintenance.

NAKAUCHI: We have not examined whether they express some P-gp. We have done rhodamine and Hoescht studies, and the results were compatible with the idea that they are rhodamine low and in the stem/progenitor cell population. I assume they express MDR genes.

SORRENTINO: It may be interesting to look at this directly, because the stem cells could be expressing other transport molecules responsible for the Hoechst-low and rhodamine-low phenotypes.

I. LEMISCHKA (*Princeton University*): I am impressed by your paired-daughter experiments. The question is since you have shown very elegantly that a single CD34⁻ cell can compete with the CD34-positives, have you done the ultimate experiment; that is, to take the two paired-daughter progeny and attempt to reconstitute mice?

NAKAUCHI: That is the experiment I will do if I have another good student. It is a very time-consuming and difficult experiment to do. I agree that it is the ultimate experiment.

LEMISCHKA: It is intriguing and somewhat counterdogmatic to the way we think about things that you can actually get these dramatic lineage segregations with one division of what is obviously a very primitive cell. I have struggled trying to figure out how that translates into molecules. The only way I can imagine it working is that whatever the key regulators are that determine lineage commitment, they must exist in titratable quantities such that you can push one cell division, and one titration can push things one way or another. The corollary of that is, if that is true, these molecules will be existing in vanishingly small quantities. The sobering part of that is that therefore they will be very difficult to identify by any kind of standard means.

D.A. WILLIAMS (*Riley Hospital for Children*): At the beginning of your talk you focused on the c-kit-positive population. What about CD34⁻c-kit-negative cells. Are they in existence, and do they contribute to early hematopoiesis?

NAKAUCHI: In mouse?

WILLIAMS: Yes.

NAKAUCHI: We could find stem cell activity only in c-kit$^+$ Sca-1$^+$ populations.

WILLIAMS: It makes you wonder. Obviously, in the W mutants which are kinase negative; there is some survival of c-kit-negative cells up to some point in time and these animals have hematopoiesis (clearly deficient hematopoiesis); so it suggests that there is a subpopulation of cells that are c-kit-negative that are able to participate in hematopoiesis.

S.J. SHARKIS (*Johns Hopkins Oncology Center*): In either of your paired-daughter cell experiments or bulk cultures where you look at exposures to cytokines, what happens to CD34 expression after exposure to the cytokines?

NAKAUCHI: *In vitro* we see appearance of CD34 expression in about 10 days. They start to express CD34 even in *in vitro* cultures.

SHARKIS: In the paired-daughter study, do you have any data that show that after a single division you can see expression of CD34?

NAKAUCHI: No, we have not done that experiment.

J.D. GRIFFIN (*Dana Farber Cancer Institute*): Is there any relationship between CD34 expression and the cell cycle?

NAKAUCHI: We have not done that experiment. We have not looked at those cells carefully, because there could be contaminating CD34$^-$ cells or there could be actual CD34 dull cells. Maybe we should do a single cell experiment using those CD34 dull cells.

GRIFFIN: In the CD34$^-$ cells, are they CD34$^-$ by RT-PCR?

NAKAUCHI: Yes. We tried the single cell RT-PCR experiment just to confirm the absence of CD34 message. Sometimes we could get that result but not always. We are not 100% sure that is why the title of my paper is CD34-low/negative. We cannot be 100% sure that message is not transcribed at all.

UNKNOWN: As you know we used the human CD34$^+$ cells in transplants and they seemed to have worked fine for the time being. Have you tried to look *in vitro* for human CD34 cells, or is there any difference?

NAKAUCHI: Of course, we did that. We spent more than 6 months extensively studying human bone marrow looking for CD34-negative stem cells, using high proliferative potential colony-forming units (HPP-CFUs). In mouse HPP-CFUs correlate well with hematopoietic stem cell activity, but we could find HPP-CFUs only in the CD34$^+$ population but not in the CD34$^-$ population in human. At that point we did not have the nonobese diabetic severe combined immunodeficiency (NOD-SCID) system. We are trying to establish a large-animal model using pigs or miniature pigs, but we do not have a sensitive enough system to answer your question yet. In our hands we have not been able to show continuing evidence for the presence of CD34$^-$ stem cells in humans.

G. KELLER (*Howard Hughes Medical Institute*): Your paired-daughter analysis is done in methylcellulose with cytokines. What is missing is some engagement of adhesion molecules. Have you considered doing the experiment in another format where you engage the adhesion molecules? Do you think that may redirect or change the kind of fluidity you are seeing?

NAKAUCHI: If we coculture the stem cells with stromal cells, it is very hard to see any change. Now we are planning the experiment using green fluorescein protein (GFP) transgenic mice.

C.J. EAVES (*Terry Fox Laboratory*): From our experience, mostly with human cells (but I understand that it is similar with murine cells), these very early cells will not proliferate in semisolid media. However, if you first expose them in liquid culture to growth factors for fairly short periods of time, even hours, they will acquire that ability. I thought you were doing your paired-daughter analysis in liquid culture. I did not realize they were in methylcellulose. Could you clarify for us which experiments were done under which conditions?

NAKAUCHI: Cells were sorted and cultured in liquid medium. As soon as the cell divided, daughter cells were put into methylcellulose medium separately by micromanipulation.

EAVES: That would then be consistent with the finding that we have, that initially the cells would not be observed to proliferate in methylcellulose even if you leave them for a week or two. Also, have you tried culturing the cells in the same cocktail of growth factors but including Flt-3 ligand? In our experience the inclusion of Flt-3 ligand has been critical in changing the kinetics of proliferation of primitive cells.

NAKAUCHI: We have not realized that.

M. OGAWA (*Medical University of South Carolina*): I was surprised that you did not find IL-3 receptor, IL-6 receptor or Flt-3 and yet you found erythropoietin receptor in the CD34-negative cells.

NAKAUCHI: The absence of IL-3 receptor α-chain gene expression is compatible with our colony-forming units in culture (CFU-C) data, because they do not respond to IL-3. I do not know why EPO-R is expressed in CD34$^-$ stem cells, while most other cytokine receptors are not. In general, these cytokine receptors are not expressed much on the cell surface. On top of that, we do not have good monoclonal antibodies against mouse EPO receptor so that the experiment you propose is not possible.

OGAWA: In the paired-daughter studies, you showed a pure macrophage colony pairing with a multilineage colony, and we have seen that in the blast cell colony replating years ago that it does not prove that the one cell division shows the stem cells committed to macrophages. It could be the result of successive progressive random commitment.

NAKAUCHI: That is a possibility.

P.M. LANSDORP (*Terry Fox Laboratory*): We have results with human CD34$^+$ CD38$^-$ fetal liver cells that are very similar to your results in the mouse in that we have documented that some of these very primitive cells generate daughter cells that differ in the amount of time they take to enter the cycle. In your liquid culture, is there any maintenance of *in vivo* repopulating cells, or are these cells differentiating and losing their repopulating potential?

NAKAUCHI: We have tried that many times with many different combinations of cytokines, but without stromal cells we cannot maintain the stem cell activity more than two weeks.

UNKNOWN: With your data showing that the entire self-renewal capacity is in the CD34$^-$ population, and assuming that this is also true for humans, would you still recommend transplanting human CD34$^+$ selected cells?

NAKAUCHI: This is a question I am asked quite frequently, and I say that if you do not want to be sued, do not be precise.

BROXMEYER: Nobody transplants only with CD34$^+$ cells, because in the cell separation procedures for isolation of CD34 cells, those populations are a mixture and always contain some CD34$^-$ cells. Thus, you have cells that are not CD34$^+$ in there, so we do not have to worry about that yet. From what we have just heard in the mouse system, it may only take one CD34$^-$ cell to get engraftment.

P.J. QUESENBERRY (*University of Massachusetts Medical Center*): The assumption is that the cytokines are evenly distributed and that your cells see the same milieu. Especially if there is a little dysynchrony in the cycle, I can envision a cell with the first hit phenomenon being that the first cytokine to hit the cell determines it. Is that not possible? It is not necessarily so that the cytokines are evenly distributed in that culture.

NAKAUCHI: What cytokine receptors are you going to hit? That is the question, because initially they do not express any cytokine receptors. Expression of cytokine receptor can also be involved in the cell fate determination, or survival of postcommitted cells.

Biology of IL-8-Induced Stem Cell Mobilization

WILLEM E. FIBBE,[a,d] JOHANNES F.M. PRUIJT,[a] GERJO A.VELDERS,[a]
GHISLAIN OPDENAKKER,[b] YVETTE VAN KOOYK,[c] CARL G. FIGDOR,[c]
AND ROEL WILLEMZE[a]

[a]*Department of Hematology, Leiden University Medical Center, Leiden, The Netherlands*
[b]*The Rega Institute, Laboratory for Molecular Immunology, Leuven, Belgium*
[c]*Department of Tumour Immunology, University of Nijmegen, Nijmegen, The Netherlands*

ABSTRACT: The CXC chemokine interleukin-8 (IL-8) has profound hematopoietic activities following systemic administration. It induces the rapid mobilization of cells with lymphomyeloid repopulating ability in mice and of
hematopoietic progenitor cells in monkeys. In this paper, evidence is presented
that stem cell mobilization in mice requires the functional expression on the β_2-
integrin leukocyte function-associated antigen-1 (LFA-1). In monkeys, systemic injection of IL-8 is followed by a significant increase in the circulating levels
of the matrix metallo proteinase gelatinase-B (MMP-9). Based on these findings, the hypothesis is discussed that mature neutrophils serve as intermediate
cells in IL-8-induced stem cell mobilization by the release of proteinases.

INTRODUCTION

Although stem cell mobilization is a property of most hematopoietic growth factors such as granulocyte colony-stimulating factor (G-CSF), granulocyte-macrophage colony-stimulating factor (GM-CSF), interleukin-3 (IL-3), stem cell factor
(SCF), and FLT-3 ligand, a relatively prolonged period of administration is required
to induce mobilization.[1,2] Few cytokines, including IL-1, IL-8 and macrophage inflammatory protein (MIP-1α) induce rapid mobilization of hematopoietic progenitor cells following a single injection. We have recently demonstrated that IL-8
induces the rapid mobilization of cells with lymphomyeloid repopulating ability in
mice and/or hematopoietic progenitor cells in monkeys.[3,4] In an attempt to explain
the mechanism underlying IL-8-induced stem cell mobilization, we have focussed
on the role of adhesion molecules and matrix metallo proteinases (MMP).

CHEMOKINES

Chemokines are a family of proinflammatory molecules that are molecularly
characterized by the conservation of four cysteine residues that play a role in maintaining the tertiary structure. Two major families have been recognized depending
on the position of the first two cysteines. These are adjacent in the cysteine cysteine
(CC) family and are separated by one residue in the CXC family. CXC chemokines

[d]Address for correspondence: Willem E. Fibbe, MD, PhD, Dept. of Hematology, University
Medical Center Leiden, PO Box 9600, Building 1:C2-R, 2300 RC Leiden, The Netherlands.
Phone, +31 71-5262271; fax, +31 71-5266755; e-mail, wfibbe@hematology.azl.nl

mainly attract and activate neutrophils, while CC chemokines are chemoattractant for monocytes, lymphocytes, basophils, eosinophils, natural killer cells and dendritic cells, but not for neutrophils.[5] Based on the presence of a Glu-Leu-Arg (ELR) motive, immediately in front of the first cysteine residue, the CXC family can be subdivided into ELR+ CXC chemokines, which include IL-8, growth-related oncogene (GROα), GROβ, GROγ, neutrophil activating protein-2 (NAP-2), epithelial cell-derived neutrophil attractant-78 (ENA-78) and granulocyte chemotactic protein-2 (GCP-2); and ELR− CXC chemokines, which include platelet factor-4 (PF-4), interferon-γ inducible protein-10 (IP-10), monokine induced by interferon-γ (MIG) and stromal cell-derived factor-1 (SDF-1).[6]

INTERLEUKIN-8

IL-8 is produced by a variety of cells including monocytes, neutrophils, fibroblasts, endothelial cells, lung epithelial cells, mast cells and keratinocytes.[5] Production of IL-8 by these cells is induced by proflammatory cytokines, i.e., tumor necrosis factor (TNFα), IL-1, and also by IL-2, IL-3 and granulocyte-macrophage colony-stimulating factor (GM-CSF).[7,8] IL-8 is chemotactic for neutrophils and induces release of metalloproteinases, i.e., elastase, gelatinase-B and β-glucuronidase. It also induces shedding of l-selectin, upregulation of the β2-integrin leukocyte function-associated antigen-1 (LFA-1) and transendothelial migration of neutrophils. High-affinity IL-8 receptors have been demonstrated on the surface of human neutrophils. Two high-affinity receptors have been identified, termed CXCR1 and CXCR2.[9,10] Neutrophils express the highest numbers of both CXCR1 and CXCR2 in an equal ratio. While CXCR1 is specific for IL-8, the CXCR2 is shared with other ELR+ CXC chemokines. The expression of receptors can be influenced by cytokines, i.e., G-CSF may upregulate both IL-8 receptors, which corresponds with increasing binding of IL-8 and enhanced neutrophil chemotaxis.[11] In mice no IL-8 homologue has been identified, but a receptor that appears to be homologous to the CXCR2 termed IL-8 receptor-homologue has been reported.[12] Candidate natural ligands for this murine IL-8 receptor homologue include the chemokines GCP-2, MIP-2 or KC. These chemokines have been reported to induce neutrophil chemotaxis, release of gelatinase-B and an increase in intracellular calcium.[13]

In vivo treatment with IL-8 in monkeys, rabbits and mice induces an instant neutropenia followed by granulocytosis, neutrophil margination and infiltration, plasma exudation and angiogenesis.[14] In rabbits, IL-8 injection induces not only granulocytosis but also an increase in immature neutrophils, suggesting recruitment from the bone marrow reservoir.[15]

METALLOPROTEINASES

The matrix metallo proteinases (MMP) family of enzymes are a group of structurally related zinc-dependent endopeptidases, which degrade component of the extracellular matrix and basement membranes.[16] The elevated activity of these MMP enzymes has been associated with a variety of physiological and pathological conditions, including wound healing, angiogenesis, as well as invasion and metastasis of solid tumors. Members of the MMP family are derived into three classes based on their substrate specificity: gelatinases, collagenases and stromelysins.[17] Besides these secreted MMP, transmembrane MMP have been described recently.[18] In man two types of gelatinases, MMP-2 (or gelatinase-A) and MMP-9 (or gelatinase-B) have been recognized. The 72-kDa form of gelatinase-A is produced constitutively by neutrophils and various other cell types including fibroblasts, endothelial cells and tumor cells. In contrast, the 92-kDa form of gelatinase-B is rapidly induced in neutrophils within 5–10 minutes following IL-8 exposure.[19] Both types of gelatinase degrade collagen type-IV as well as gelatin. Gelatinase activity in cell cultured supernatants can be detected by sodium dodecylsulfate polyacrylamide gel electrophoresis (SDS-PAGE) zymography using gelatin as a substrate.

MMP are synthesized as inactive proenzymes that require the removal of an 80-acid amino terminal domain for activation.[20] The activity of MMP appears to be dependent on the balance between the production of latent enzymes, activation of latent enzyme and production of the naturally occurring inhibitors, most notably the tissue inhibitors of metallo proteinases (TIMP). It is apparent that this balance of MMP activity and TIMP expression is a critical determinant of the invasive potential of many solid tumors.[16] In addition to blocking MMP activity, TIMP may also have growth promoting properties. Both TIMP-1 and TIMP-2 have been demonstrated to have erythroid potentiating activity, as measured in the burst-formation assay.[21] TIMP-1 also has growth-promoting properties for the erythroid hematopoietic cell line K-562.

ADHESION MOLECULES

Hematopoietic progenitor cells express a variety of cell adhesion molecules including integrins, selectins and members of the immunoglobulin superfamily.[22] A number of reports indicate a decreased expression of the β1-integrin very late antigen-4 (VLA-4: CD49d/CD29) and of c-kit on hematopoietic progenitor cells.[23] One of the most direct lines of evidence supporting a role of these molecules in mobilization is the observation that anti-VLA-4 antibodies induce mobilization of progenitor cells.[24] In contrast, antibodies to the common β2- integrin chain CD18 failed to induce mobilization. In addition to an altered expression of cell adhesion molecules on progenitor cells, functional changes may occur in the absence of altered expression. For instance, CD34+ cells in steady state bone marrow have been reported to express β1-integrins VLA-4 and VLA-5 in an inactive state.[25] Following treatment with mobilization-inducing cytokines (SCF, M-CSF), a dose-dependent increase in ligand binding properties was observed. Expression of c-kit, the ligand for stem cell factor, appears to be downregulated following mobilization induced by IL-3, GM-CSF and SCF, suggesting that hematopoietic cell mobilization is mediated via a common cytokine network that ultimately results in altered c-kit expression.[26] It has also been reported that the chemokine MIP-2 may downmodulate the interaction between hematopoietic progenitor cells (HPC) and the bone marrow stroma by reducing the expression of L-selectin on HPC and that this process causes the rapid mobilization into the peripheral blood.[27]

IL-8-INDUCED STEM CELL MOBILIZATION IN MICE

Following a single injection of IL-8 at doses ranging from 0.1–100 µg per mouse, an immediate neutropenia is observed within 5 minutes after injection, which is followed by neutrophilia at several hours. Coinciding with the neutropenia an increase in the number of circulating colony-forming cells is observed that peaks between 15 and 30 minutes after a single injection.3 Injection of 30 µg IL-8 resulted in a mean 20-fold increment in the number of granulocyte/macrophage colony-forming units (CFU-GM) per ml blood, peaking at 15 minutes after a single interperitoneal (i.p.) injection. At 60 minutes after injection, the number of circulating colony-forming cells returned to baseline levels. A higher dose of 100 µg IL-8 per animal did not result in a further increment in numbers of colony-forming cells. To assess the radioprotective capacity of mobilized cells, lethally (8.5 Gy)-irradiated recipient mice were transplanted with 5×10^5 blood-derived mononuclear cells obtained at 15–30 minutes after IL-8 injection. Seventy percent of recipient mice transplanted with IL-8 mobilized cells were radio protected at 3 months after transplantation versus 22% for animals transplanted with an equal number of nonprimed steady state blood-derived mononuclear cells. By increasing the number of transplanted mononuclear cells to 1.5×10^6 per recipient, a 100% radioprotection rate was reached.3 Pretreatment with stem cell factor prior to mobilization induced by IL-8 resulted in an increased number of progenitor cells in comparison with mobilization induced by IL-8 only.[28] To assess the long-term repopulating ability of the mobilized cell population, female recipients of IL-8-mobilized blood cells derived from male donors were sacrificed at 6 months after transplantation, and chimerism was assessed for myeloid cells in the bone marrow, B-cells in the spleen and T-cells in the thymus using a Y-chromosome-specific probe and fluorescent in-situ hybridization. The large majority of bone marrow, spleen and thymus cells were of donor origin, showing that the IL-8-mobilized cells had lymphomyeloid long-term repopulating ability. These experiments indicate that IL-8 induces mobilization of stem cells following a single injection and that these cells are able to completely and permanently repopulate lethally irradiated hosts.[3]

EFFECT OF ANTI-LFA-1 BLOCKING ANTIBODIES ON STEM CELL MOBILIZATION

To study the role of β2-integrins in mobilization, we have treated Balb-C mice with intraperitoneal injections of anti-LFA-1 antibody (H154.163).[29] IL-8-induced mobilization of progenitor cells was completely blocked by treatment with the anti-LFA-1 antibody, while IL-1-induced mobilization was partially inhibited. In contrast, anti-VLA-4 antibodies had no effect on mobilization (FIG. 1). Addition of LFA-1 antibody to colony cultures had no inhibitory effect, showing that the antibody did not interfere with colony formation in vitro. Transplantation of mobilized mononuclear cells derived from animals pretreated with anti-LFA-1 antibody of saline protected 19% and 95% of lethally irradiated recipient mice, respectively (FIG. 2). These results indicate that anti-LFA-1 antibodies completely prevent the rapid mobilization of colony-forming cells and of cells exhibiting radioprotective capacity

Treatment

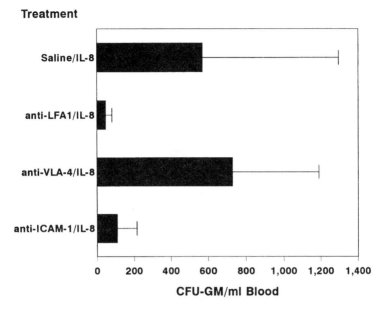

CFU-GM/ml Blood

FIGURE 1. Effect of pretreatment with blocking anti-LFA-1 antibodies on IL-8-induced progenitor cell mobilization. Mice were pretreated with a single i.p. injection of 100 µg anti-LFA-1 antibody, 300 µg anti-ICAM-1 or anti VLA-4 antibody, or saline. After 24 hours IL-8 was administered as a single i.p. injection 20 minutes before harvesting peripheral blood cells. (From Pruijt *et al.*[29] Reprinted by permission from *Blood*.)

and indicate a major role for the β2-integrin LFA-1 in the mechanism of IL-8-induced stem cell mobilization.

EXPRESSION OF LFA-1 ON MURINE HEMATOPOIETIC STEM CELLS

The β2-integrin LFA-1 has been reported to be expressed on some populations of human hematopoietic progenitor cells, although more primitive cells as determined in the long-term bone marrow culture system were found to be LFA-1 negative.[30] It has been suggested that LFA-1 is expressed by default on human HPCs and that binding of progenitor cells in the bone marrow microenvironment results in the active suppression of LFA-1 on HPCs.[31]

In an attempt to explain the blocking effects of anti-LFA-1 antibodies on stem cell mobilization, we studied the expression of LFA-1 on murine hematopoietic progenitor cells and stem cells.[32] First, bone marrow-derived mononuclear cells from Balb-C mice were incubated with anti-LFA-1 CD11a antibody (H154.163) and goat-anti-rat phycoerythrin (PE) (GaRa-Pe) and analyzed by fluorescence-activated cell sorter (FACS). In the bone marrow ±50% of the mononuclear cells (MNC) were LFA-1 negative. Culture supplemented with GM-CSF/IL-1/IL-3/IL-6/SCF and erythropoi-

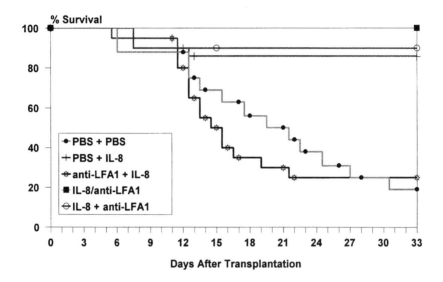

FIGURE 2. Survival of recipient mice transplanted with 5×10^5 blood-derived mononuclear cells from IL-8-mobilized animals pretreated with anti-LFA-1 antibodies or saline. To exclude the possibility that the antibodies interfered with homing of progenitor cells, mobilized blood cells were incubated with antibodies prior to transplantation (IL-8/LFA-1). Recipient mice were also injected with antibodies prior to transplantation (IL-8 + anti-LFA-1). (From Pruijt et al.[29] Reprinted by permission from *Blood*.)

etin (EPO) of 7,500 sorted cells indicated that the LFA-1-negative cell fraction contained the majority of the colony-forming cells (CFU) (LFA-1-negative 154 ± 164 versus LFA-1-positive 22 ± 13, mean $\pm$ SD, $n = 5$). To assess the radioprotective capacity, lethally irradiated recipient mice were transplanted with increasing numbers of BM-derived LFA-1-negative or LFA-1-positive MNC. The radioprotective capacity resided almost entirely in the LFA-1-negative cell fraction, the radioprotection rate after transplantation of 10^3, 3×10^3, 10^4 and 3×10^4 cells being 80, 80, 100 and 100%, respectively. In contrast, after transplantation of 3×10^3, 10^4 and 3×10^4 LFA-1-positive cells, a radioprotection rate of 11, 0 and 30% was obtained. Subsequently, BM-derived sorted wheat germ agglutinin (WGA)-positive/Lin-negative cells were stained with Rhodamine (Rho) (100 ng/ml 201, 37°C), followed by incubation in Rho-free medium (20^1, 37°C). Rho-negative cells were isolated and incubated with anti-LFA-1 antibody and GaRa-Pe. More than 95% of the Rho-negative cells were LFA-1 negative. Cultures of 750 sorted cells showed that the LFA-1-negative fraction contained all CFU (247 versus 1, mean, $n = 4$). Transplantation of 150 Rho-negative LFA-1-negative or up to 600 Rho-negative LFA-1-positive cells protected 100 and 0% of lethally irradiated recipient mice, respectively. These results show that HPC with colony-forming or radioprotective capacity in steady state BM do not express LFA-1. Similar results have been obtained using HPC derived from IL-8- or G-CSF-mobilized blood.[32]

NEUTROPENIC MICE LACK IL-8-INDUCED
STEM CELL MOBILIZATION

Since stem cell mobilization in mice and monkeys could be blocked by anti-LFA-1 antibodies and anti-gelatinase B antibodies (see below), respectively, we hypothesized the existence of an intermediate cell expressing LFA-1 and receptors for IL-8 and being capable of releasing gelatinase-B. Specifically, we hypothesized that neutrophils would serve as mediators for stem cell mobilization. To further substantiate this, mice were rendered neutropenic by administration of anti-neutrophil (anti-Gr-1) antibodies.[33,34] Following a single i.p. injection of 250 µg antibodies, mice became neutropenic for approximately 3 days with neutrophil counts <0.1 × 10⁹/L. At day 4 or 5 after antibody administration, neutrophil counts increased to baseline levels. However, at day 7 to 9 after antibody injection, a rebound granulocytosis was observed (8–10 × 10⁹/L). At various time intervals after antibody injection, stem cell mobilization was induced by injecting IL-8. Mobilization of progenitor cells was completely blocked in neutropenic animals and recovered concomitant with the recurrence of circulating neutrophils. Moreover, the IL-8-induced mobilizing capacity appeared to be proportional to the absolute number of circulating neutrophils. In granulocytotic mice, the mobilizing effect of IL-8 was significantly increased proportial with the degree of granulocytosis. To test the possibility that a lack of mobilizing capacity was due to a decrease in the number of progenitor cells in the bone marrow, progenitor cell pools were quantitated in bone marrow and spleen. In accordance with published results,[34] no reduction was observed in either organ after administration of antibody. The results points toward circulating neutrophils as major regulators in IL-8-induced stem cell mobilization.

MOBILIZING CAPACITY OF IL-8 IN RHESUS MONKEYS

In view of its potential application in humans, we continued the studies on IL-8 mobilization in nonhuman primates.[4] Recombinant human IL-8 was administered as a single intravenous injection in rhesus monkeys at doses ranging from 10–100 µg/kg bodyweight. Blood samples were collected at various time intervals after injection ranging from 1 minute to 8 hours after administration. A time controlled bolus injection of IL-8 at a dose of 100 µg/kg resulted in IL-8 plasma levels of up to 5 µg/ml. From these data, the calculated half-life of free IL-8 was 9.9 ± 2.2 minutes. Similar to the data observed in mice, IL-8 injection resulted in instant neutropenia. This was likely related to pulmonary sequestration of neutrophils as shown by the accumulation of radioactivity over the lungs after injection of radiolabeled neutrophils. At 30 minutes after injection, neutrophilia was observed up to 10-fold over baseline levels. The number of hematopoietic progenitor cells increased from 45/ml to almost 1,400/ml at 30 minutes after injection of 100 µg IL-8/kg bodyweight. In individual animals, up to a 100-fold increase in the number of circulating progenitor cells was observed. After 4–8 hours these numbers returned to pretreatment levels. Based on the numbers that are commonly used in blood stem cell transplantation in humans (20 × 10⁴ CFU-GM per kilogram bodyweight) a leukapheresis procedure processing

300 ml blood would be sufficient for autologous stem cell transplantation in these animals.

INVOLVEMENT OF METALLOPROTEINASES AS MEDIATORS OF STEM CELL MOBILIZATION

To study a possible role for MMP in stem cell mobilization, circulating levels of gelatinase-B were determined by zymoghrapic analysis in rhesus monkeys injected with IL-8. MMP enzyme levels increased up to 1,000-fold within minutes after injection concomitant with the increase in the number of HPC. Rhesus monkeys were then injected with inhibitory monoclonal anti-gelatinase-B antibodies (Rega-3G12) prior to IL-8 injection. A dose of 1 mg/kg anti-gelatinase-B antibody completely inhibited the IL-8-induced mobilization of progenitor cells. Zymographic analysis indicated that the induction of gelatinase-B protein was not inhibited by the antibody. Thus, IL-8 induced the rapid release of gelatinase-B with the concurrent mobilization of HPC that could be prevented by blocking gelatinase-B enzyme activity. These data indicate the involvement of gelatinase-B as a mediator of the IL-8 induced mobilization of hematopoietic progenitor cells in rhesus monkeys.[35] However, in mice gelatinase-B levels remain low following IL-8-induced mobilization, suggesting involvement of other MMPs.

DISCUSSION

The preliminary data presented in this report indicate that mobilization of hematopoietic progenitor cells induced by IL-8 requires the functional expression of LFA-1. Although it can be speculated that this is mediated by a direct effect of the antibody on LFA-1 expressed on hematopoietic progenitor cells, it was demonstrated that murine hematopoietic stem cells do not express the $\beta2$-integrin LFA-1. The majority of colony-forming cells from murine steady state bone marrow reside in the LFA-1-negative cell fraction. Similarly, the radioprotective capacity resided almost entirely in the LFA-1-negative fraction. Thus, hematopoietic progenitor cells with both colony-forming or radioprotective capacity do not appear to express LFA-1, and therefore these cells are unable to function as direct targets for the blocking antibody.

Experiments with neutralizing antibodies directed against gelatinase-B suggest that this metalloproteinase may serve as a mediator of IL-8-induced stem cell mobilization. Experiments in mice indicate that IL-8 is a weak inducer of gelatinase-B, and therefore it is likely that in addition to gelatinase-B other enzymes play an important role in the induction of stem cell mobilization. However, the data indicate a prominent role for MMPs as a group of enzymes that degrade matrix molecules during the induction of mobilization. Accordingly, it was recently demonstrated that neutropenic mice lacking the G-CSF receptor are unable to mobilize progenitor cells in response to IL-8.[36] This mobilization defect appeared to be due to a failure to release progenitor cells, rather than to an impaired stem cell pool, since the numbers of colony-forming cells in the bone marrow were not decreased. In selected animals, a lack of IL-8-induced mobilization was observed in the presence of almost normal numbers of neutrophils, indicating other mechanisms or the involvement of functionally defective neutrophils unable to release MMP in response to activation.

Integrins, in particular Mac-1 (CD11b/CD18) and LFA-1 (CD11a/CD18), have also been implicated in neutrophil migration.[37] Antibody studies have shown that both CD11a/CD18 and CD11b/CD18 as well as their counterreceptor intercellular adhesion molecule-1 (ICAM- 1) participate in controlling neutrophil migration across endothelial monolayers in response to chemotactic agents.[38] Neutrophils isoloated from mice deficient for Mac-1 were defective in adherence to glass and in homotypic aggregation. When challenged by thioglycollate, Mac-1- deficient mice had similar levels of neutrophil accumulation in the peritoneal cavity. Treatment with monoclonal antibodies to LFA-1 blocked 78% of neutrophil accumulation in these deficient mice and 58% in wild type mice. These data indicate that neutrophil migration is more dependent upon LFA-1 and that Mac-1 does not play a critical role herein. Indeed, peritoneal lavage after thioglycollate treatment in mice lacking CD11a resulted in a decreased infiltrate of neutrophils in the peritoneal cavity, indicating that LFA-1 is also important in the extravasation of neutrophils into the peritoneum in response to inflammatory stimuli.[39] Whether neutrophil degranulation is also defective in LFA-1-deficient mice has not been reported.

Taken together, our results are consistent with the hypothesis that neutrophils that express LFA-1 release metalloproteinases upon stimulation by IL-8 and that this process is influenced by antibodies against LFA-1. It remains to be demonstrated that enzyme release is indeed affected by these antibodies. Our data point towards a prominent role for neutrophils as regulators in IL-8-induced stem cell mobilization. Although gelatinase-B can be detected in the plasma of healthy donors undergoing G-CSF-induced stem cell mobilization (unpublished observations), the role of neutrophils in the induction of mobilization by other growth factors, in particular G-CSF, is still unclear and will be the subject of future studies.

REFERENCES

1. SHERIDAN, W.P., C.G. BEGLEY, C.A. JUTTNER, J. SZER, T.B. TO, D. MAHER, K.M. MCGRATH , G. MORSTYN & R.M. FOX. 1992. Effect of peripheral blood progenitor cells mobilized by filgrastim (G-CSF) on platelet recovery after high doses chemotherapy. Lancet **339:** 640.
2. GIANNI, A.M., S. SIENA, M. BREGNI, C. TARELLA, A.C. STERN, A. PILER & G. BONADONNA. 1989. Granulocyte-macrophage colony-stimulating factor to harvest circulating hematopoietic stem cells for autotransplantation. Lancet **2:** 580.
3. LATERVEER, L., I.J.D. LINDLEY, M.S. HAMILTON, R. WILLEMZE & W.E. FIBBE. 1995. Interleukin-8 induces rapid mobilization of hematopoietic progenitor cells with radioprotective capacity and long-term lymphomyeloid repopulating ability. Blood **85**(8): 2269–2275.
4. LATERVEER, L., I.J.D. LINDLEY, D.P.M. HEEMSKERK, J.A.J KAMPS, E.K.J. PAUWELS, R. WILLEMZE & W.E. FIBBE. 1996. Rapid mobilization of hematopoietic progenitor cells in rhesus monkeys by a single intravenous injection of interleukin-8. Blood **87:** 781–788.
5. VAN DAMME, J. 1994. Interleukin-8 and related chemotactic cytokines. 1994. The Cytokine Handbook. 2nd edit. A. Thomson, Ed.: 185–208. Academic Press. London.
6. LUSTER, A.D. 1998. Chemokines—chemotactic cytokines that mediate inflammation. N. Engl. J. Med. **338**(7): 436–445.

7. STRIETER, R.M., S.L. KUNKEL, H.J. SHOWELL, D.G. REMICK, S.H. PHAN, P.A. WARD & R.M. MARKS. 1989. Endothelial cell gene expression of a neutrophil chemotactic factor by TNF-α, LPS and IL-1β. Science **243:** 1467–1469.

8. MATSUSHIMA, K. & J.J. OPPENHEIM. 1989. Interleukin-8 and MCAF: novel inflammatory cytokines inducible by IL-1 and TNF. Cytokine **1:** 2–13.

9. HOLMES, W.E., J. LEE, W.J. KUANG, G.C. RICE & W.I. WOOD. 1991. Structure and functional expression of a human interleukin-8 receptor. Science **253:** 1278–1280.

10. MURPHY, P.M. & H.L. TIFFANY. 1991. Cloning of complementary DNA encoding a functional human interleukin-8 receptor. Science **253:** 1280–1283.

11. LLOYD, A.R., A. BIRAGYN, J.A. JOHNSTON, D.D. TAUB, L. XU, D. MICHIEL, H. SPRENGER, J.J. OPPENHEIM & D.J. KELVIN. 1995. Granulocyte colony-stimulating factor and lipopolysaccharide regulate the expression of interleukin-8 receptors on polymorphonuclear leukocytes. J. Biol. Chem. **270:** 28188–28192.

12. CACALANO, G., J. LEE, K. KIKLY, A.M. RYAN, S. PITTS-MEEK, B, HULTGREN, W.I. WOOD & M.W. MOORE. 1994. Neutrophil and B cell expansion in mice that lack the murine IL-8 receptor homolog. Science **265:** 682–684.

13. WUYTS, A., A. HAELENS, P. PROOST, J.-P. LENAERTS, R. CONINGS, G. OPDENAKKER, & J. VAN DAMME. 1996. Identification of mouse granulocyte chemotactic protein-2 (GCP-2) from fibroblasts and epithelial cells: functional comparison with natural KC and MIP-2. J. Immunol. **157:** 1736–1743.

14. VAN ZEE, K.J., E. FISCHER, A.S. HAWES, C.A. HEBERT, T.G. TERRELL, J.B. BAKER, S.F. LOWRY & L.L. MOLLDAWER. 1992. Effect of intravenous IL-8 administration in nonhuman primates. J. Immunol. **148:** 1746–1752.

15. JAGELS, M.A. & T.E. HUGLI. 1992. Neutrophil chemotactic factors promote leukocytosis. J. Immunol. **148:** 1119–1128.

16. GOETZL, E.J., M.J. BANDA & D. LEPPERT. 1996. Matrix metalloproteinases in immunity. J. Immunol. **156:** 1–4.

17. MATRISIAN, L.M. 1992. The matrix-degrading metalloproteinases. Bioessays **14:** 455–463.

18. SATO, H., T. TAKINO, Y. OKADA, J. CAO, A. SHINAGAWA, E. YAMAMOTO & M. SEIKI 1994. A matrix metalloproteinase expressed on the surface of invasive tumor cells. Nature **370:** 361.

19. MASURE, S., P. PROOST, J. VAN DAMME & G. OPDENAKKER. 1991. Purification and identification of 91-kDa neutrophil gelatinase. Release by the activating peptide interleukin-8. Eur. J. Biochem. **198:** 391–398.

20. KLEINER, D. & W. STETLER-STEVENSON. 1993. Structural biochemistry and activation of matrix metalloproteinases. Curr. Opin. Cell Biol. **5:** 891.

21. CHESLER, L., D.W. GOLDE, N. BERSCH & M.D. JOHNSON. 1995. Metalloproteinase inhibition and erythroid potentiation are independent activities of tissue inhibitor of metalloproteinases-1. Blood **86:** 4506–4515.

22. SIMMONS, P., A. ZANNETTINO, S. GRONTHOS & D LEAVESLEY. 1994. Potential adhesion mechanisms for localisation of hematopoietic progenitors to bone marrow stroma. Leuk. Lymphoma **12:** 353–363.

23. TO, L.B., D.N. HAYLOCK, T. DOWSE, P.J. SIMMONS, S. TRIMBOLI, L.K. ASHMANN & C.A. JUTTNER. 1994. A comparative study of the phenotype and proliferative capacity of peripheral blood (PB) CD34⁻ cells mobilized by four different protocols and those of steady-phase PB and bone marrow CD34⁺ cells. Blood **84:** 2930–2935.

24. PAPAYANNOPOULOU, T. & B. NAKAMOTO. 1993. Peripheralisation of hemapoietic progenitors in primates treated with anti-VLA-4 integrin. Proc. Natl. Acad. Sci. **90:** 9374–9378.

25. KERST, J.M., J.B. SANDERS, I.C.M. SLAPER-CORTENBACH, M.C. DOORAKKERS, B. HOOIBRINK, R.H.J. VAN OERS, A.E.G.KR. VON DEM BORNE & C.E. VAN DER

SCHROOT. 1993. 4 1 and 5 1 are differentially expressed during myelopoiesis and mediate the adherence of human CD34$^+$ cells to fibronectin in an activation-dependent way. Blood **81**: 344.

26. LEVESQUE, J.P., D.I. LEAVESLEY, S. NIUTTA, M. VADAS & P.J. SIMMONS. 1995. Cytokines increase human hematopoietic cell adhesiveness by activation of very late antigen (VLA)-4 and VLA-5 integrins. J. Exp. Med. **181**: 1805–1815.

27. WANG, J., N. MUKAIDA, Y. ZHANG, T. ITO, S. NAKAO & K. MATSUSHIMA. 1997. Enhanced mobilization of hematopoietic progenitor cells by mouse MIP-2 and granulocyte colony-stimulating factor in mice. J. Leuk. Biol. **62**: 503–509.

28. LATERVEER, L., J.M.J.M. ZIJLMANS, I.J.D. LINDLEY, M.S. HAMILTON, R. WILLEMZE & W.E. FIBBE. 1996. Improved survival of lethally irradiated recipient mice transplanted with circulating progenitor cells mobilized by IL-8 after pretreatment with stem cell factor. Exp. Hematol. **24**: 1387–1393.

29. PRUIJT, J.F.M., Y. VAN KOOYK, C.G. FIGDOR, I.J.V. LINDLEY, R. WILLEMSE & W.E. FIBBE. 1998. Anti-lymphocyte function-associated-1 blocking antibodies prevent mobilization of hematopoietic progenitor cells induced by interleukin-8. Blood **91**: 4099–4105.

30. GUNJI, Y., M. NAKAMURA, T. HAGIWARA, K. HAYAKAWA, H. MATSUSHITA, H. OSAWA, K. NAGAYOSHI, H. NAKAUCHI, M. YANAGISAWA, Y. MIURA & T. SUDA. 1992. Expression and function of adhesion molecules on human hematopoietic stem cells: CD34+ LFA-1- cells are more primitive than CD34$^+$ LFA-1$^+$ cells. Blood **80**: 429–436.

31. TORENSMA, R., R.A. RAYMAKERS, Y. VAN KOOYK & C.G. FIGDOR. 1996. Induction of LFA-1 on pluripotent CD34+ bone marrow cells does not affect lineage commitment. Blood **87**: 4120–4128.

32. PRUIJT, J.F.M., C.G. FIGDOR, Y. VAN KOOYK, R. WILLEMZE & W.E. FIBBE. 1997. No expression of LFA-1 on murine hematopoietic progenitor cells with colony-forming or radioprotective capacity. Blood **90**(10): abstr. 1640.

33. CZUPRYNSKI, C.J., J.F. BROWN, N. MAROUSHEK, R.D. WAGNER & H. STEINBERG. 1994. Administration of anti-granulocyte antibody Mab RB6-8C5 impairs the resistance of mice to Listeria monocytogenes infection. J. Immunol. **152**: 1836–1846.

34. HESTDAL, K., F. RUSCETTI, J. IHLE, S.E. JACOBSEN, C.M. DUBOIS, W.C. KOPP, D.L. LONGO & J.R. KELLER. 1991. Characterization and regulation of RB6-8C5 antigen expression on murine bone marrow cells. J. Immunol. **147**: 22–28.

35. PRUIJT, J.F.M., W.E. FIBBE, L. LATERVEER, R. WILLEMZE, S. MASURE, L. PAEMEN & G. OPDENAKKER. 1996. Prevention of interleukin-8-induced mobilization of hematopoietic progenitor cells in rhesus monkeys by antibodies to the metalloproteinase gelatinase-B. Blood **88**(I): 455a.

36. LIU, F., J. POURSINE-LAURENT & D.C. LINK. 1997. The granulocyte colony-stimulating factor receptor is required for the mobilization of murine hematopoietic progenitors into peripheral blood by cyclophosphamide or interleukin-8 but not Flt-3 ligand. Blood **90**: 2522–2528.

37. LU, H., C.W. SMITH, J. PERRARD, D. BULLARD, L. TANG, S.B. SHAPPELL, M.L. ENTMAN, A.L. BEAUDET & C.M. BALLANTYNE. 1997. LFA-1 is sufficient in mediating neutrophil emigration in Mac-1-deficient mice. J. Clin. Invest. **99**: 1340–1350.

38. FURIE, M., M.C.A. TANCINCO & C.W. SMITH. 1991. Monoclonal antibodies to leukocyte integrins CD11a/CD18 and CD11b/CD18 or intercellular adhesion molecule-1 inhibit chemoattractant-stimulated neutrophil transendothelial migration in vitro. Blood **78**: 2089–2097.

39. SCHMITS, R., T.M. KÜNDIG, D.M. BAKER, G. SHUMAKER, J.L. SIMARD, G. DUNCAN, A. WAKEHAM, A. SHAHINIAN, A. VAN DER HEIDEN, M.F. BACHMANN, P.S. OHASHI,

T.W. MAK & D.D. HICKSTEIN. 1996. LFA-1-deficient mice show normal CTL responses to virus but fail to reject immunogenic tumor. J. Exp. Med. **183:** 1415–1426.

DISCUSSION

D. METCALF (*P. O. Royal Melbourne Hospital*): Is there a common mechanism involved with G-CSF mobilization and mobilization by other agents?

FIBBE: I have no conclusive data yet, but we have a hypothesis that could perhaps explain the delay that you see between G-CSF injection and mobilization. Following injection of G-CSF you will see immediate peripheral neutrophilia, but if you look in the bone marrow there is a neutropenia because of this shift. It may be that what you need is neutrophils that are formed in the marrow and that are bound to proteoglycans in the marrow microenvironment. Following treatment with G-CSF for several days you get maturing cells in the marrow. Since they are bound to the microenvironment, they may be better targets for degranulation. After 3–4 days when they mature and get gelatanase-B granules, they may release enyzmes. We are currently doing studies in this neutropenia model to study if G-CSF mobilization is affected by neutrophils.

T. PAPAYANNOPOULOU (*University of Washington*): The common thread in both the G-CSF and the IL-8 mobilization is the target cells, i.e., the normal neutrophil. Unless you have a normal functioning neutrophil, there will not be any mobilization in either of these agents.

FIBBE: In the clinical setting you always see neutrophilia concurrent with mobilization with G-CSF.

PAPAYANNOPOULOU: In your case, there are differences. The first injection of IL-8 induces neutropenia. Yet during the neutrophilic phase with the second injection, you do see mobilization.

(R)Evolutionary Considerations in Hematopoietic Development

DONNA D. COOPER AND GERALD J. SPANGRUDE[a]

Departments of Oncological Sciences and Medicine, Division of Hematology/Oncology, University of Utah, Salt Lake City, Utah 84132, USA

ABSTRACT: Evolutionary aspects of three characteristics of the mammalian hematopoietic system are considered in the context of both established and recent data. First, the lineage relationships among early members of the hematopoietic hierarchy are reconsidered in a tripartite model proposing lineage segregation based on vascular function, innate immunity, and acquired immunity on an evolutionary time scale. Second, the observation of two stem cell populations that differ in cell cycle status is considered as an evolved mechanism to enhance survival of the species in response to exposure to environmental toxins. Finally, the mobilization of hematopoietic stem cells into the peripheral circulation is proposed to be a mechanism for rapid dissemination of myeloid function during acute bacterial infections. These revolutionary hypotheses challenge some conventional concepts of stem cell biology, and provide an evolutionary context for considering mammalian hematopoiesis.

INTRODUCTION

The current concept of hematopoietic lineage relationships is the result of classical *in vitro* culture experiments that established patterns of mature myeloid, erythroid, and megakaryocyte development in clonal populations derived from progenitor cells. The conventional hematopoietic hierarchy depicts a totipotent hematopoietic stem cell (HSC) undergoing an early division into two types of committed progenitor cells: myeloid and lymphoid. In this model, an initial cohort of multipotent progenitor cells gives rise to a second level of progenitor cells, which are committed to specific lineages. The myeloid lineage produces megakaryocytes, myeloid cells, and erythrocytes, whereas the lymphoid lineage gives rise to B and T cells. However, there is emerging evidence that contradicts the accuracy of the traditional model. For example, several laboratories have reported isolation of lymphoid progenitor cells that are also capable of giving rise to macrophages and dendritic cells.[1,2] Subsequent studies have established the existence of two lineages of dendritic cells, one with predominantly myeloid characteristics with respect to cytokine responsiveness and cell surface phenotype, and a separate lineage that is derived from lymphoid progenitors.[3,4]

Further evidence suggesting inaccuracies in the conventional hematopoietic hierarchy comes from a series of embryologic studies of hematopoietic development.

[a]Corresponding author: Gerald J. Spangrude, Department of Oncological Sciences, Room 5C334 SOM, University of Utah, Salt Lake City, UT 84132. Phone, 801/585-5544; fax, 801/585-3778; e-mail, DrBlood@medschool.med.utah.edu

This work focuses on the question of the embryonic origin of hematopoiesis, and challenges the long-standing view that HSCs originate as a committed lineage within the extraembryonic yolk sac.[5,6] Although still controversial, recent studies suggest that prior to the onset of circulation, HSCs capable of lymphoid differentiation can only be isolated from the aortic region of the embryo proper.[7] In contrast, primitive erythroid potential is prominent in the developing yolk sac. Transplant studies have demonstrated a stepwise acquisition of spleen and marrow homing potential by yolk sac- and embryonic body-derived cells,[8,9] suggesting that the questions of lineage potential and commitment are complicated by variable, age-dependent interactions of HSCs with stromal environments. At a minimum, these studies demonstrate that hematopoietic lineages are more complex than suggested by the classical hematopoietic model.[10]

A TRIPARTITE MODEL OF HEMATOPOIETIC DEVELOPMENT

Undoubtedly our understanding of the hematopoietic hierarchy is incomplete, and emerging evidence also suggests it is actually incorrect with respect to the relationship between the granulocytic myeloid lineages and the erythroid and megakaryocytic lineages. Evidence suggesting there is a need to reorder this aspect of the hematopoietic hierarchy comes from a variety of sources, which will be reviewed here.

Experiments probing the molecular biology of HSC have utilized targeted mutation of a variety of transcription factors to reveal a number of molecules involved in differentiation of specific hematopoietic lineages. Among these, several mutations selectively effect the erythroid and megakaryocytic lineages. For example, mutation of c-myb has been shown to block definitive hematopoiesis in the fetal liver without interrupting primitive yolk sac hematopoiesis (predominantly erythroid and macrophage lineages) or the development of megakaryocytes.[11] In contrast, targeted mutation of PU.1 abolishes myeloid and lymphoid development, leaving erythroid and megakaryocytic development relatively intact.[12] Further, SCL/TAL1, which is indispensable in hematopoietic development,[13] selectively enhances megakaryocyte and erythroid development when overexpressed in normal human CD34+ hematopoietic cells.[14] Although transcription factor mutation studies cannot be directly interpreted in the context of lineage relationships due to variable expression patterns in different hematopoietic lineages and to complex interactions between individual domains of different proteins,[15] these observations nonetheless support the concept of an erythroid/megakaryocytic component of hematopoiesis that may include a separate bipotent progenitor.

Yolk sac hematopoiesis primarily supplies two elements essential to early embryogenesis, the vascular primordium and primitive erythropoiesis. The existence of a common progenitor for these two lineages, the hemangioblast, has long been proposed and recently supported by a number of studies.[16–18] A correlative hypothesis in adult hematopoiesis is that a progenitor for the vascular lineages (in the adult, the megakaryocyte and erythroid lineages without an endothelial progenitor) may exist as a separate precursor from other myeloid lineages. Integrating the concept of a separate vascular lineage into the existing myeloid and lymphoid paradigm gives rise to a tripartite model (FIG. 1), in which the most primitive HSCs differentiate into three branches of committed progenitor cells: the vascular, myeloid, and lymphoid lineages. These three lineages correspond to an evolutionary emergence of vascular function, innate immunity, and acquired immune responses. The vascular lineage predominantly produces cells associated with maintenance of the circulatory system and nutrient and waste exchange: erythrocytes, megakaryocytes, and macrophages. The myeloid lineage produces the cells associated with innate immunity: granulocytes, macrophages, mast cells, and dendritic cells. Finally, the lymphoid lineage gives rise to cells associated with antigen-specific acquired immunity: B and T cells, natural killer cells, dendritic cells, and macrophages. Unlike the traditional model of hematopoietic development, the tripartite model as proposed in FIGURE 1 does not require some cell populations, specifically macrophages and dendritic cells, to be the product of a single progenitor cell lineage. This aspect of the tripartite model accounts for the observations of macrophage and dendritic cell potential in otherwise lymphoid-committed progenitors as noted above.[1,2]

Additional evidence supporting the model shown in FIGURE 1 comes from a variety of published studies. The most novel aspect of this model, the common progenitor for erythroid, megakaryocytic, and macrophage lineages, has been suggested repeatedly.[19] For example, a large number of studies have documented structural and

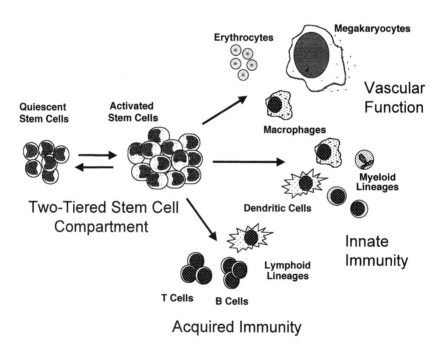

FIGURE 1. A tripartite model of mammalian hematopoiesis that proposes an early segregation of lineages based on the evolution of vascular function, innate immunity, and acquired immunity. A key element in this model is that specific cell populations, such as macrophages and dendritic cells, can arise from different lineage-committed progenitors. See the text for further details.

functional homologies between the two major regulators of the erythroid and mega-karyocytic lineages, erythropoietin and thrombopoietin.[20,21] In addition, these two cytokines utilize receptors that activate common signal transduction pathways.[22–24] Numerous studies have documented progenitor cells that are restricted to erythroid and megakaryocytic lineages, with macrophages as the only other lineage detected. Johnson and Metcalf demonstrated that 60% of the mixed erythroid/megakaryocytic colonies derived from mouse fetal liver cells contained macrophages as the only oth-er cell lineage.[25] Bipotent erythroid/megakaryocytic progenitors were identified in mouse yolk sac,[26] and isolated by phenotype from human bone marrow.[27] In addi-tion, numerous continuous cell lines with the characteristics of a bipotent progenitor for these two lineages have been described.[28,29] Taken together with the results from targeted mutation of transcription factors as noted above, these studies strongly sup-port the idea of a separate vascular progenitor in the hematopoietic lineage.

EVOLUTIONARY ASPECTS OF THE TRIPARTITE MODEL

At the simplest level, the result of hematopoiesis is to provide an animal with two systems: vascular function and immunity. As animals increase in complexity, the de-mands on these systems and their structural complexity increases. It is therefore en-lightening to envision the lineages of hematopoiesis in the context of the larger process of evolution and development; such an analysis provides additional evidence supporting the tripartite model of hematopoiesis as shown in FIGURE 1. The cladis-tic-based analysis of any organ system or developmental process presupposes that the characteristics of the system are modified in the descendants of the ancestor, and that the process of modification can include either loss or expansion of the system. A review of the products of hematopoiesis suggests that expansion has been the pri-mary evolutionary mechanism operative in this system.

As multicellular organisms evolved, a mechanism for transporting elemental gas-ses, nutrients, and wastes to and from sites distant from the environmental interface became necessary. The evolution of a fluid-based circulatory system meets these re-quirements and introduces others, such as the need to maintain the system's integrity by a clotting activity. The cells of the vascular lineage in the tripartite model, eryth-rocytes and megakaryocytes, are capable of meeting these needs and probably co-evolved early. This prediction is strengthened by several experimental observations: the existence of a common erythroid/megakaryocytic progenitor as discussed above, the coincidental timing of erythrocytes and megakaryocytes very early in embryo-genesis, and the presence of numerous bipotent progenitors for these two lineages in the embryonic yolk sac.[26]

As animals were evolving from single- into multicellular organisms, a mecha-nism for eliminating potentially pathogenic organisms would have enhanced surviv-al. The evolution of innate immunity introduces additional requirements, because in order to eliminate pathogens an animal must be capable of distinguishing "self" from "nonself." This ability is the defining characteristic of immunity. Animals with even the most primitive immune systems are able to isolate and destroy pathogens by ph-agocytosis. The cellular elements of the second arm of the tripartite model, the cells of the myeloid lineage, provide the first line of defense against infections. Cells similar to macrophages and granulocytes are present in the simplest multicellular organisms, including sponges and tunicates. Although one can point to simple organisms with open circulatory systems containing macrophages as evidence that innate immunity was established before circulation in evolution, this timeline has not been definitively established. However, given that none of the invertebrates has the advantage conferred by immunological memory, it is virtually certain that innate immunity evolved before antigen-specific immunity. Classic immunoglobulin molecules do not appear until the emergence of the vertebrates. Molecules similar to members of the immunoglobulin family and other molecules capable of distinguishing self from nonself are present in invertebrates; however, these molecules do not have the high-specificity epitope recognition characteristic of vertebrate antibodies. This function is filled by the cellular elements of the third arm of the tripartite model, the B and T cells of the lymphoid lineage.

Recent results from several laboratories have demonstrated a distinct segregation of the progenitors of acquired immunity from those involved in vascular function or innate immunity. In our laboratory, we have utilized the selection scheme shown in FIGURE 2 to define the cell surface antigen expression of mouse bone marrow cells committed to either the myeloid or lymphoid lineages. The vast majority of mouse stem and progenitor cells can be found among bone marrow cells that lack expression of a series of differentiation antigens termed "lineage" markers; depletion of

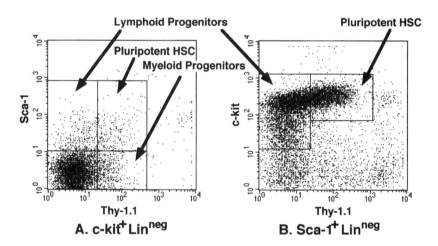

FIGURE 2. Isolation of mouse hematopoietic stem and progenitor cells by surface antigen phenotype. Normal mouse bone marrow cells were reacted with monoclonal antibodies specific for antigens expressed by differentiated blood cells, and these mature cells were removed by immunomagnetic selection. The remaining cells (10% of the initial bone marrow cell population) were reacted with fluorescent antibodies specific for the Sca-1, Thy-1.1, and c-kit surface antigens and analyzed by flow cytometry. **(A)** Cells expressing c-kit (60% of the total) are displayed with respect to Sca-1 and Thy-1.1 expression, while in **(B)** cells expressing Sca-1 (5% of the total) are displayed with respect to c-kit and Thy-1.1 expression. The phenotype of pluripotent hematopoietic stem cells, lymphoid-committed progenitors, and myeloid-committed progenitors, as determined in our laboratory by transplant and cell culture assays, is indicated.

these cells by immunomagnetic technology enriches for hematopoietic stem and progenitor cells approximately 10-fold. Among these "lineage-negative" (Lin^{neg}) cells, we can demonstrate several distinct populations by immunofluorescent staining of the surface antigens Thy-1.1, Sca-1, and c-kit (FIG. 2). By selecting only c-kit-positive cells from the Lin^{neg} pool of cells (FIG. 2A), the hematopoietic cells with potential to differentiate into all hematopoietic lineages are segregated into the subset that expresses both Sca-1 and Thy-1.1. Cells committed to lymphoid lineages express c-kit and Sca-1 but differ from multipotent cells by the loss of the Thy-1.1 antigen. In contrast, cells committed to the myeloid lineages are positive for Thy-1.1 and c-kit but have lost Sca-1 expression.

Because Sca-1 expression is restricted to a smaller subset of Lin^{neg} bone marrow cells than is c-kit expression, evaluation of the $Sca-1^{+}$ subset of Lin^{neg} cells shows the distinction between pluripotent HSCs and committed lymphoid progenitors more distinctly (FIG. 2B). While transplantation of the $Thy-1.1^{+}c-kit^{+}$ subset of $Sca-1^{+}Lin^{neg}$ cells results in hematologic rescue and long-term reconstitution of lethally irradiated mice,[30] the $Thy-1.1^{neg}$ subset reconstitutes only the T and B lymphoid lineages and a low level of macrophages. Because transplant recipients do not recover erythroid or platelet lineages after these transplants, the animals are not rescued from hematopoietic failure and do not survive beyond 30 days. Similar results have been reported by Kondo et al.[31] in experiments where the lymphoid-specific receptor for interleukin (IL)-7 was used as a selection of $Sca-1^{+}c-kit^{+}$ cells. These experiments confirm the existence of a progenitor cell committed to the acquired immunity lineage of hematopoiesis as shown in FIGURE 1, and extend to mouse bone marrow the observation of lymphoid/macrophage bipotent progenitors in mouse fetal liver.[1]

MOBILIZATION AND SELF-RENEWAL: IS THERE AN EVOLUTIONARY BASIS?

Another characteristic of the mammalian hematopoietic hierarchy not usually depicted in conventional lineage diagrams is the existence of two distinct pluripotent cell populations within the HSC compartment;[32] this is depicted in FIGURE 1 as a two-tiered stem cell compartment comprised of quiescent and activated subsets of stem cells. Transplantation studies have demonstrated that only the quiescent subset of HSCs can contribute to long-term engraftment,[33] even though both the quiescent and activated subsets are comprised of pluripotent cells requiring complex mixtures of cytokines in order to proliferate.[34] Recently, Bradford et al. have utilized continuous bromo-deoxyuridine (BrdU) labeling to demonstrate the turnover kinetics of these two stem cell populations;[35] the results show that while virtually all cells within the activated population undergo cell division over a period of a few days, the quiescent subset requires continuous labeling for almost 30 days in order to label most of the cells.

Why would the mammalian hematopoietic system include quiescent stem cells in addition to activated stem cells? Due to the extensive turnover of peripheral blood cells, the HSC compartment must include an actively cycling component. These cycling cells are highly vulnerable to genetic injury mediated by plant toxins and other noxious substances normally found in nature. While one interpretation of the two-tiered HSC compartment depicted in FIGURE 1 may be that the quiescent component of the system is responsible for slow but sustained self-renewing cell divisions, another perspective would be that self-renewal occurs normally as part of the function of the proliferating component of the stem cell compartment and that the quiescent component exists for another reason.

One can identify a selective pressure that coincidentally favors the two-tiered structure of the mammalian stem cell compartment, and perhaps also the modern process of peripheral blood stem cell mobilization and transplantation. Foraging animals, such as our evolutionary ancestors, would occasionally be expected to encounter and ingest toxic plant or animal substances found in their environment. Such substances abound in nature, and are often sources of medicinal products; for example, the chemotherapeutic drugs taxol and vincristine were originally extracted from plants. The search for food in the environment is a strong potential source of selective pressure, as is the need for plants and some animals to evolve toxic defense mechanisms as protection against extinction. Hematopoietic progenitor cells present optimal targets for cell-cycle specific poisons, which in order to be effective, must mediate their toxic effects in a relatively short period of time prior to detoxification by the liver. Therefore, some of the most pronounced acute effects of metabolic poisons are observed as a failure in hematopoietic function.

The two-tiered nature of the HSC compartment seems ideally adapted to tolerate episodes of poisoning. The metabolically quiescent HSCs are relatively resistant to the direct effects of cycle-active toxins like 5-fluorouracil,[36] while the second tier of HSCs is highly vulnerable to toxic poisoning due to its high proliferative rate (FIG. 1). The loss of the proliferating progenitor compartment would quickly prove fatal to the organism in the absence of a compensatory mechanism. In this context, it is not difficult to understand how evolutionary pressures would favor a two-tiered hematopoietic compartment, and that the catastrophic depletion of the actively cycling compartment would result in a rapid mobilization of the quiescent component to ensure replacement of a functional hematopoietic system.

Stem cells mobilized from the bone marrow into the peripheral blood are now commonly utilized for stem cell rescue following high-dose chemotherapy in both autologous and allogenic transplant settings. Chemotherapeutic agents such as cyclophosphamide and taxol cause mobilization by inducing large numbers of stem cells to enter the peripheral blood. The magnitude of the mobilization can be amplified by the administration of cytokines such as granulocyte colony-stimulating factor (G-CSF) following chemotherapy. Mobilized stem cells are predominantly noncycling as they enter the circulation, but evidence suggests that once mobilized, HSCs will readily respond to cytokine stimulation and grow *in vitro*.[37] Taken together, this evidence suggests that mobilized HSCs are predominantly in the G_1 phase of the cell cycle, rather that the G_0 phase, which is characteristic of the cells in the normal bone marrow stem cell compartment. One recent study utilized orally administered BrdU labeling to demonstrate that most mobilized stem cells have recently undergone cell division, suggesting that the population of cells is essentially synchronized in the G_1 phase by selective release of stem cells into the circulation just after mitosis.[38] Hematopoietic recovery after transplantation of peripheral blood stem cells is rapid and predictable, likely due in part to the blood-to-blood transport protocol, which selects for cells that are able to respond well to an intravenous infusion.

Did evolutionary pressure to maintain a toxin-resistant, quiescent HSC population serendipitously serve to make stem cell mobilization effective as a transplant protocol? Obviously, any selective pressure favoring transplantation of hematopoietic function could not have been direct. An example of an evolutionary selection with profound additional consequences is the major histocompatibility system, which evolved to provide an efficient mechanism for the immune system to distinguish normal somatic cells from those infected by viruses or genetically transformed by mutation. It is an unfortunate coincidence that the evolution of this advanced immune function also resulted in a formidable barrier to medical intervention in the form of organ transplantation. The mobilization of primitive progenitors into the peripheral blood following chemotherapy exactly mirrors a natural process that may have evolved as a mechanism to compensate for toxic poisoning. Transplantation of these cells after high-dose chemotherapy completely recapitulates the process one might expect to see in nature as a compensatory process to help ensure survival. This hypothesis also accounts for the observation that mammalian bone marrow contains far more stem cells than are needed during the normal lifespan of the organism. Taken to its extreme, this concept may even provide a basis for the success of conventional bone marrow transplantation, since in this case it is known that the cells most effective at reconstituting hematopoiesis in a transplant setting are the members of the quiescent first tier of the hierarchy, rather than the activated stem cells that drive day-to-day hematopoietic function.[33,39]

Animal transplant experiments suggest that the first tier of HSCs is largely depleted after transplantation.[40,41] In spite of this depletion, transplant recipients live a normal life span with normal hematopoietic function. This observation suggests that the primary role of the quiescent first tier of HSCs is not self-renewal as a mechanism for maintaining hematopoietic function. The evidence is more consistent with the hypothesis that the first tier is simply a reserve supply, or "savings account," of stem cells that is maintained by a very low but constant amount of cell division, and whose main role is to be rapidly recruited to replace the second tier should the need arise. An extension of this hypothesis suggests that self-renewal of hematopoietic function predominantly occurs at the second tier, where proliferation is rapid and sustained. The unique ability of quiescent HSCs to function as self-renewing stem cells in a transplant setting in no way proves that they are the same cells that fulfill this function in normal, unperturbed hematopoiesis.[42]

An additional evolutionary pressure selecting for HSC mobilization from marrow reserves can also be identified, primarily as a result of the work of Fibbe and colleagues.[43] In these studies, it has been demonstrated that degranulating neutrophils release matrix metalloproteases, including gelatinase B, which degrade the extracellular matrix components of connective tissues that are important in maintaining cell adherence in the marrow cavities. This process can lead to rapid mobilization of leukocytes, including HSCs, into the peripheral blood. Rapid mobilization by the chemokine IL-8 has been used to model the kinetically slower process of clinical mobilization of HSCs following low-dose chemotherapy and G-CSF stimulation.[44] The involvement of neutrophils in the rapid mobilization of HSCs from marrow stores can be coupled with the observation that *in vitro*, primitive HSCs preferentially differentiate as large colonies of macrophages and neutrophils.[34,45] These observations suggest the hypothesis that acute bacterial infections can induce HSC mobilization, both directly via bacterial products such as lipopolysaccharide, and indirectly through the activation of neutrophils, which release matrix-degrading enzymes in the marrow. The result of this mobilization of HSCs from marrow stores into the peripheral blood is a circulating pool of progenitor cells that can be chemotactically recruited into tissue sites of infection. Under the influence of cytokines produced by mature myeloid cells already present in the inflammatory site, the recruited progenitors could rapidly proliferate and differentiate to result in large, localized populations of myeloid cells in specific sites of infection. This mechanism would provide a means to rapidly deliver far more neutrophils to an inflammatory tissue site than could be recruited from circulating pools of mature cells, and would reduce the risk of collateral damage to normal tissues at sites distant to the infection, since the circulating progenitor of the neutrophil burst would require additional activating signals within the inflammatory site to result in large-scale neutrophil production.

An interesting corollary to this hypothesis is the long-known but poorly understood propensity of HSCs to proliferate in response to proinflammatory cytokines such as IL-1 and IL-6 in combination with other cytokines,[46–48] and to respond to G-CSF by both proliferation and mobilization.[49] Thus, in the context of a rapid response to acute infection, the mobilization of HSCs via mechanisms mediated by neutrophils is an attractive mechanism to explain many of the observations surrounding peripheral blood stem cell transplantation. This would include the mobilization process itself as well as the rapid neutrophil recovery observed in clinical transplants of peripheral blood stem cells.[50]

Contemplation of experimental observations in any biological system can often be greatly enhanced by evolutionary considerations. While the results of the present contemplations may seem somewhat revolutionary in the context of modern hematopoiesis research, the hypotheses that have been developed here can explain a number of recent as well as long-standing biologic observations in experimental and clinical hematology. Many of the proposals put forth here are amenable to experimental testing, which will certainly lead to a number of interesting new observations and further questions.

REFERENCES

1. CUMANO, A. *et al.* 1992. Bipotential precursors of B cells and macrophages in murine fetal liver. Nature **356:** 612–615.
2. ARDAVIN, C. *et al.* 1993. Thymic dendritic cells and T cells develop simultaneously in the thymus from a common precursor population. Nature **362:** 761–763.
3. INABA, K. *et al.* 1993. Granulocytes, macrophages, and dendritic cells arise from a common major histocompatibility complex class-II-negative progenitor in mouse bone marrow. Proc. Natl. Acad. Sci. USA **90:** 3038–3042.
4. SHORTMAN, K. & C. CAUX. 1997. Dendritic cell development: multiple pathways to nature's adjuvants. Stem Cells **15:** 409–419.
5. MOORE, M.A.S. & D. METCALF. 1970. Ontogeny of the haemopoietic system: yolk sac origin of *in vivo* and *in vitro* colony forming cells in the developing mouse embryo. Br. J. Haematol. **18:** 279–296.
6. WEISSMAN, I., V. PAPAIOANNOU & R. GARDNER. 1978. Fetal hematopoietic origins of the adult hematolymphoid system. *In* Differentiation of Normal and Neoplastic Hematopoietic Cells. B. Clarkson *et al.*, Eds. : 33–47. Cold Spring Harbor Laboratory Press. Cold Spring Harbor, NY.

7. CUMANO, A., F. DIETERLEN-LIEVRE & I. GODIN. 1996. Lymphoid potential, probed before circulation in mouse, is restricted to caudal intraembryonic splanchnopleura. Cell **86:** 907–916.
8. SANCHEZ, M.J. *et al.* 1996. Characterization of the first definitive hematopoietic stem cells in the AGM and liver of the mouse embryo. Immunity **5:** 513–525.
9. YODER, M.C., K. HIATT & P. MUKHERJEE. 1997. *In vivo* repopulating hematopoietic stem cells are present in the murine yolk sac at day 9.0 postcoitus. Proc. Natl. Acad. Sci. USA **94:** 6776–6780.
10. DZIERZAK, E., A. MEDVINSKY & M. DE BRUIJN. 1998. Qualitative and quantitative aspects of haematopoietic cell development in the mammalian embryo. Immunol. Today **19:** 228–236.
11. MUCENSKI, M.L. *et al.* 1991. A functional c-myb gene is required for normal murine fetal hepatic hematopoiesis. Cell **65:** 677–689.
12. SCOTT, E.W. *et al.* 1997. PU.1 functions in a cell-autonomous manner to control the differentiation of multipotential lymphoid-myeloid progenitors. Immunity **6:** 437–447.
13. ROBB, L. *et al.* 1996. The scl gene product is required for the generation of all hematopoietic lineages in the adult mouse. EMBO J. **15:** 4123–4129.
14. ELWOOD, N.J. *et al.* 1998. Enhanced megakaryocyte and erythroid development from normal human CD34(+) cells: consequence of enforced expression of SCL. Blood **91:** 3756–3765.
15. PETROVICK, M.S. *et al.* 1998. Multiple functional domains of AML1: PU.1 and C/EBPalpha synergize with different regions of AML1. Mol. Cell. Biol. **18:** 3915–3925.
16. CHOI, K. *et al.* 1998. A common precursor for hematopoietic and endothelial cells. Development **125:** 725–732.
17. VISVADER, J.E., Y. FUJIWARA & S.H. ORKIN. 1998. Unsuspected role for the T-cell leukemia protein SCL/tal-1 in vascular development. Genes Dev. **12:** 473–479.
18. EICHMANN, A. *et al.* 1997. Ligand-dependent development of the endothelial and hemopoietic lineages from embryonic mesodermal cells expressing vascular endothelial growth factor receptor 2. Proc. Natl. Acad. Sci. USA **94:** 5141–5146.
19. MCDONALD, T.P. & P.S. SULLIVAN. 1993. Megakaryocytic and erythrocytic cell lines share a common precursor cell. Exp. Hematol. **21:** 1316–1320.
20. PARK, H. *et al.* 1998. Identification of functionally important residues of human thrombopoietin. J. Biol. Chem . **273:** 256–261.
21. PORTEU, F. *et al.* 1996. Functional regions of the mouse thrombopoietin receptor cytoplasmic domain: evidence for a critical region which is involved in differentiation and can be complemented by erythropoietin. Mol. Cell. Biol. **16:** 2473–2482.
22. PARGANAS, E. *et al.* 1998. Jak2 is essential for signaling through a variety of cytokine receptors. Cell **93:** 385–395.
23. NAGATA, Y., E. NISHIDA & K. TODOKORO. 1997. Activation of JNK signaling pathway by erythropoietin, thrombopoietin, and interleukin-3. Blood **89:** 2664–2669.
24. KIERAN, M.W. *et al.* 1996. Thrombopoietin rescues *in vitro* erythroid colony formation from mouse embryos lacking the erythropoietin receptor. Proc. Natl. Acad. Sci. USA **93:** 9126–9131.
25. JOHNSON, G.R. & D. METCALF. 1977. Pure and mixed erythroid colony formation *in vitro* stimulated by spleen conditioned medium with no detectable erythropoietin. Proc. Natl. Acad. Sci. USA **74:** 3879–3882.
26. ERA, T. *et al.* 1997. Thrombopoietin enhances proliferation and differentiation of murine yolk sac erythroid progenitors. Blood **89:** 1207–1213.
27. PAPAYANNOPOULOU, T. *et al.* 1996. Insights into the cellular mechanisms of erythropoietin-thrombopoietin synergy. Exp. Hematol. **24:** 660–669.
28. BONSI, L. *et al.* 1997. An erythroid and megakaryocytic common precursor cell line (B1647) expressing both c-mpl and erythropoietin receptor (Epo-R) proliferates and modifies globin chain synthesis in response to megakaryocyte growth and development factor (MGDF) but not to erythropoietin (Epo). Br. J. Haematol. **98:** 549–559.

29. KOMATSU, N. *et al.* 1997. *In vitro* development of erythroid and megakaryocytic cells from a UT-7 subline, UT-7/GM. Blood **89:** 4021–4033.
30. SPANGRUDE, G.J., S. HEIMFELD & I.L. WEISSMAN. 1988. Purification and characterization of mouse hematopoietic stem cells. Science **241:** 58–62.
31. KONDO, M., I.L. WEISSMAN & K. AKASHI. 1997. Identification of clonogenic common lymphoid progenitors in mouse bone marrow. Cell **91:** 661–672.
32. SPANGRUDE, G.J. & G.R. JOHNSON. 1990. Resting and activated subsets of mouse multipotent hematopoietic stem cells. Proc. Natl. Acad. Sci. USA **87:** 7433–7437.
33. NIBLEY, W.E. & G.J. SPANGRUDE. 1998. Primitive stem cells alone mediate rapid marrow recovery and mulitlineage engraftment after transplantation. Bone Marrow Transplant. **21:** 345–354.
34. LI, C.L. & G.R. JOHNSON. 1992. Rhodamine123 reveals heterogeneity within murine Lin⁻, Sca-1⁺ hemopoietic stem cells. J. Exp. Med. **175:** 1443–1447.
35. BRADFORD, G.B. *et al.* 1997. Quiescence, cycling, and turnover in the primitive hematopoietic stem cell compartment. Exp. Hematol. **25:** 445–453.
36. HODGSON, G.S. & T.R. BRADLEY. 1979. Properties of haematopoietic stem cells surviving 5-fluorouracil treatment: evidence for a pre-CFU-S cell? Nature **281:** 381–382.
37. R.M. *et al.* 1997. Cycling status of CD34⁺ cells mobilized into peripheral blood of healthy donors by recombinant human granulocyte colony-stimulating factor. Blood **89:** 1189–1196.
38. MORRISON, S.J., D.E. WRIGHT & I.L. WEISSMAN. 1997. Cyclophosphamide/granulocyte colony-stimulating factor induces hematopoietic stem cells to proliferate prior to mobilization. Proc. Natl. Acad. Sci. USA **94:** 1908–1913.
39. ZIJLMANS, J.M. *et al.* 1998. The early phase of engraftment after murine blood cell transplantation is mediated by hematopoietic stem cells. Proc. Natl. Acad. Sci. USA **95:** 725–729.
40. ROSS, E.A., N. ANDERSON & H.S. MICKLEM. 1982. Serial depletion and regeneration of the murine hematopoietic system. Implications for hematopoietic organization and the study of cellular aging. J. Exp. Med. **155:** 432–444.
41. HARRISON, D.E. & C.M. ASTLE. 1982. Loss of stem cell repopulating ability upon transplantation. Effects of donor age, cell number, and transplantation procedure. J. Exp. Med. **156:** 1767–1779.
42. LORD, B.I. & T.M. DEXTER. 1995. Which are the hematopoietic stem cells? or: Don't debunk the history. Exp. Hematol. **23:** 1237–1241.
43. OPDENAKKER, G., W.E. FIBBE & J. VAN DAMME. 1998. The molecular basis of leukocytosis. Immunol. Today **19:** 182–189.
44. PRUIJT, J.F. *et al.* 1998. Anti-LFA-1 blocking antibodies prevent mobilization of hematopoietic progenitor cells induced by interleukin-8. Blood **91:** 4099–4105.
45. HEIMFELD, S. *et al.* 1991. The *in vitro* response of phenotypically defined mouse stem cells and myeloerythroid progenitors to single or multiple growth factors. Proc. Natl. Acad. Sci. USA **88:** 9902–9906.
46. BARTELMEZ, S.H. *et al.* 1989. Interleukin 1 plus interleukin 3 plus colony-stimulating factor 1 are essential for clonal proliferation of primitive myeloid bone marrow cells. Exp. Hematol. **17:** 240–245.
47. IKEBUCHI, K. *et al.* 1987. Interleukin 6 enhancement of interleukin 3-dependent proliferation of multipotential hemopoietic progenitors. Proc. Natl. Acad. Sci. USA **84:** 9035–9039.
48. JACOBSEN, S.E. *et al.* 1994. Distinct and direct synergistic effects of IL-1 and IL-6 on proliferation and differentiation of primitive murine hematopoietic progenitor cells *in vitro*. Exp. Hematol. **22:** 1064–1069.
49. MOLINEUX, G. *et al.* 1991. The effects on hematopoiesis of recombinant stem cell factor (ligand for c-kit) administered *in vivo* to mice either alone or in combination with granulocyte colony-stimulating factor. Blood **78:** 961–966.
50. SMITH, T.J. *et al.* 1997. Economic analysis of a randomized clinical trial to compare filgrastim-mobilized peripheral-blood progenitor-cell transplantation and autologous bone marrow transplantation in patients with Hodgkin's and non-Hodgkin's lymphoma. J. Clin. Oncol. **15:** 5-10.

Stem Cell Gene Therapy for the β-Chain Hemoglobinopathies

Problems and Progress[a]

DAVID W. EMERY AND GEORGE STAMATOYANNOPOULOS[b]

Division of Medical Genetics, University of Washington Department of Medicine, Seattle, Washington 98195, USA

ABSTRACT: Virus vectors hold great promise for the stem cell gene therapy of β-chain hemoglobinopathies. However, conventional vectors suffer from low gene transfer rates, low expression levels, and inconsistent or short-lived expression *in vivo*. In this review we summarize the current status of vector systems for the transduction of hematopoietic stem cells, including the development of novel vector systems and methods for selection of transduced stem cells *in vivo*. We also summarize efforts to achieve therapeutic expression levels of transferred globin genes with retrovirus vectors, including the manipulation of transcription cassettes, the use of globin gene enhancers, and advances in the use of chromatin insulators for improving the frequency of gene expression following hematopoietic stem cell transduction.

INTRODUCTION

The main obstacles to achieving effective hematopoietic stem cell (HSC) gene therapy include: 1) The rarity of long-term reconstituting HSC; 2) the low density of receptors for commonly used gene delivery vectors on this population of cells; 3) the inefficiency of commonly used gene delivery vectors at gene transfer; 4) the inadequate levels of gene expression in the target cells; and 5) the silencing and extinction of expression due to position effects. The issues of receptor density and progress in acquiring HSC through cytokine mobilization are described in the paper of Orlic *et al.* (this volume). In this paper we summarize the current status of vector systems for the transduction of HSC, efforts to achieve therapeutic expression levels of transferred globin genes, and recent advances in the use of chromatin insulators for improving gene expression following HSC transduction.

VECTOR SYSTEMS

Recombinant vectors based on onco-retroviruses are currently being used for the delivery of genes into hematopoietic stem cells (as reviewed in Ref. 1). The first vec-

[a]This work was supported by grant HL 53750 from the National Institutes of Health.

[b]Corresponding author: George Stamatoyannopoulos, M.D., Dr.Sci., Head, Division of Medical Genetics, University of Washington, Box 357720, Seattle, WA 98195. Phone, 206/543-3526; fax, 206/543-3050; e-mail: gstam@u.washington.edu

tors of this type made use of murine leukemia viruses (MLV) (as reviewed in Ref. 2). In these vectors, all the structural genes were removed but all the critical *cis*-regulatory elements needed for efficient vector production and provirus integration, such as the long terminal repeats (LTRs) and packaging Ψ site, were retained. Virus particles are generated using packaging lines engineered to express the virus structural genes in *trans*, effectively generating replication-defective vectors, which are only capable of one-step infection (as reviewed in Ref. 3). These vectors are able to carry upwards of 7 kb of heterologous sequences, and frequently include drug selection genes to assist in the generation of vector-producer lines. Alternative vectors have been generated using LTR sequences from other onco-retroviruses, such as the murine embryonic stem cell virus (MESV) used to generate the murine stem cell virus (MSCV)-based vectors.[4] In other cases the original MLV vectors have been directly modified to increase expression or reduce the incidence of temporal expression extinction *in vivo*, as for the recently reported MND vector.[5]

Although the recombinant retrovirus vectors provide a highly efficient method of stable gene transfer into eukaryotic cells,[6] provirus integration requires the target cell to divide, a phenomenon thought to be dependent on the breakdown of the nuclear membrane during mitosis.[7] Unfortunately, only a small fraction of the most primitive HSC are in cycle at any given time,[8,9] limiting the clinical utility of this class of vectors for stem cell gene therapy. More recently, chimeric vectors containing sequences from conventional MLV vectors and the human lentivirus HIV have been introduced, which reportedly can transduce quiescent cells *in vivo*.[10] Further work will be required to determine the clinical applicability of this class of vectors.

Two new types of vectors are being developed by our colleagues at the Markey Molecular Medicine Center of the University of Washington. Vectors based on the human foamy virus (HFV), developed in the laboratory of D.W. Russell,[11] have the ability to transduce nondividing cells at least in culture, and are nonpathogenic in humans. HFV-based vectors have been found to transduce transformed cell lines and primary hematopoietic progenitors from mice, baboons, and humans. A packaging system capable of generating replication-defective HFV vector stocks has recently been generated,[12] and reconstitution studies with transduced HSC in mice have been initiated.

In another system developed in the laboratory of A. Lieber, elements from the double stranded DNA viruses adenovirus (Ad) and adeno-associated virus (AAV) were used to form a chimeric vector exhibiting desirable traits from both components. In particular, these vectors use the E1/E3-deleted Ad vector sequences needed for large capacity, high titer, and efficient infectivity, flanked by the AAV indirect terminal repeats (ITRs) responsible for vector integration.[13] The resulting deleted vector (ΔAd.AAV) is devoid of all virus genes and therefore is not associated with toxicity and immunogenicity. This ΔAd.AAV vector has been found to efficiently integrate into the chromosomes of cultured cell lines in the absence of cell division as expected for AAV-based vectors.[14] To date this ΔAd.AAV vector has only been tested by packaging in Ad5 capsids, which are incapable of infecting HSC; studies are underway to screen other adenovirus strains for HSC-tropism to be used in this chimeric vector system.

IN VIVO SELECTION

As an alternative approach to increasing the frequency of cells that contain vector provirus following HSC transduction and transplantation, transduced cells can be selected *in vivo*. In the most common application, a minor population of genetically modified cells are enriched through the introduction of a drug resistance gene and subsequent administration of the corresponding cytotoxic drug *in vivo*. In order to achieve a persistent change, it is necessary that the drug of choice exert selective pressure at the level of the HSC, a prerequisite that has been problematic.[15,16] In the case of the cytotoxic drugs taxol, navelbine, and vinblastine used in conjunction with the dominant selectable marker multi-drug resistance gene 1 (MDR1), *in vivo* toxicity at the level of primitive hematopoietic progenitors could only be achieved by pretreatment of the recipient with the early-acting cytokine stem cell factor (SCF).[15] In the case of folate analogs, such as methotrexate, used in conjunction with the dominant selectable marker dihydrofolate reductase (DHFR), nucleoside transport inhibitors were found to be necessary to achieve *in vivo* selection at the primitive hematopoietic level.[17]

In another approach for *in vivo* selection being developed by one of our colleagues in the Markey Molecular Medicine Center at the University of Washington, C.A. Blau, vector-transduced HSC are induced to expand in response to a pharmacological agent by including in the vector a chimeric gene containing a signaling domain for cell expansion that is dependent on dimerization and a binding domain for dimerization.[18] By using a signaling domain from mpl, the receptor for thrombopoietin, and a binding domain for the pharmacological dimerizer FK1012, it has been possible to achieve a specific, sustained, and completely reversible expansion of transduced mouse bone marrow cells *ex vivo* with a nearly 600,000-fold expansion of myeloid progenitors over 42 days of culture.[19] Further studies will be required to determine whether similar results can be achieved with human marrow and whether this approach can be used to expand transduced HSC *in vivo*.

DEVELOPMENT OF VECTORS FOR GENE THERAPY OF THE HEMOGLOBINOPATHIES

Currently Available Vectors

Retrovirus vectors for human β- and $^A\gamma$-globin are actively being developed for the stem cell gene therapy of the β-chain hemoglobinopathies, sickle cell disease and homozygous β-thalassemia. This approach has been limited in part by the restricted size of these vectors and the effect of globin gene and enhancer sequences on vector titer and stability. In the case of retrovirus vectors for β-globin, these problems have been addressed to some degree by introducing several genetic alterations in both coding and virus sequence and by including regulatory elements from the β-globin locus control region (LCR),[20,21] although consistent, robust expression in mice is still limited.[22,23] Initial studies[24] with retrovirus vectors for the human $^A\gamma$-globin gene revealed two important problems: 1) At best only modest expression could be achieved using genomic $^A\gamma$-globin coding and cis-regulatory sequences alone; and 2) High titers could only be achieved by fully deleting at least intron 2 of the $^A\gamma$-

globin expression cassette, which resulted in a further decrease in expression. Increased expression has been reported[25] by using the HS-40 enhancer from the α-globin locus to flank a retrovirus vector containing an intact $^A\gamma$-globin gene using a 'double-copy'[26] approach. However, the ability of this vector to generate high titers has been difficult to confirm,[27] and the role of the HS-40 enhancer has not been directly tested.

Because of the efficient anti-sickling properties of hemoglobin F (HbF, as reviewed in Ref. 28) and the therapeutic impact of even moderate HbF levels in homozygous β thalassemia (as reviewed in Ref. 29), we have sought to develop optimal retrovirus vectors for $^A\gamma$-globin. This has involved the development of an optimal expression cassette for $^A\gamma$-globin using expression plasmids,[30] the development of a novel composite LCR and its use in retrovirus vectors containing the optimal $^A\gamma$-globin expression cassette,[31] and the systematic analysis of $^A\gamma$-globin expression elements and various α-globin HS-40 enhancer configurations directly in retrovirus vectors.[27]

Development of an Optimal Expression Cassette for γ-Globin[30]

The goal of these studies was to identify a promoter/enhancer combination with sufficient sequences to direct therapeutic expression levels of γ-globin, yet small enough for inclusion in retrovirus vectors.[30] Sequences in the second intron of the γ-globin gene responsible for reducing vector titers without effecting expression were removed. The sequence requirements and strengths of the γ- and β-globin promoters were tested, activities of various erythroid-specific enhancer elements were compared, and the influence of 3′ flanking sequences on globin gene expression was examined. The optimal cassette developed in these studies (FIG. 1) consists of a truncated β-globin promoter and a γ-globin gene containing a large internal deletion of intron 2 ($\beta_{pr.}{}^A\gamma 1^+2^\Delta$). When linked to a single copy of the α-globin HS-40 enhancer, γ-globin expression levels for this cassette averaged 105% of murine α-globin mRNA per copy.[30]

Testing of a Composite nanoLCR[31]

When a version of this expression cassette with a truncated 3′ UT region and no enhancer was inserted in a standard MLV-based vector (FIG. 1, second diagram), the resulting recombinant vector was genetically stable and capable of generating virus titers well in excess of those reported for similar vectors with intron 2 intact. In order to increase expression, we first turned to a composite enhancer containing core elements from the β-globin LCR, termed a nLCR. This composite was developed using a drug-resistance colony assay in erythroid cell lines, and was capable of enhancing β-globin gene expression in stably transfected MEL585 cells to 82% per copy of mouse α-globin.[31] However, inclusion of this nLCR in retrovirus vectors containing the optimal $\beta_{pr.}{}^A\gamma 1^+2^\Delta$ cassette (FIG. 1, third diagram) resulted in extreme genetic instability and reduced titers. Specific deletions were abrogated by removing homologous sequences, but random recombinations were still observed at significant frequencies. In transduced MEL585 cells containing intact provirus, $^A\gamma$-globin mRNA produced by this vector was only 2-fold higher compared to the same vector without the nLCR. These data suggest that vector elements, such as the enhancers and pro-

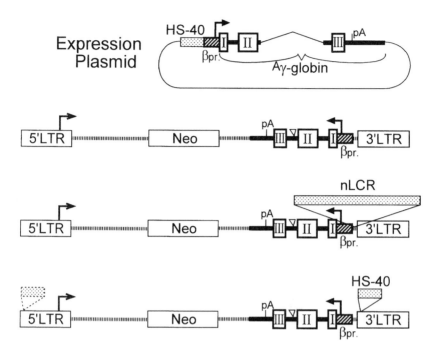

FIGURE 1. Development of retrovirus vectors for γ-globin. As seen in the top diagram, an optimal expression cassette first developed in an expression plasmid[30] consists of a truncated β-globin promoter and a genomic coding fragment for human ^{A}γ-globin with a large internal deletion of intron 2. Maximal expression of this cassette could be achieved by linkage to the HS-40 enhancer element from the α-globin locus. This cassette was included in MLV-based retrovirus vectors either in the absence of an exogenous enhancer (top vector),[31] with a composite nLCR enhancer (middle vector),[31] or the HS-40 enhancer in a 'double-copy' configuration (bottom vector).[27]

moters in the virus LTRs, detract from the ability of the nLCR to enhance expression of the $\beta_{pr.}{}^A\gamma1^+2^\Delta$ cassette.

Development of a New γ-Globin Vector[27]

In a separate series of studies, we also investigated several combinations of ^{A}γ-globin intron deletions and β- and ^{A}γ-globin promoters directly in retrovirus vectors flanked with the γ-globin HS-40 enhancer.[27] Optimal expression and titer could be achieved using an expression cassette consisting of a truncated β-globin promoter and a large internal deletion of intron 2 (FIG. 1, bottom diagram). When used to transduce the murine erythroleukemia cell line MEL585, this vector expressed ^{A}γ-globin mRNA at 46 ± 19% of endogenous β-globin per copy, with a range in 12 clones of 18–75%. High-level, uniform γ-globin protein expression was confirmed in these clones by immunofluorescent staining and flow cytometry using an antibody specific for human γ-globin chain. Although the average level of expression for these

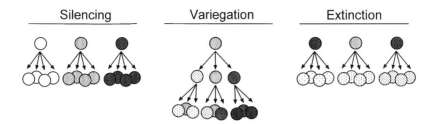

FIGURE 2. Three different patterns of gene expression have been attributed to position effects. In the case of silencing, expression is variable between clones, with the complete absence of expression frequently observed. In the case of position-effect variegation, expression variation is observed within the progeny of a single clone. In the case of extinction, expression is downregulated over time. Note that multiple patterns are frequently observed for vector-transduced genes.

clones is promising, the moderately high degree of variation in expression indicates sensitivity to negative position effects at the interclonal level.

In order to test expression in primary cells, mouse bone marrow cells were transduced, and erythroid burst-forming unit (BFU-E) colonies grown under G418 selection were analyzed by flow cytometry. Mouse marrow was chosen because of the lack of endogenous γ-globin gene expression. High-level expression of human γ-globin protein was detected in 6 out of 6 mouse erythroid progenitor colonies; γ-globin expression was heterocellular. Although such heterocellular expression might be expected for a γ-globin gene in adult-stage cells, it is also possible that this pattern reflects a high degree of position effect variegation as described below.

POSITION EFFECTS ON THERAPEUTIC GENES

Virtually all currently available systems for stable gene transfer lead to integration of the transferred genes into random sites of the target cell chromosomes. Because the vast majority of these sites, especially those near telomers or centromers, are usually not transcriptionally active, expression of the transferred genes is frequently compromised by the flanking chromatin (as reviewed in Ref. 32). As indicated in the left diagram of FIGURE 2, this can lead to highly variable expression between clones, with a significant fraction of clones that are transcriptionally silent from the start. In addition, position effects can be manifested by expression variegation, wherein the progeny of a single clone containing a unique integration event can be affected by the surrounding chromatin to varying degrees (FIG. 2, middle diagram). Such 'position effect variegation' is thought to result from a stochastic and ultimately heritable epigenetic silencing of gene expression, and is frequently associated with transgenes integrated at the boundary of euchromatin and heterochromatin.[33] Finally, there can be temporal extinction, wherein a transferred gene is initially active but becomes inactive over time (FIG. 2, right diagram).

In the case of retrovirus vectors, the problems of position effects have led to striking variations in expression both *in vitro* and *in vivo* (as reviewed in Ref. 34). Retro-

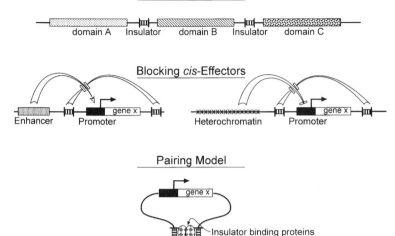

FIGURE 3. Functions of insulators. As indicated in the top diagram, chromatin insulators function as domain boundaries, protecting independent domains from the regulatory influences of adjacent domains. As indicated in the middle diagram, these elements have been found to block *cis*-effectors such as positive enhancers and negative heterochromatin in a polar fashion, i.e., when interposed between the *cis*-effector and the gene promoter. As indicated in the bottom diagram, chromatin insulators are thought to work in pairs and interact with specific binding proteins in order to form looped nucleoprotein complexes.

virus vectors for globin genes in particular seem to be profoundly sensitive to position effects (as reviewed in Ref. 23), with a high incidence of integrated provirus, which are transcriptionally silent, and evidence of clonal expression variation, variegation, and temporal extinction observed *in vitro* and *in vivo*. This has been reported for vectors containing β-globin genes linked to β-globin LCR elements,[22,23] and observed in our studies of vectors containing $^A\gamma$-globin genes linked to an α-globin HS-40 enhancer. As discussed above, attempts have been made to overcome these problems by either genetically modifying the virus LTRs to remove sequences thought to be involved in temporal quiescence,[5,35] or by using LTR sequences from alternative viruses.[4] Below we describe an alternative approach for protecting retrovirus vectors from position effects through the use of chromatin insulators.

PREVENTION OF POSITION EFFECTS: CHROMATIN INSULATORS

Properties of Insulators

The size of mammalian genomes dictates that some mechanism be in place to prevent the promiscuous interaction of genetic loci with neighboring positive and negative cis-regulatory effectors. This can be accomplished by breaking the genome into chromosomal domains with autonomous regulatory elements capable of specifying appropriate levels and patterns of gene expression. Current evidence indicates that there is a hierarchy of chromatin organization that is used in part to accomplish this task. At the gross level, scaffold attachment regions (SARs), or matrix attachment regions (MARs), anchor the chromatin fibers to the chromosome scaffold matrix, physically delineating the structural chromatin domains (as reviewed in Ref. 36). As described below, some loci, such as that for the β-globin-like genes, contain LCRs that function both structurally and functionally to open the chromatin during precise stages of development and differentiation. Finally, some loci make use of sequences that function as chromatin insulators. These elements, first described in *Drosophila*, are thought to shield promoters from the negative influence of surrounding chromatin, and as such are ideal candidates for reducing the incidence or severity of negative position effects on expression of retrovirus vectors for globin and other genes.

Chromatin insulator elements have historically been defined by function. As described above and diagrammed at the top of FIGURE 3, it is thought that their function in the cell is to separate chromosomal domains. Such a function would be critical if two adjacent loci were expressed at different developmental stages or in different tissues. In many cases, such expression patterns are dictated by strong transcriptional enhancers that normally function over large distances, or by the silencing of whole regions through heterochromatinization. As diagrammed in the bottom of FIGURE 3, insulators can block both of these cis-regulatory functions in a polar manner (see examples below). In fact, several insulators have been identified and characterized predominantly using enhancer-promoter blocking assays.[37–39] Such assay systems have also been used to demonstrate that insulators do not have stimulatory or inhibitory effects on transcriptional activity on their own, distinguishing them from classical enhancers[40] and silencers such as that for ε-globin gene.[41]

Examples of Chromatin Insulators

The *Drosophila* suppressor of hairy wing (su(Hw)) protein and its cognate binding sites in the retrotransposon *gypsy* constitute the best studied insulator system to date. In the presence of su(Hw), the cognate binding site from *gypsy* is able to block promoter-enhancer interactions when placed physically between these elements, and can also insulate genes from the repressive effects of flanking heterochromatin.[42,43] Most of the insulator function in *gypsy* is restricted to a 340-bp sequence containing a total of 12 cognate binding sites for the su(Hw).[44]

Palindromic sequences flanking the 87A1 heat shock locus of *Drosophila*, termed scs and scs', have also been found to exhibit insulator properties such as enhancer-promoter blocking and prevention of negative position effects.[45,46] In *Drosophila*, the function of scs' is thought to be mediated though binding of boundary element-associated factor of 32 kD (BEAF-32), a protein that is present in many interband regions of polytene chromosomes, suggesting a general role in defining boundaries. The boundary elements scs and scs' have also been found to function in human T cells,[38] indicating a high degree of species conservation in this system.

Although SAR elements do not appear to function in enhancer-promoter blocking assays,[46] they have been reported to enhance expression of heterologous genes *in vitro*[47,48] and in transgenic mice.[49,50] They also have been reported to confer position-independent expression to linked genes in transgenic mice,[47,49] a hallmark of

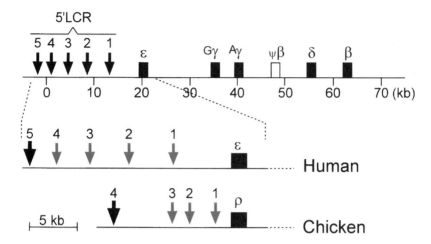

FIGURE 4. The human β-globin gene cluster consists of 5 expressed genes arranged in order of developmental expression and a 5′ locus control region (LCR) consisting of 5 DNase-I hypersensitive sites (HS) as indicated by vertical arrows. As indicated in the bottom diagram, the chicken 5′ LCR consists of only 4 DNase-I hypersensitive sites. Chromatin insulting activity has been ascribed to both human HS5 and chicken HS4.

chromatin insulators. In one recent report, inclusion of a SAR from the β-interferon locus in a retrovirus vector reportedly enhanced expression in transduced primary T cells in an orientation-dependent manner.[51] Although the SAR in this study did not confer position-independent expression, it did prevent the expression extinction that otherwise occurred as the transduced cells became quiescent.

Use of Insulators in Retrovirus Vectors

Regulation of the β-globin loci is accomplished in large part by well defined and characterized regulatory elements, the β-locus control region (β-LCR, as reviewed in Ref. 52). As diagrammed in FIGURE 4, this regulatory LCR is located 6 to 20 kb upstream of the cluster of five functional β-globin-like genes in humans,[53] and consists of five DNase I hypersensitive sites (HS), designated HS5 to HS1.[54–56] The β-LCR has been shown to mediate the activation of the β-locus domain, the developmental switch in β-globin-like genes, and the very high level of expression during terminal erythroid differentiation.[52,53,57] It has also been shown to confer high-level, erythroid-restricted expression to linked globin[53,57] and heterologous promoters[58] in a copy number-dependent, position-independent fashion. Of the five DNase I hypersensitive sites of the LCR, only HS5 has been reported to contain promoter-enhancer blocking properties in murine erythroid leukemia (MEL) cell assays,[59] but not in transgenic mice.[60]

As diagrammed in FIGURE 4, a regulatory element similar to the human β-globin LCR is found in the chicken β-globin locus.[61] One of the HS elements of the chicken LCR, HS4, is constitutively present in erythroid and nonerythroid tissues. This element has been shown to contain potent enhancer-promoter blocking activity and the

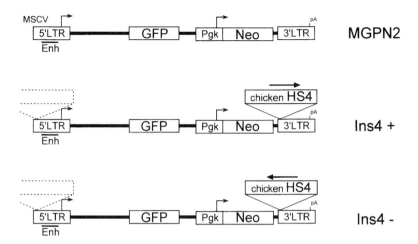

FIGURE 5. Reporter retrovirus vectors were generated using the MSCV-based vector MGPN2,[63] which expresses green fluorescence protein (GFP) from the LTR promoter and Neo from an internal Pgk promoter. A 1.2-kb fragment containing chicken HS462 was inserted into the NheI site of the vector 3′ LTR in the indicated orientations (Ins4+ and Ins4−), where it is copied into the 5′ LTR during reverse transcription (dotted lines). In the resulting provirus, the chicken HS4 fragment flanks the 5′ LTR enhancer and both the GFP and Neo expression cassettes.

ability to shield the *white* minigene from position effects in *Drosophila*.[62] Subsequent analysis of this element revealed that much of the activity is contained in a 250-bp fragment that includes the HS core.[37] This element has also been found to prevent temporal expression extinction in cell lines, although this latter point is still controversial.

We are investigating whether chromatin insulators can be used to reduce or prevent the sensitivity of retrovirus vectors to position effects. As diagrammed in FIG-URE 5, we are making use of an MSCV-based reporter vector, called MGPN2,[63] which expresses green fluorescence protein (GFP) from the LTR promoter and the drug-selection gene neomycin phosphotransferase (Neo) from an internal phosphoglycerate kinase (Pgk) promoter. A 1.2-kb fragment containing the chicken HS4 insulator element was inserted in the 3′ LTR of this vector in either orientation in order to create the vectors Ins4+ and Ins4−. During provirus integration, these elements are copied into the 5′ LTR, essentially flanking the vector in a 'double-copy' configuration.[26] High titer producer clones have been generated and fully characterized for each of these vectors. Using Southern analysis of transduced pools and clones, we found that the insulated vectors are genetically stable, an important criterion for any element included in such vectors. Using standard end-point titration methods,[64] we also found that the inserted elements had no adverse effect on virus titers, another important criterion for their inclusion in therapeutic vectors. These vectors have been used for *in vitro* and *in vivo* studies in order to test the ability of chicken HS4 to insulate expression of a GFP reporter gene. Preliminary studies in mice transplanted with vector-transduced marrow suggest that the 1.2-kb chicken insulator element may serve to reduce the incidence of temporal expression extinction *in vivo* (studies in progress).

ACKNOWLEDGMENTS

We would like to thank G. Felsenfeld both for the chicken HS4 insulator element and for helpful discussions, and Dr. L. Cheng for the MGPN2 vectors.

REFERENCES

1. VERMA, I.M. & N. SOMIA. 1997. Gene therapy—promises, problems and prospects. Nature **389:** 239–242.
2. MILLER, A.D. & G.J. ROSMAN. 1989. Improved retroviral vectors for gene transfer and expression. BioTechniques **7:** 980–890.
3. MILLER, A.D., D.G. MILLER, J.V. GARCIA & C.M. LYNCH. 1993. Use of retroviral vectors for gene transfer and expression. Methods Enzymol. **217:** 581–599.
4. HAWLEY, R.G., F.H.L. LIEU, A.Z.C. FONG & T.S. HAWLEY. 1994. Versatile retroviral vectors for potential use in gene therapy. Gene Ther. **1:** 136–138.
5. ROBBINS, P.B., D.C. SKELTON, X.-J. YU, S. HALENE, E.L. LEONARD & D.B. KOHN. 1998. Consistent, persistent expression from modified retroviral vectors in murine hematopoietic stem cells. Proc. Natl. Acad. Sci. USA **95:** 10182–10187.
6. MILLER, A.D. 1990. Progress toward human gene therapy. Blood **76:** 271–278.
7. ROE, T., T.C. REYNOLDS, G. YU & P.O. BROWN. 1993. Integration of murine leukemia virus DNA depends on mitosis. EMBO J. **12:** 2099–2108.
8. KIM, M., D.D. COOPER, S.F. HAYES & G.J. SPANGRUDE. 1998. Rhodamine-123 staining in hematopoieti stem cells in young mice indicates mitochondrial activation rather than dye efflux. Blood **91:** 4106–4117.
9. GOODELL, M.A., K. BROSE, G. PARADIS, A.S. CONNER & R.C. MULLIGAN. 1996. Isolation and functional properties of murine hematopoietic stem cells that are replicating *in vivo.* J. Exp. Med. **183:** 1797–1806.
10. NALDINI, L., U. BLOMER, F.H. GAGE, D. TRONO & I.M. VERMA. 1996. Efficient transfer, integration, and sustained long-term expression of the transgene in adult rat brains injected with a lentiviral vector. Proc. Natl. Acad. Sci. USA **93:** 11382–11388.
11. HIRATA, R.K., A.DD. MILLER, R.G. ANDREWS & D.W. RUSSELL. 1996. Transduction of hematopoietic cells by foamy virus vectors. Blood **88:** 3654–3461.
12. TROBRIDGE, G.D. & D.W. RUSSELL. 1998. Helper-free foamy virus vectors. Hum. Gene Ther. **9.** In press.
13. RUTLEDGE, E.A. & D.W. RUSSELL. 1997. Adeno-associated virus vector integration junctions. J. Virol. **71:** 8429–8436.
14. LIEBER, A. & M.A. KAY. An integrating andeno-AV hybrid vetor devoid of all viral genes. Submitted.
15. BLAU, C.A., T. NEFF & T. PAPAYANNOPOULOU. 1997. Cytokine prestimulation as a gene therapy stratagy: implications for using the MDR1 gene as a dominant selectable marker. Blood **89:** 146–154.
16. BLAU, C.A., T. NEFF & T. PAPAYANNOPOULOU. 1996. The hematological effects of folate analogs: implications for using the dihydrofolate reductase gene for *in vivo* selection. Hum. Gene Ther. **7:** 2069–2078.

17. ALLAY, J.A., D.P. PERSONS, J. GALIPEAU, J.M. RIBERDY, R.A. SHMUN, R.L. BLAKLEY & B.P. SORRENTINO. 1998. *In vivo* selection of retrovirally transduced hematopoietic stem cells. Nat. Med. **4:** 1136–1143.

18. BLAU, C.A., K.R. PETERSON, J.G. DRACHMAN & D.M. SPENCER. 1997. A proliferative switch for genetically modified cells. Proc. Natl. Acad. Sci. USA **94:** 3076–3081.

19. JIN, L., N SIRITANARATKUL, D.W. EMERY, R.E. RICHARDS, K. KAUSHANSKY, T. PAPAYANNOPOULOU & C.A. BLAU. 1998. Targeted expansion of genetically modified bone marrow cells. Proc. Natl. Acad. Sci. USA **95:** 8093–8097.

20. LEBOULCH, P., G.M.S. HUANG, R.K. HUMPHRIES, Y.H. OH, C.J. EAVES, D.Y. TUAN & I.M. LONDON. 1994. Mutagenesis of retroviral vectors transducing human β-globin gene and β-globin locus control region derivatives results in stable transmission of an active transcription structure. EMBO J. **13:** 3065–3076.

21. SADELAIN, M., C.H. WANG, M. ANTONIOU, F. GROSVELD & R.C. MULLIGAN. 1995. Generation of a high-titer retroviral vector capable of expressing high levels of the human β-globin gene. Proc. Natl. Acad. Sci. USA **92:** 6728–6732.

22. RAFTOPOULOS, H., M. WARD, P. LEBOULCH & A. BANK. 1997. Long-term transfer and expression of the human β-globin gene in a mouse transplant model. Blood **90:** 3414–3422.

23. RIVELLA, S. & M. SADELAIN. 1998. Genetic treatment of sever hemoglobinopathies: the combat against transgene variegation and transgene silencing. Semin. Hematol. **35:** 112–125.

24. RIXON, M.W., E.A. HARRIS & R.E. GELINAS. 1990. Expression of the human γ-globin gene after retroviral transfer to transformed erythroid cells. Biochemistry **29:** 4393–4400.

25. REN, S., B.Y. WONG, J. LI, X.N. LUO, P.M. WONG & G.F. ATWEH. 1996. Production of genetically stable high-titer retroviral vectors that carry a human γ-globin gene under the control of the γ-globin locus control region. Blood **87:** 2518–2524.

26. HANTZOPOULOS, P.A., B.A. SULLENGER, G. UNGERS & E. GILBOA. 1989. Improved gene expression upon transfer of the adenosine deaminase minigene outside the transcriptional unit of the retroviral vector. Proc. Natl. Acad. Sci. USA **86:** 3519–3523.

27. EMERY, D.W., F. MORRISH, Q. LI & G. STAMATOYANNOPOULOS. Development of an optimal ^Aγ-globin expression cassette in retrovirus vectors. Hum. Gene Ther. In press.

28. BUNN, H.F. 1994. Sickle hemoglobin and other hemoglobin mutants. *In* The Molecular Basis of Blood Diseases. 2nd edit. G. Stamatoyannopoulos, A.W. Nienhuis, P.W. Majerus & H. Varmus, Eds.: 207–256. W.B. Saunders Company. Philadelphia, PA.

29. WEATHERALL, D.J. 1994. The thalassemias. *In* The Molecular Basis of Blood Diseases. 2nd edit. G. Stamatoyannopoulos, A.W. Nienhuis, P.W. Majerus & H. Varmus, Eds.: 157–206. W.B. Saunders Company. Philadelphia, PA.

30. LI, Q., D.W. EMERY, M. FERNANDEZ, H. HAN & G. STAMATOYANNOPOULOS. Development of viral vectors for gene therapy of β chain hemoglobinopathies: Optimization of an ^Aγ-globin gene expression cassette. Blood. In press.

31. EMERY, D.W., H. CHEN, Q. LI & G. STAMATOYANNOPOULOS. 1998. Development of a condensed locus control region cassette and testing in retrovirus vectors for ^Aγ-globin. Blood Cells Mol. Dis. **24:** 322–339.

32. KARPEN, G.H. 1994. Position-effect variegation and the new biology of heterochromatin. Curr. Opin. Genet. Dev. **4:** 281–291.

33. KARPEN, G.H. & A.C. SPALDING. 1992. Analysis of subtelomeric heterochromatin in *Drosophila* minichromosome Dp1187 by simple P element insertional mutagenesis. Genetics **3:** 737–753.

34. NEFF, T., F. SHOTKOSKI & G. STAMATOYANNOPOULOS. 1997. Stem cell gene therapy, postion effects and chromatin insulators. Stem Cells 15(Suppl. 1): 265–271.
35. DENG, H., Q. LIN & P.A. KHAVARI. 1997. Sustainable cutaneous gene delivery. Nat. Biotechnol. 15: 1388–1391.
36. DAVIE, J.R. 1996. Histone modifications, chromatin structure, and the nuclear matrix. J. Cell. Biochem. 62: 149–157.
37. CHUNG, J.H., A.C. BELL & G. FELSENFELD. 1997. Characterization of the chicken β-globin insulator. Proc. Natl. Acad. Sci., USA 94: 575–580.
38. Zhong, X.P. & M.S. Krangel. 1997. An enhancer-blocking element between α and δ gene segments within the human T cell receptor α/δ locus. Proc. Natl. Acad. Sci. USA 94: 5219–5224.
39. PALLA, F., R. MELFI, L. ANELLO, M. DI-BERNARDO & G. SPINELLI. 1997. Enhancer blocking activity located near the 3' end of the sea urchin early H2A histone gene. Proc. Natl. Acad. Sci. USA 94: 2272–2277.
40. TREISMAN, R. & T. MANIATIS. 1985. Simian virus 40 enhancer increases number of RNA polymerase II molecules on linked DNA. Nature 315: 73–75.
41. RAICH, N., T. PAPAYANNOPOULOU, G. STAMATOYANNOPOULOS & T. ENVER. 1992. Demonstration of a human ε-globin gene silencer with studies in transgenic mice. Blood 79: 861–864.
42. GEYER, P.K. & V.G. CORCES. 1992. DNA position-specific repression of transcription by a Drosophila zink finger protein. Genes Dev. 6: 1865–1873.
43. ROSEMAN, R.R., V. PIRROTTA & P.K. GEYER. 1993. The su(Hw) protein insulates expression of the Drosophila melanogaster white gene from chromosomal position-effects. EMBO J. 12: 435–442.
44. ROSEMN, R.R., E.A. JOHNSON, C.K.RODESCH, M. BJERKE, R.N. NAGOSHI & P.K. GEYER. 1995. A P element containing suppressor of hairy-wing binding regions has novel properties for mutagenesis in Drosophila. Genetics 141: 1061–1074.
45. KELLUM, R. & P. SCHEDL. 1991. A position-effect assay for boundaries of higher order chromosomal domains. Cell 64: 941–950.
46. KELLUM, R. & P. SCHEDL. 1992. A group of scs elements function as domain boundaries in an enhancer-bloking assay. Mol. Cell. Biol. 12: 2424–2431.
47. KALOS, M. & R.E. FOURNIER. 1995. Position-independent transgene expression mediated by boundary elements from the apolipoprotein B chromatin domain. Mol. Cell. Biol. 15: 198–207.
48. POLJAK, L., C. SEUM, T. MATTIONI & U.K. LAEMMLI. 1994. SARs stimulate but do not confer position independent gene expression. Nucleic Acids Res. 22: 4386–4394.
49. MCKNIGHT, R.A., A. SHAMAY, L. SANKARAN, R.J. WALL & L HENNIGHAUSEN. 1992. Matrix-attachment regions can impart position-independent regulation of a tissue-specific gene in transgenic mice. Proc. Natl. Acad. Sci. USA 89: 6943–6947.
50. THOMPSON, E.M., E. CHRISTIANS, M.G. STINNAKRE & J.P. RENARD. 1994. Scaffold attachment regions stimulate HSP70.1 expression in mouse preimplantation embryos but not in differentiated tissues. Mol. Cell. Biol. 14: 4694–4703.
51. AGARWAL, M., T.W. AUSTIN, F. MOREL, J. CHEN, E. BOHNLEIN & I. PLAVEC. 1998. Scaffold attachment region-mediated enhancement of retroviral vector expression in primary T cells. J. Virol. 72: 3720–3728.
52. STAMATOYANNOPOULOS, G. & A.W. NIENHUIS. 1994. Hemoglobin switching. In The Molecular Basis of Blood Diseases. 2nd edit. G. Stamatoyannopoulos, A.W. Nienhuis, P.W. Majerus & H. Varmus, Eds.: 107–155. W.B. Saunders Company. Philadelphia, PA.
53. GROSVELD, F., G. BLOM VAN ASSENDELFT, D.R. GREAVES & G. KOLLIAS. 1987. Position-independent, high-level expression of the human ß-globin gene in transgenic mice. Cell 51: 975–985.

54. TUAN, D., W. SOLOMON, Q. LI & I.M. LONDON. The "β-like globin" gene domain in human erythroid cells. Proc. Natl. Acad. Sci. USA **82:** 6384–8388.
55. FORRESTER, W.C., C. THOMPSON, J.T. ELDER & M. GRUDINE. 1986. A developmentally stable chromatin structure in the human ß-globin gene cluster. Proc. Natl. Acad. Sci. USA **83:** 1359–1363.
56. FORRESTER, W.C., S. TAKEGAWA, T. PAPAYANNOPOULOU, G. STAMATOYANNOPOULOS & M. GRUDINE. 1987. Evidence for a locus activation region: The formation of developmentally stable hypersensitive sites in globin-expressing hybrids. Nucleic Acids Res. **15:** 10159–10177.
57. TALBOT, D., P COLLIS, M. ANTONIOU, M. VIDAL, F. GROSVELD & D.R. GREAVES. 1989. A dominant control region from the human ß-globin locus conferring integration site-independent gene expression. Nature **338:** 352–355.
58. VAN ASSENDELFT, G.B., O. HANSCOMBE, F. GROSVELD & R. GREAVES. 1989. The β-globin dominant control region activates homologous and heterologous promoters in a tissue-specific manner. Cell **56:** 969–977.
59. LI, Q. & G. STAMATOYANNOPOULOS. 1994. Hypersensitive site 5 of the human β locus control region funtions as a chromatin insulator. Blood **84:** 1399–1401.
60. ZAFARANA, G., S. RAGUZ, S. PRUZINA, F. GROSVELD & D. MEIJER. 1994. The regulation of human β-globin gene expression: The analysis of hypersensitive site 5 (HS%) in the LCR. *In* Molecular Biology of Hemoglobin Switching. Vol. 1. G. Stamatoyannopoulos, Ed.: 39–44. Intercept Limited. Andover, United Kingdom.
61. REITMAN, M. & G. FELSENFELD. 1990. Developmental regulation of topoisomerase II sites and DNase I-hypersensitive sites in the chicken β-globin locus. Mol. Cell. Biol. **10:** 2774–2786.
62. CHUNG, J.H., M. WHITELEY & G. FELSENFELD. 1993. A 5' element of the chicken β-globin domain serves as an insultor in human erythroid cells and protects against position effect in *drosophila*. Cell **74:** 505–514.
63. CHENG, L., C. DU, D. MURRAY, X. TONG, Y.A. ZHANG, B.P. CHEN & R.G. HAWLEY. 1997. A GFP reporter system to assess gene transfer and expression in human hematopoietic progenitor cells. Gene Ther. **4:** 1013–1022.
64. BODINE, D.M., K.T. MCDONAGH, S.J. BRANDT, P.A. NEY, B. AGRICOLA, E. BYRNE & A.W. NIENHUIS. 1990. Development of a high-titer retrovirus producer cell line capable of gene transfer into rhesus monkey hematopoietic stem cells. Proc. Natl. Acad. Sci. USA **87:** 3738–3742.

DISCUSSION

H.E. BROXMEYER (*Indiana University*): I thought that one of the problems with the use of adenoviruses as vectors was a heavy immune response. If you use an adeno-AAV vector, do you anticipate there are going to be problems with that? Also will immune responses block the capacity of these new vectors to work in a gene therapy setting?

STAMATOYANNOPOULOS: As far as the immune response to products of the viral genes is concerned, there will be none, because there are no viral genes in the deleted adeno-AAV vectors. All the genes have been deleted. As for an immune response against the capsid proteins, yes, there will be such a response. However, you should proceed under the assumption that you will transduce only once; you will transduce all the stem cells, and therefore you will not need to transduce again. If the vectors become, for the hematopoietic stem cell, as efficient as they are in the liver, you will not need to repeat the transduction again and again. You will be able to infect all your cells with just one manipulation and to have the AAV vector integrating into the stem cell. So if Andre Lieber, who is a terrifc scientist and probably one the best we have in our center, succeeds in producing deleted adeno-AAV vectors with stem cell tropism, I think the vectors will be used very efficiently for stem cell transduction.

D.M. BODINE (*National Human Genome Research Institute/NIH*): Is the chicken HS4 erythroid specific in your assays? I think you will say no, because you are seeing it in granulocyte/macrophage-colony forming units (CFU-GM). Have you looked at that?

STAMATOYANNOPOULOS: I think that the chicken HS4 is erythroid specific, but I am not sure. Probably it is a boundary. This is the beauty of this sequence, because the chromatin is DNAse-1 sensitive downstream, and it is totally resistent upstream. I cannot answer the question whether HS-4 or the retroviral vector is erythroid lineage specific or not. (*Note added in proof*: My answer to Dr. Bodine should have been that HS4 is not erythroid specific, because it works as an insulator in *Drosophila*.)

Retroviral-Fibronectin Interactions in Transduction of Mammalian Cells

DAVID A. WILLIAMS[a]

Section of Pediatric Hematology/Oncology, Herman B Wells Center for Pediatric Research, Riley Hospital for Children, Howard Hughes Medical Institute, Indiana University School of Medicine, 1044 W. Walnut Street -R4 402, Indianapolis, Indiana 46202, USA

ABSTRACT: Hematopoiesis occurs in a complex environment in the medullary cavity in close proximity to stromal cells, fibroblasts, endothelial cells and matrix molecules. Hematopoietic cell interactions in this environment appear to involve both integrin and proteoglycan-mediated cell-cell and cell-matrix interactions. Genetic transduction of hematopoietic cells via retroviral vectors has been hampered by low efficiency of gene transfer. Recently, hematopoietic stem cell adhesion to the extracellular matrix molecule fibronectin has been shown to increase transduction of these target cells using retrovirus vectors. The mechanism of increased transduction appears to involve colocalization of virus particles and target cells. These data are reviewed in this paper.

Hematopoiesis occurs in a complex hematopoietic microenvironment made up of endothelial cells, fibroblasts, macrophages and matrix proteins.[1] Hematopoietic cell adhesion in this environment is mediated via several cell-cell and cell-matrix interactions, which can involve both integrin- and proteoglycan-mediated processes. Primitive hematopoietic stem cells capable on long-term reconstitution *in vivo* adhere to the extracellular matrix molecule fibronectin (FN) via the integrins very late antigen (VLA)-4[2–4] and VLA-5,[4a] and also via cell surface proteoglycans.[5] Sequences mediating adhesion via VLA-5 are located in the central cell binding domain of fibronectin, while VLA-4 interacts with a sequence termed connecting segment-1 (CS-1) expressed via an alternative spliced mRNA of fibronectin. Cell surface proteoglycans are known to interact with heparin binding domains located in type III repeats 12–14 (FIG. 1).

Genetic transduction of more primitive hematopoietic stem cells of large animals via retroviral vectors has previously been inefficient, limiting the application of gene transfer methods to therapeutic trials.[6] Inefficient transduction of these cells is likely due to multiple properties of hematopoietic stem cells, including the presence of a large number of these cells in quiescent state, a low density of receptors for the binding of retroviruses and the inability to manipulate stem cells *in vitro* for prolonged periods of time without loss of repopulating capacity. In this regard, new approaches to gene transfer into hematopoietic stem cells of large animals have included: 1) the use of different viral pseudotypes in an effort to utilize viruses with increased recep-

[a]Phone, 317/274-8960; fax, 317/274-8679; e-mail, dwilliam@iupui.edu

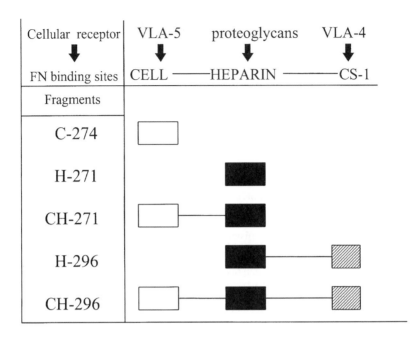

FIGURE 1. Composition of recombinant FN fragments derived from sequences located within the A chain of FN. The binding sites for the integrins VLA-5 and VLA-4 are marked as CELL and CS-1, respectively. The CS-1 site is composed of the first 25 amino acids of the alternatively spliced IIICS region. The binding site for proteoglycans is marked as HEPARIN for the heparin-binding domain spanning the type III repeats 12–14 (III 12–14).

tor density on the target cells; 2) the use of viruses that do not require cell division for integration; 3) the use of *in vivo* selection methods to select and amplify a small population of transduced cells; 4) methods to increase the level of viral receptor expression on target cells; and 5) methods to improve ex vivo manipulation of cells and/or modify virus/cell interactions.

Previous work by Moore *et al.*[7] and by Nolta *et al.*[8] has shown increased gene transfer into hematopoietic cells adherent to bone marrow-derived stromal cells, although the mechanism of this increased transduction is unclear. In other cell systems, integrin-mediated inside-out signaling has been shown to affect the proliferation of cells. Since our laboratory[2] and other investigators[3,4] have demonstrated expression of integrins on primitive hematopoietic cells, we have examined the effect of the adhesion of hematopoietic and other cells to fibronectin on gene transfer efficiency. Human CD34+ bone marrow or peripheral blood cells adhere to fibronectin fragments that contain the central cell binding domain, CS-1, and type III repeats 12–14 called CH-296 (FIG. 1). Infection of cells adherent to this fragment increases transduction 4–5-fold compared to nonadherent cells.[9] This increase in transduction requires prestimulation with cytokines, apparently to increase the number of cells in cycle, but also to increase the binding of the target cells to CH-296. By using this method, transduction of $CD34^+$ bone marrow cell-derived colony-forming units (CFU) reaches 80%, while transduction of granulocyte colony-stimulating factor mobilized peripheral blood CD34-derived progenitors is as high as 70%.[10] More primitive $CD34^+$, $CD38^-$ cells, a fraction believed to contain long-term repopulating cells, is transduced at a frequency of 10–15%, based on CFU analysis.

Although these assays demonstrate a significant improvement in transduction of progenitor and primitive cell populations analyzed *in vitro*, a more difficult target population for retroviral infection and integration is the *in vivo* repopulating cell. To analyze transduction of cells in this hematopoietic compartment, bone marrow cells derived from 5-fluorouracil-treated mice were either cocultivated directly on retroviral producer cell lines, infected with supernatant virus in the absence of producer cells or infected with supernatant after the target cells were adhered to the carboxy-terminal fragment of fibronectin containing the CS-1 sequence and the type III repeats 12–14. The vector used, phosphoglycerate kinase–human adenosine deaminase (PGK-hADA), expresses the hADA cDNA via the phosphoglycerate kinase promoter.[11] Expression of the hADA transgene can be detected by *in situ* gel analysis and the level of expression compared to endogenous murine ADA expression. Infected cells were harvested and infused into lethally irradiated mice. One year after transplantation, no expression of hADA was detectable in mice transplanted with cells infected with supernatant alone. In contrast, expression of hADA was easily detectable in mice transplanted with cells infected either by cocultivation or by the use of supernatant on FN-adherent cells.[12] Thus these studies demonstrate that efficient infection of long lived stem cells is possible in the presence of FN without the need for cocultivation. Recently, Keim *et al.*[13] extended these studies and demonstrated that FN is superior to cocultivation in the transduction of primate repopulating cells.

In addition to a FN fragment containing the CS-1 sequence and type III repeats, we also utilized recombinant FN fragments that contain combinations of all three cell binding domains. Surprisingly, we found that transduction of murine stem cells was facilitated on a fragment, CH-271, containing only the cell binding domain and type III repeats, but not on a fragment, H-271, containing the type III repeats.[14] These data, along with our previous data showing that colocalization of target cells and virus is the mechanism by which FN facilitates gene transfer, suggested that repopulating murine stem cells adhere to the cell binding domain of FN. Such binding has not previously been demonstrated for reconstituting stem cell populations. Adhesion assays were performed using recombinant FN fragments with either murine bone marrow or granulocyte colony-stimulating factor (G-CSF) mobilized peripheral blood cells. Analysis of adherent cells populations included colony-forming unit (CFU) and nonobese diabetic/severe combined immunodeficiency (NOD/SCID) engraftment assays (human) and high proliferative potential–colony-forming cells (HPP-CFC) and competitive long-term repopulation assays (mouse). Data from these experiments demonstrate that both CFU and HPP-CFC largely adhere to the type III repeats in combination with CS-1, as previously demonstrated for murine and human cells. Surprisingly, however, a population of NOD/SCID engrafting human cells and long-term repopulating murine cells adhere to the cell binding domain. This adhesion was specific and via VLA-5, since inhibition of adhesion could be demonstrated with anti-VLA-5 monoclonal antibodies.[4a]

Additional studies in both CD34[+] primary cells and hematopoietic cell lines show that transduction of cell targets on FN is not affected by the apparent multiplicity of infection (titer of virus: cell number) over several logs. This result, and the ability to pre-incubate virus on FN, increasing the apparent titer subsequently presented to the target cells ('pre-loading') suggests that saturation of the retroviral receptor while using FN is possible. In addition, specific targeting of cells within a mixed population may also be possible by exploiting unique cell surface receptors present on the target cell and utilizing chimeric FN fragments containing both retoviral binding sequences and cell-specific ligands. These applications are currently being investigated in our laboratory. For instance, cells that express VLA-4 but not VLA-5 are transduced when CS-1, but not the cell binding domain is present in on the FN molecule; while cells expressing VLA-5 but not VLA-4 are transduced on FN containing the cell binding domain but not CS-1.[14] Finally, incubation of primary T lymphocytes with antibodies to CD3 and CD28 increases the adhesion of these cells to both VLA-5 and VLA-4. By utilizing a FN fragment that contains both ligands (CH-296), up to 90% of primary T cells can be transduced, eliminating the need for selection.[15]

Since adhesion via integrins may affect cell cycle progression, or the position in cell cycle may affect adhesion, the interaction of stem cells with FN during retroviral infection requires further analysis to investigate the affects of adhesion on stem cell survival and repopulating capacity. However, the data presented here demonstrate highly efficient transduction of human and murine hematopoietic cells, routinely yielding transduction efficiencies of 50–70%, and eliminating the use of cocultivation, polycations and extended exposure to growth factors and stroma. The use of recombinant FN is currently being studied in human Phase I trials.

REFERENCES

1. YODER, M.C. & D.A. WILLIAMS. 1995. Matrix molecule interactions with hematopoietic stem cells. Exp. Hematol. **23:** 961–967.
2. WILLIAMS, D.A., M. RIOS, C. STEPHENS & V. PATEL. 1991. Fibronectin and VLA-4 in haematopoietic stem cell–microenvironment interactions. Nature **352:** 438–441.
3. VERFAILLIE, C.M., J.B. MCCARTHY & P.B. MCGLAVE. 1991. Differentiation of primitive human nultipotent hematopoietic progenitors is accompanied by alterations in their interaction with fibronectin. J. Exp. Med. **174:** 693–703.
4. PAPAYANNOPOULOU, T. & B. NAKAMOTO. 1993. Peripheralization of hematopoietic progenitors in primates treated with anti-VLAÃ Ã4Ã Ä integrin. Proc. Natl. Acad. Sci. USA **90:** 9374–9378.
4a. VAN DER LOO, J.C., X. XIAO, D. MCMILLIN, K. HASHINO, I. KATO & D.A. WILLIAMS. 1998. VLA-5 is expressed by mouse and human long-term repopulating hematopoietic cells and mediates adhesion to extracellular matrix protein fibronectin. J. Clin. Invest. **102:** 1051–1061.
5. MINGUELL, J.J., C. HARDY & M. TAVASSOLI. 1992. Membrane associated chondroitin sulfate proteoglycan and fibronectin mediate the binding of hemopoietic progenitor cells to stromal cells. Exp. Cell Res. **201:** 200–207.
6. MORITZ, T. & D.A. WILLIAMS. 1994. Somatic gene therapy. In Scientific Basis of Transfusion Medicine. K. Anderson, Ed.: 872–888. Churchill Livingstone. Philadelphia.
7. MOORE, K.A., A.B. DEISSEROTH, C.L. READING, D.E. WILLIAMS & J.W. BELMONT. 1992. Stromal support enhances cell-free retroviral vector transduction of human bone marrow long-term culture-initiating cells. Blood **79:** 1393–1399.

8. NOLTA, J.A., E.M. SMOGORZEWSKA & D.B. KOHN. 1995. Analysis of optimal conditions for retroviral-mediated transduction of primitive human hematopoietic cells. Blood **86:** 101–110.

9. MORITZ, T., V.P. PATEL & D.A. WILLIAMS. 1994. Bone marrow extracelolular matrix molecules improve gene transfer into human hematopoietic cells via retroviral vectors. J. Clin. Invest. **93:** 1451–1457.

10. HANENBERG, H., K. HASHINO, H. KONISHI, R.A. HOCK, I. KATO & D.A. WILLIAMS. 1997. Optimization of fibronectin-assisted retroviral gene transfer into human CD34+ hematopoietic cells. Hum. Gene Ther. **8:** 2193–2206.

11. LIM, B., D.A. WILLIAMS & S. H. ORKIN. 1987. Retrovirus-mediated gene transfer of human adenosine deaminase: Expression of functional enzyme in murine hematopoietic stem cells *in vivo*. Mol. Cell. Biol. **7:** 3459–3465.

12. MORITZ, T., P. DUTT, X.L. XIAO, D. CARSTANJEN, T. VIK, H. HANENBERG & D.A. WILLIAMS. 1996. Fibronectin improves transduction of reconstituting hematopoietic stem cells by retroviral vectors: evidence of direct viral binding to chymotryptic carboxy-terminal fragments. Blood **88:** 855–862.

13. KIEM, H.P., J. MORRIS, S. HEYWARD, L. PETERSON, J. POTTER, A.D. MILLER & R. G. ANDREWS. 1997. Gene transfer into baboon hematopoietic repopulating cells using recombinant human fibronectin fragment CH-296. Blood **90**(Suppl.): 236a.

14. HANENBERG, H., X.L. XIAO, D. DILLOO, K. HASHINO, I. KATO & D.A. WILLIAMS. 1996. Colocalization of retrovirus and target cells on specific fibronectin fragments increases genetic transduction of mammalian cells. Nat. Med. **2**(8): 876–882.

15. POLLOK, K.E., H. HANENBERG, T.W. NOBLITT, W.L. SCHROEDER, I. KATO, D. EMANUEL & D.A. WILLIAMS. 1998. High-efficiency gene transfer into normal and adenosine deaminase-deficient T-lymphocytes is mediated by transduction on recombinant fibronectin fragments. J. Virol. **72:** 4882–4892.

DISCUSSION

G. KELLER (*Howard Hughes Medical Institute*): Does binding to fibronectin induce a signal in the cell?

WILLIAMS: We cannot answer that directly yet. That is what Gillian Bradford, who joined the laboratory from Ivan Bertincello's group, is examining. But based on other cell systems, that is what you would hypothesize. Binding of the integrin itself probably sends a signal that relates to differentiation and proliferation, but probably the binding actually colocalizes signaling molecules related to growth factor receptors. Therefore, one would hypothesize that this probably is an important and complex system by which the cell amplifies signals from growth factors. That is clearly where we are fucusing our studies right now. We have some evidence that this is an important interaction. If one takes cells in the murine system, Sca$^+$Lin$^-$ cells, and incubates them *in vitro* either on or off fibronectin and very low concentrations of growth factor, i.e., not the concentrations you normally would use to do progenitor assays, and then tests to see how long the reconstituting cells survive, it is clear that with cells adherent to fibronectin, survival is maintained for prolonged periods *in vitro* versus nonadherent cells. That is the key observation in our laboratory that tells us that this is an important aspect of biology to look at.

T. PAPAYANNOPOULOU (*University of Washington*): Does the CH-296 induce mobilization of stem/progenitor cells into the blood?

WILLIAMS: We looked at the spleen, but we have not looked at the blood. We decided to look at the spleen of these animals. CH-296 injected *in vivo* does perturb hematopoiesis in the spleen, increasing the number of CFUs contained within the spleen.

Amphotropic Retrovirus Transduction of Hematopoietic Stem Cells

DONALD ORLIC,[a,c] LAURIE J. GIRARD,[a] STACIE M. ANDERSON,[a] STEPHANE BARRETTE,[a] HAL E. BROXMEYER,[b] AND DAVID M. BODINE[a]

[a]Hematopoiesis Section, Genetics and Molecular Biology Branch, National Human Genome Research Institute, NIH, Bethesda, Maryland, USA

[b]Departments of Microbiology/Immunology and Medicine, and the Walther Oncology Center, Indiana University School of Medicine, Indianapolis, Indiana, USA

ABSTRACT: Mice treated with cytokines for 5 days have large numbers of hematopoietic stem cells (HSCs) in their peripheral blood and bone marrow at 1 and 14 days after the last injection. We fractionated the HSCs from the bone marrow of these mice using elutriation at flow rates of 25, 30 and 35 ml/min. The subpopulations of HSCs from cytokine-treated mice show a 3- to 8-fold higher level of mRNA encoding the amphotropic retrovirus receptor (amphoR) compared with the corresponding HSC subpopulation from untreated mouse bone marrow. In an earlier study with mouse HSCs we showed a direct correlation between high levels of amphoR mRNA and efficient retrovirus transduction. We have now utilized our gene transfer protocol to assay amphotropic retrovirus transduction efficiency using HSCs from the bone marrow of mice treated with granulocyte-colony stimulating factor/stem cell factor (G-CSF/SCF). To extend these findings to a more clinically relevant protocol we analyzed the amphoR mRNA levels in HSCs from human cord blood and adult bone marrow. The amphoR mRNA level in HSCs from human bone marrow and fresh cord blood was detectable at an extremely low level compared with the HSC population in cryopreserved cord blood samples. The 12- to 22-fold increase in amphoR mRNA in HSCs from cryopreserved cord blood renders these HSCs likely candidates for high efficiency, gene transfer.

INTRODUCTION

Hematopoietic stem cells (HSCs) have the capacity to self-renew and to differentiate into all blood cell lineages. HSCs are present in bone marrow at a frequency of 1/10,000 to 1/100,000 cells. This rare population of HSCs can be enriched 1,000-fold with purification procedures that utilize monoclonal antibodies to subtract specific blood cell lineages and flow cytometry for positive selection based on expression of specific HSC surface markers.[1,2] HSCs are desirable target cells for gene therapy because a therapeutic gene integrated into the genome of a HSC will be transferred to all HSC-derived progeny, and the correction should be permanent. However, human clinical trials have not achieved major progress largely because HSCs appear to be highly refractory to retrovirus transduction.

Retrovirus binding to target cells followed by cell division are two factors recognized to be important for retrovirus transduction (FIG. 1). Each of the currently used retroviruses has its host range determined by its envelope protein.[3–6] Ecotropic retroviruses bind to an amino acid transport protein on mouse bone marrow cells. Al-

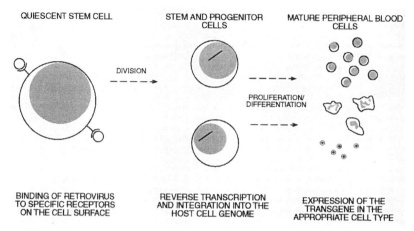

FIGURE 1. Each of the commonly used retroviruses, including ecotropic, amphotropic and gibbon ape leukemia virus, recognizes a specific protein on the surface of its target cell. After binding to its specific receptor the vector enters the cell and the RNA genome is converted to cDNA. Transduction of a quiescent hematopoietic stem cell requires that the cell undergo cell division during which the reverse transcribed viral cDNA integrates into the host cell's DNA. Self-renewal of transduced stem cells will assure a continued presence of the provirus in this primitive cell population. Differentiation of stem/progenitor cells should result in all mature blood cells carrying the therapeutic gene. If expression of the transgene can be regulated so that expression occurs only in the appropriate cell type, this would result in a highly desirable outcome for gene therapy.

though ecotropic retroviruses transduce mouse HSCs with an efficiency approaching 40%, they are murine specific and cannot transduce human HSCs. In contrast, amphotropic retroviruses utilize a phosphate transport protein present on cells of many species, and they can transduce HSCs across species barriers. However, their transduction efficiency is less than 1% when cocultured with mouse, monkey or human bone marrow HSCs. Based on the differences between ecotropic and amphotropic retrovirus transduction efficiencies, we propose that the number of amphotropic retrovirus receptors (amphoRs) is low and that this may be the primary block to transduction using this vector. We have tested this hypothesis by comparing the level of mRNA encoding the amphoR with transduction efficiency in several fractionated subpopulations of HSCs from untreated and cytokine-treated mice and HSCs from human bone marrow.

RETROVIRUS TRANSDUCTION OF HETEROGENEOUS POPULATIONS OF MURINE HEMATOPOIETIC STEM CELLS.

Long-term repopulating stem cells in mouse bone marrow can be isolated on the basis of size by counterflow centrifugal elutriation[7,8] using flow rates (FR) of 25, 30 and 35 ml/min, followed by lineage subtraction (Lin$^-$) and fluorescence-activated cell sorting (FACS) based on high c-kit (c-kit^{High}) expression.[9] The small FR25 Lin$^-$ c-kit^{High}, intermediate FR30 Lin$^-$ c-kit^{High} and large FR35 Lin$^-$ c-kit^{High} stem cells

TABLE 1. RT-PCR analysis of amphoR mRNA levels in HSCs from bone marrow from untreated and cytokine-treated mice[a]

	Unfr. BM	FR25 Lin⁻ c-kit^High	FR30 Lin⁻ c-kit^High	FR35 Lin⁻ c-kit^High	NIH-3T3
Untreated BM	0.49 ± 0.12^b	0.05 ± 0.04	0.12 ± 0.04	0.14 ± 0.02	1.0
G-CSF/ SCF Treated	0.86 ± 0.23	0.39 ± 0.37	0.30 ± 0.20	0.39 ± 0.06	1.0

[a]Unfractionated bone marrow (Unfr. BM) and bone marrow elutriated at flow rates (FR) of 25, 30 and 35 ml/min, lineage subtracted (Lin⁻) and sorted by flow cytometry based high c-kit (c-kit^High) expression. Bone marrow was assayed 14 days after the last cytokine injection.

[b]Mean + SD. All values were normalized to the receptor mRNA level in NIH- 3T3 cells.

were assayed by reverse transcriptase–polymerase chain reaction (RT-PCR) for ecotropic receptor (ecoR) mRNA levels. Each of these three stem cell-enriched populations showed a high level of ecoR mRNA when their values were normalized relative to the level in the positive control NIH-3T3 cells (TABLE 1). In contrast, the amphotropic receptor (amphoR) mRNA level was nearly undetectable in FR25 Lin⁻ c-kit^High cells but somewhat higher in both FR30 Lin⁻ c-kit^High and FR35 Lin⁻ c-kit^High HSC populations (TABLE 1). Each of these several HSC populations showed lower levels of amphoR mRNA than any of 4 independent isolates of unfractionated bone marrow. Since unfractionated bone marrow consists of 95% to 98% Lin⁺ cells, it seems likely that most of the amphoR mRNA in unfractionated bone marrow is present in the Lin⁺ cells.

In order to obtain stem cells with higher levels of amphoR mRNA, splenectomized mice were injected daily for 5 days with granulocyte-colony stimulating factor (G-CSF) and stem cell factor (SCF).[10] At 14 days after the last injection, bone marrow was harvested, and the three c-kit^High stem cell-enriched populations were purified. Each population showed a significant increase in the level of amphoR mRNA compared with the corresponding HSC population found in untreated bone marrow. The most remarkable increase was observed in the FR25 Lin⁻ c-kit^High population, which is highly enriched for HSCs and largely devoid of comtaminating progenitor cells. This population showed an 8-fold increase in amphoR mRNA compared with the level found in the corresponding HSC fraction in untreated adult mice (TABLE 1).

In order to relate amphoR mRNA levels to receptor formation and retrovirus-transduction, we established the following protocol. Enriched HSC populations purified as indicated above were exposed for 96 hours to supernatant containing equivalent titers of ecotropic (Ψ-CRE MFG-lacZ) and amphotropic (Ψ-CRIP MFG-NLSlacZ) retroviruses and interleukin-3 (IL-3), IL-6 and SCF. The two retroviral sequences differed by a 21 base pair nuclear localizing sequence (NLS) in the amphotropic retrovirus genome. After transduction, the cells were injected into a lateral tail vein of young adult female *W/W^v* recipients. At 16 weeks posttransplant, peripheral blood cells were harvested and their DNA purified and analyzed by PCR for proviral integration. We used a primer pair that recognized a sequence in the lacZ gene and a sequence in the proviral backbone.[11] The PCR-amplified amphotropic fragment spanned the NLS sequence and was resolved as a 310-nucleotide fragment 21 nucleotides larger than the amplified ecotropic proviral fragment. The combined results of two separate transduction experiments indicated that the efficiency of ecotropic and amphotropic retroviruses was directly related to the levels of ecoR and amphoR mRNA in each subpopulation of stem cells. Only I of 13 W/W^v recipients of transduced FR25 Lin⁻ c-kit^High HSCs was positive for amphotropic provirus, whereas 6 of 11 recipients of FR35 Lin⁻ c-kit^High HSCs were positive for amphotropic provirus. The transduction efficiency of these two HSC populations correlated closely with their level of amphoR mRNA. Our results agree with the findings of others that suggest that inefficient amphotropic retrovirus gene transfer into murine hematopoietic stem cells and fetal liver cells may be related to low levels of amphoR mRNA.[12,13]

Although these studies were designed to identify HSC populations that could be efficiently transduced by amphotropic retroviruses, the simultaneous exposure to ecotropic retroviruses enabled us to monitor the transduction efficiency of both vec-

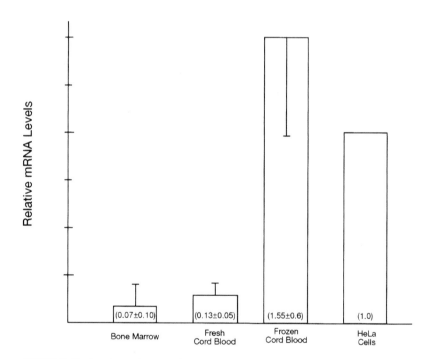

FIGURE 2. Amphotropic retrovirus receptor mRNA levels in human HSC-enriched Lin⁻ CD34⁺ CD38⁻ populations. The level of receptor mRNA in each cell population was determined by comparing the cell's receptor mRNA level with the level of β2-microglobulin mRNA, a constitutively expressed gene in all cell populations. The receptor mRNA level in HeLa cells, which are efficiently transduced by amphotropic retroviruses, was adjusted to 100% (1.0) and the other receptor mRNA values were normalized to the mRNA level in HeLa cells. The high level of receptor mRNA in the HSC from cryopreserved cord blood was significantly higher than the level in the HSC form normal bone marrow and fresh cord blood.

tors. Nearly all recipients (22 of 24) of transduced FR25 and FR35 Lin$^-$ c-kit^{High} HSCs were marked with the ecotropic provirus. This high level of transduction efficiency suggested that the HSCs were cycling at the time of exposure to the combined retrovirus supernatants. Based on these results, we propose that the low efficiency of amphotropic retrovirus transduction of stem cells compared with ecotropic retrovirus transduction is not a result of noncycling in the HSC population, but rather is a consequence of the low level of expression of amphoR mRNA and subsequent low numbers of amphotropic retrovirus receptors.

ANALYSIS OF RETROVIRUS RECEPTOR mRNA EXPRESSION IN HUMAN HSCs FROM BONE MARROW

Expression of retrovirus receptor mRNAs was analyzed in two populations of human primitive hematopoietic cells. Bone marrow cells coexpressing the CD34 and CD38 antigens (CD34$^+$ CD38$^+$) are enriched for progenitor cells, while CD34$^+$ CD38$^-$ cells are enriched for more primitive cells.[14,15] mRNA of the human homologue of the ecotropic retrovirus receptor was expressed at high levels in CD34$^+$ CD38$^+$ cells and at low but detectable levels in CD34$^+$ CD38$^-$ cells. Although mRNA encoding this amino acid transporter protein was assayed by us, it should be noted that it does not serve as a receptor for the ecotropic retrovirus on human cells due to changes in the virus binding site. mRNA encoding the phosphate transport protein, which is a functional amphoR in human cells, is expressed in CD34$^+$ CD38$^+$ cells. However, the amphoR mRNA level in the HSC-enriched CD34$^+$ CD38$^-$ population was present at only 7% of the level observed in the positive control HeLa cells (FIG. 2). This pattern was similar to the pattern of expression seen in mouse FR25 Lin$^-$ c-kit^{High} HSCs.

ANALYSIS OF RETROVIRUS RECEPTOR mRNA EXPRESSION IN HUMAN HSCs FROM CORD BLOOD

HSCs in human cord blood have been transduced in a gene therapy protocol with amphotropic retroviruses carrying the adenosine deaminase cDNA but at less than 1% efficiency.[16] In our efforts to isolate subpopulations of HSCs with high levels of amphoR mRNA we used flow cytometry to enrich for Lin$^-$ CD34$^+$ CD38$^-$ cells from fresh and frozen cord blood. The HSC population in fresh cord blood contained 13% of the level of amphoR mRNA present in HeLa cells and was not significantly higher than the level observed in HSCs from fresh bone marrow. In contrast, the HSC-enriched Lin$^-$ CD34$^+$ CD38$^-$ population in cryopreserved cord blood had 22-fold more amphoR mRNA compared with the HSC population in fresh bone marrow and 12-fold higher levels of amphoR mRNA compared with the same cell fraction in fresh cord blood samples. Furthermore, this population of cord blood HSCs had a 1.5-fold higher level of amphoR mRNA than the positive control HeLa cells. We conclude that the freeze/thaw cycle or exposure to one or more components of the freezing media induced this high level of mRNA expression in cord blood HSCs. The increased expression found in cryopreserved cord blood cells may be related to exposure to dimethyl sulfoxide (DMSO), and we are currently investigating the possible effects of DMSO on HSCs maintained in standard culture media.

AMPHOTROPIC RETROVIRUS BINDING ASSAY

This assay involved amphotropic retrovirus binding to target cells followed by monoclonal antibody staining as described previously by others[17,18] and by us.[19,20]

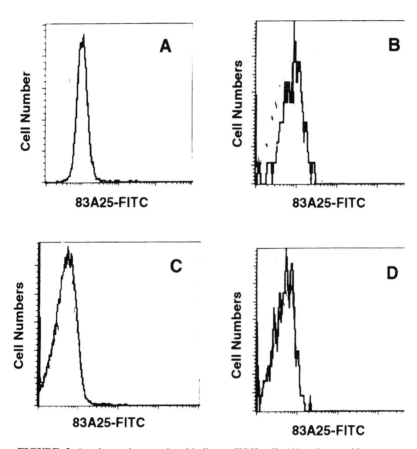

FIGURE 3. Amphotropic retrovirus binding to K562 cells (**A**) and normal bone marrow cells which were sorted into three populations based on CD38 expression (**B, C and D**). The cells were cultured in supernatant containing retrovirus for 40 minutes at 37°C, followed by staining with the mAb 83A25-FITC, which is specific for the viral envelope protein gp70. The *thin gray trace* represents background levels on cells exposed to the retrovirus and non-specific isotype-FITC antibody. The *thick black trace* represents retrovirus binding on this cell population. Substantial retrovirus binding was always observed in the positive control K562 cells. The highest level of retrovirus binding to bone marrow cells occurred in the Lin⁻ CD34⁺ CD38^{High} population (B) with undetectable levels of binding in cells of the phenotypes Lin⁻ CD34⁺ CD38$^{Intermediate/Low}$ and Lin⁻ CD34⁺ CD38^{Negative}.

Briefly, K562 cells, which have a high transduction efficiency, were used as a positive control. Enriched populations of CD34$^+$ cells were obtained from bone marrow of untreated normal adults (Poietic Technologies, Inc., Gaithersburg, MD). Cells were incubated at a concentration of 1 X 10^6/ml at 37°C for 40 minutes with supernatant from the A721 MFG-NLSlacZ producer cell line. The cells were collected and washed with 10% rat serum in phosphate-buffered saline (PBS). They were then incubated with fluorescein isothiocyanate (FITC)-conjugated 83A25, a rat monoclonal antibody (mAb) specific for the virus envelope protein gp70, at 4°C for 30 minutes. The K562 cells were then analyzed by flow cytometry using a FACStar instument (Becton-Dickinson, San Jose, CA). The bone marrow cells were further stained with anti-CD34-Cy5PE and anti-CD38-PE mAbs (Becton-Dickinson, San Jose, Ca). Controls consisted of cells incubated with FITC-conjugated rat isotype antibodies. Finally, the CD34$^+$ (Cy5PE$^+$) cells were fractionated into CD38^{High} (highest 2%), CD38$^{Intermediate/Low}$ and CD38^{Negative} (lowest 2%) fractions and each fraction was analyzed for virus binding (FITC$^+$).

The bone marrow hematopoietic cell populations were not able to bind amphotropic retrovirus at the high level obtained with the positive control K562 cells (Fɪɢ. 3). Of the three bone marrow populations, the progenitor-enriched Lin$^-$ CD34$^+$ CD38^{High} cells showed the highest capacity for binding amphotropic retrovirus. The pattern of virus binding displayed by the Lin$^-$ CD34$^+$ CD38^{High} cells occurred within a normal distribution. No retrovirus binding was observed in Lin$^-$ CD34$^+$ CD38$^{Intermediate/Low}$ and Lin$^-$ CD34$^+$ CD38^{Negative} bone marrow cells.

In summary, we have shown that it is possible to isolate subpopulations of HSCs from bone marrow of cytokine-treated mice that express high levels of amphoR mRNA and are efficiently transduced by amphotropic retrovirus vectors. Based on these findings we plan to extend our studies to include analysis of human HSCs in peripheral blood and bone marrow of individuals treated with cytokines such as G-CSF. If populations of human HSCs expressing higher levels of amphoR mRNA can be isolated and efficiently transduced by amphotropic retroviruses, this may be of benefit for gene therapy protocols. We will also assay retroviral transduction of human HSCs in cryopreserved cord blood, which have the highest level of amphoR mRNA of all human HSC populations assayed by us to date. Clinical trials indicate that cytokine-mobilized peripheral blood HSCs and cord blood HSCs are both effective in transplant recipients, and both have been identified as likely candidates for efficient gene transfer using retroviral vectors.[21–25]

ACKNOWLEDGMENTS

This work was supported in part by NIH Grants RO1 HL 54037 and RO1 HL 46416, and by a project in NIH Grant PO1 HL 53586 (to H.E.B.).

REFERENCES

1. Sᴘᴀɴɢʀᴜᴅᴇ, G.J., S. Hᴇɪᴍғᴇʟᴅ & I.L. Wᴇɪssᴍᴀɴ. 1988. Purification and characterization of mouse hematopoietic stem cell. Science **241:** 58–62.

2. OGAWA, M., Y. MATSUZAKI, S. NISHIKAWA, S-I. HAYASHI, T. KUNISADA, T. SUDO, T. KINA, H. NAKAUCHI & S-I. NISHIKAWA. 1991. Expression and function of c-kit in hemopoietic progenitor cells. J. Exp. Med. **174:** 63–71.

3. O'HARA, B., S.V. JOHANN, H.P. KLINGER, D.G. BLAIR, H. RUBINSON, K.J. DUNN, P. SASS, S.M. VITEK & T. ROBINS. 1990. Characterization of a human gene conferring sensitivity to infection by gibbon ape leukemia virus. Cell. Growth Differ. **1:** 119–127.

4. MILLER, D.G., R.H. EDWARDS & A.D. MILLER. 1994. Cloning of the cellular receptor for amphotropic murine retroviruses reveals homology to that for gibbon ape leukemia virus. Proc. Natl. Acad. Sci. USA **91:** 78–82.

5. VAN ZEIJL, M., S.V. JOHANN, E. CLOSS, J. CUNNINGHAM, R. EDDY, T.B. SHOWS & B. O'HARA. 1994. A human amphotropic retrovirus receptor is a second member of the gibbon ape leukemia virus receptor family. Proc. Natl. Acad. Sci. USA **91:** 1168–1172.

6. KAVANAUGH, M.P, D.G. MILLER, W. ZHANG, W. LAW, S.L. KOZAK, D. KABAT & A.D. MILLER. 1994. Cell-surface receptors for gibbon ape leukemia virus and amphotropic murine retrovirus are inducible sodium-dependent phosphate symporters. Proc. Natl. Acad. Sci. USA **91:** 7071–7075 .

7. JONES, R.J., J.E. WAGNER, P. CELANO, M.S. ZICHA & S.J. SHARKIS. 1990. Separation of pluripotent hematopoietic stem cells from spleen colony-forming cells. Nature **347:** 188–189.

8. ORLIC, D. & D.M. BODINE. 1992. Pluripotent hematopoietic stem cells of low and high density can repopulate W/W^v mice. Exp. Hematol. **20:** 1291–1295.

9. ORLIC, D., R. FISCHER, S-I. NISHIKAWA, A.W. NEINHUIS & D.M. BODINE. 1993. Purification and characterization of heterogeneous pluripotent hematopoietic stem cell populations expressing high levels of c-kit receptor. Blood **82:** 762–770.

10. BODINE, D.M., N.E. SEIDEL & D. ORLIC. 1996. Bone marrow collected 14 days after *in vivo* administration of granulocyte colony-stimulating factor and stem cell factor to mice has 10-fold more repopulating ability than untreated bone marrow. Blood **88:** 89–97.

11. ORLIC, D., L.J. GIRARD, C.T. JORDAN, S.M. ANDERSON, A.P. CLINE & D.M. BODINE. 1996. The level of mRNA encoding the amphotropic retrovirus receptor in mouse and human hematopoietic stem cells is low and correlates with the efficiency of retroviral transduction. Proc. Natl. Acad. Sci. USA **93:** 11097–11102.

12. OSBORNE, W.R.A., R.A. HOCK, M. KALEKO & A.D. MILLER. 1990. Long-term expression of human adenosine deaminase in mice after transplantation of bone marrow infected with amphotropic retroviral vectors. Hum. Gene Ther. **1:** 31–41.

13. Richardson, C. & A. Bank. 1996. Developmental-stage-specific expression and regulation of an amphotropic retroviral receptor in hematopoietic cells. Mol. Cell. Biol. **16:** 4240–4247.

14. TERSTAPPEN, L.W.M.M., S. HUANG, M. SAFFORD, P.M. LANSDORP & M.R. LOKEN. 1991. Sequential generations of hematopoietic colonies derived from single non-lineage-committed CD34+ CD38− progenitor cells. Blood **77:** 1218–1227.

15. BAUM, C.M., I.L. WEISMANN, A.S. TSUKAMOTO, A. BUCKLE & B. PEAULT. 1992. Isolation of a candidate human hematopoietic stem cell population. Proc. Natl. Acad. Sci. USA **89:** 2804–2808.

16. KOHN, D.B., K.I. WEINBERG, J.A. NOLTA, L.N. HEISS, C. LENARSKY, G.M. CROOKS, M.E. HANLEY, G. ANNETT, J.S. BROOKS, A. EL-KHOUREIY, K. LAWRENCE, S. WELLS, R.C. MOEN, J. BASTIAN, D.E. WILLIAMS-HERMAN, M. ELDER, D. WARA, T. BOWEN, M.S. HERSHFIELD, C.A. MULLEN, R.M. BLAESE & R. PARKMAN. 1995. Engraftment of gene-modified umbilical cord blood cells in neonates with adenosine deaminase deficiency. Nature Med. **1:** 1017–1023.

17. KADAN, M.J., S. STURM, W.F. ANDERSON & M.A. EGLITIS. 1992. Detection of receptor murine leukemia virus binding to cells by immunofluorescence analysis. J. Virol. **66:** 2281–2287.

18. CROOKS, G.M. & D.B. KOHN. 1993. Growth factors increase amphotropic retrovirus binding to human CD34+ bone marrow progenitor cells. Blood **82:** 3290–3297.

19. ORLIC, D., L.J. GIRARD, S.M. ANDERSON, L.C. PYLE, M.C. YODER, H.E. BROXMEYER & D.M. BODINE. 1998. Identification of human and mouse hematopoietic stem cell populations expressing high levels of mRNA encoding retrovirus receptors. Blood **91**: 3247–3254.
20. SABATINO, D.E., Q.D. BAO-KHNAH, L.J. GIRARD, L.C. PYLE, C.T. JORDAN, D. ORLIC & D.M. BODINE. 1997. Increased amphotropic and Gibbon ape leukemia virus (GaLV) retrovirus transduction correlates with increased expression of amphotropic and GaLV receptor in cell lines and HL60 cells treated with PMA or interleukin-1a. Blood Cells Mol. Dis. **23**: 422–433.
21. MORITZ, T., D.C. KELLER & D.A. WILLIAMS. 1993. Human cord blood cells as targets for gene transfer: potential use in gene therapies of severe combined immunodeficiency disease. J. Exp. Med. **178**: 529–536.
22. LU, L., M. XIAO, D.W. CLAPP, Z-H. LI & H.E. BROXMEYER. 1993. High efficiency retroviral mediated gene transduction into single isolated immature and replatable CD34[+++] hematopoietic stem/progenitor cells from human umbilical cord blood. J. Exp. Med. **178**: 2089–2096.
23. BODINE, D.M., N.E. SEIDEL, M.S. GALE, A.W. NEINHUIS & D. ORLIC. 1994. Efficient retrovirus transduction of mouse pluripotent hematopoietic stem cells mobilized into the peripheral blood by treatment with granulocyte-colony stimulating factor and stem cell factor. Blood **84**: 1482–1491.
24. DUNBAR, C.E., N.E. SEIDEL, S. DOREN, S. SELLERS, A.P. CLINE, M.E. METZGER, B.A. AGRICOLA, R.E. DONAHUE & D.M. BODINE. 1996. Improved retroviral gene transfer into murine and rhesus peripheral blood or bone marrow repopulating cells primed *in vivo* with stem cell factor and granulocyte colony-stimulating factor. Proc. Natl. Acad. Sci. USA **93**: 11871–11876.
25. WHITWAM, T., N.E. SEIDEL, M.E. HASKINS, S.M. ANDERSON, P.S. HENTHORN, D.M. BODINE & J.M. PUCK. 1996. Marking of canine hematopoietic progenitors in cytokine stimulated bone marrow with retroviruses containing the IL2RG gene. Blood **88**: 275a.

DISCUSSION

G. KELLER (*Howard Hughes Medical Institute*): It seems like Dr. Broxmeyer's freezing medium might be important for upregulation. Have you looked at frozen peripheral blood mobilized cells?

ORLIC: We have not assayed frozen mobilized peripheral blood cells. However, we have recently assayed frozen/thawed murine bone marrow stem cells, but the results are ambiguous.

W.E. FIBBE (*University Medical Center Leiden*): Have you looked at the composition of the cells after thawing them? One of the possible explanations may be that you have selected a population that by itself was already positive. For instance, your CD38[+] cells had significantly higher levels of mRNA. If you have enriched after thawing for these cells, that may explain it.

ORLIC: I think we controlled for that by looking at fresh CD38[−] cells as well as frozen CD38[−] cells. The fresh stem cell mRNA levels matched the low mRNA levels in stem cell populations in untreated bone marrow, so we really do not think that we are dealing with a select population of CD38[−] cells in cord blood. We believe the CD38[−] cells are somehow modified by the freeze/thaw cycle. After thawing, the protocol for staining and sorting requires several hours, during which mRNA expression may occur.

K. WELTE (*Hannover Medical School*): Also following up on this issue. Did you test the cells in the freezing medium containing DMSO before freezing them? If you add the freezing medium to the cells and wash it away and then test the cells without freezing, do you find an increase in receptor mRNA?

ORLIC: We have not done that. However, we have incubated murine stem cells with 1% DMSO. In one instance we found a slight increase in receptor mRNA but the results are not definitive.

R. HOFFMAN (*University of Illinois College of Medicine*): The studies with myelopoietin, a unique receptor agonist molecule, are exciting. Can such effects be recapitulated with *ex vivo* treatment rather than *in vivo* administration to the primates?

ORLIC: We have not done any *in vitro* analyses using myelopoietin.

Effects of Retroviral-Mediated MDR1 Expression on Hematopoietic Stem Cell Self-Renewal and Differentiation in Culture[a]

KEVIN D. BUNTING,[b] JACQUES GALIPEAU,[b] DAVID TOPHAM,[c] ELY BENAIM,[b] AND BRIAN P. SORRENTINO[b,d,e]

[b]Division of Experimental Hematology, [c]Department of Immunology, and [d]Department of Biochemistry, St. Jude Children's Research Hospital, Memphis, Tennessee 38105, USA

ABSTRACT: *Ex vivo* expansion of hematopoietic stem cells would be useful for bone marrow transplantation and gene therapy applications. Toward this goal, we have investigated whether retrovirally-transduced murine stem cells could be expanded in culture with hematopoietic cytokines. Bone marrow cells were transduced with retroviral vectors expressing either the human multidrug resistance 1 gene (HaMDR1), a variant of human dihydrofolate reductase (HaDHFR), or both MDR1 and DHFR in an internal ribosomal entry site (IRES)-containing bicistronic vector (HaMID). Cells were then expanded for 15 days in cultures stimulated with interleukin (IL)-3, IL-6, and stem cell factor. When very low marrow volumes were injected into lethally irradiated recipient mice, long-term reconstitution with 100% donor cells was seen in all mice injected with HaMDR1- or HaMID-transduced cells. By contrast, engraftment with HaDHFR- or mock-transduced cells ranged from partial to undetectable despite injection of significantly larger marrow volumes. In addition, mice transplanted with expanded HaMDR1- or HaMID-transduced stem cells developed a myeloproliferative disorder that was characterized by an increase in abnormal peripheral blood leukocytes. These results show that MDR1-transduced stem cells can be expanded *in vitro* with hematopoietic cytokines, but indicate that an increased stem cell division frequency can lead to stem cell damage.

INTRODUCTION

Hematopoietic stem cells are capable of maintaining multilineage production of mature blood cells over the lifetime of an animal. A single stem cell can thus provide a large number of progeny during hematopoietic maturation and differentiation. Due

[a]Supported in part by National Heart, Lung, and Blood Institute Program Project Grant No. P01 HL 53749, The James S. McDonnell Foundation Grant No. 94-50, US Public Health Service Grant No. P01 CA 31922, Cancer Center Support Grant No. P30 CA 21765, and the American Lebanese Syrian Associated Charities (ALSAC).

[e]Address correspondence to: Brian P. Sorrentino, M.D., Dept. of Biochemistry and Hematology/Oncology, St. Jude Children's Research Hospital, 332 N. Lauderdale, Memphis, TN 38105. Phone, 901/495-2727; fax, 901/495-2176; e-mail: brian.sorrentino@stjude.org

to the low frequency of stem cells in normal bone marrow,[1,2] efforts to isolate enriched stem cell fractions have provided information about the identifying physical characteristics of stem cells. Human stem cells have been identified primarily by cell surface marker expression,[3] functional characteristics,[4,5] and long-term culture initiating cell (LTC-IC) assays.[6] But these *in vitro* assays can be unreliable for quantitating the true human pluripotent hematopoietic stem cell.[7] Development of *in vivo* severe combined immunodeficiency (SCID) mouse repopulating assays has been a significant advance for studying human stem cells.[8–11] The stem cell content of mouse bone marrow can be assayed by either competitive repopulation or limiting dilution analysis in lethally irradiated recipient mice. Due to the advantage that these assays provide for quantitation of stem cell numbers, significant progress has been made in murine stem cell isolation. For example, it has been shown that 1 out of 20 Thy1.1^{low}Sca1$^+$Lin$^-$ purified mouse bone marrow cells are capable of long-term lymphomyeloid reconstitution following transplantation.[12]

Despite a large increase in the understanding of the murine stem cell phenotype, little is known about the mechanisms that regulate hematopoietic stem cell self-renewal divisions. For gene therapy applications, 5-fluorouracil (5-FU) treatment[13,14] followed by interleukin-3 (IL-3), IL-6, and stem cell factor (SCF) culture[15–17] facilitates retroviral gene transfer by stimulating stem cell cycling during a 4-day *ex vivo* manipulation. Screening large numbers of hematopoietic cytokines has also yielded other combinations with modest activity regarding murine stem cell expansion.[18] However, no single cytokine has been identified that is capable of providing a continuous stem cell amplification. Attempts to further amplify stem cells during *ex vivo* cultures greater than 4 days have been unsuccessful. Cytokine-stimulated bone marrow grafts obtain a repopulating defect[9,20] following extended culture times. Stem cells likely either undergo differentiative cell divisions following stimulation[21] or enter apoptotic cell death pathways.[22] As a result, the stem cell content is quantitatively depleted during *ex vivo* culture.

We previously described a novel approach for *in vitro* stem cell amplification that leads to large increases in the number of murine stem cells over a 12-day culture period.[23] Exogenous expression of human MDR1 by retroviral-mediated gene transfer allowed stem cell self-renewal divisions to occur at a remarkable rate, with increases in stem cell content of at least 13-fold over 12 days in culture. The data presented here now extend those results to include another MDR1 vector design in which MDR1 is expressed from a Harvey (Ha) murine sarcoma virus-based bicistronic construct containing a human dihydrofolate reductase variant (HaMID). Mice were transplanted with extremely low donor volumes of either HaMDR1 or HaMID-transduced bone marrow that had been cultured *ex vivo* for 15 days. Despite the low donor volumes injected, all mice showed 100% engraftment with donor cells. Also, mice engrafted with expanded HaMDR1- or HaMID-transduced bone marrow cells developed a myeloproliferative disorder characterized by large increases in the peripheral blood leukocyte count, splenomegaly, and increased progenitor content in the blood and spleen. The results presented here demonstrate that the human MDR1 gene has important effects on murine stem cell self-renewal and differentiation processes, and suggest a role for this gene in controlling stem cell fate decisions.

MATERIALS AND METHODS

Retroviral Producer Cell Lines and Vector Constructs

The Harvey (Ha)MDR1, HaDHFR, and HaMID vectors and ecotropic producer cell lines were generated as described previously.[24,25] The MDR1 cDNA encodes the wild-type protein containing glycine at amino acid 185. The MDR1 cDNA has also been modified as previously described[24] to reduce aberrant splicing of viral RNA,[26] allowing enhanced expression of P-glycoprotein (P-gp) in target cells. The DHFR cDNA contains a leucine to tyrosine mutation at codon 22 (L22Y) that has been described previously.[25]

Retroviral-Mediated Bone Marrow Cell Transduction

Bone marrow cells were flushed from both hind limbs of a single C57/Bl6 (C57) mouse (day -4) and prestimulated for 48 hours in Dulbecco's modified essential medium (DMEM; BioWhittaker, Walkersville, MD) supplemented with 15% fetal bovine serum, 100 units/ml penicillin, and 100 ng/ml streptomycin (P/S; Gibco-BRL). Cells were cultured in liquid suspension culture in the presence of the following growth factors; 20 ng/ml murine IL-3 (Amgen), 50 ng/ml human IL-6 (Amgen), and 50 ng/ml murine SCF (Amgen and R & D Systems). Following prestimulation (day -2), cells were divided into 4 separate groups for coculture on irradiated (1500 rads) GP + E86[27] ecotropic producer cell lines or naive GP + E86 cells (mock-infected control). Transductions were done for 48 hours in the same cultures as above except with added 6 µg/ml polybrene (Sigma, St. Louis, MO).

Ex Vivo Culture and Expansion of Myeloid Progenitors

Following transduction (day 0), cells were cultured in the presence of growth factors at the same concentrations as listed above. Cells were resuspended at 1×10^6 cells/ml every 3 days for a total of 15 days of expansion. The percentage of drug-resistant myeloid progenitors on day 0 was calculated by plating cells in methylcellulose (Stem Cell Technologies, Vancouver, Canada) in the presence of selective concentrations of drugs. HaMDR1-transduced progenitors were resistant to 50 nM taxol (Bristol-Myers Squib Co., Princeton, NJ) and HaDHFR-transduced progenitors were resistant to 25 nM trimetrexate (Drug Synthesis and Chemistry Branch, Developmental Therapeutics Program, Division of Cancer Treatment, NCI.). HaMID-transduced progenitors were resistant to taxol or trimetrexate at the same concentrations as listed above.

Quantitation of Progenitor Enrichment by Flow Cytometry

Murine bone marrow cells that had been cultured for 12 days were stained with a stem cell antigen-1 (Sca-1) phycoerythrin (PE)-linked antibody and with a mixture of lineage-specific fluorescein isothiocyanate (FITC)-linked antibodies. Included in the FITC lineage cocktail were antibodies to the lymphoid markers CD4 (L3T4), CD8 (Ly-2), B220 (CD45R), and myeloid markers GR-1 (Ly-6G), and MAC-1 (CD11b). Also, a biotinylated antibody to TER-119 was used to detect erythroid progenitors. All antibodies were obtained from Pharmingen (San Diego, CA) unless otherwise indicated. Cells were stained in a final volume of 100 μl of phosphate-buffered saline (PBS) for 10 minutes on ice, followed by 2 washes in 500 μl PBS, and incubation with streptavidin-FITC to detect TER-119. Stained cells were fixed using fluorescence-activated cell sorter (FACS) lysing solution (Becton Dickinson, San Jose, CA) and analyzed by flow cytometry. For negative controls, isotype immunoglobulin G2a (IgG2a) and IgG2b antibodies were incubated separately at the same ratios as above.

Bone Marrow Transplant

Recipient B6.C-H1/BY (HW80) mice were lethally-irradiated with 1100 rads of γ-irradiation from a Cs^{137} source. Donor C57 cells, which had been expanded in culture for 15 days, were harvested and cell doses ranging from $1–6 \times 10^6$ cells/mouse were injected via the tail vein in a volume of 0.5 ml. These cell doses represented original donor hind limb volumes ranging from 0.007 to 0.44%. Mice transplanted with *ex vivo* expanded bone marrow grafts survived long-term and were analyzed at 16 weeks for engraftment. The percentage of donor cells was determined by hemoglobin electrophoresis on cellulose acetate gels (Helena Laboratories, Beaumont, TX) and was quantitated by densitometry (Alpha Innotech Corporation).

Detection of Human P-gp on Murine Peripheral Blood Leukocytes

Murine whole blood was diluted in 10 mL of PBS and centrifuged at 1100 rpm for 5 minutes. Cells were then resuspended in 2 ml Hank's balanced salt solution (HBSS)/0.1% bovine serum albumin (BSA), and red blood cells were lysed following addition of 6 ml Gey's solution. Leukocytes were pelleted by centrifugation, washed in PBS twice, and blocked with normal mouse serum in a final volume of 50 μL PBS/0.1% BSA on ice for 30 minutes. Leukocyte suspensions were split into two equal 20-μL aliquots, and an equal volume of FITC-labeled murine monoclonal anti-human P-gp, 4E3-FITC (Signet Laboratories Inc., Dedham, MA) or isotype control was added. Cell/antibody mixtures were incubated for 30 minutes on ice, washed twice in PBS, and resuspended in 500 μL PBS. Stained cells were fixed in 1% paraformaldehyde and stored at 4°C prior to analysis.

RESULTS

MDR1 Gene Transfer Allows Cytokine-Mediated Stem Cell Expansion

Ex vivo expanded bone marrow cells have often shown an engraftment defect following extended culture. By contrast, we have previously shown that introduction of the MDR1 gene by retroviral-mediated gene transfer removes a block to stem cell self-renewal divisions *in vitro* and allows large increases in retrovirally-transduced stem cells over a 12-day culture period.[23] As a result, mice transplanted with expanded cells showed much higher levels of engraftment than would have been predicted. FIGURE 1 summarizes these results in which HaMDR1-transduced stem cells (filled circles, top) were expanded following *ex vivo* culture. Subsequent analysis of MDR1 gene marking in spleen colony-forming units (CFU-S) from secondary recipient mice revealed that all primitive repopulating cells were MDR1 positive.[23] This

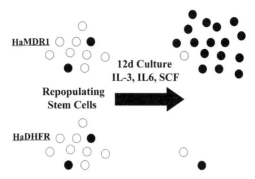

FIGURE 1. *Ex vivo* expansion of MDR1-transduced hematopoietic stem cells. Harvey (Ha) murine sarcoma virus based-retroviral vectors expressing either MDR1 or a DHFR variant were introduced into bone marrow cells isolated from the same C57 donor mouse. Following transduction, cells were cultured for 12 days in the presence of stimulatory growth factors and assayed by competitive repopulation versus fresh bone marrow. Circles represent individual transduced (filled) or nontransduced (open) stem cells in the pool of cultured bone marrow. At the end of 12 days there was a large increase in the number of stem cells obtained from the HaMDR1 cultures, but a depletion in the stem cell content resulted in the HaDHFR cultures. The expansion of HaMDR1 stem cells allowed for much higher levels of engraftment in transplanted mice than would have been predicted even from freshly isolated cells. In addition, expanded primitive cells remaining after 12 days in culture were highly MDR1 vector positive.

indicated that only those stem cells that expressed the exogenous MDR1 gene were capable of surviving and amplifying during *ex vivo* culture. By contrast, HaDHFR-transduced stem cells (filled circles, bottom) and nontransduced stem cells (open circles) were reduced as a consequence of the expansion culture conditions.

We next wanted to determine whether the stem cell expansion phenotype could be obtained using another independently derived producer cell clone expressing the MDR1 gene. A bicistronic vector was generated containing the human MDR1 cDNA

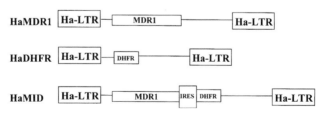

FIGURE 2. Retroviral vector constructs utilized for bone marrow transduction and expansion. High-titer ecotropic retroviral producer cell lines were generated from a series of Harvey (Ha) murine sarcoma virus-based–retroviral vectors. These vector designs included either the MDR1 gene, a resistance-conferring DHFR variant, or both MDR1 and DHFR. In the bicistronic vector, DHFR expression is initiated from an internal ribosomal entry sequence (IRES). Transcription from all three retroviral vectors is driven off the retroviral long-terminal repeat (LTR), and the upstream genes are all inserted into the SacII/XhoI restriction site. All three vectors also contain endogenous rat virus-like 30 (VL-30) sequences that are critical for generation of high viral titers.

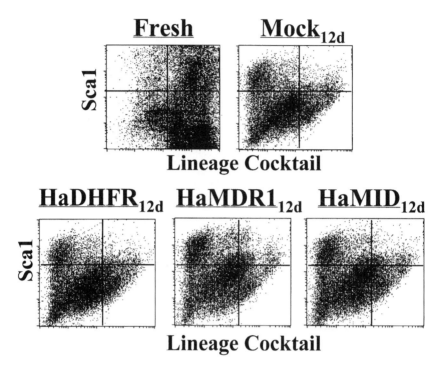

FIGURE 3. Flow cytometry analysis of fresh and 12-day expanded bone marrow cells. Bone marrow cells were stained with a panel of lineage-specific markers and an antibody to Sca-1. Freshly isolated bone marrow cells showed a low percentage of Sca-1+Lin− cells. To determine the effects of *ex vivo* expansion on this phenotype, cells were expanded in culture for 12 days and then analyzed by flow cytometry. Cells were analyzed from mock, HaDH-FR, HaMDR1, and HaMID groups. In all cases, there was a shift in the population of cells from mostly lineage positive to mostly lineage negative. A unique population of Sca-1+Lin-cells appeared in these cultures, representing the progenitor enrichment and expansion typically obtained during *ex vivo* culture with IL-3, IL-6, and SCF. No significant differences were seen between MDR1-transduced cells and the DHFR or mock groups.

upstream of an internal ribosomal entry site (IRES) driving expression of a DHFR cDNA. For the studies reported here, three vector designs were compared, all of which utilized the Harvey murine sarcoma virus long-terminal repeat to drive expression of the upstream gene (FIG. 2). The only difference between the HaMDR1 and HaMID vectors was the presence of the IRES-DHFR sequences. Expression of both genes from the bicistronic vector and the ability to confer resistance to both anti-folate and MDR1-effluxed drugs has been previously documented.[24]

Long-Term Reconstitution with Very Low Hind Limb Volumes of MDR1-Transduced Bone Marrow Cells Expanded for 15 days

Mouse bone marrow cells were obtained from a single C57/Bl6 mouse and retrovirally transduced by previously described methods.[26] Cells were divided into 4 experimental groups that included mock-infected cells and cells transduced with the

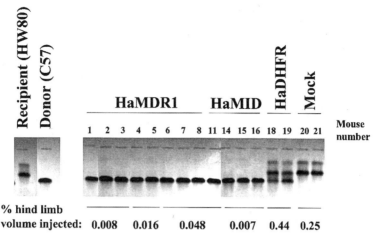

FIGURE 4. Hematopoietic reconstitution of recipient mice with low donor hind limb volumes of 15-day expanded bone marrow cells. Following flow cytometry analysis on day 12, cells were cultured for an additional 3 days and then injected into lethally irradiated HW80 mice on day 15. Mice were analyzed for engraftment with donor marrow by hemoglobin electrophoresis at 16 weeks posttransplant. Shown on the left are donor C57 (single) and recipient HW80 (diffuse) hemoglobin patterns. All mice injected with donor hind limb volumes ranging from 0.007 to 0.048% of HaMDR1 or HaMID-transduced bone marrow showed 100% reconstitution with donor cells. By contrast, mice injected with much higher donor volumes of HaDHFR cells, showed only partial donor reconstitution, and mice injected with mock bone marrow showed no engraftment with donor cells.

HaDHFR, HaMDR1, or HaMID vectors. Progenitor transduction percentages as determined by drug resistance in semisolid media for 3 separate transductions were: HaDHFR (47 ± 6%), HaMDR1 (33 ± 7%), and HaMID (8 ± 4%). Following coculture, cells were put into liquid suspension culture with IL-3, IL-6, and SCF for 12 days and then analyzed by flow cytometry. Sca-1$^+$Lin$^-$ cells were quantitated to examine the effects of *ex vivo* culture on this primitive but heterogeneous population of cells (FIG. 3). Freshly isolated bone marrow cells showed a very low percentage of Sca-1$^+$Lin$^-$ cells (1–2%). Expanded bone marrow cells showed an increased Sca-1$^+$Lin$^-$ percentage irrespective of the vector used, reflecting the enrichment in myeloid progenitors during *ex vivo* culture with IL-3, IL-6, and SCF. Quantitation of this increase in the percentage of total cells with colony-forming ability by methylcellulose assay showed an average 13-fold enrichment for all expansion groups relative to fresh bone marrow. This increased progenitor frequency was also maintained throughout the *ex vivo* expansion culture period (data not shown).

To determine whether the previously described expansion of stem cells would be sufficient to allow engraftment of mice with relatively low hind limb volumes of donor marrow, small percent donor volumes from the 15-day expanded grafts were injected into HW80 recipient mice. The volumes injected for these experiments were 100- to 300-fold lower than those used previously in competitive repopulation studies.[23] Engraftment was monitored using hemoglobin polymorphisms as previously

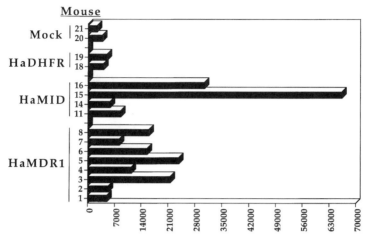

Peripheral blood leukocytes/μl

FIGURE 5. Peripheral blood leukocyte counts in mice 16 weeks following bone marrow transplant. Some mice from the HaMDR1 or HaMID groups that engrafted with expanded stem cells developed an abnormal increase in the peripheral blood leukocyte numbers by 16 weeks posttransplant. All mice injected with HaDHFR- or mock-transduced cells, however, maintained normal peripheral blood hematology. All 12 of the mice from the HaMDR1 and HaMID groups eventually died from elevated leukocyte counts by 6 months following transplant. Counts were quantitated using a coulter counter and are represented as the number of leukocytes per μl of whole blood.

described.[28] Mice transplanted with doses as low as 0.007% donor volume of HaMDR1 or HaMID cells showed 100% donor reconstitution at 16 weeks following transplant (FIG. 4). By contrast, mice receiving HaDHFR or mock cells showed partial to undetectable levels of engraftment despite injection of much higher donor hind limb volumes. This result indicates that the HaMID vector allows stem cell expansion at a level comparable to HaMDR1, thus demonstrating that expansion is not specific to a particular vector configuration or producer cell clone. The failure of the HaDHFR or mock grafts to fully reconstitute recipient mice also demonstrates that the Sca-1$^+$Lin$^-$ enrichment of the expanded cells was not predictive of the hematopoietic repopulating potential of the expanded graft and more accurately reflects the progenitor enrichment.

A Myeloproliferative Disorder Results in Mice Engrafted with Expanded HaMDR1- or HaMID-Transduced Stem Cells

Mice were analyzed long-term for peripheral blood leukocyte counts, differential counts, and any potential adverse effects of stem cell expansion. As seen previously, a myeloproliferative disorder occurred in mice engrafted with expanded HaMDR1-tranduced cells. The disorder was also detected here in mice transplanted with expanded HaMID-transduced bone marrow. FIGURE 5 shows the peripheral blood leukocyte counts in mice analyzed at 16 weeks following transplant. Abnor-

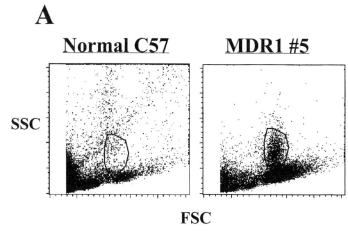

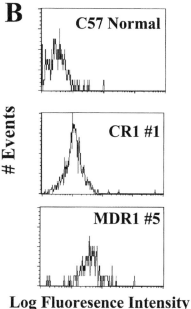

FIGURE 6. Flow cytometry analysis of expression of human P-glycoprotein on abnormal peripheral blood leukocytes. Peripheral blood from mice transplanted with MDR1-transduced and expanded stem cells was analyzed by flow cytometry. (A) The forward scatter (FSC) and side scatter (SSC) profile for a normal C57 mouse is shown (*left*). The profile from a mouse with the myeloproliferative syndrome showed an increase in an abnormal population of cells (*right*). Gates were drawn on the abnormal population and analyzed for expression of P-gp. (B) Expression of human P-gp was detected in all mice examined, but the levels of expression showed marked heterogeneity. CR1 #1 and MDR1 #5 are representative mice from competitive repopulation experiments described in FIG. 1. A normal C57 mouse is shown at the top and serves as a negative control for expression of human P-gp.

mally high counts developed in mice transplanted with either HaMDR1- or Ha-MID-transduced bone marrow at this time point. At later times, leukocyte counts for these mice were detected at levels as high as 190,127 cells/µl. All 12 of the HaMDR1 and HaMID mice ultimately died from the disorder by 6 months posttransplant, whereas 3 out of 4 of the HaDHFR and mock mice remained alive. Analysis of the peripheral blood from diseased mice revealed the presence of a large abnormal cell population (FIG. 6A). Gating on this population and analysis for expression of human P-glycoprotein (P-gp) by flow cytometry demonstrated that the abnormal cells were expressing the transferred MDR1 gene (FIG. 6B). In addition, the percentages of taxol resistant progenitors ranged from 24 to 85% in peripheral blood, bone marrow, and spleen from diseased HaMID mice. P-gp expression in these abnormal cells tightly links the disorder to transduction with the MDR1 vector. Also, the abnormal cell population was polyclonal as determined by Southern blot analysis of peripheral blood DNA (data not shown). The progenitor content was elevated ranging from 300- to 700-fold above normal in the peripheral blood and spleen. Splenomegaly was also evident with spleen weights as high as 715 mg. No instance of this disease was seen in mice receiving HaDHFR or mock grafts or previously in mice receiving unexpanded bone marrow that had been transduced with the HaMDR1 or HaMID vectors. This indicates that the abnormal myeloproliferation is specific to MDR1-transduced cells that had been expanded in culture for 15 days, but is not directly caused by MDR1 transduction per se, given that the disorder does not occur in the absence of *ex vivo* expansion.

DISCUSSION

In summary, we have demonstrated that *ex vivo* stem cell expansion can be achieved following retroviral-mediated gene transfer of MDR1. This expansion was seen with two viral constructs, a monocistronic vector containing MDR1 (HaMDR1) and a bicistronic construct containing both MDR1 and DHFR genes (HaMID). Despite lower levels of expression of both genes following transduction with the HaMID virus,[24] clear evidence of stem cell expansion was obtained with the HaMID vector. For these reconstitution experiments, the original donor volumes injected into recipient mice were extremely low. A percent donor hind limb volume of 0.007%, the lowest amount transplanted, represents a cell dose of approximately 3000 initial freshly harvested bone marrow cells. Since the frequency of long-term repopulating stem cells in fresh mouse bone marrow has been estimated to be 1 per 10,000 cells,[1,2] it would not be predicted that engraftment could be obtained at high frequency unless stem cell amplification had occurred. In addition, the cells had been cultured for 15 days, which is known to be detrimental to overall stem cell survival. Not only did mice engraft, but also all recipients of low donor volumes of HaMDR1 or HaMID bone marrow showed 100% donor reconstitution at 16 weeks. The degree of stem cell expansion that would account for this increase, could potentially be highly useful for bone marrow transplant where donor cells are often available in limited supply.

The phenotypic markers defining the murine stem cell have been extensively characterized. Freshly isolated Sca-1$^+$Lin$^-$Thy1.1^{low} bone marrow cells are relatively enriched for long-term reconstituting activity.[29] High-level expression of c-kit has also been shown to be a marker of primitive stem cell subsets.[30] The dyes rhodamine 123[31–34] and Hoechst 33342[35] have provided the means to further subfractionate stem cell activity. Rhodamine 123 exclusion has proved to be a highly specific marker of primitive stem cells. One out of 5 Thy1.1^{low}Lin$^-$Sca-1$^+$Rh123^{low} cells is capable of long term reconstitution following transplant.[36] Interestingly, both rhodamine 123 and Hoechst 33342 are substrates for P-gp, and staining profiles indicate an increased P-gp efflux activity in the most primitive hematopoietic cells. Thus it can be speculated that P-gp efflux function may be a determinant of stem cell activity. Although mice deficient in both MDR1a and MDR1b do not demonstrate any obvious hematologic defects[37] and display normal viability, the stem cell population in the MDR1a/1b −/− mouse has not been formally analyzed. Thus a stem cell defect in the MDR1 knockout mouse cannot be excluded at this time.

Enforced expression of exogenous P-gp in the murine stem cell could result in dysregulated MDR1 expression. Overexpression of MDR1 above the levels of the endogenous mouse protein has been documented with retroviral gene transfer.[26] Thus, if MDR1 expression is developmentally regulated during hematopoiesis, constitutive expression may perturb the normal stem cell maturation pathway. It is not known whether this effect is specific for the introduced human MDR1 gene or whether this function can be generalized to all MDR efflux pumps. In addition, the MDR1 cDNA used for these experiments contained the wild-type codon 185. Amino acid substitutions can change the relative substrate affinity of MDR1 proteins,[38,39] thus codon 185 could be a critical residue for the stem cell expansion function.

P-gp has been most extensively characterized as a drug detoxifying enzyme.[40,41] Thus, P-gp may play a role in protecting stem cells from potential toxic compounds.

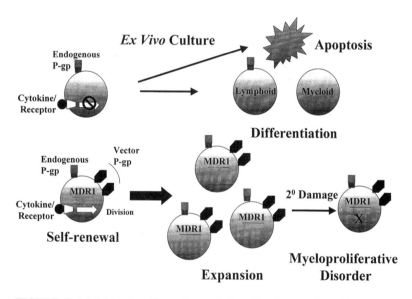

FIGURE 7. Model for the effects of retroviral-mediated expression of human P-gp on murine hematopoietic stem cells during *ex vivo* expansion culture. Cytokine manipulation of hematopoietic stem cells stimulates cells to enter distinct differentiation or apoptotic cell death pathways. Either of these two stem cell fates results in a decrease in the absolute stem cell number present in the culture. By contrast, expression of human P-gp on murine stem cells allows stem cell self-renewal divisions to occur at high frequency. As a result, the number of MDR1-transduced stem cells increases in culture, and these cells maintain long-term repopulating capacity. A secondary event, possibly DNA damage accumulated during rapid cell division, leads to development of a myeloproliferative disorder at time points following initial engraftment.

A P-gp lipid translocase activity, allowing for reorganization of membrane phospholipids,[42] could play a potential role in modulating phosphatidylserine accumulation on the surface of apoptotic cells.[43,44] Another potential role for P-gp in protection against apoptosis could be reduction of ceramide levels within the cell. Ceramide is a potent inducer of apoptosis[45] and has recently been shown to be a substrate for MDR1.[42] In fact, treatment of a human leukemia cell line with the P-gp blocker PSC 833 ([3'-keto-Bmt-1]-[Val-2]-cyclosporin) has been effective in restoring TNF-α-induced ceramide production, plasma membrane sphingomyelinase distribution, and subsequent apoptosis.[46] Also, transfection of P-gp into Chinese hamster ovary cells has shown an antiapoptotic effect.[47] Since apoptosis of hematopoietic stem cells in culture can result in depletion of the repopulating activity of the bone marrow graft, this mechanism may be relevant to the effects seen during *ex vivo* marrow culture.

FIGURE 7 summarizes our current working model for MDR1-mediated stem cell expansion. Cultured murine stem cells not expressing human MDR1 are highly sensitive to apoptosis or undergo terminal differentiation at the expense of self-renewal. MDR1 gene transfer removes an as yet unidentified block to stem cell expansion, but this later results in an uncontrolled proliferation. Consistent with this hypothesis, are the high levels of engraftment of some HaMDR1 and HaMID mice at 16 weeks with maintenance of normal peripheral blood leukocyte counts. Since the number of stem cell divisions has been dramatically increased over the culture period, it is possible that replication errors could have accumulated, and these effects were not seen until a later time. Indeed, mice that have died from this disease have been exclusively those that have shown engraftment with *ex vivo* expanded stem cells when competed against fresh bone marrow at an unfavorable ratio. Recent data have shown, however, that this disease can occur following transplant of nonexpanded marrow (data not shown). No adverse consequences of retroviral-mediated MDR1 expression have been reported previously in mice transplanted with nonexpanded bone marrow.[23,26,48–50] Since MDR1 gene therapy is currently being tested clinically for bone marrow chemoprotection, the safety of this approach may need reexamination. Despite the potential negative consequences of this disease, the ability of MDR1 gene transfer to influence the self-renewal decisions of hematopoietic stem cells is a new concept, and further study may provide valuable information about the regulatory mechanisms critical for stem cell self-renewal and differentiation.

SUMMARY

These results demonstrate that retrovirally expressed MDR1 can alter the response of murine hematopoietic stem cells to cytokine stimulation *in vitro*. As a result, stem cells obtain the ability to undergo extensive self-renewal divisions and increase in number by greater than 1 log over a 12-day expansion culture. However, as a consequence of this expansion transplanted mice developed an abnormal myeloproliferative disorder. This finding illustrates the potential adverse consequences that can be associated with rapid stem cell division and serves as the basis for future studies aimed at determining the mechanism of action of human P-gp in conferring this effect.

REFERENCES

1. MORRISON, S.J. & I.L. WEISSMAN. 1994. The long-term repopulating subset of hematopoietic stem cells is deterministic and isolatable by phenotype. Immunity 1: 661–673.

2. HARRISON, D.E., C.M. ASTLE & C. LERNER. 1988. Number and continuous proliferative pattern of transplanted primitive immunohematopoietic stem cells. Proc. Natl. Acad. Sci. USA **85**: 822–826.

3. HAO, Q.L., A.J. SHAH, F.T. THIEMANN, E.M. SMOGORZEWSKA & G.M. CROOKS. 1995. A functional comparison of CD34+CD38- cells in cord blood and bone marrow. Blood **86**: 3745–3753.

4. BERARDI, A.C., A. WANG, J.D. LEVINE, P. LOPEZ & D.T. SCADDEN. 1995. Functional isolation and characterization of human hematopoietic stem cells. Science **267**: 104–108.

5. LERNER, C. & D.E. HARRISON. 1990. 5-Fluorouracil spares hemopoietic stem cells responsible for long-term repopulation. Exp. Hematol. **18**: 114–118.

6. PETZER, A.L., P.W. ZANDSTRA, J.M. PIRET & C.J. EAVES. 1996. Differential cytokine effects on primitive (CD34+CD38−) human hematopoietic cells: novel responses to Flt3-ligand and thrombopoietin. J. Exp. Med. **183**: 2551–2558.

7. ORLIC, D. & D.M. BODINE. 1994. What defines a pluripotent hematopoietic stem cell (PHSC): will the real PHSC please stand up! Blood **84**: 3991–3994.

8. LAROCHELLE, A., J. VORMOOR, H. HANENBERG, J.C. WANG, M. BHATIA, T. LAPIDOT, T. MORITZ, B. MURDOCH, X.L. XIAO, I. KATO, D.A. WILLIAMS & J.E. DICK. 1996. Identification of primitive human hematopoietic cells capable of repopulating NOD/SCID mouse bone marrow: implications for gene therapy. Nat. Med. **2**: 1329–1337.

9. NOLTA, J.A., M.B. HANLEY & D.B. KOHN. 1994. Sustained human hematopoiesis in immunodeficient mice by cotransplantation of marrow stroma expressing human interleukin-3: analysis of gene transduction of long-lived progenitors. Blood **83**: 3041–3051.

10. NAMIKAWA, R., K.N. WEILBAECHER, H. KANESHIMA, E.J. YEE & J.M. MCCUNE. 1990. Long-term human hematopoiesis in the SCID-hu mouse. J. Exp. Med. **172**: 1055–1063.

11. CASHMAN, J.D., T. LAPIDOT, J.C. WANG, M. DOEDENS, L.D. SHULTZ, P. LANSDORP, J.E. DICK & C.J. EAVES. 1997. Kinetic evidence of the regeneration of multilineage hematopoiesis from primitive cells in normal human bone marrow transplanted into immunodeficient mice. Blood **89**: 4307–4316.

12. SMITH, L.G., I.L. WEISSMAN & S. HEIMFELD. 1991. Clonal analysis of hematopoietic stem-cell differentiation *in vivo*. Proc. Natl. Acad. ci. USA **88**: 2788–2792.

13. HARRISON, D.E. & C.P. LERNER. 1991. Most primitive hematopoietic stem cells are stimulated to cycle rapidly after treatment with 5-fluorouracil. Blood **78**: 1237–1240.

14. BODINE, D.M., K.T. MCDONAGH, N.E. SEIDEL & A.W. NIENHUIS. 1991. Survival and retrovirus infection of murine hematopoietic stem cells *in vitro*: effects of 5-FU and method of infection. Exp. Hematol. **19**: 206–212.

15. BODINE, D.M., S. KARLSSON & A.W. NIENHUIS. 1989. Combination of interleukins 3 and 6 preserves stem cell function in culture and enhances retrovirus-mediated gene transfer into hematopoietic stem cells. Proc. Natl. Acad. Sci. USA **86**: 8897–8901.

16. BODINE, D.M., D. ORLIC, N.C. BIRKETT, N.E. SEIDEL & K.M. ZSEBO. 1992. Stem cell factor increases colony-forming unit-spleen number *in vitro* in synergy with interleukin-6, and *in vivo* in Sl/Sld mice as a single factor. Blood 79: 913–919.

17. LUSKEY, B.D., M. ROSENBLATT, K. ZSEBO & D.A. WILLIAMS. 1992. Stem cell factor, interleukin-3, and interleukin-6 promote retroviral-mediated gene transfer into murine hematopoietic stem cells. Blood **80**: 396–402.

18. MILLER, C.L. & C.J. EAVES. 1997. Expansion *in vitro* of adult murine hematopoietic stem cells with transplantable lympho-myeloid reconstituting ability. Proc. Natl. Acad. Sci. USA **94:** 13648–13653.
19. PETERS, S.O., E.L. KITTLER, H.S. RAMSHAW & P.J. QUESENBERRY. 1996. *Ex vivo* expansion of murine marrow cells with interleukin-3 (IL-3), IL-6, IL-11, and stem cell factor leads to impaired engraftment in irradiated hosts. Blood **87:** 30–37.
20. TRAYCOFF, C.M., K. CORNETTA, M.C. YODER, A. DAVIDSON & E.F. SROUR. 1996. *Ex vivo* expansion of murine hematopoietic progenitor cells generates classes of expanded cells possessing different levels of bone marrow repopulating potential. Exp. Hematol. **24:** 299–306.
21. WILLIAMS, D.A. 1993. *Ex vivo* expansion of hematopoietic stem and progenitor cells—robbing Peter to pay Paul? Blood **81:** 3169–3172.
22. TRAYCOFF, C.M., A. ORAZI, A.C. LADD, S. RICE, J. MCMAHEL & E.F. SROUR. 1998. Proliferation-induced decline of primitive hematopoietic progenitor cell activity is coupled with an increase in apoptosis of *ex vivo* expanded CD34+ cells. Exp. Hematol. **26:** 53–62.
23. BUNTING, K.D., J. GALIPEAU, D. TOPHAM, E. BENAIM & B.P. SORRENTINO. 1998. Transduction of murine bone marrow cells with an MDR1 vector enables *ex vivo* stem cell expansion, but these expanded grafts cause a myeloproliferative syndrome in transplanted mice. Blood **92:** 2269–2279
24. GALIPEAU, J., E. BENAIM, H.T. SPENCER, R.L. BLAKLEY & B.P. SORRENTINO. 1997. A bicistronic retroviral vector for protecting hematopoietic cells against antifolates and P-glycoprotein effluxed drugs. Hum. Gene Ther. **8:** 1773–1783.
25. SPENCER, H.T., S.E. SLEEP, J.E. REHG, R.L. BLAKLEY & B.P. SORRENTINO. 1996. A gene transfer strategy for making bone marrow cells resistant to trimetrexate. Blood **87:** 2579–2587.
26. SORRENTINO, B.P., K.T. MCDONAGH, D. WOODS & D. ORLIC. 1995. Expression of retroviral vectors containing the human multidrug resistance 1 cDNA in hematopoietic cells of transplanted mice. Blood **86:** 491–501.
27. MARKOWITZ, D., S. GOFF & A. BANK. 1988. A safe packaging line for gene transfer: separating viral genes on two different plasmids. J. Virol. **62:** 1120–1124.
28. ALLAY, J.A., H.T. SPENCER, S.L. WILKINSON, J.A. BELT, R.L. BLAKLEY & B.P. SORRENTINO. 1997. Sensitization of hematopoietic stem and progenitor cells to trimetrexate using nucleoside transport inhibitors. Blood **90:** 3546–3554.
29. SPANGRUDE, G.J., S. HEIMFELD & I.L. WEISSMAN. 1988. Purification and characterization of mouse hematopoietic stem cells. Science **241:** 58–62.
30. ORLIC, D., R. FISCHER, S. NISHIKAWA, A.W. NIENHUIS & D.M. BODINE. 1993. Purification and characterization of heterogeneous pluripotent hematopoietic stem cell populations expressing high levels of c-kit receptor. Blood **82:** 762–770.
31. SPANGRUDE, G.J. & G.R. JOHNSON. 1990. Resting and activated subsets of mouse multipotent hematopoietic stem cells. Proc. Natl. Acad. Sci.USA **87:** 7433–7437.
32. ZIJLMANS, J.M., J.W. VISSER, K. KLEIVERDA, P.M. KLUIN, R. WILLEMZE & W.E. FIBBE. 1995. Modification of rhodamine staining allows identification of hematopoietic stem cells with preferential short-term or long-term bone marrow-repopulating ability. Proc. Natl. Acad. Sci. USA **92:** 8901–8905.
33. UCHIDA, N., J. COMBS, S. CHEN, E. ZANJANI, R. HOFFMAN & A. TSUKAMOTO. 1996. Primitive human hematopoietic cells displaying differential efflux of the rhodamine 123 dye have distinct biological activities. Blood **88:** 1297–1305.
34. CHAUDHARY, P.M. & I.B. RONINSON. 1991. Expression and activity of P-glycoprotein, a multidrug efflux pump, in human hematopoietic stem cells. Cell **66:** 85–94.

35. GOODELL, M.A., K. BROSE, G. PARADIS, A.S. CONNER & R.C. MULLIGAN. 1996. Isolation and functional properties of murine hematopoietic stem cells that are replicating *in vivo*. J. Exp. Med. **183:** 1797–1806.

36. SPANGRUDE, G.J., D.M. BROOKS & D.B. TUMAS. 1995. Long-term repopulation of irradiated mice with limiting numbers of purified hematopoietic stem cells: *in vivo* expansion of stem cell phenotype but not function. Blood **85:** 1006–1016.

37. SCHINKEL, A.H., U. MAYER, E. WAGENAAR, C.A. MOL, L. VAN DEEMTER, J.J. SMIT, M.A. VAN DER VALK, A.C. VOORDOUW, H. SPITS, O. VAN TELLINGEN, J.M. ZIJL-MANS, W.E. FIBBE & P. BORST. 1997. Normal viability and altered pharmacokinetics in mice lacking mdr1-type (drug-transporting) P-glycoproteins. Proc. Natl. Acad. Sci. USA **94:** 4028–4033.

38. GROS, P., R. DHIR, J. CROOP & F. TALBOT. 1991. A single amino acid substitution strongly modulates the activity and substrate specificity of the mouse mdr1 and mdr3 drug efflux pumps. Proc. Natl. Acad. Sci. USA 88: 7289–7293.

39. RONINSON, I.B., J.E. CHIN, K.G. CHOI, P. GROS, D.E. HOUSMAN, A. FOJO, D.W. SHEN, M.M. GOTTESMAN & I. PASTAN. 1986. Isolation of human mdr DNA sequences amplified in multidrug-resistant KB carcinoma cells. Proc. Natl. Acad. Sci. USA **83:** 4538–4542.

40. SCHINKEL, A.H. & P. BORST. 1991. Multidrug resistance mediated by P-glycoproteins. Sem. Cancer Biol. **2:** 213–226.

41. BORST, P. 1991. Genetic mechanisms of drug resistance. A review. Acta Oncol. **30:** 87–105.

42. VAN HELVOORT, A., A.J. SMITH, H. SPRONG, I. FRITZSCHE, A.H. SCHINKEL, P. BORST & G. VAN MEER. 1996. MDR1 P-glycoprotein is a lipid translocase of broad specificity, while MDR3 P-glycoprotein specifically translocates phosphatidylcholine. Cell **87:** 507–517.

43. MARTIN, S.J., D.M. FINUCANE, G.P. AMARANTE-MENDES, G.A. O'BRIEN & D.R. GREEN. 1996. Phosphatidylserine externalization during CD95-induced apoptosis of cells and cytoplasts requires ICE/CED-3 protease activity. J. Biol. Chem. **271:** 28753–28756.

44. MARTIN, S.J., C.P. REUTELINGSPERGER, A.J. MCGAHON, J.A. RADER, R.C. VAN SCHIE, D.M. LAFACE & D.R. GREEN. 1995. Early redistribution of plasma membrane phosphatidylserine is a general feature of apoptosis regardless of the initiating stimulus: inhibition by overexpression of Bcl-2 and Abl. J .Exp. Med. **182:** 1545–1556.

45. HANNUN, Y.A. & L.M. OBEID. 1997. Mechanisms of ceramide-mediated apoptosis. Adv. Exp. Med. Biol. **407:** 145–149.

46. BEZOMBES, C., N. MAESTRE, G. LAURENT, T. LEVADE, A. BETTAIEB & J.P. JAFFREZOU. 1998. Restoration of TNF-alpha-induced ceramide generation and apoptosis in resistant human leukemia KG1a cells by the P-glycoprotein blocker PSC833. FASEB J. **12:** 101–109.

47. ROBINSON, L.J., W.K. ROBERTS, T.T. LING, D. LAMMING, S.S. STERNBERG & P.D. ROEPE. 1997. Human MDR 1 protein overexpression delays the apoptotic cascade in Chinese hamster ovary fibroblasts. Biochemistry **36:** 11169–11178.

48. PODDA, S., M. WARD, A. HIMELSTEIN, C. RICHARDSON, E. DE LA FLOR-WEISS, L. SMITH, M. GOTTESMAN, I. PASTAN & A. BANK. 1992. Transfer and expression of the human multiple drug resistance gene into live mice. Proc. Natl. Acad. Sci. USA **89:** 9676–9680.

49. WARD, M., C. RICHARDSON, P. PIOLI, L. SMITH, S. PODDA, S. GOFF, C. HESDORFFER & A. BANK. 1994. Transfer and expression of the human multiple drug resistance gene in human CD34+ cells. Blood **84:** 1408–1414.

50. HANANIA, E.G. & A.B. DEISSEROTH. 1994. Serial transplantation shows that early hematopoietic precursor cells are transduced by MDR-1 retroviral vector in a mouse gene therapy model. Cancer Gene Ther. **1:** 21–25.

DISCUSSION

J.W. ADAMSON (*New York Blood Center*): You analzyed your animals at a certain point for clonality. Have you analyzed the peripheral white cells later on in the course of the development of the leukocytosis? Do they remain polyclonal at that point or are the circulating cells at that point monoclonal?

SORRENTINO: We have done what you just asked in a relatively limited number of mice where we have sacrificed them and actually looked at sorted myeloid and lymphoid cells. They do have different patterns of integration sites. Even when this myeloproliferative syndrome develops, it is not derived from a single stem cell clone. We have looked in a relatively few animals, and perhaps as we look at more animals, we will modify that interpretation. It appears that even as the syndrome develops, hematopoiesis is at least oligoclonal at that point.

W.E. FIBBE (*University Medical Center Leiden*): If your experiments are related to one of the substrates for P-gp, you could try to modify it by trying to block P-gp function using one of the well-known blockers such as cyclosporin or verapamil? Have you tried to do that?

SORRENTINO: We are in the process of doing that. The fact that all the spleen colony-forming units (CFU-S) from engrafted animals have the MDR-1 virus does tightly link at least transduction per se to expansion and to the syndrome. However, we have not formally proved that P-gp function is required for both those outcomes, so we are going to do blocking experiments.

J.D. GRIFFIN (*Dana Farber Cancer Institute*): Are you sure that the nonexpanded but MDR-1-transduced cells do not cause this myeloproliferative syndrome? Has anyone taken a mouse where the stem cells are transduced with MDR-1, and given that mouse repeated courses of cytokines?

SORRENTINO: To my knowledge, that has not been done, but let me point out another interesting fact that addresses that question. Al Deisseroff had a paper some years ago showing that if you transduced with MDR-1, no expansion, and go straight into recipient mice, one can serially transplant that marrow through six secondary receipients while the control dies out at about two or three. His interpretation was that MDR-1 transduction was increasing the self-renewal of stem cells *in vivo*. That may generalize our findings beyond the *ex vivo* expansion into an *in vivo* context. We are going to do similar experiments. It is still unproved whether what we are describing is related only to the *ex vivo* expansion culture or whether P-gp is modulating stem cell behavior *in vivo*. It is a critical thing. Al's data suggest that it is generalizable but that it is clearly an area that needs more exploration. In terms of just administering cytokines and seeing if the cells are disregulated, to my knowledge that experiment has not been done.

C.J. EAVES (*Terry Fox Laboratory*): Have you or anybody looked at any other cell surface component to see if simply overexpressing a cell-surface molecule that might disturb the geography of the cell surface could have a similar effect, or is the finding you have made really specific for MDR-1?

SORRENTINO: Yes, we are going to try to get at that. There is a question whether the membrane fluidity or composition is changed by this big transmembrane protein. There are functionally dead MDR-1 mutants; there are two adenosine diphosphate (ADP) hydrolosis sites, and you can knock those out and P-gp no longer pumps substrates. So if it were simply a membrane effect then, these MDR-1 dead mutants should give the same phenotype.

K. WELTE (*Hannover Medical School*): Did you test the lifespan of these cells in the myeloproliferative syndrome?

SORRENTINO: I do not understand exactly what you mean by lifespan.

WELTE: With regard to the time of survival of granulocytes in these mice, is it longer in your mice compared to normal mice?

SORRENTINO: The half-life of the circulating cells has not been determined. What is remarkable is that these animals are completely healthy with white counts of 400,000. Probably we discovered it late because of that. As opposed to other mouse leukemias we have seen, the animals seem to tolerate it quite well. It almost acts like a chronic myelogenous leukemia (CML) in chronic phase. However, unlike CML in chronic phase, we do not think it is a monoclonal disorder.

Effects of CC, CXC, C, and CX3C Chemokines on Proliferation of Myeloid Progenitor Cells, and Insights into SDF-1-Induced Chemotaxis of Progenitors[a]

HAL E. BROXMEYER,[b–e,g] CHANG H. KIM,[b,d,e] SCOTT H. COOPER,[b,d,e] GIAO HANGOC,[b,d,e] ROBERT HROMAS,[c–e] AND LOUIS M. PELUS[f]

Departments of [b]Microbiology/Immunology and [c]Medicine and the [d]Walther Oncology Center, Indiana University School of Medicine, Indianapolis, Indiana 46202, USA
[e]The Walther Cancer Institute, Indianapolis, Indiana 46208, USA
[f]Department of Molecular Virology and Host Defense, SmithKline Beecham Pharmaceuticals, Collegeville, Pennsylvania 19426, USA

ABSTRACT: Chemokines have been implicated in the regulation of stem/progenitor cell proliferation and movement. The purpose of the present study was to assess a number of new chemokines for suppressive activity and to delve further into SDF-1-mediated chemotaxis of progenitor cells. This report extends the list of chemokines that have suppressive activity against immature subsets of myeloid progenitors stimulated to proliferate by multiple growth factors to include: MCP-4/CKβ-10, MIP-4/CKβ-7, I-309, TECK, GCP-2, MIG and lymphotactin. The suppressive activity of a number of other chemokines was confirmed. Additionally, pretreatment of the active chemokines with an acetylnitrile solution enhanced specific activity of a number of these chemokines. The new chemokines found to be lacking suppressive activity include: MCP-2, MCP-3, eotaxin-1, MCIF/HCC-1/CKβ-1, TARC, MDC, MPIF-2/eotaxin-2/CKβ-6, SDF-1 and fractalkine/neurotactin. Overall, 19 chemokines, crossing the CC, CXC, and C subgroups, have now been found to be myelosuppressive, and 14 chemokines crossing the CC, CXC and CX3C subgroups have been found to lack myelosuppressive activity under the culture conditions of our assays. Because of the redundancy in chemokine/chemokine receptor interactions, it is not yet clear through which chemokine receptors many of these chemokines signal to elicit suppressive activities. It was also found that SDF-1-induced chemotaxis of progenitors can occur in the presence of fibronectin (FN) and extracellular matrix components and that FN effects involve activation of β_1-, and possibly α_4-, integrins.

[a]This work was supported by Public Health Service Grants R01 DK53674, R01 HL56416, and R01 HL54037 and by a project in P01 HL53586 from the National Institutes of Health to Hal E. Broxmeyer.

[g]Address correspondence to: Hal E. Broxmeyer, Ph.D., Walther Oncology Center, Indiana University School of Medicine, 1044 W. Walnut Street, Room 302, Indianapolis, IN 46202-5254. Phone, 317/274-7510; fax, 317/274-7592; e-mail: hbroxmey@iupui.edu

142

INTRODUCTION

The production and movement of hematopoietic stem and progenitor cells reflect the interacting roles of stromal cells, other accessory cells, cytokines produced by these cells, and extracellular matrix (ECM) components.[1]

Among the increasing list of cytokines that can influence blood cell production and movement are members of the chemokine family.[2–7] Chemokines were originally named based on their functions as *chemo*attractant cyto*kines* for mature blood cell types. Although chemokines are a relatively new family of proteins in terms of our full understanding of the actual number of these cytokines and their receptors, over 50 chemokines have been identified. Chemokines fall into at least four different subgroups. These include those proteins with position invariant cysteine cysteine (CC), CXC (where X can be any amino acid), C or CX_3C motifs near the N-terminal portion of the molecule.[2–5]

The first member of the chemokine family to be implicated in the proliferation of myeloid progenitor cells was macrophage inflammatory protein (MIP)-1α,[8,9] a CC chemokine. MIP-1α enhanced proliferation of the more mature members of the granulocyte-macrophage (CFU-GM) and macrophage (CFU-M) progenitor cell subsets, which responded to stimulation by a single growth factor, respectively, such as granulocyte-macrophage colony-stimulating factor (GM-CSF) and macrophage (M)-CSF.[8,9] MIP-1α was subsequently found to act as a suppressor molecule for mature subsets of stem cells[10] and for the immature subsets of CFU-GM, erythroid (BFU-E, erythroid burst-forming unit) and multipotential (CFU-GEMM, granulocyte, erythroid, macrophage, megakaryocyte–colony-forming unit) progenitor cells that proliferate in response to multiple growth factors, such as erythropoietin (Epo), interleukin (IL)-3, GM-CSF and steel factor (SLF).[9,11–20] The suppressive effects of MIP-1α were direct acting on the stem/progenitor cells[12,15] and appeared to be mediated during the DNA synthesis (S)-phase of the cell cycle.[13,14] MIP-1α was also active *in vivo* and administration of MIP-1α to mice resulted in a dose-dependent, time-related, and reversible suppression of the cycling status and absolute numbers of CFU-GM, BFU-E and CFU-GEMM in the marrow and spleen.[21,22] An analogue of MIP-1α BB10010,[23] was found to suppress progenitor cell proliferation in patients on a phase I clinical trial.[24] The myelosuppressive effects of MIP-1α *in vitro* and *in vivo* were later found to be mimicked by a number of other chemokines of the CC and CXC groups.[12,14,25–40] However, not all chemokines tested were myelosuppressive.[9,11,12,14] Those chemokines that were myelosuppressive *in vitro* were myelosuppressive *in vivo* and those chemokines lacking suppressive activity *in vitro* were without suppressive effects when administered to mice.[14,21,22]

The first member of the chemokine family to demonstrate the capacity for directed movement (chemotaxis) of myeloid progenitor cells was stromal cell-derived factor (SDF)-1.[41–43] Presently, only two other chemokines, of a large number assayed, have been demonstrated to cause chemotaxis of progenitor cells, and these chemokines, MIP-3β[44] and exodus-2,[34] have a more restricted target cell population confined to CFU-M.

The aims of the study presented herein were to determine if a number of new chemokines, not previously assessed for effects on proliferation of myeloid progenitor cells, had suppressive activity on immature subsets of myeloid progenitors from normal human bone marrow that respond to the stimulating effects of a combination of growth factors. Additionally, since it has been reported that the specific activity of some chemokines can be enhanced by pretreating the chemokines with an acetylnitrile (ACN) solution,[13,14] we tested whether this enhancing activity of ACN treatment was apparent with a number of additional chemokines that crossed chemokine subgroups. Lastly, we evaluated the roles of fibronectin (FN) and ECM components on the chemotactic effects of SDF-1 for migration of progenitor cells, and assessed the involvement of integrins on this movement.

MATERIALS AND METHODS

Cytokines

Chemokine designations are usually given in abbreviated form and the same chemokine may have a number of different names. TABLE 1 lists the commonly used chemokine abbreviations and their full names. The following purified recombinant human chemokines were purchased from R&D Systems (Minneapolis, MN): MIP-1α, I-309, TECK, MCP-2, MCP-3, eotaxin-1, TARC, MDC, MIG, lymphotactin, SDF-1β, MCP-4 and fractalkine/neurotactin. SDF-1α was a kind gift from Dr. Ian Clark-Lewis (University of British Columbia, Vancouver, BC, Canada).[44] The following purified recombinant chemokines were kind gifts from SmithKline Beecham Pharmaceuticals (Collegeville, PA): MCP-4/CKβ-10, MIP-3α/LARC/exodus 1/CKβ-4, exodus- 2/6Ckine/SLC/CKβ-9, MIP-3β/ELC/exodus-3/CKβ-11,[34,44] MIP-4/CKβ-7, MPIF-1/CKβ-8, MCIF/HCC-1/CKβ-1 and MPIF-2/eotaxin-2/CKβ-6. ENA-78 was a kind gift from Dr. M.-S. Chang (Amgen Corp., Thousand Oaks, CA). Another preparation of MIP-3α/LARC/exodus-1/CKβ-4 was also prepared as described.[26] The exodus-2/6Ckine/SLC/CKβ-9 preparation used in the present study was not the same as the preparation made at the Indiana University School of Medicine and used as described in Hromas *et al.*,[27] and the preparation of MPIF-1/CKβ-8 used for the present study was not the same preparation as used and described in the study by Youn *et al.*[31] It is noted that two different preparations of MCP-4 were used in the present study. One was purchased from R&D and one was a gift from SmithKline Beecham. Some of the chemokines were pretreated in an ACN solution as previously described.[13,14] Recombinant human Epo was purchased from Amgen Corp., and the recombinant human preparations of GM-CSF, IL-3 and SLF and the murine preparation of SLF were kind gifts of Immunex Corp. (Seattle, WA).

Colony Assays

Human bone marrow cells were collected from normal volunteer donors after receiving informed consent. Murine bone marrow cells were obtained from C57Bl/6 mice after sacrifice of the mice. Murine bone marrow was used without further separation, while low-density human bone marrow cells were used after density cut separation on Ficoll-Hypaque (Pharmacia, Piscataway, NJ) gradients (density, 1.070 gm/cm^3). Human and murine bone marrow cells were plated at 5×10^4 cells/ml. Human bone marrow was plated either in 0.3% agar culture medium with 10% fetal bovine serum (FBS; Hyclone, Logan, UT) for colony formation by CFU-GM stimulated by human GM-CSF (100 U/ml) plus human SLF (50 ng/ml), or in 1% me-

TABLE 1. Commonly used chemokine abbreviations[a]

Abbreviations	Full Names
CKβ	chemokine β
ELC	EBI (EBV-induced gene) 1-ligand chemokine
ENA	epithelial-derived neutrophil attractant
GCP	granulocyte chemotactic protein
GRO	growth-related oncogene
HCC	HCC
I-309	I-309
IL-8	interleukin-8
IP	γ-interferon-inducible protein
LARC	liver and activation–regulated chemokine
LKN	leukotactin
LMC	lymphocyte and monocyte chemoattractant
MCIF	macrophage colony-inhibitor factor
MCP	monocyte chemoattractant protein
MDC	macrophage-derived chemokine
MIG	monokine induced by γ-interferon
MIP	macrophage inflammatory protein
MPIF	myeloid progenitor inhibitor factor
NAP	neutrophil-activating *p* Peptide
PF4	platelet factor-4
RANTES	regulated on activation of normal T cell expressed and secreted
SDF	stromal cell-derived factor
SLC	secondary lymphoid-tissue chemokine
TARC	thymus and activation-regulated chemokine
TECK	thymus-expressed chemokine

[a]There are a number of different MIPs (e.g., MIP-1α, MIP-1β, MIP-2α, MIP-2β, MIP-3α, MIP-3β, MIP-4 and MIP-5) and MCPs (MCP-1 to MCP-5). Additionally, there are a number of other chemokines such as eotaxin-1 and eotaxin-2, lymphotactin and fractalkine/neurotactin, exodus, and 6CKine, which are not abbreviated.

thylcellulose culture medium with 30% FBS for colony formation by CFU-GM, BFU-E and CFU-GEMM with Epo (1 U/ml), IL-3 (100 U/ml), human SLF (50 ng/ml) with or without GM-CSF (100 U/ml). The effects of chemokines were the same on colony formation by CFU-GM in agar or methylcellulose, so the CFU-GM data were pooled, and the effects of chemokines on colony formation by myeloid progenitor cells forming colonies in methylcellulose were the same in the absence and presence of GM-CSF so the data accumulated from cultures containing Epo, IL-3, SLF

−/+ GM-CSF were pooled for calculation. Murine bone marrow cells were plated in methylcellulose under the same condition as for human cells except that cells were stimulated by human Epo (1 U/ml), murine SLF (50 ng/ml) and 5% vol/vol pokeweed mitogen mouse spleen cell conditioned medium (prepared as previously described)[45] and 0.1 mM hemin (Eastman Kodak Co., Rochester, NY). Human and murine bone marrow colonies were respectively scored after 14 and 7 days' incubation at 5% CO_2 and lowered (5%) O_2 in a BNP-210 incubator (Tabai ESPEC Corp., South Plainfield, NJ). Detailed descriptions of the colony assays can be found elsewhere.[45]

Chemotaxis Assays

Chemokine-dependent chemotaxis of human growth factor-dependent M07e cells and magnetic bead-separated primary CD34$^+$ human cord blood cells was determined as previously described[34,42,44] using Costar Transwells (6.5 mm diameter, 5 μM pore size, polycarbonate membrane) with the modifications described in the legend to FIGURE 4. The cord blood was obtained with institutional review board approval for samples scheduled for discard.

Statistical Analysis

Student's *t* test was used to analyze the data. *P* values <0.05 were considered to designate significant differences between test points.

RESULTS

Influence of Chemokines on Colony Formation by Human Bone Marrow Cells Stimulated to Proliferate by Multiple Cytokines

A number of CC and CXC chemokines have been assessed for their effects on the proliferation of myeloid progenitor cells. Some have demonstrated suppressive activity. In the present studies, 16 different members of the CC chemokine family, 3 different members of the CXC chemokine family and the one known member each of the C and the CX_3C chemokine families were evaluated for their effects on colony formation by bone marrow CFU-GM, BFU-E and CFU-GEMM (FIG. 1). As shown in FIGURE 1A–C, the following CC chemokines manifested significant dose-dependent suppressive activity against the myeloid progenitors, with maximal activity usually apparent at concentrations of 50 to 100 ng/ml, and with suppressive effects titering out between 6.25 and 25 ng/ml: MCP-4/CKβ-10 (with two different preparations manifesting equivalent activity), MIP-4/CKβ-7, MPIF-1/CKβ-8, I-309, TECK, MIP-3β/ELC/exodus-3/CKβ-11, 6Ckine/exodus-2/SLC/CKβ-9, MIP-1α and exodus-1/CKβ-4. The suppressive effects of all CC chemokines on CFU-GM colony formation were significant to at least *p* <0.01 at chemokine concentrations of 25 to 100 ng/ml (Fig. 1A). Similar significant suppression was seen against BFU-E (FIG. 1B) and CFU-GEMM (FIG. 1C) for these chemokines, except that I-309 suppression was only significant at the 50- and 100-ng/ml concentrations. The following CC chemokines did not significantly suppress colony formation (*p* >0.05) at concentrations of 50 or 100 ng/ml: MCP-2, MCP-3, eotaxin-1, MCIF/HCC-1/CKβ-1, TARC, MDC, and MPIF-2/eotaxin-2/CKβ-6.

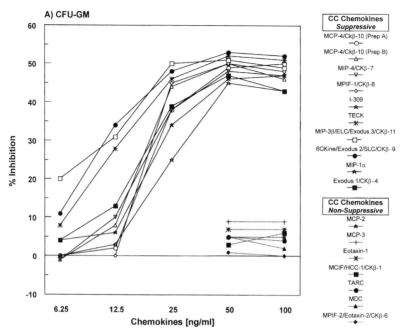

FIGURE 1. Influence of human CC **(Parts A–C)**, CXC, C, and CX_3C **(Parts D–F)** chemokines on colony formation by immature subsets of myeloid progenitor cells in normal human bone marrow stimulated to proliferate by recombinant human preparations of Epo, IL-3, SLF –/+ GM-CSF. Results are shown as mean percent inhibition for a total of 2 to 8 different experiments in which control colony numbers (mean ± 1 SEM) for CFU-GM were: 34 ± 2, 34 ± 3, 44 ± 4, 54 ± 2, 55 ± 3, 115 ± 3, 151 ± 7, 174 ± 5; for BFU-E were: 44 ± 1, 55 ± 3, 57 ± 2, 81 ± 3, 84 ± 4, 89 ± 6; and for CFU-GEMM were: 15 ± 1, 16 ± 1, 18 ± 2, 22 ± 1, 24 ± 1, 36 ± 2. Those chemokines manifesting significant suppressive activity (to at least $p <0.01$) at the 50–100-ng/ml concentrations and those chemokines without significant activity ($p >0.05$) are listed to the right of each figure as part of the figure key.

Of the CXC chemokines assessed for activity (FIG. 1D–F), MIG and GCP-2 had significant suppressive activity at 25 to 100 ng/ml (p at least <0.01) with suppression lost or almost lost at 6.25 ng/ml. Of the three CXC chemokines tested in this study, only SDF-1 was without activity. Both SDF-1α and SDF-1β were tested, and since results were the same for these chemokines, the data reflect a pooled composite of both. The C chemokine, lymphotactin, had the same significant suppressing activity (p at least <0.01) as the active CC and CXC chemokines, but the CX_3C chemokine fractalkine/neurotactin was without significant activity ($p >0.05$) in this assay (FIG. 1D–F).

As reported in a number of our other papers,[9,11–14] chemokine suppression was only partial (45–55% at optimal concentration of chemokines) for total colony formation, but it was complete or near complete inhibition of the enhanced colony formation induced by the combination of growth factors that included SLF, compared

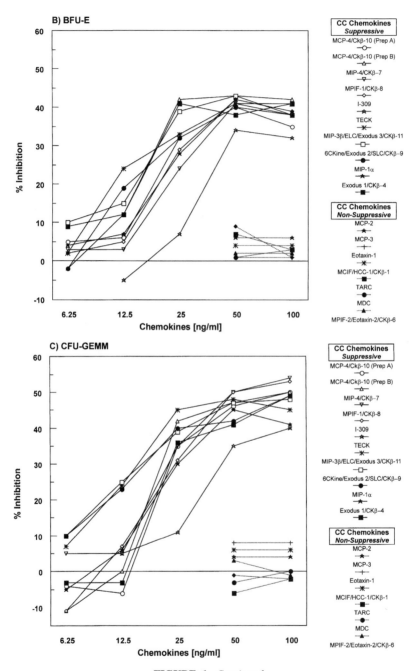

FIGURE 1. *Continued*

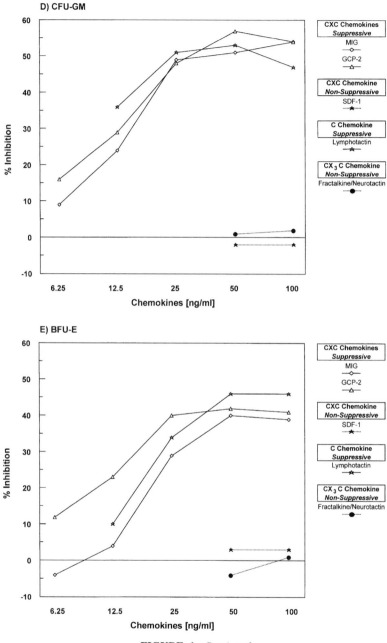

FIGURE 1. *Continued*

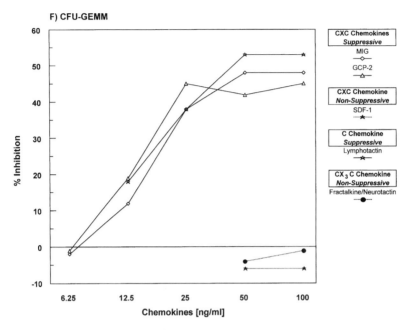

FIGURE 1. *Continued*

to the lack of suppressive effects on colonies stimulated by a single growth factor, such as Epo for BFU-E, and GM-CSF or IL-3 for CFU-GM (data not shown).

Comparative Influence of Chemokines on Colony Formation by Myeloid Progenitors in Human and Mouse Bone Marrow

A number of human chemokines of the CC and CXC groups have suppressive activity on the proliferation of myeloid progenitor cells in both human and mouse bone marrow, and have suppressive effects *in vivo* when administered to mice.[14,21–23] Eight CC, two CXC and the one C chemokine were compared at a concentration of 100 ng/ml for their effects on proliferation of progenitors in human and mouse bone marrow (FIG. 2A–C). MIP-1α, MCP-4/CKβ-10 (two different preparations), MPIF-1/CKβ-8, MIP-3β/ELC/exodus-3/CKβ-11, exodus-1/CKβ-4, MIP-4/CKβ-7, MIG and lymphotactin were equally suppressive (*p* at least <0.01) against CFU-GM (FIG. 2A), BFU-E (FIG. 2B), and CFU-GEMM (FIG. 2C) in human and mouse bone marrow. MCIF/HCC-1/CKβ-1, MPIF-2/eotaxin-2/CKβ-6 and SDF-1 were not suppressive (*p* >0.05) against the myeloid progenitors in either human or mouse marrow (FIG. 2A–C).

Influence of ACN on the Suppressive Activity of Chemokines

Pretreatment of MIP-1α,[13,14,22] MIP-2α, PF4, IL-8, MCP-1 and IP-10[14] with ACN solution significantly enhanced the suppressive activity of the chemokines both *in vitro* and *in vivo* such that significant suppression could be seen at lower

A) CFU-GM

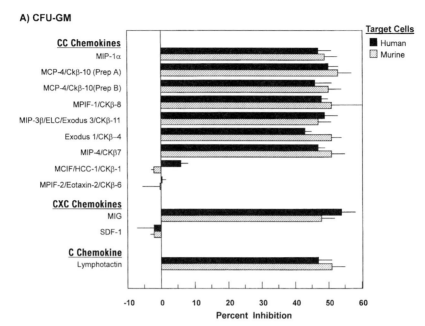

FIGURE 2. Comparative effects of human chemokines on colony formation by immature subsets of myeloid progenitor cells in normal human and C57Bl/6 mouse bone marrow. Human bone marrow cells were stimulated to proliferate by recombinant human preparations of Epo, IL-3, SLF −/+ GM-CSF, and mouse bone marrow cells were stimulated to proliferate by human Epo, murine SLF, PWMSCM and hemin. Results are shown as mean ± 1 SEM. Effects on human bone marrow cells are based on a total of 2 to 8 different experiments, and effects on mouse bone marrow cells are based on a total of 3 different experiments. Control colony numbers (mean ± 1 SEM) for human cells are the same as those given in the legend to FIGURE 1, while those for mouse CFU-GM were: 75 ± 3, 96 ± 7, 86 ± 4; for mouse BFU-E were: 11 ± 1, 8 ± 1, 11 ± 1; and for mouse CFU-GEMM were: 7 ± 1, 6 ± 1, 6 ± 1.

chemokine concentrations/doses than with the non-ACN-treated chemokines. To determine if the enhancement in chemokine suppression was a more general phenomenon than previously shown by us, two other CC chemokines (MCP-4/CKβ-10, the R&D preparation, and MIP-3α/LARC/exodus-1/CKβ-4, the Indiana University preparation[26]), two other CXC chemokines (MIG and ENA-78) and the one C chemokine (lymphotactin) were tested as previously described,[13,14] with and without ACN-pretreatment for 16 hr, for effects on colony formation by human bone marrow cells in agar culture medium stimulated to proliferate by GM-CSF and SLF (FIG. 3). The diluent control for the ACN-pretreated chemokines contained the same final concentration of ACN as the ACN-treated chemokines, and as seen in FIGURE 3, the ACN-diluent control had no effect on colony formation different from the same diluent without ACN. In all cases tested in this present study, the suppressive activity of the ACN-pretreated chemokines was manifest at significantly lower concentrations than the chemokines not pretreated with ACN. Pretreatment of chemok-

B) BFU-E

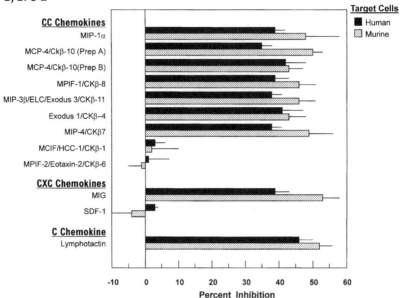

C) CFU-GEMM

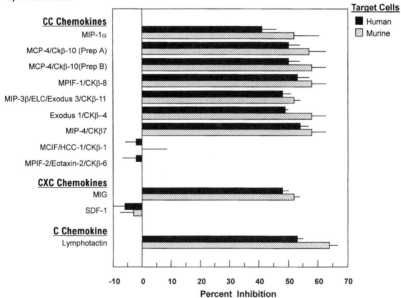

FIGURE 2. *Continued*

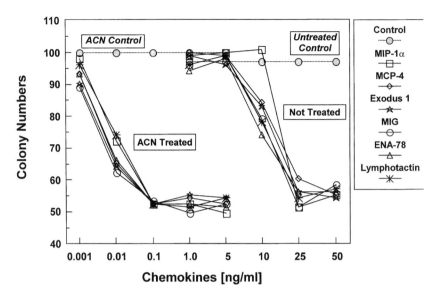

FIGURE 3. Comparison of the suppressive activities of recombinant human CC, CXC, and C chemokines on colony formation by immature subsets of granulocyte macrophage progenitor cells (CFU-GM) in normal human bone marrow with and without pretreatment of chemokines in an acetylnitrile (ACN) solution . Results for one of two reproducible experiments shown are the mean number of colonies per 5×10^4 low-density bone marrow cells plated in agar culture medium in the presence of recombinant GM-CSF and SLF.

ines with ACN, as previously reported,[13,14] enhanced the specific activity for chemokine suppression by over 1000-fold, such that one could see suppressive activity using over 1000-fold less ACN-pretreated chemokine compared with the use of that chemokine not pretreated with ACN.

Influence of SDF-1α on Chemotaxis of M07e and CD34+ Cord Blood Cells in the Presence of Fibronectin and ECM Components

SDF-1 is a potent chemoattractant for M07e cells[42,44] and for CD34+ bone marrow or cord blood cells.[41–44] The chemotactic effects of SDF-1 for M07e cells and for CD34+ cells have been assessed using bare polycarbonate membranes,[41,42,44] while CD34+ cells have also been studied for migration responses to SDF-1 through a bone marrow endothelial cell layer.[43] In the present study, we evaluated the migration of M07e cells and CD34+ bone marrow cells in response to SDF-1 through membranes coated with either FN or ECM components (FIG. 4).

As seen in FIGURE 4A, SDF-1 was a potent chemoattractant for M07e cells through FN-, and even more so through ECM-coated membranes, compared to membranes coated with BSA, which barely supported chemotaxis to SDF-1. Under these conditions, the SDF-1-induced migration of M07e cells (FIG. 4B) and CD34+ cord blood cells (FIG. 4C) through FN-coated membranes was nearly completely

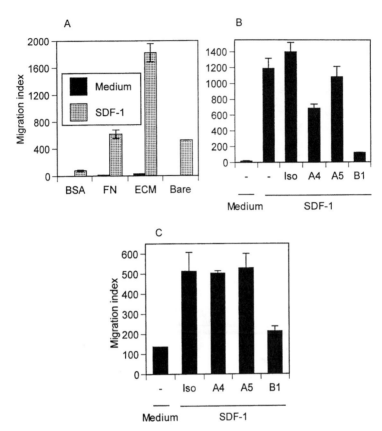

FIGURE 4. Role of fibronectin and extracellular matrix proteins in chemotaxis of M07e cells and CD34+ cells in response to SDF-1. **(A)** The upper side of bare transwell membranes were coated with BSA (Calbiochem, La Jolla, CA), fibronectin (FN, Collaborative Biomedical, Bedford, MA), or human extracellular matrix proteins (ECM, Collaborative Biomedical) at 50 μg/ml in PBS, pH 7.3 at 4°C or not coated (Bare) for chemotaxis experiments and left for 14 hr prior to use. 2×10^5 M07e cells in chemotaxis buffer (RPMI 1640 media supplemented with 0.5% BSA) were added to the upper chamber, and SDF-1 was added at 100 ng/ml to the lower chamber of transwells to attract cells. Cells migrating to the lower chamber for 4 hr were counted by FACScan for 20 s, and these cell numbers were used to calculate the migration index. **(B)** Bare transwells were coated with fibronectin, isotype control antibody, or neutralizing antibodies to integrins $\alpha 4$ (VLA-4, A4), $\alpha 5$ (VLA-5, A5), or $\beta 1$(CD29, B1) (all antibodies from Immunotech, France) were added to both chambers at 10 μg/ml final concentration to evaluate potential blocking of chemotaxis of M07e cells to SDF-1 (100 ng/ml). **(C)** 10^5 cord blood CD34+ cells, isolated as previously described,[42,44] were used instead of M07e cells for the chemotaxis experiments as in (B). Each experiment was performed in triplicate, and results are expressed as mean ± SD.

blocked with antibodies to β_1-integrin. The SDF-1-induced migration of M07e cells through the FN-coated membranes was partially blocked by antibodies to α_4-, but not α_5-, integrin (FIG. 4B). Neither α_4- nor α_5-integrins alone blocked SDF-1-induced migration of $CD34^+$ cord blood cells. Thus, SDF-1 chemotactic effects on M07e and $CD34^+$ cord blood cells are manifest in the presence of FN and ECM components and β_1-, and possibly α_4-, integrins present on M07e, and $CD34^+$ cells are involved in the SDF-1/FN migration effects

DISCUSSION

Chemokines have a number of diverse functions including chemotaxis of leukocytes, suppression of HIV infection, regulation of angiogenesis, regulation of the immune system, antitumor effects and regulation of hematopoiesis.[2-8] In the context of hematopoietic cell regulation, a number of chemokines have been implicated in suppression of the proliferation of subsets of mature stem cells and immature progenitor cells.[9-40] The present report now extends the list of chemokines that have suppressive activity on the proliferation of myeloid progenitor cells that respond to the proliferative effects of combinations of growth factors such as Epo, IL-3, GM-CSF and SLF. This report also extends the list of chemokines that do not have suppressive effects under the culture conditions utilized by us. TABLE 2 lists the chemokines tested by us, and evaluated by us and others for myelosuppressive activity and includes chemokines whose actions have been previously reported and those assessed as part of the current study. Overall, nineteen chemokines, crossing three chemokine subgroups (CC, CXC, and C) have been found to be myelosuppressive, and fourteen chemokines, crossing the CC, CXC and CX_3C subgroups were inactive as suppressor molecules for CFU-GM, BFU-E and CFU-GEMM proliferating under our culture conditions. The new chemokines shown to be suppressive in our assay include, among the CC chemokines: MCP-4/CKβ-10, MIP-4/CKβ-7, I-309, and TECK, among the CXC chemokines: GCP-2 and MIG, and in the C chemokine group: lymphotactin. The new chemokines found to lack suppressive activity in our assays include among the CC group: MCP-2, MCP-3, eotaxin-1, MCIF/HCC-1/CKβ-1, TARC, MDC and MPIF-2/eotaxin-2/CKβ-6, among the CXC group SDF-1α and SDF-1β, and for the CX_3C group: fractalkine/neurotactin. It was found that different preparations of the same chemokine manifested the exact same effects in our assay system. However, it is possible that some of the chemokines shown to be inactive as a suppressive molecule in our study may have suppressive activities for myeloid progenitors under other culture conditions. For example, MPIF-2/eotaxin-2/CKβ-6 has been shown by others to suppress high proliferative potential colony-forming cells from mouse bone marrow with some activity on human marrow CFU-GM and CFU-Mix.[38] Under the culture conditions utilized in our study, the preparation of MPIF-2/eotaxin-2/CKβ-6 we used was consistently inactive as a suppressor of progenitors in human (FIG. 1A–C) and mouse bone marrow (FIG. 2A–C). Other differences noted between groups include the larger range of suppressive activities noted for MPIF-1/CKβ-8 in a previous study of ours,[31] reproduced herein with another preparation of MPIF-1/CKβ-8, in which CFU-GM, BFU-E and CFU-GEMM were suppressed, compared to that of another group[38] that had only seen suppression on low proliferative potential colony- forming cells of the CFU-GM type. Our observations of the suppressive effects of MIG complement and add to the report of others.[40] Interestingly, we previously noted that while GRO-α has no myelosuppressive activity on

TABLE 2. Chemokines assessed by authors for their capacity to suppress colony formation by immature subsets of myeloid progenitor cells in normal human bone marrow low-density cells stimulated to proliferate by multiple growth factors

CC Chemokine	CXC Chemokine
*MIP-1α ([a]9–20)[b]	*GRO-β/MIP-2α ([a]12,14)
*MCP-1 ([a]12,14)	*IL-8/NAP-1 ([a]12,14,39)
*MCP-4/CKβ-10[b]	*PF-4 ([a]12,14,35–37)
*LKN-1/MIP-5/HCC2 ([a]30)	*IP-10 ([a]14,28,40)[d]
*MIP-3α/LARC/exodus-1/CKβ-4 ([a]26)[b]	*MIG ([a]40)[b,d]
*Exodus-2/6Ckine/SLC/CKβ-9 ([a]27,34)[b]	
*MIP-3β/exodus-3/ELC/CKβ-11 ([a]34)[b]	⊗ GRO-α ([a]12,14)[e]
*MIP-4/CKβ-7[b]	⊗ GRO-γ/MIP-2β ([a]12,14)
*MPIF-1/CKβ-8 ([a]31,38)[b]	⊗ NAP-2 ([a]12)
*CKβ-8-1 (splicing variant) ([a]31)	⊗ SDF-1[b]
*I-309[b]	
*TECK[b]	
*LMC ([a]32)	
⊗ MIP-1α ([a]9,11,14)	C Chemokine
⊗ RANTES ([a]12,14)	*Lymphotactin[b]
⊗ MCP-2[b]	
⊗ MCP-3[b]	CX₃C Chemokine
⊗ Eotaxin-1[b]	⊗ Fractalkine/neurotactin[b]
⊗ MCIF/HCC-1/CKβ-1[b]	
⊗ TARC[b]	
⊗ MDC[b]	
⊗ MPIF-2/eotaxin-2/CKβ-6[b,c]	

*Suppressive chemokines.
⊗ Nonsuppressive chemokines.
[a]Reference number for published reports on suppressive/nonsuppressive effects of chemokines on proliferation of myeloid progenitor cells.
[b]Effects are reported in present paper.
[c]While we did not note inhibition in our assay system with MPIF-2/eotaxin-2/CKβ-6, others[38] have noted suppressive effects under different culture conditions.
[d]Reference 40 describes MIG suppression of IGF-II-dependent enhancement of CFU-GM and LTC- IC, and IL-3 and SLF enhancement of CFU-GM.
[e]While we did not note inhibition in our assay with GRO-α, others[39] have reported the suppressive effects of GRO-α on IL-3-dependent proliferation of the murine 32D cell line.

primary progenitor cells, it does block the myelosuppressive activity of other chemokines including IL-8 and PF-4.[12] Reports by others suggest that GRO-α has a similar suppressive activity to IL-8 on proliferation of the murine 32D cell line in response to IL-3 stimulation.[39] Whether GRO-α will have suppressive activity on primary progenitor cells under different culture conditions than that used by us remains to be determined.

Of the human chemokines tested in the present study, the myelosuppressive effects on human and mouse bone marrow progenitors were similar, suggesting that human MIP-1α, MCP-4/CKβ-10, MPIF-1/CKβ-8, MIP-3β/ELC/exodus- 3/CKβ-11, exodus-1/CKβ-4, MIP-4/CKβ-7, MIG and lymphotactin recognize and can signal through chemokine receptors on both human and mouse target cells. This adds to the list of human chemokines that have effects on mouse cells and allows the testing of these new chemokines for effects on myelopoiesis *in vivo* in mice. Such preclinical studies could lead to testing in human clinical trials. MIP-1α,[46,47] IL-8[48] and PF-4[48,49] have shown myeloprotective effects in the context of chemotherapy in mice and an analogue of MIP-1α, BB10010 has been tested in mice[23] and in human clinical trial for activity.[24] While BB10010 had myelosuppressive activity on the progenitors, myeloprotection in the context of chemotherapy has not yet been seen. Perhaps other chemokines, such as those reported here, will be more effective, alone or in combination, as myeloprotective agents.

Whether the effects of chemokines resulting in suppression of myeloid progenitor cell proliferation are always direct acting on the progenitors themselves needs to be evaluated for each of the new active chemokines. While there is strong evidence from studies on the effects of chemokines on single isolated progenitors that the actions of some chemokines are direct,[15] this does not rule out the possibility of suppression also being mediated indirectly through actions on accessory or stromal cells, a possibility especially difficult to rule out in studies *in vivo*.

Regardless of whether the myelosuppressive effects are direct or indirect acting, the actions are mediated through chemokine receptors. Which specific chemokine receptors mediate the suppressive effects of the individual chemokines is not clear and is complicated because of the known redundancy of some chemokine/chemokine receptor interactions. Some chemokines bind more than one receptor, and some receptors bind more than one chemokine.[6,7] Of those chemokines found to bind only one receptor so far, there is still the possibility that other receptors will be identified that bind these chemokines.

Chemokine receptors are cell surface proteins with 7-transmembrane domains coupled to heterotrimeric G-proteins; nine CC receptors (designated CCR1 to CCR9), five CXC receptors (designated CXCR1 to CXCR5), one CX_3C receptor (designated CX_3CR1) and one C receptor (designated XCR1) have been identified (reviewed in Refs. 6,7). CCR1 binds MIP-1α, RANTES, MCP-3, LKN-1 and MPIF-1; CCR2 binds MCP-1 to MCP-5; CCR3 binds eotaxin, RANTES, MCP-2, MCP-3, MCP-4, MPIF-2 and LKN-1; CCR4 binds TARC and MDC; CCR5 binds RANTES, MIP-1α and MIP-1β; CCR6 binds MIP-3α; CCR7 binds MIP-3β and exodus-2; CCR8 binds I-309, TARC and MIP-1α; CCR9 promiscuously binds a number of CC chemokines but does not appear to signal in response to them; CXCR2 binds IL-8, GRO-α, GRO-β, GRO-γ, GCP-2, ENA-78 and other ELR chemokines; CXCR3 binds IP-10 and MIG; CXCR4 binds SDF-1; CXCR5 binds BCA-1/BLC; CX_3CR1 binds fractalkine; and XCR1 binds lymphotactin.

It is likely that chemokine receptors dominant for mediating the suppressive and other hematopoietic effects of chemokines will have to be identified by studies in which the specific chemokine receptors have been 'knocked-out'/functionally deleted. Use of 'gene knock-out' mice has suggested that IL-8 or a murine equivalent of IL-8, such as murine MIP-2, mediate their suppressive effects through CXCR2,[50] and MCP-1 mediates its effects through CCR2.[51,52] CCR1 does not appear to be a dominant receptor mediating the myelosuppressive effects of MIP-1α, although it appears to be a dominant receptor that mediates the enhancing effects of MIP-1α on more mature subsets of CFU-GM.[53] Further delineation of the dominant chemokine receptors involved in mediating the suppressive effects of chemokines awaits the production of viable mice in which chemokine receptors have been functionally deleted, or of progenitor cells in which specific receptors have been deleted.

In contrast to the numbers of different chemokines that can mediate myelosuppression, the numbers of chemokines that mediate chemotaxis of progenitor cells is rather limited and is currently confined to three: SDF-1,[41–44] MIP-3β/exodus-3/ELC/CKβ-11,[34,44] and exodus-2/6Ckine/SLC/CKβ-9.[34] SDF-1 has the broadest range of activities and attracts CFU-GM, BFU-E and CFU-GEMM, while MIP-3β and exodus-2 attract mainly macrophage progenitors (CFU-M). To answer the question whether other chemokines will be found to attract stem or progenitor cells or subsets of these cells requires additional work, but the identification of such chemokines could impact stem cell transplantation in a positive way. Studies have demonstrated that only a small percentage of stem cells that are infused into mice actually home to an environment conducive to the growth of these cells. Being able to direct or enhance direction of stem and progenitor cells to their appropriate microenvironmental niches *in vivo* could increase the engraftment potential of these cells, and possibly allow the use of fewer cells for optimal engraftment. Identification of a chemokine that could attract the earliest subsets of stem cells with long-term marrow repopulating capacity would be especially useful in the context of stem cell transplantation.

Not much is known regarding the conditions under which SDF-1 induces chemotaxis of progenitor cells, or the mechanisms involved in this specific chemoattraction. SDF-1 has been shown to attract progenitor cells through bare membranes, and also through a bone marrow endothelial cell line layer. In the present paper we have added additional information by demonstrating the effects of SDF-1-mediated chemotaxis through membranes coated with FN and ECM components. Interestingly, migration of M07e cells in response to SDF-1 was more active under the conditions in which ECM components were used, compared to that of FN and BSA. It is not yet known whether this is true for primary CD34+ cells or what integrins are involved in this adhesion and movement. However, for FN, both M07e and CD34+ cord blood cells are utilizing β1-integrins. This area warrants further investigation, especially as to the intracellular mechanisms involved in the 'inside-out' and 'outside-in' signaling shown to be involved in FN adhesion studies using other cytokines.[54–57]

ACKNOWLEDGMENTS

The authors thank Becki Miller for preparation of the manuscript.

REFERENCES

1. BROXMEYER, H.E. 1998. The hematopoietic system: Principles of therapy with hematopoietically active cytokines. *In* Cytokines in the Treatment of Hematopoietic Failure. A. Ganser & D. Hoelzer, Eds.: 1–37. Marcel Dekker. New York.
2. BAGGIOLINI, M. 1998. Chemokines and leukocyte traffic. Nature **392**: 565–568.
3. MURPHY, P.M. 1996. Chemokine receptors: Structure, function and role in microbial pathogenesis. Cytokine Growth Factor Rev. **7**: 47–64.
4. ROLLINS, B.J. 1997. Chemokines. Blood **90**: 909–928.
5. BAGGIOLINI, M., B. DEWALD & B. MOSER. 1997. Human chemokines: An update. Annu. Rev. Immunol. **15**: 675–705.
6. BROXMEYER, H.E. & C.H. KIM. 1998. Chemokines and hematopoiesis. In Chemokines and Cancer. B.J. Rollins, Ed. Humana Press. Totowa, NJ. In press.
7. KIM, C.H. & H.E. BROXMEYER. 1998. Chemokines for immature blood cells: Effects on migration, proliferation and differentiation. In Chemokines and Diseases. M.E. Rothenberg, Ed. Marcel Dekker. New York. In press.
8. BROXMEYER, H.E., B. SHERRY, L. LU, S. COOPER, C. CAROW, S.D. WOLPE & A. CERAMI. 1989. Myelopoietic enhancing effects of murine macrophage inflammatory proteins 1 and 2 *in vitro* on colony formation by murine and human bone marrow granulocyte-macrophage progenitor cells. J. Exp. Med. **170**: 1583–1594.
9. BROXMEYER, H.E., B. SHERRY, L. LU, S. COOPER, K.-O. OH, P. TEKAMP-OLSON, B.S. KWON & A. CERAMI. 1990. Enhancing and suppressing effects of recombinant murine macrophage inflammatory proteins on colony formation *in vitro* by bone marrow myeloid progenitor cells. Blood **76**: 1110–1116.
10. GRAHAM, G.J., E.G. WRIGHT, R. HEWICK, S.D. WOLPE, N.M. WILKIE, D. DONALDSON, S. LORIMORE & I.B. PRAGNELL. 1990. Identification and characterization of an inhibitor of haemopoietic stem cell proliferation. Nature **344**: 442–444.
11. BROXMEYER, H.E., B. SHERRY, S. COOPER, F.W. RUSCETTI, D.E. WILLIAMS, P. AROSIO, B.S. KWON & A. CERAMI. 1991. Macrophage inflammatory protein (MIP)-1b abrogates the capacity of MIP-1a to suppress myeloid progenitor cell growth. J. Immunol. **147**: 2586–2594.
12. BROXMEYER, H.E., B. SHERRY, S. COOPER, L. LU, R. MAZE, M.P. BECKMANN, A. CERAMI & P. RALPH. 1993. Comparative analysis of the suppressive effects of the human macrophage inflammatory protein family of cytokines (chemokines) on proliferation of human myeloid progenitor cells. J. Immunol. **150**: 3448–3458.
13. MANTEL, C., Y.-J. KIM, S. COOPER, B. KWON & H.E. BROXMEYER. 1993. Polymerization of murine macrophage inflammatory protein-1a inactivates its myelosuppressive effects *in vitro*. The active form is monomer. Proc. Natl. Acad. Sci. USA **90**: 2232–2236.
14. BROXMEYER, H.E., S. COOPER, N. HAGUE, L. BENNINGER, A. SARRIS, K. CORNETTA, S. VADHAN-RAJ, P. HENDRIE & C. MANTEL. 1995. Human chemokines: Enhancement of specific activity and effects *in vitro* on normal and leukemic progenitors and a factor dependent cell line and *in vivo* in mice. Ann. Hematol. **71**: 235–246.
15. LU, L., M. XIAO, S. GRIGSBY, W.X. WANG, B. WU, R.-N. SHEN & H.E. BROXMEYER. 1993. Comparative effects of suppressive cytokines on isolated single CD34^{+++} stem/progenitor cells from human bone marrow and umbilical cord blood plated with and without serum. Exp. Hematol. **21**: 1442–1446.
16. CLEMENTS, J.M., S. CRAIG, A.J.H. GEARING, M.G. HUNTER, C.M. HEYWORTH, T.M. DEXTER & B.I. LORD. 1992. Biological and structural properties of MIP-1α expressed in yeast. Cytokine **4**: 76–82.
17. GRAHAM, G.J., M.G. FRESHNEY, D. DONALDSON & I.B. PRAGNELL. 1992. Purification and biochemical characterisation of human and murine stem cell inhibitors (SCI). Growth Factors **7**: 151–160.
18. KELLER, J.R., S.H. BARTELMEZ, E. SITNICKA, F.W. RUSCETTI, M. ORTIZ, J.M. GOOYA & S.E.W. JACOBSEN. 1994. Distinct and overlapping direct effects of macrophage

inflammatory protein-1α and transforming growth factor β on hematopoietic progenitor/stem cell growth. Blood **84:** 2175–2181.

19. MAYANI, H., M.T. LITTLE, W. DRAGOWSKA, G. THORNBURY & P.M. LANSDORP. 1995. Differential effects of the hematopoietic inhibitors MIP-1α, TGF-β, and TNF-α on cytokine–induced proliferation of subpopulations of CD34$^+$ cells purified from cord blood and fetal liver. Exp. Hematol. **23:** 422–427.

20. SU, S.B., N. MUKAIDA, J.B. WANG, Y. ZHANG, A. TAKAMI, S. NAKAO & K. MATSUSHIMA. 1997. Inhibition of immature erythroid progenitor cell proliferations by macrophage inflammatory protein-1α by interacting mainly with a C-C chemokine receptor, CCR1. Blood **90:** 605–611.

21. MAZE, R., B. SHERRY, B.S. KWON, A. CERAMI & H.E. BROXMEYER. 1992. Myelosuppressive effects *in vivo* of purified recombinant murine macrophage inflammatory protein-1 alpha. J. Immunol. **149:** 1004–1009.

22. COOPER, S., C. MANTEL & H.E. BROXMEYER. 1994. Myelosuppressive effects *in vivo* with very low dosage of monomeric recombinant murine macrophage inflammatory protein-1α. Exp. Hematol. **22:** 186–193.

23. HUNTER, M.G., L. LAWDEN, D. BROTHERTON, S. CRAIG, S. CRIBBES, L.G. CZAPLEWSKI, T.M. DEXTER, A.H. DRUMMOND, A.H. GEARING, C.M. HEYWORTH, B.I. LORD, M. MCCOURT, P.G. VARLEY, L.M. WOOD, R.M. EDWARDS & P.J. LEWIS. 1995. BB-10010: An active variant of human macrophage inflammatory protein-1α with improved pharmaceutical properties. Blood **86:** 4400–4408.

24. BROXMEYER, H.E., A. ORAZI, N.L. HAGUE, G.W. SLEDGE, JR., H. RASMUSSEN & M.S. GORDON. 1998. Myeloid progenitor cell proliferation and mobilization effects of BB10010, a genetically engineered variant of human macrophage inflammatory protein-1α, in a phase I clinical trial in patients with relapsed/refractory breast cancer. Blood Cells Mol. Dis. **24:**14–30.

25. DALY, T.J., G.J. LAROSA, S. DOLICH, T.E. MAIONE, S. COOPER & H.E. BROXMEYER. 1995. High activity suppression of myeloid progenitor proliferation by chimeric mutants of interleukin 8 and platelet factor 4. J. Biol. Chem. **270:** 23282–23292.

26. HROMAS, R., P.W. GRAY, D. CHANTRY, M. KRATHWOHL, K. FIFE, G.I. BELL, J. TAKEDA, S. ARONICA, M. GORDON, S. COOPER, H.E. BROXMEYER & M. KLEMSZ. 1997. Cloning and characterization of exodus, a novel b-chemokine. Blood **89:** 3315–3322.

27. HROMAS, R., C.H. KIM, M. KLEMSZ, M. KRATHWOHL, K. FIFE, S. COOPER, C. SCHNIZLEIN-BICK & H.E. BROXMEYER. 1997. Isolation and characterization of exodus-2, a novel C-C chemokine with a unique 37 amino acid carboxy terminal extension. J. Immunol. **159:** 2554–2558.

28. SARRIS, A.H., H.E. BROXMEYER, U. WIRTHMUELLER, N. KARASAVVAS, J. KRUEGER & J.V. RAVETCH. 1993. Human interferon inducible protein 10: Expression and purification of recombinant protein demonstrate inhibition of early human hematopoietic progenitors. J. Exp. Med. **178:** 1127–1132.

29. YOUN, B.S., I.-K. JANG, H.E. BROXMEYER, S. COOPER, N.A. JENKINS, D.J. GILBERT, N.G. COPELAND, T.A. ELICK, M.J. FRASER, JR. & B.S. KWON. 1995. A novel chemokine, macrophage inflammatory protein-related protein-2, inhibits colony formation of bone marrow myeloid progenitors. J. Immunol. **155:** 2661–2667.

30. YOUN, B.S., S.M. ZHANG, E.K. LEE, D.H. PARK, H.E. BROXMEYER, P.M. MURPHY, M. LOCATI, J.E. PEASE, K.K. KIM, K. ANTOL & B.S. KWON. 1997. Molecular cloning of leukotactin-1: A novel human b-chemokine, a chemoattractant for neutrophils, monocytes and lymphocytes, and a potent agonist at CC chemokine receptors 1 and 3. J. Immunol. **159:** 5201–5205.

31. YOUN, B.S., S.M. ZHANG, H.E. BROXMEYER, S. COOPER, K. ANTOL, M. FRASER & B.S. KWON. 1998. Characterization of CKβ-8 and CKβ8-1: Two alternatively

spliced forms of human β-chemokine, chemoattractants for neutrophils, monocytes and lymphocytes, and potent agonists at CC chemokine receptor 1. Blood **91:** 3118–3126.

32. YOUN, B.S., S. ZHANG, H.E. BROXMEYER, K. ANTOL, M.J. FRASER, JR., G. HANGOC & B.S. KWON. 1998. Isolation and characterization of LMC, a novel lymphocyte and monocyte chemoattractant human CC chemokine with myelosuppressive activity. Biochem. Biophys. Res. Commun. **247:** 217–222.

33. BROXMEYER, H.E., S. COOPER, Z.H. LI, L. LU, A. SARRIS, M.H. WANG, C. METZ, M.S. CHANG, D.B. DONNER & E.J. LEONARD. 1996. Macrophage-stimulating protein, a ligand for the RON receptor protein tyrosine kinase, suppresses myeloid progenitor cell proliferation and synergizes with vascular endothelial cell growth factor and members of the chemokine family. Ann. Hematol. **73:** 1–9.

34. KIM, C.H., L.M. PELUS, E. APPELBAUM, K. JOHANSON & H.E. BROXMEYER. 1998. Functional comparision of the two ligands of CC chemokine receptor CCR7, SLC/6Ckine/Exodus 2 and CKβ-11/MIP-3β/ELC. Submitted for publication.

35. GEWIRTZ, A.M., B. CALABRETTA, B. RUCINSKI, S. NIEWIAROWSKI & W.Y. XU. 1988. Inhibition of human megakaryocytopoiesis *in vitro* by platelet factor 4 (PF4) and a synthetic COOH-terminal PF4 peptide. J. Clin. Invest. **83:** 1477–1486.

36. GEWIRTZ, A.M., J. ZHANG, J. RATAJCZAK, M. RATAJCZAK, K.S. PARK, C. LI, Z. YAN & M. PONCZ. 1995. Chemokine regulation of human megakaryocytopoiesis. Blood **86:** 2559–2567.

37. HAN, Z.C., L. SENSEBE, J.F. ABGRALL & J. BRIERE. 1990. Platelet factor 4 inhibits human megakaryocytopoiesis *in vitro*. Blood **75:** 1234.

38. PATEL, V.P., B.L. KREIDER, Y. LI, H. LI, K. LEUNG, T. SALCEDO, B. NARDELLI, V. PIPPALLA, S. GENTZ, R. THOTAKURA, D. PARMELEE, R. GENTZ & G. GAROTTA. 1997. Molecular and functional characterization of two novel human CC chemokines as inhibitors of two distinct classes of myeloid progenitors. J. Exp. Med. **185:** 1163–1172.

39. SANCHEZ, X., K. SUETOMI, B. COUSINS-HODGES, J.K. HORTON & J. NAVARRO. 1998. CXC chemokines suppress proliferation of myeloid progenitor cells by activation of the CXC chemokine receptor 2. J. Immunol. **160:** 906–910.

40. SCHWARTZ, G.N., F. LIAO, R.E. GRESS & J.M. FARBER. 1997. Suppressive effects of recombinant human monokine induced by IFN-((rHuMig) chemokine on the number of committed and primitive hematopoietic progenitors in liquid cultures of CD34+ human bone marrow cells. J. Immunol. **159:** 895–904.

41. AIUTI, A., I.J. WEBB, T. SPRINGER & J.C. GUTIERREZ-RAMOS. 1997. The chemokine SDF-1 is a chemoattractant for human CD34+ hematopoietic progenitor cells and provides a new mechanism to explain the mobilization of CD34+ progenitors to peripheral blood. J. Exp. Med. **185:** 111–120.

42. KIM, C.H & H.E. BROXMEYER. 1998. *In vitro* behavior of hematopoietic progenitor cells under the influence of chemoattractants: Stromal cell-derived factor-1, steel factor and the bone marrow environment. Blood **91:** 100–110.

43. MÖHLE, R., F. BAUTZ, S. RAFII, M.A.S. MOORE, W. BRUGGER & L. KANZ. 1998. The chemokine receptor CXCR-4 is expressed on CD34+ hematopoietic progenitors and leukemic cells and mediates transendothelial migration induced by stromal cell-derived factor-1. Blood **91:** 4523–4530.

44. KIM, C.H., L.M. PELUS, J.R. WHITE & H.E. BROXMEYER. 1998. CKb-11/MIP-3b/ELC, a CC chemokine, is a chemoattractant with a specificity for macrophage progenitors amongst myeloid progenitor cells. J. Immunol. **161:** 2580–2585.

45. COOPER, S. & H.E. BROXMEYER. 1996. Measurement of interleukin-3 and other hematopoietic growth factors, such as GM-CSF, G-CSF, M-CSF, erythropoietin and the potent co-stimulating cytokines steel factor and Flt-3 ligand. In Current

Protocols in Immunology. J.E. Coligan, A.M. Kruisbeek, D.H. Margulies, E.M. Shevach, W. Strober & R. Coico, Eds. Suppl **18:** 6.4.1–6.4.12. John Wiley & Sons, Inc. New York.

46. DUNLOP, D.J., E.G. WRIGHT, S. LORIMORE, G.J. GRAHAM, T. TOLYOAKE, D.J. KERR, S.D. WOLPE & I.B. PRAGNELL. 1992. Demonstration of stem cell inhibition and myeloprotective effects of SCI/rhMIP-1α *in vivo.* Blood **79:** 2221–2225.

47. LORD, B.I., T.M. DEXTER, J.M. CLEMENTS, M.A. HUNTER & A.J.H. GEARING. 1992. Macrophage-inflammatory protein protects multipotent hematopoietic cells from the cytotoxic effects of hydroxyurea *in vivo.* Blood **79:** 2605–2609.

48. BROXMEYER, H.E., S. COOPER, T. MAIONE, M. GORDON & T. DALY. 1995. Myeloprotective effects of the chemokines interleukin-8 and platelet factor 4 in a mouse model of cytosine arabinoside (ARA-C) chemotherapy [abstract]. Exp. Hematol. **23:** 900.

49. HAN, Z.C., M. LU, J. LI, M. DEFARD, B. BOVAL, N. SCHLEGEL & J.P. CAEN. 1997. Platelet-factor 4 and other CXC chemokines support the survival of normal hematopoietic cells and reduce the chemosensitivity of cells to cytotoxic agents. Blood **89:** 2328–2335.

50. BROXMEYER, H.E., S. COOPER, G. CACALANO, N.L. HAGUE, E. BAILISH & M.W. MOORE. 1996. Interleukin-8 receptor is involved in negative regulation of myeloid progenitor cells *in vivo*: Evidence from mice lacking the murine IL-8 receptor homolog. J. Exp. Med. **184:** 1825–1832.

51. BORING, L., J. GOSLING, S.W. CHENSUE, S.L. KUNKEL, R.V. FARESE, JR., H.E. BROXMEYER & I.F. CHARO. 1997. Impaired monocyte migration and reduced type 1 (Th1) cytokine responses in C-C chemokine receptor 2 knockout mice. J. Clin. Invest. **100:** 2552–2561.

52. REID, S., A. RITCHIE, L. BORING, S. COOPER, G. HANGOC, I.F. CHARO & H.E. BROXMEYER. 1999. Enhanced myeloid progenitor cell cycling and apoptosis in mice lacking the chemokine receptor, CCR2. Blood. In press.

53. BROXMEYER, H.E., S. COOPER, G. HANGOC, J.L. GAO & P.M. MURPHY. 1997. Chemokine receptor CCR1 acts as a dominant receptor for MIP-1a enhancement of proliferation of mature progenitors *in vitro*, MIP-1a mobilization of progenitors *in vivo*, and MIP-1a enhancement of G-CSF induced mobilization, but not for MIP-1a suppression of immature progenitors *in vitro*: Effects elucidated using CCR1 knock-out mice [abstract]. Blood **90** (Suppl. 1, Part 1): 571a.

54. TAKAHIRA, H., A. GOTOH, A. RITCHIE & H.E. BROXMEYER. 1997. Steel factor enhances integrin-mediated tyrosine phosphorylation of focal adhesion kinase (pp125FAK) and paxillin. Blood **89:** 1574–1584.

55. GOTOH, A., H. TAKAHIRA, R.L. GEAHLEN & H.E. BROXMEYER. 1997. Cross-linking of integrins induces tyrosine phosphorylation of proto-oncogene product vav and protein tyrosine kinase Syk in a human factor-dependent myeloid cell line. Cell Growth & Differ. **8:** 721–729.

56. GOTOH, A., A. RITCHIE, H. TAKAHIRA & H.E. BROXMEYER. 1997. Thrombopoietin and erythropoietin activate inside-out signal of integrin and enhance adhesion to immobilized fibronectin in human growth-factor-dependent hematopoietic cells. Ann. Hematol. **75:** 207–213.

57. SHIBAYAMA, H., N. ANZAI, A. RITCHIE, S. ZHANG, C. MANTEL & H.E. BROXMEYER. 1998. Interleukin-3 and Flt3-ligand induce adhesion of Baf3/Flt3 precursor B-lymphoid cells to fibronectin via activation of VLA-4 and VLA-5. Cell. Immunol. **187:** 27–33.

DISCUSSION

D. METCALF (*P. O. Royal Melbourne Hospital*): I am puzzled by your cell cycle data on progenitor cells from +/+ mice. You showed figures of 10% of progenitors being in S phase in normal marrow. That is an unusually low figure.

BROXMEYER: In my experience, a lot of the knock-out animals have been bred on backgrounds where the proliferation of the progenitor cells is not very high. Many of the wild-type littermate control mice of the knock-out mice I have had the opportunity to work with over the past three years have slowly cycling cells. A good number of the wild-type littermate controls of the knock-outs, especially the ones on the C57Bl/6 background, have progenitor cells that do not show very much cyclying when assayed by the tritiated thymidine kill assay. The cycling is consistent within the mice from the different knock-out experiments.

METCALF: We have never seen that in about 30 strains that we have looked at. I am surprised.

BROXMEYER: Cycling rates may relate to the degree of mouse strain crossings and back-crossings that generate the knock-out and littermate controls. Most importantly, results are all consistent internally, which is what matters.

Y. REISNER (*Weizmann Institute of Science*): Have you tried to look at the effect *in vivo* of these two chemokines that you were showing?

BROXMEYER: We have begun experiments with SDF-1. It works the same as IL-8 and MIP-1α, but the mobilization is very modest. At best we are getting a twofold increase in progenitor cells being mobilized by SDF-1. Mobilization is seen within 15–30 minutes, and within an hour you do not see it. We just do not have enough CKβ-11 with which to do these same experiments at this time.

REISNER: But you said you hoped it would improve engraftment rather than look at mobilization. Have you tried to look at engraftment?

BROXMEYER: No. I believe, and I know that my graduate student Chang Kim believes, that what you see in the movement of cells depends on where these materials are really being expressed—the amount that is in the marrow versus the amount that you are putting into the animals and the amounts in the other organs. We are beginning to work with making transgenic mice where we are trying to either express the genes in all the cells or trying limiting expression to the thymus especially for the thymic migration. A problem is just getting enough material to do the kinds of experiments we really want to do.

W.E. FIBBE (*University Medical Center Leiden*): I want to come back to one of your experiments in the CCR1 knock-out mice where you have observed this increase in mobilization in response to G-CSF. Is there any difference between these animals in other respects? For instance, in white blood cell counts or neutrophils or progenitors in the marrow ?

BROXMEYER: There is not a lot of difference in mature cells in the CCR1 knockouts versus the littermate controls. There are differences in the movement of progenitor cells between the organs. We do not see differences in the numbers of progenitors or neutrophils in the marrow.

Dissecting the Marrow Microenvironment

BEVERLY TOROK-STORB,[a] MINEO IWATA, LYNN GRAF, JOANN GIANOTTI,
HEIDI HORTON, AND MICHAEL C. BYRNE

*Clinical Research Division, Fred Hutchinson Cancer Research Center, Seattle,
Washington, USA and Genetics Institute, Cambridge, Massachusetts, USA*

ABSTRACT: Cloned human stromal cell lines representing functionally distinct cellular components of the marrow microenvironment were generated to serve as tools for identifying gene products that regulate hematopoiesis. Oligonucleotide arrays, or "gene chips" were used to provide a comprehensive comparison of gene expression among the cell lines. One line, designated HS-5, was found to secrete large amounts of cytokines, and conditioned media from this line was found to support the *ex vivo* expansion of both immature and mature progenitors. In contrast, a second line, designated HS-27a, does not secrete known cytokines but does support cobblestone area formation by CD34+/38lo cells. HS-27a, but not HS-5, was also found to express h.Jagged1, a ligand for Notch1, which may function to influence cell fate decisions of hematopoietic precursors. Both cell lines are currently being used to identify other gene products that regulate hematopoiesis and to generate reagents that will allow more formal evaluation of the putative role of h.Jagged1 in hematopoietic cell fate decisions.

It is generally agreed that maintenance of an undifferentiated stem cell pool is critical for long-term hematopoiesis, yet the mechanisms responsible for preventing hematopoietic stem cell differentiation have not been identified. Studies conducted to understand this phenomenon suggest that regulatory signals involve cellular interactions that require direct cell:cell contact as well as indirect interactions mediated by factors or matrix, both of which occur within the marrow microenvironment (ME). The hematopoietic ME is defined largely by function as a complex of cells and factors critical for the maintenance and regulation of stem cells and their progeny. For several decades primary long-term cultures (LTCs) of marrow stroma have been used to approximate the ME. The functional complex as defined by this system consists of several heterogeneous populations of cells, including endothelial cells, fibroblasts, fat cells, adventitial reticular cells, and macrophages. A properly functioning LTC is capable of maintaining a population of stem cells for several months and at the same time supporting proliferation and at least myeloid differentiation. A large body of work in this area has resulted in the identification of many gene products produced by stromal cells that have very definite effects on the proliferation and maturation rates of progenitor cells (reviewed in Ref. 1). Therefore, while it is clear that cytokines like interleukin-6 (IL-6), granulocyte colony-stimulating factor (G-CSF), and granulocyte/macrophage colony-stimulating factor (GM-CSF) made in LTC

[a]Address all correspondence to: Beverly Torok-Storb, Ph.D., Fred Hutchinson Cancer Research Center, 1100 Fairview Avenue N., D1-100, P.O. Box 19024, Seattle, WA 98109-1024. Phone, 206/ 667-4549; fax, 206/667-5978, e-mail, btorokst@fhcrc.org

TABLE 1. Variable characteristics of five human stromal (HS) lines

	HS-5	HS-17	HS-21	HS-23	HS-27a
Constitutive factor secretion	++++	–	+++	+	–
Inducible factor secretion	ND	+++	ND	+++	+
Constitutive VCAM-1	–	+	+	+	++++
Cobblestone support	–	–	–	–	+++
Collagen I	+	–	–	–	+
Collagen III	+++	ND	+	+++	++
Collagen IV	+++	+++	+	+++	++
Constitutive ICAM-1	+++	ND	++	+	++
Inducible ICAM-1	+++	ND	+++	+++	+++
CD34$^+$ cell proliferation	++++	–	–	–	–

Abbreviations: ICAM, intercellular adhesion molecule; VCAM, vascular cell adhesion molecule.

contribute to myelopoiesis,[2] it is less clear what gene products are responsible for the maintenance of stem cells.

During steady-state hematopoiesis most stem cells are thought to be quiescent. Historically this quiescence has been interpreted as an absence of sufficient positive stimulating signals and/or the presence of inhibitory signals. Considerable effort has been directed towards identifying signals that can inhibit hematopoiesis, and several have been identified. Transforming growth factor-β (TGF-β), macrophage inflammatory protein-1α (MIP-1α), interferon (IFN), and tumor necrosis factor (TNF) have all been shown to inhibit hematopoiesis in various *in vitro* assays and, in some cases, when administered to mice they can inhibit the cycling activity of progenitors *in vivo*.[3–7] Whether these activities play a role in maintaining the undifferentiated state of stem cells, as well as preventing cell division, is not clear. Inhibitory signals have been detected in LTCs, but given the complexity of this assay system, the source of these activities, how their expression is controlled, and how they work in the context of other ME signals is unknown.[8,9]

More recently several groups have used cloned stromal cell lines in an effort to identify individual ME components.[10–15] We used a recombinant retrovirus to transduce normal human stromal cells with the E6/E7 genes of the human papilloma virus.[16] The E6/E7 gene products interfere with the cell cycle regulators p53 and Rb, respectively, resulting in immortalized cells that appear to retain a relatively normal mature phenotype. In our initial studies, over 30 clones were isolated, expanded and screened for hematopoietic supporting activity. Detailed studies have been conducted on five of these cell lines chosen on the basis of morphology, surface phenotype and function. Functions of interest are those that mimic characteristics of primary LTCs. They include the ability to support the formation of cobblestone areas by CD34$^+$ cells, the production of activities to support the proliferation and differentiation of CD34$^+$ cells, and the ability to upregulate cytokine production in response to IL-1. A brief description of these five human stromal (HS) lines is summarized in TABLE 1.

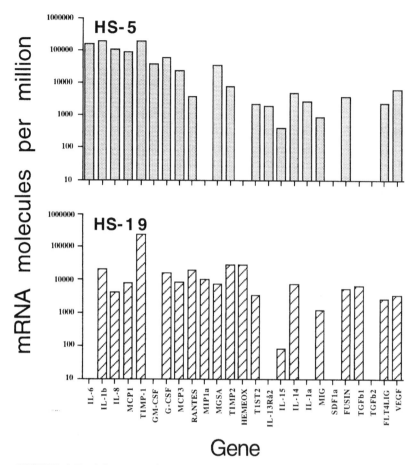

FIGURE 1. Partial summary from the oligonucleotide arrays ("gene chips") representing mRNA molecules per million for 25 of the known RNA sequences analyzed.

Our overall strategy has been to develop cloned stromal cell lines that represent functionally distinct cell types of the ME and then determine which expressed genes, known and unknown, are associated with each specific function. Known genes of interest were first addressed using enzyme-linked immunosorbent assay (ELISA)-based assays to detect proteins of interest. These results, already reported, did not provide a sufficiently comprehensive analysis to discriminate among lines.[16] For this reason, we initiated a collaboration with Drs. Steve Clark and Michael Byrne of Genetics Institute to use oligonucleotide arrays ("gene chips")[17] to screen simultaneously for differential expression of 250 human genes that play a role in hematopoiesis and immunology. A partial summary showing differential expression of 25 known genes is provided in FIGURE 1. These data serve to confirm our hypothesis that these cell lines are distinct; they also help to focus our studies on molecules that may be associated with particular functions. As shown in FIGURE 1, HS-5 and

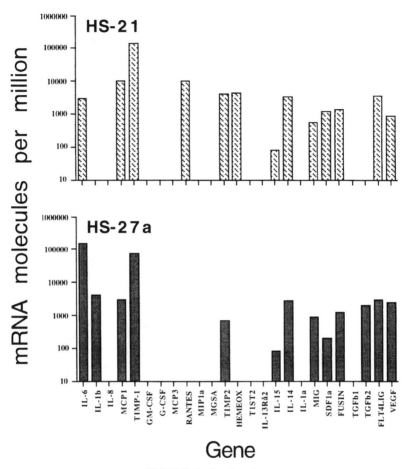

FIGURE 1. Continued.

HS-27a, which have very distinct functions, also have very different expressed gene profiles. A more detailed discussion of these two lines is provided below.

The HS-5 stromal line can be distinguished grossly from HS-27a by the absence of contact inhibition of cell growth and the production of a visible layer of extracellular matrix. As mentioned above, HS-5 cells can also be distinguished on a functional level by their constitutive production of known cytokines. A detailed comparison of HS-5 conditioned media (CM) with various cocktails of recombinant factors indicated that HS-5 CM plus one additional cytokine, either kit ligand (KL) or flt3-ligand, produces the highest fold increase in colony-forming units (CFUs) from CD34[+] cells.[18] In particular, the combination of HS-5 CM plus flt3-ligand not only increases CFUs but also maintains stem cells capable of long-term repopulation as measured by serial transplantation in fetal sheep.[19] These observations have led to the development of a Phase I clinical protocol to use HS-5 CM plus flt3-ligand for

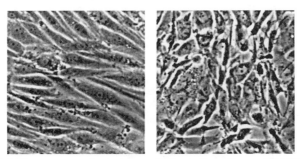

FIGURE 2. Phase contrast photomicrograph of growing cultures of HS-27a cells on the *left* and HS-5 cells on the *right*. The image was obtained using an inverted Nikon Biophot microscope with direct camera attachment. Original magnification was 400×.

ex vivo expansion of CD34$^+$ cells in an autologous transplantation model. Our goal is to use HS-5 CM plus flt3-ligand to expand progenitors and stem cell numbers in situations where cell dose is limiting. Ultimately, we want to identify the activities in HS-5 CM responsible for the *ex vivo* expansion.

In contrast to HS-5, initial screening studies indicated that HS-27a supported the formation of cobblestone areas by CD34$^+$ 38^{lo} cells. However, it did not support the proliferation and differentiation of CD34$^+$ cells in serum-free media. HS-27a can also be distinguished morphologically from HS-5 as shown in FIGURE 2. The fact that HS-27a supported cobblestone area formation made it reasonable to speculate that this cell line may prove useful for isolating gene products associated with that function. For this purpose a number of monoclonal antibodies have been generated that distinguish HS-27a from HS-5. Of greater interest was the fact that the gene for hJagged1, recently cloned in collaboration with Dr. Linheng Li of the University of Washington, was expressed by HS-27a.[20] Both Western and Northern analyses indicated that HS-27a, but not HS-5, expresses this gene (FIG. 3).

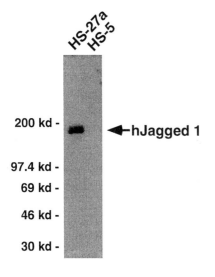

FIGURE 3. Antibody J89, which recognizes an intracellular domain of hJagged1, specifically recognized a 180-kD protein detected in HS-27a cells but not HS-5 cells. The J89 antibody was developed and characterized as previously described.[20]

hJagged1 is a homolog for rat Jagged1, which is known to interact with Notch1, a surface receptor that, when activated, plays a role in cell-fate decisions.[21–27] In collaboration with Dr. Laurie Milner, also of the Fred Hutchinson Cancer Research Center, we have shown that hJagged1 expressed by HS-27a cells activates Notch1 expressed by 32D cells and prevents G-CSF-induced differentiation of the 32D cells. These observations suggest that hJagged1 expressed on marrow stroma cells may function as a ligand for Notch1 and that the interaction between Jagged1 ligand and Notch1 receptor may play a role in mediating cell-fate decisions for human hematopoietic progenitors. However, whether hJagged1 expressed on HS-27a cells plays a role in cobblestone area formation remains to be determined. Studies to address this possibility require reagents capable of blocking or mimicking the hJagged function. Our efforts to generate such reagents are underway. Critical to this process is the identification of a simple and fast assay to detect Notch/Jagged signaling. Our recent efforts to identify such an assay are summarized briefly in the following paper by Tanaka *et al.*

ACKNOWLEDGMENTS

This work was supported in part by Grants DK34431, DK51417, HL36444, and CA18221 from the National Institutes of Health, Bethesda, MD, USA.

REFERENCES

1. MOORE, M.A.S. 1991. Clinical implications of positive and negative hematopoietic stem cell regulators. Blood **78:** 1–19.
2. BROXMEYER, H.E., D.E. WILLIAMS, G. HANGOC *et al.* 1987. Synergistic myelopoietic actions *in vivo* after administration to mice of combinations of purified natural murine colony-stimulating factor 1, recombinant murine interleukin 3, and recombinant murine granulocyte/macrophage colony-stimulating factor. Proc. Natl. Acad. Sci. USA **84:** 3871–3875.
3. BROXMEYER, H.E., B. SHERRY, L. LU *et al.* 1990. Enhancing and suppressing effects of recombinant murine macrophage inflammatory proteins on colony formation *in vitro* by bone marrow myeloid progenitor cells. Blood **76:** 1110–1116.
4. BROXMEYER, H.E., D.E. WILLIAMS, L. LU *et al.* 1986. The suppressive influences of human tumor necrosis factors on bone marrow hematopoietic progenitor cells from normal donors and patients with leukemia: synergism of tumor necrosis factor and interferon-gamma. J. Immunol. **136:** 4487–4495.
5. CASHMAN, J.D., A.C. EAVES, U.H. KOSZINOWSKI, R. ROSS & C.J. EAVES. 1990. Mechanisms that regulate the cell cycle status of very primitive hematopoietic cells in long-term human marrow cultures. I. Stimulatory role of a variety of mesenchymal cell activators and inhibitory role of TGF-beta. Blood **75:** 96–101.
6. GOEY, H., J.R. KELLER, T. BACK, D.L. LONGO, F.W. RUSCETTI & R.H. WILTROUT. 1989. Inhibition of early murine hemopoietic progenitor cell proliferation after *in vivo* locoregional administration of transforming growth factor-beta 1. J. Immunol. **143:** 877–880.
7. MOSES, H.L., E.Y. YANG & J.A. PIETENPOL. 1990. TGF-beta stimulation and inhibition of cell proliferation: new mechanistic insights [review]. Cell **63:** 245–247.
8. VERFAILLIE, C.M. 1993. Soluble factor(s) produced by human bone marrow stroma increase cytokine-induced proliferation and maturation of primitive hematopoietic progenitors while preventing their terminal differentiation. Blood **82:** 2045–2053.

9. VERFAILLIE, C.M., P.M. CATANZARRO & W.N. LI. 1994. Macrophage inflammatory protein 1 alpha, interleukin 3 and diffusible marrow stromal factors maintain human hematopoietic stem cells for at least eight weeks *in vitro*. J. Exp. Med. **179:** 643–649.
10. TSAI, S., S.G. EMERSON, C.A. SIEFF & D.G. NATHAN. 1986. Isolation of a human stromal cell strain secreting hemopoietic growth factors. J. Cell. Physiol. **127:** 137–145.
11. NOVOTNY, J.R., U. DUEHRSEN, K. WELCH, J.E. LAYTON, J.S. CEBON & A.W. BOYD. 1990. Cloned stromal cell lines derived from human Whitlock/Witte-type long-term bone marrow cultures. Exp. Hematol. **18:** 775–784.
12. SLACK, J.L., J. NEMUNAITIS, D.F. ANDREWS & J.W. SINGER. 1990. Regulation of cytokine and growth factor gene expression in human bone marrow stromal cells transformed with simian virus 40. Blood **75:** 2319–2327.
13. SINGER, J.W., P. CHARBORD, A. KEATING *et al.* 1987. Simian virus 40-transformed adherent cell lines from human long-term marrow cultures: cloned cell lines produce cells with stromal and hematopoietic characteristics. Blood **70:** 464–474.
14. THALMEIER, K., P. MEISSNER, G. REISBACH, M. FALK, A. BRECHTEL & P. DORMER. 1994. Establishment of two permanent human bone marrow stromal cell lines with long-term post irradiation feeder capacity. Blood **83:** 1799–1807.
15. WILLIAMS, D.A., M.F. ROSENBLATT, D.R. BEIER & R.D. CONE. 1988. Generation of murine stromal cell lines supporting hematopoietic stem cell proliferation by use of recombinant retrovirus vectors encoding simian virus 40 large T antigen. Mol. Cell. Biol. **8:** 3864–3871.
16. ROECKLEIN, B.A. & B. TOROK-STORB. 1995. Functionally distinct human marrow stromal cell lines immortalized by transduction with the human papilloma virus E6/E7 genes. Blood **85:** 997–1005.
17. LOCKHART, D.J., H.L. DONG, M.C. BYRNE *et al.* 1996. Expression monitoring by hybridization to high-density olignocleotide arrays. Nat. Biotechnol. **14:** 1675–1680.
18. ROECKLEIN, B.A., J. REEMS, S. ROWLEY & B. TOROK-STORB. 1998. *Ex vivo* expansion of immature 4-hydroperoxycyclophosphamide resistant progenitor cells from G-CSF mobilized peripheral blood. Biol. Blood Marrow Transplant. In press.
19. ROECKLEIN, B., G. ALMAIDA-PORADA, B. TOROK-STORB *et al.* 1997. Serial xenogeneic transplantation of *ex vivo* expanded human CD34+ cells [abstract #1750]. Blood **90** (Suppl. 1): 393a.
20. LI, L., L.A. MILNER, Y. DENG *et al.* 1998. The human homolog of *rat Jagged1* expressed by marrow stroma inhibits differentiation of 32D cells through interaction with Notch1. Immunity **8:** 43–55.
21. ARTAVANIS-TSAKONAS, S., K. MATSUNO & M.E. FORTINI. 1995. Notch signaling. Science **268:** 225–232.
22. NYE, J.S. & R. KOPAN. 1995. Developmental signaling. Vertebrate ligands for Notch. Curr. Biol. **5:** 966–969.
23. SIMPSON, P. 1995. Developmental genetics. The Notch connection. Nature **375:** 736–737.
24. ELLISEN, L.W., J. BIRD, D.C. WEST *et al.* 1991. TAN-1, the human homolog of the *Drosophila* notch gene, is broken by chromosomal translocations in T lymphoblastic neoplasms. Cell **66:** 649–661.
25. ROBEY, E., D. CHANG, A. ITANO *et al.* 1996. An activated form of Notch influences the choice between CD4 and CD8 T cell lineages. Cell **87:** 483–492.
26. MILNER, L.A., R. KOPAN, D.I.K. MARTIN & I.D. BERNSTEIN. 1994. A human homologue of the *Drosophila* developmental gene, *Notch*, is expressed in CD34+ hematopoietic precursors. Blood **83:** 2057–2062.
27. MILNER, L.A., A. BIGAS, R. KOPAN, C. BRASHEM-STEIN, I.D. BERNSTEIN & D.I.K. MARTIN. 1996. Inhibition of granulocytic differentiation by *m*Notch1. Proc. Natl. Acad. Sci. USA **93:** 13014–13019.

Stromal Inhibition of Myeloid Differentiation

A Possible Role for hJagged1

JUNJI TANAKA, MINEO IWATA, LYNN GRAF, IAN GUEST, AND
BEVERLY TOROK-STORB[a]

*Clinical Research Division, Fred Hutchinson Cancer Research Center, Seattle,
Washington 98109-1024, USA*

Cloned human stromal cell lines, HS-27a and HS-23, were established in our laboratories as previously described.[1] HS-27a, unlike HS-23, supports the formation of cobblestone areas from immature $CD34^{+}/38^{-}$ cells. Recently we reported that HS-27a expresses a human homolog for rat Jagged1 (hJagged1), a ligand for Notch1, which may play a role in cell-fate decisions that prevent differentiation and allow cobblestone area formation.[2] The purpose of the current study was to develop a model for investigating whether hJagged1 can prevent myeloid differentiation. Towards this end we used U937 cells, which can be induced to differentiate by exposure to *all trans* retinoic acid (ATRA). This model was attractive because the induction of differentiation could be easily followed by the expression of CD11b on the surface of the differentiating cells. Critical to the model was the observation that U937 cells do express considerable amounts of mRNA for Notch1 (data not shown), suggesting that the receptor may be present on these cells.

Based on the observations that Notch/Jagged interactions induce several genes that have the recombination binding protein Jκ (RBPJκ) consensus sequence, we first used electrophoretic mobility shift assays (EMSA) to detect the induction of nuclear protein binding to this consensus sequence in U937 cells before and after they were cultured on either hJagged1-expressing HS-27a cells or hJagged1-negative HS-23 cells. The data shown in FIGURE 1 indicate that the EMSA assay is specific for the DNA binding protein and, further, that nuclear protein binding to the RBPJκ consensus sequence was increased when Notch-expressing cells were cultured with HS-27a, but not after coculturing with HS-23. This strongly suggested that Notch/Jagged signaling occurs in the U937 cells, although it is possible that some other, as yet undefined, molecule on HS-27a cells is responsible for inducing the increase in DNA binding protein.

We next hypothesized that if Notch/Jagged signaling prevented U937 from differentiating in response to ATRA, this block would result in the failure of U937 cells to express CD11b, which is uniformly induced during differentiation. To test this hypothesis, U937 cells were cultured in ATRA alone or in the presence of HS-23 or HS-27a cells. After 4 days the nonadherent and adherent U937 cells were harvested separately and analyzed by fluorescence-activated cell sorter (FACS) for expression of CD11b. FIGURE 2 shows that U937 cells exposed to ATRA alone or in the pres-

[a]Address all correspondence to: Beverly Torok-Storb, Ph.D., Fred Hutchinson Cancer Research Center, 1100 Fairview Avenue North, D1-100, P.O. Box 19024, Seattle, WA 98109-1024. Phone, 206/667-4549; fax, 206/667-5978; e-mail, btorokst@fhcrc.org

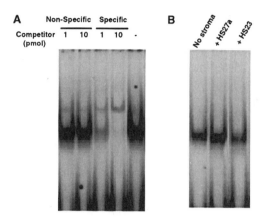

FIGURE 1. (**A**) The addition of unlabeled specific probe (Cp: ACACGCC<u>GTGGGA</u> <u>AAAAATTT</u>, RBPJκ consensus sequence is underlined) inhibited the induction of nuclear protein binding to the RBPJκ consensus sequence in a dose-dependent manner. The addition of nonspecific probe, however, did not interfere with binding; establishing the specificity of the assay. (**B**) Nuclear protein binding to the RBPJκ consensus sequence was increased after culturing the Notch1-expressing cells on HS-27a but not after culturing on HS-23 cells.

ence of HS-23 cells uniformly increase their expression of CD11b reflecting their differentiation process. In contrast, 30–40% of the U937 cells that adhered to HS-27a did not show increased expression of CD11b, suggesting they did not differentiate. By sorting and reculturing these CD11b^{lo} U937 cells, it was possible to establish that they were viable and could be induced to differentiate after a second exposure to ATRA (data not shown).

These data suggest that U937 cells in contact with HS-27a cells are blocked in ATRA-induced differentiation. Whether this is mediated by hJagged 1 or some other molecule is not clear from these studies. However, measuring the induction of differentiation by flow analysis of CD11b expression provides a quick way to detect inhibition of differentiation. Therefore, this model should prove useful for identifying antibodies that block this regulatory effect or peptides that mimic it.

REFERENCES

1. ROECKLEIN, B.A. & B. TOROK-STORB. 1995. Functionally distinct human marrow stromal cell lines immortalized by transduction with the human papilloma virus E6/E7 genes. Blood **85:** 997–1005.
2. LI, L., L.A. MILNER, Y. DENG, M. IWATA, A. BANTA, L. GRAF, S. MARCOVINA, C. FRIEDMAN, B.J. TRASK, L. HOOD & B. TOROK-STORB. 1998. The human homolog of *rat Jagged1* expressed by marrow stroma inhibits differentiation of 32D cells through interaction with Notch1. Immunity **8:** 43–55.

DISCUSSION

S.J. SHARKIS (*Johns Hopkins Oncology Center*): You told us that the HS-5 cells with Flt-3 ligand or maybe stem cell factor (SCF) might be potentially very exciting

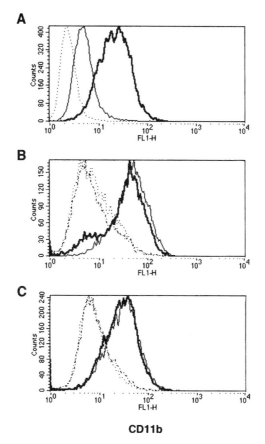

CD11b

FIGURE 2. **(A)** CD11b expression of U937 cells cultured for 4 days in the presence (bold line) or absence (thin line) of 25 μM ATRA. The dotted line represents U937 cells labeled with an isotype control IgG1a antibody. **(B)** CD11b expression of U937 cells cultured on HS-27a cells in the presence of ATRA (solid lines) or in the absence of ATRA (dotted lines). The solid bold line represents the adherent population retrieved after treatment with ethylenediaminetetraacetic acid (EDTA). The thin solid line represents the nonadherent population. **(C)** represents the same groups cultured on HS-23 cells.

with activity for expansion of long-term repopulating cells. You said you do not know what that factor might be in HS-5 cells. On the other hand, do you know what it is not in terms of known cytokines?

TOROK-STORB: Yes. Once we knew the profile of known cytokines that were expressed, we tried to reconstruct that mix using recombinant cytokines. However, we could not mimic the effect. It could be that we did not have things in the right proportion. Our suspicion, and the suspicion of our collaborators, is that there is an as yet undefined activity that is responsible. It may have some IL-3-like activity, but it is not IL-3. IL-3 is not made by HS-5 cells.

SHARKIS: It is interesting, because a recent report in Blood (March, 1998) shows that thrombopoietin (TPO), SCF and Flt -3 ligand seem to be the best combination for expansion activity. So I was particularly interested in whether or not you looked for TPO as a possibility.

TOROK-STORB: We have looked for TPO, and it is there at low levels. But we have not been able to demonstrate that TPO is responsible for the effect.

D.A. WILLIAMS (*Riley Hospital for Children*): If it is an IL-3-like activity that is not IL-3, couldn't you use a read out on an IL-3 cell line, then eliminate IL-3 clones that you picked up? This is the way we did the IL-11 cloning.

TOROK-STORB: We probably can. The functional expression cloning that is being done now for that activity is being done at Genetics Institute. However, the assay itself is proprietary, so I am not allowed to speak to it.

WILLIAMS: I apologize to Dr. Zipori in advance, because I cannot remember the name of the negative regulator that he identified from stromal cells. But it reminds me of your data. Do you know whether that is a similar activity or not?

TOROK-STORB: I do not know. If I remember correctly, he did not have a sequence for that activity. If he had a sequence, it would be quite easy to find out.

WILLIAMS: He had an activity.

TOROK-STORB: Yes, he had an activity, and you are right, it was very similar.

G. STAMATOYANNOPOULOS (*University of Washington*): What are the initial cells you transduced? Fibroblast?

TOROK-STORB: No. It was a primary long-term stromal culture. It was only 2 weeks old, and had many different cell types in it.

STAMATOYANNOPOULOS: So they were primary cells?

TOROK-STORB: It was a primary long-term stromal culture.

STAMATOYANNOPOULOS: After transduction you came out with 250 clones.

TOROK-STORB: We came out with a lot of clones, but only worked up about 100.

STAMATOYANNOPOULOS: You showed examples of clones with tremendous differences in phenotype.

TOROK-STORB: Yes.

STAMATOYANNOPOULOS: Is this expected for primary cells?

TOROK-STORB: Yes.

STAMATOYANNOPOULOS: Do you think that these are epigenetic effects?

TOROK-STORB: In primary long-term cultures, at least in the ones we grow, there are endothelial cells, there are macrophages, there are fibroblasts, there are reticular cells, there are adipocytes. There are many different kinds of cells.

STAMATOYANNOPOULOS: So there are different lineages?

TOROK-STORB: Yes, many represent different lineages.

P.M. LANSDORP (*Terry Fox Laboratory*): How exactly did you document expansion to justify clinical trials?

TOROK-STORB: We had done a lot of in vitro studies, looking at various combinations of cytokine cocktails. We decided, based on the data set that I showed you, that HS-5 cells with kit ligand (KL) or Flt-3 ligand gave us the best expansion. Then we collaborated with Esmail Zanjani to determine if our expanded cells would still provide long-term hematopoiesis in sheep. He did serial transplantation in fetal sheep and demonstrated that he did get long-term hematopoiesis.

LANSDORP: But was that better or worse than the cells without expansion?

TOROK-STORB: We did not test the cells without expansion, but in our clinical protocol, we are not giving expanded cells only. It is a phase 1 trial where we give expanded cells together with unmanipulated product. It is just a toxicity trial, so we are not yet at the stage where we would use expanded cells exclusively.

I. LEMISCHKA (*Princeton University*): I would like to make a comment that gets to Dr. Sharkis's point and also to yours. In our hands when we look at stromal cell lines that are absolutely dead negative in terms of supporting any primitve activity and compare them to lines that are very, very good, at least at the RNA level, all of them express SCF, Flt-3 ligand and TPO. Therefore, at least at that level your point is very well taken that there are likely to be other activities. Have you done a gain-of-function experiment and put Jagged into a cell line that normally does not express it and see if you can restore any activity? And also, have you looked at the cells that are expanded in response to the Jagged-expressing line and demonstrated that in fact they express Notch?

TOROK-STORB: We are doing the gain-of-function experiment now, because it was strongly suggested to us. The reason we hesitated to do it, was because I had a bias that Jagged operates in the context of other molecules expressed by HS-27a cells. The functional readout may be influenced by other molecules, like vascular cell adhesion molecule-1 (VCAM-1), which are uniquely expressed by HS-27a cells. In addition, the absence of factors like granulocyte colony-stimulating factor (G-CSF) may also be critical for the functional assay. HS-27a cells do not make G-CSF, and I think that in some assays G-CSF could override the Jagged-mediated inhibition. So I was reluctant to do the gain-of-function experiment. I was concerned that if we expressed Jagged in HS-5 cells, we might not get the same effect because of the large quantities of cytokines expressed by HS-5 cells and the fact that HS-5 cells do not express VCAM-1. What I wanted to do was knock out Jagged in HS-27a cells. We had proposed to do homologous recombination. Phil Sorriano was going to help us with a strategy to recycle the vectors to knock out both copies. But we found out that HS-27a cells actually have 3 copies of Jagged instead of 2, because they have a dicentric chromosome 20 and Jagged is on 20. So it was going to be quite difficult to knock it out this way. We still want to do the loss-of-function experiment. We shall probably use a retrovirus and just do a shotgun approach with different antisense sequences to try to knock it out. However, we are doing the gain-of-function experiment, but I am very apprehensive about the interpretation of these studies for the reasons I have just given. We have made the gain-of-function construct, we have expression, but we do not yet have a functional read out.

G. KELLER (*Howard Hughes Medical Institute*): What function are you interested in? It seemed that this cell line was less interesting than your HS-5 cell line.

TOROK-STORB: The reason we focused on the HS-27a cell line was because it supported cobblestone area formation, and the other stromal lines did not.

KELLER: Does the one that supports the expansion of CD34 cells express Jagged? That was not clear.

TOROK-STORB: No, it does not.

Regulation of Transendothelial Migration of Hematopoietic Progenitor Cells

ROBERT MÖHLE,[a,d] FRANK BAUTZ,[a] SHAHIN RAFII,[b] MALCOLM A.S. MOORE,[c] WOLFRAM BRUGGER,[a] AND LOTHAR KANZ[a]

[a]Department of Medicine II, University of Tübingen, Tübingen, Germany
[b]Cornell University Medical College, Division of Hematology & Oncology, New York, New York, USA
[c]Laboratory of Developmental Hematopoiesis, Sloan-Kettering Institute, New York, New York, USA

ABSTRACT: Transendothelial migration of hematopoietic progenitor cells occurs in the bone marrow during mobilization and homing, and may therefore play a key role in the trafficking of hematopoietic stem cells. We hypothesize that adhesion molecules, chemokines, and paracrine cytokines are involved in this multifactorial process. As suggested in several studies, downregulation of adhesion molecules (e.g., integrins) may contribute to mobilization of progenitors due to a decreased avidity to bone morrow stromal and endothelial cells, which express the corresponding ligands. Using an *in vitro* model of transendothelial migration, we have shown that only a small number of more mature, committed progenitors migrates spontaneously under the control of adhesion molecules of the beta-2-integrin family and their corresponding endothelial/stromal ligands. However, transendothelial migration of progenitors *in vitro* is substantially enhanced by the chemokine stromal cell-derived factor-1 (SDF-1), which is constitutively produced by bone marrow stromal cells. More primitive progenitors also respond to this chemokine. In addition, the ligand for SDF-1, the chemokine receptor CXCR-4, is expressed in greater levels on bone marrow CD34+ cells as compared to mobilized progenitors, suggesting that downregulation of chemokine receptors occurs during progenitor mobilization. Indeed, bone marrow CD34+ cells migrate more avidly in response to SDF-1 than mobilized progenitors. Paracrine cytokines may also play a role in hematopoietic stem cell trafficking, since growth factor-stimulated hematopoietic cells produce cytokines that act on endothelial cells (e.g., vascular endothelial growth factor, VEGF), modifying their proliferation, motility, permeability, and fenestration. We conclude that transendothelial migration of hematopoietic progenitor cells is regulated by adhesion molecules, paracrine cytokines, and chemokines. Cytotoxic therapy as well as exogenously administered hematopoietic growth factors may affect adhesion molecule expression, the local cytokine and chemokine milieu, and chemokine receptor expression, which indirectly results in mobilization of hematopoietic stem cells.

[d]Address for correspondence: Robert Möhle, M.D., Dept. of Medicine II, University of Tübingen, Otfried-Müller-Str. 10, 72076 Tübingen, Germany. Phone, +49-7071-2982726; fax, +49-7071-293671; e-mail, robert.moehle@med.uni-tuebingen.de

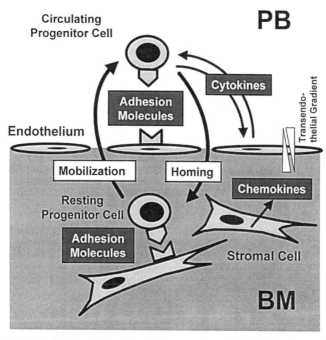

FIGURE 1. Trafficking of hematopoietic progenitor cells. Mobilization and homing of hematopoietic progenitor cells are multifactorial processes that involve interactions via adhesion molecules, chemokines, and paracrine cytokines. Transendothelial migration most likely plays a key role in hematopoietic progenitor cell trafficking. Adhesion molecules expressed on progenitor and bone marrow endothelial cells may regulate transition from the resting to the circulating progenitor cell compartment and *vice versa*. Chemokines produced in the bone marrow stroma build up transendothelial gradients that may either support or inhibit migration of progenitor cells across the endothelial layer. In addition, endothelial cells can produce cytokines that influence proliferation and motility of progenitors, and hematopoietic progenitor cells may also produce cytokines that act on endothelial cells.

MOBILIZATION AND HOMING OF HEMATOPOIETIC PROGENITOR CELLS: A MULTIFACTORIAL PROCESS

The mechanisms regulating mobilization and homing of hematopoietic stem and progenitor cells are still poorly understood. Since endothelial cells separate the resting from the circulating progenitor cell compartment,[1] we hypothesize that progenitor cell trafficking is at least partially regulated at the level of the bone marrow microvascular endothelium. Indeed, migration across bone marrow endothelium occurs *in vivo* during both mobilization and homing of progenitor cells. As suggested particularly by *in vivo* studies, progenitor cell mobilization is a multifactorial process, involving adhesion molecules, paracrine cytokines, and chemokines (FIG. 1). Adhesion molecules expressed on progenitors recognize their corresponding ligands on stromal and endothelial cells, while stromal cells produce cytokines acting on progenitors. Also endothelial and stromal cells may be influenced by progenitor cell-derived cytokines. Moreover, transendothelial gradients of chemokines (cytokines with chemotactic activity) produced by stromal cells could control direction and efficacy of progenitor cell migration.

THE ROLE OF ADHESION MOLECULES IN PROGENITOR CELL TRAFFICKING

It has been shown in previous studies that hematopoietic progenitor cells from the bone marrow and peripheral blood express adhesion molecules (selectins, selectin ligands, integrins, CD44, and PECAM[2–5]). However, none of these adhesion molecules is specific for progenitor cells. In mature leukocytes, selectins, integrins, and PECAM mediate the sequential steps of leukocyte extravasation in inflamed tissues, which involves reversible attachment ("rolling"), firm adhesion, and finally transendothelial migration.[6] Interestingly, it has been shown that bone marrow microvascular endothelium *in vivo* expresses adhesion molecules such as vascular cell adhesion molecule (VCAM, ligand for the beta-1-integrin very late activation-antigen-4, VLA-4) and E-selectin in the absence of inflammation,[7,8] suggesting that integrins and selectins may also play a role in progenitor cell trafficking. Moreover, it has been shown that the adhesion molecule PECAM is involved in transendothelial progenitor cell migration *in vitro*[9] similar to studies using mature leukocytes (monocytes).[10]

Several studies have shown that the beta-1-integrin VLA-4 and the beta-2-integrin LFA-1 (leukocyte function antigen-1) are downregulated on circulating progenitors, suggesting a role for these integrins in stem cell mobilization and homing.[11,12] *In vivo*-administration of antibodies to VLA-4 has been shown to mobilize progenitors,[13] while antibodies to VLA-4 and VCAM interfere with stem cell homing to the bone marrow.[14] These studies further support the idea that integrins play an important role in stem cell trafficking. Ligands for integrins (VCAM-1 and ICAM-1 (intercellular adhesion molecule-1)) are found on bone marrow stromal and endothelial cells.[7,15] In addition, extracellular matrix proteins (e.g., fibronectin) have also been shown to act as as integrin ligands.[16]

Cytokines and cytokine receptors may also act as adhesion molecules. It has been reported that stem cell factor (SCF, c-kit ligand) is expressed as a membrane-bound molecule on bone marrow stromal and endothelial cells.[17,18] The corresponding cytokine receptor (c-kit) is found on hematopoietic progenitor cells. Interestingly, circulating progenitors express a lower level of c-kit as compared to bone marrow CD34+ cells, which suggests a role in progenitor mobilization similar to the integrins LFA-1 and VLA-4, which are also downmodulated on circulating progenitors.[19]

We and other groups have described methods for the isolation of primary bone marrow endothelial cells and the generation of bone marrow endothelial cell lines, and have developed *in vitro* models of transendothelial progenitor cell migration.[20–23] In our *in vitro* model, the immortalized human bone marrow endothelial cell line BMEC-1 (bone marrow endothelial cell-1), grown on 3-μm microporous transwell membranes, separates an upper from a lower chamber in a 6-well tissue culture plate.[23] CD34+ hematopoietic progenitor cells from bone marrow or peripheral blood are added to the upper chamber of the transmigration system and incubated for

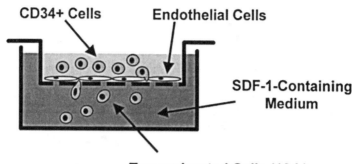

CD34+ Cells   **Endothelial Cells**

SDF-1-Containing Medium

Transmigrated Cells (10 h)

FIGURE 2. An *in vitro* model of transendothelial migration of hematopoietic progenitor cells. The human bone marrow endothelial cell line BMEC-1[22,23] was grown to confluency on 3-µm microporous transwell membrane inserts, separating upper from lower chambers in 6-well tissue culture plates. CD34$^+$ progenitor cells were added to the upper chamber of the transmigration system. Transmigrated progenitors could be recovered from the lower chamber after incubation for 10 h at $37°C/5\%$ CO_2. This system allows quantification of transendothelial migration as well as characterization of transmigrated and nonmigrating cells. The effect of chemokines added to the lower chamber (e.g., SDF-1), which build up a transendothelial gradient, can also be assessed.

10 hours. Transmigrated progenitor cells can be recovered from the lower chamber and quantified (FIG. 2).

We have shown that only a small number of hematopoietic progenitor cells migrates spontaneously across bone marrow endothelium *in vitro*.[23] More primitive, CD34$^+$/CD38$^-$ progenitors could not be detected in the transmigrated fraction. These studies support the hypothesis that in addition to adhesion molecules, paracrine cytokines and locally secreted chemokines are required for efficient progenitor cell migration in the hematopoietic microenvironment of the bone marrow stroma, particularly for migration across bone marrow endothelium.

CHEMOKINES CONTROL TRANSENDOTHELIAL MIGRATION OF HEMATOPOIETIC PROGENITORS

Chemokines are cytokines with direct chemotactic effect on specific target cells expressing the corresponding chemokine receptor. While mature leukocytes respond to a variety of chemokines, only stromal cell derived factor-1 (SDF-1), which is produced by bone marrow stromal cells (but also by stromal cells of other tissues), has chemotactic activity in hematopoietic progenitor and stem cells.[24,25] SDF-1 is a member of the CXC chemokine family, which is characterized by an intervening residue separating the first two cystein residues within a conserved motif.[26] *In vivo*, a transendothelial gradient of SDF-1 could contribute to the avidity of progenitor cells for the bone marrow stroma and thus contribute to the homing process. This idea is supported by the phenotype of SDF-1-deficient mice, which do not develop hematopoiesis in the bone marrow, while fetal liver hematopoiesis is unaffected.[27] In our

Nonmigrating Cells

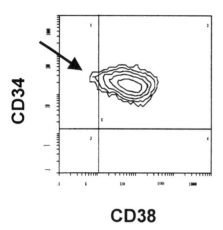

Transmigrated Cells

FIGURE 3. Phenotype of cells migrating in response to the chemokine SDF-1. Peripheral blood CD34+ cells were added to the upper chamber of the transmigration system (FIG. 2). SDF-1-containing conditioned medium from the stromal cell line MS-5 was added to the lower chamber. After 10 h, nonmigrating cells were recovered from the upper, and transmigrated cells from the lower chamber. The phenotype of the progenitor cells was analyzed by flow cytometry. In contrast to spontaneous transendothelial migration, which is confined to more committed CD34+/CD38+ progenitors,[23] there was no difference between transmigrated and nonmigrating cells. More primitive, CD34+/CD38− progenitors were found in both fractions (*arrow*).

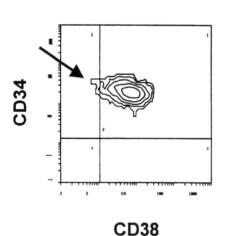

transmigration system (FIG. 2), addition of SDF-1 containing conditioned medium from the stromal cell line MS-5 or recombinant SDF-1 increased the number of CD34+ peripheral blood progenitor cells migrating across bone marrow endothelium more than 10-fold.[28] Also, in contrast to spontaneous transendothelial migration, more primitive, CD34+/CD38− progenitor cells are found in the transmigrated fraction (FIG. 3). The phenotype of migrating and nonmigrating CD34+ cells was virtually identical.

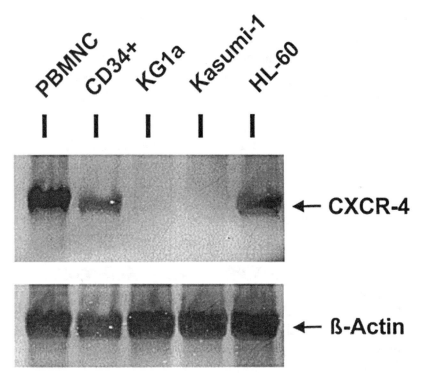

FIGURE 4. mRNA expression of the chemokine receptor CXCR-4. Total RNA was isolated from peripheral blood mononucelar cells (PBMNC) and circulating CD34+ cells. A 484-bp DNA fragment was amplified from CXCR-4 cDNA by polymerase chain reacion (PCR)[28] and used as a probe in a Northern blot analysis (for RNA blotting and probing, standard techniques were employed). RNA from KG1a and Kasumi cells was used as a negative, and RNA from HL60 cells as a positive control. As a control for equal RNA loading, a 513-bp beta-actin probe was generated by PCR amplification.[29] Expression of CXCR-4 mRNA was weaker in circulating CD34+ cells as compared to peripheral blood mononuclear cells.

We could demonstrate that the ligand for SDF-1, the chemokine receptor CXCR-4, is expressed in circulating CD34+ cells at the mRNA level (FIG. 4). However, the amount of CXCR-4 mRNA is low in the CD34+ cells as compared to peripheral blood mononuclear cells. This finding suggests that CXCR-4 is downregulated in mobilized, circulating CD34+ cells. Indeed, cell surface expression of CXCR-4 as measured by flow cytometry is substantially lower on circulating progenitors as compared to progenitors from normal bone marrow (FIG. 5). Moreover, bone marrow CD34+ cells migrate more efficiently in response to SDF-1 as compared to mobilized, peripheral blood CD34+ cells (FIG. 5). Similar to data from malignant hematopoietic cells.[28] the cell surface density of CXCR-4 on hematopoietic progenitor cells might correlate with the ability to respond to SDF-1. Downregulation of CXCR-4

CXCR- 4 Expression

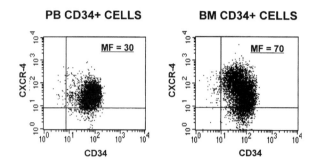

Transendothelial Migration (10 h)

PB CD34+ CELLS   BM CD34+ CELLS

<u>2.81 %</u>   **<u>7.85 %</u>**

FIGURE 5. Cell surface expression of CXCR-4 on peripheral blood and bone marrow CD34[+] progenitor cells and transendothelial migration in response to SDF-1. CD34[+] cells were stained with CD34-FITC (fluorescein isothiocyanate) and CXCR-4-PE (phycoerythrin), and analyzed by flow cytometry as described previously.[28] The expression level of CXCR-4 (expressed as mean fluorescence, MF) was lower on mobilized peripheral blood (PB) CD34[+] cells as compared to bone marrow (BM)-derived CD34+ cells. In accordance with the flow cytometry data, the percentage of PB progenitors migrating in response to SDF-1 (assay shown in Fig. 2) was lower compared to BM CD34[+] cells.

during mobilization could decrease the avidity of progenitors to the bone marrow stroma and thus facilitate circulation.

PARACRINE CYTOKINES MAY SUPPORT HEMATOPOIETIC PROGENITOR CELL MOBILIZATION

We have shown previously that proliferating hematopoietic cells produce cytokines that act on endothelial cells.[29] For example, megakaryocytic precursors stimulated with hematopoietic growth factor (interleukin-3, thrombopoietin) produce vascular endothelial growth factor (VEGF), which specifically acts on endothelial cells. The fact that VEGF-deficient mice do not develop hematopoiesis at all suggests a global role for this cytokine in the establishment and maintenence of hematopoiesis.[30] VEGF not only supports endothelial proliferation, but also increases endothelial fenestration.[31–33] VEGF released in the bone marrow microenvironment during hematopoietic regeneration after cytotoxic therapy or in response to exogenously administered cytokines may thus facilitate the release of progenitors. In reverse, VEGF induces production of hematopoietic cytokines in endothelial cells without inflammatory endothelial activation, resulting in a paracrine loop.[34] The release of VEGF in the bone marrow microenvironment may also explain expression of E-selectin on bone marrow endothelium in the absence of inflammation,[8] because it induces a specific endothelial phenotype which includes expression of E-selectin.[35]

CONCLUSIONS

Mobilization and homing of hematopoietic progenitor cells is a multifactorial process that is regulated at least partially at the level of the bone marrow endothelium. Regulatory mechanisms involve adhesion molecules, chemokines, and paracrine cytokines. Downregulation of adhesion molecules (integrins) and chemokine receptors (CXCR-4) expressed on progenitor cells may facilitate the egress of progenitors from the bone marrow. Cytokines acting on endothelial cells (e.g., VEGF) could support progenitor migration by increasing endothelial fenestration and permeability. Conditions that favor progenitor cell circulation such as cytotoxic therapy and exogenously administered hematopoietic growth factors most likely act indirectly, affecting the cytokine and chemokine milieu in the bone marrow microenvironment, the expression and/or avidity of adhesion molecules, chemokine and cytokine receptors on hematopoietic, endothelial, and stromal cells. Thus, the altered microenvironment supports the shift from the resting to the circulating progenitor cell compartment.

ACKNOWLEDGMENTS

This work was supported by grants from the Deutsche Forschungsgemeinschaft (SFB 510) to R.M., F.B., W.B., and L.K.; by NIH Grant KO8-HL-02926, the Dorothy Rodbell Cohen Foundation for Sarcoma Research, and the Rich Foundation (S.R.); and by the Gar Reichman Fund of the Cancer Research Institute and the Rosemary Breslin Fund (M.A.S.M.) We thank Alexandra Schüller and Petra Mayer for excellent techical assistance.

REFERENCES

1. WEISS, L. 1976. The hematopoietic microenvironment of the bone marrow: an ultrastructural study of the stroma in rats. Anat. Rec. **186:** 161–184.
2. LUND-JOHANSEN, F. & L.W.M.M. TERSTAPPEN. 1993. Differential surface expression of cell adhesion molecules during granulocyte maturation. J. Leukoc. Biol. **54:** 47–55.
3. SAELAND, S., V. DUVERT, C. CAUX, D. PANDRAU, C. FAVRE, A. VALLE, I. DURAND, P. CHARBORD, J. DEVRIES & J. BANCHEREAU. 1992. Distribution of surface-membrane molecules on bone-marrow and cord blood CD34+ hematopoietic cells. Exp. Hematol. **20:** 24–33.

 4. ZANNETTINO, A.C.W., M.C. BERNDT, C. BUTCHER, E.C. BUTCHER, M.A. VADAS &
    P.J. SIMMONS. 1995. Primitive human hematopoietic progenitors adhere to P-selectin
    (CD62P). Blood **85:** 3466–3477.
 5. WATT, S.M., J. WILLIAMSON, H. GENEVIER, J. FAWCETT, D.L. SIMMONS, A.
    HATZFELD, S.A. NESBITT & D.R. COOMBE. 1993. The heparin binding PCAM-1
    adhesion molecule is expressed by CD34$^+$ hematopoietic precursor cells with early
    myeloid and B-lymphoid phenotypes. Blood **82:** 2649–2663.
 6. CARLOS, T.M. & J.M. HARLAN. 1994. Leukocyte-endothelial adhesion molecules.
    Blood **84:** 2068–2101.
 7. JACOBSEN, K., J. KRAVITZ, P.W. KINCADE & D.G. OSMOND. 1996. Adhesion receptors
    on bone marrow stromal cells: *in vivo* expression of vascular cell adhesion mole-
    cule-1 by reticular cells and sinosoidal endothelium in normal and gamma-irradiated
    mice. Blood **87:** 73–82.
 8. SCHWEITZER, K.M., A.M. DRAGER, P. VANDERVALK, S.F. THIJSEN, A. ZEVENBERGEN,
    A.P. THEIJSMEIJER, C.E. VANDERSCHOOT & M.M. LANGENHUIJSEN. 1996. Constitu-
    tive expression of E-selectin and vascular cell adhesion molecule-1 on endothelial
    cells of hematopoietic tissues. Am. J. Pathol. **148:** 165–175.
 9. YONG, K.L., M.J. WATTS, N. SHAUNTHOMAS, A. SULLIVAN, S. INGS & D.C. LINCH.
    1998. Transmigration of CD34$^+$ cells across specialized and nonspecialized endothe-
    lium requires prior activation by growth factors and is mediated by PECAM-1. Blood
    91: 1196–1205.
10. MULLER, W.A. & S.A. WEIGL. 1992. Monocyte-selective transendothelial migration:
    dissection of the binding and transmigration phases by an *in vitro* assay. J. Exp.
    Med. **176:** 819–828.
11. MÖHLE, R., S. MUREA, M. KIRSCH & R. HAAS. 1995. Differential expression of
    L-selectin, VLA-4, and LFA-1 on CD34$^+$ progenitor cells from bone marrow and
    peripheral blood during G-CSF enhanced recovery. Exp. Hematol. **23:** 1535–1542.
12. DERCKSEN, M.W., W.R. GERRITSEN, S. RODENHUIS, M.K. DIRKSON, I.C. SLA-
    PER-CORTENBACH, W.P. SCHAASBERG, H.M. PINEDO, A.E.G.K. VONDEMBORNE &
    C.E. VANDERSCHOOT. 1995. Expression of adhesion molecules on CD34$^+$ cells:
    L-selectin$^+$ cells predict a rapid platelet recovery after peripheral blood stem cell
    transplantation. Blood **85:** 3313–3319.
13. PAPAYANNOPOULOU, T. & B. NAKAMOTO. 1993. Peripheralization of hemopoietic
    progenitors in primates treated with anti-VLA4 integrin. Proc. Natl. Acad. Sci.
    USA **90:** 9374–9378.
14. PAPAYANNOPOULOU, T., C. CRADDOCK, B. NAKAMOTO, G.V. PRIESTLEY & N.S. WOLF.
    1995. The VLA-4/VCAM-1 adhesion pathway defines contrasting mechanisms of
    lodgement of transplanted murine hemopoietic progenitors between bone marrow
    and spleen. Proc. Natl. Acad. Sci. USA **92:** 9647–9651.
15. TEIXIDO, J., M.E. HEMLER, J.S. GREENBERGER & P. ANKLESARIA. 1992. Role of ß1
    and ß2 integrins in the adhesion of human CD34^{hi} stem cells to bone marrow
    stroma. J. Clin. Invest. **90:** 358–367.
16. ROSEMBLATT, M., M.H. VUILLET-GAUGLER, C. LEROY & L. COULOMBEL. 1991. Coex-
    pression of two fibronectin receptors, VLA-4 and VLA-5, by immature human
    erythroblastic precursor cells. J. Clin. Invest. **87:** 6–11.
17. FLANAGAN, J.G., D.C. CHAN & P. LEDER. 1991. Transmembrane form of kit ligand
    growth factor is determined by alternative splicing and is missing in the Sld
    mutant. Cell **64:** 1025–1035.
18. FLEISCHMAN, R.A., F. SIMPSON, T. GALLARDO, X.L. JIN & S. PRKINS. 1995. Isolation
    of endothelial-like stromal cells that express kit ligand and support *in vitro*
    hematopoiesis. Exp. Hematol. **23:** 1407–1416.
19. MÖHLE, R., R. HAAS & W. HUNSTEIN. 1993. Expression of adhesion molecules and
    c-kit on CD34$^+$ hematopoietic progenitor cells: comparison of cytokine-mobilized
    blood stem cells with normal bone marrow and peripheral blood. J. Hematother. **2:**
    483–489.
20. RAFII, S., F. SHAPIRO, J. RIMARACHIN, R.L. NACHMAN, B. FERRIS, B. WEKSLER,
    M.A.S. MOORE & A. ASCH. 1994. Isolation and characterization of human bone

marrow microvascular endothelial cells: hematopoietic progenitor cell adhesion. Blood **84:** 10–19.

21. SCHWEITZER, C.M., C.E. VANDERSCHOOT, A.M. DRÄGER, P. VANDERVALK, A. ZEVEN-BERGEN, B. HOOIBRINK, A.H. WESTRA & M.M.A.C. LANGENHUIJSEN. 1995. Isolation and culture of human bone marrow endothelial cells. Exp. Hematol. **23:** 31–48.

22. CANDAL, F.J., S. RAFII, J.T. PARKER, E.W. ADES, B. FERRIS, R.L. NACHMAN & K.L. KELLAR. 1996. BMEC-1: a human bone marrow microvascular endothelial cell with primary cell characteristics. Microvasc. Res. **52:** 221–234.

23. MÖHLE, R., M.A.S. MOORE, R.L. NACHMAN & S. RAFII. 1997. Transendothelial migration of CD34$^+$ and mature hematopoietic cells: an *in vitro* study using a human bone marrow endothelial cell line. Blood **89:** 72–80.

24. NAGASAWA, T., H. KIKUTANI & T. KISHIMOTO. 1994. Molecular cloning and structure of a pre-B-cell growth-stimulating factor. Proc. Natl. Acad. Sci. USA **91:** 2305–2309.

25. AIUTI, A., I.J. WEBB, C. BLEUL, T. SPRINGER & J.C. GUTIERREZ-RAMOS. 1997. The chemokine SDF-1 is a chemoattractant for human hematopoietic progenitor cells and provides a new mechanism to explain the mobilization of CD34$^+$ progenitors to peripheral blood. J. Exp. Med. **185:** 111–120.

26. WELLS, T.N., C.A. POWER, M. LUSTI-NARASIMHAN, A.J. HOOGEWERF, R.M. COOKE, C.W. CHUNG, M.C. PEITSCH & A.E. PROUDFOOT. 1996. Selectivity and antagonism of chemokine receptors. J. Leukocyte Biol. **59:** 53–60.

27. NAGASAWA, T., S. HIROTA, K. TACHIBANA, N. TAKAKURA, S. NISHIKAWA, Y. KITA-MURA, N. YOSHIDA, H. KIKUTANI & T. KISHIMOTO. 1996. Defects of B-cell lymphopoiesis and bone marrow myelopoiesis in mice lacking the CXC chemokine PBSF/SDF-1. Nature **382:** 635–638.

28. MÖHLE, R., F. BAUTZ, S. RAFII, M.A.S. MOORE, W. BRUGGER & L. KANZ. 1998. The chemokine receptor CXCR-4 is expressed on CD34$^+$ hematopoietic progenitors and leukemic cells and mediates transendothelial migration induced by stromal cell-derived factor-1. Blood **91:** 4523–4530.

29. MÖHLE, R., D. GREEN, M.A.S. MOORE, R.L. NACHMAN & S. RAFII. 1997. Constitutive production and thrombin-induced release of vascular endothelial growth factor by human megakaryocytes and platelets. Proc. Natl. Acad. Sci. USA **94:** 663–668.

30. FERRARA, N., K. CARVER-MOORE, H. CHEN, M. DOWD, L. LU, K.S. O'SHEA, L. POW-ELL-BRAXTON, K.J. HILLAN & M.W. MOORE. 1996. Heterozygous embryonic lethality induced by targeted inactivation of the VEGF gene. Nature **380:** 439–442.

31. CONNOLLY, D.T., D.M. HEUVELMAN, R. NELSON, J.V. OLANDER, B.L. EPPLEY, J.J. DELFINO, N.R. SIEGEL, R.M. LEIMGRUBER & J. FEDER. 1989. Tumor vascular permeability factor stimulates endothelial growth and angiogenesis. J. Clin. Invest. **84:** 1470–1478.

32. DVORAK, H.F., L.F. BROWN, M. DETMAR & A.M. DVORAK. 1995. Vascular permeability factor/vascular endothelial growth factor, microvascular hyperpermeability, and angiogenesis. Am. J. Pathol. **146:** 1029–1039.

33. ROBERTS, W.G. & G.E. PALADE. 1995. Invreased microvascular permeability and endothelial fenestration induced by vascular endothelial growth factor. J. Cell Sci. **108:** 2369–2379.

34. MÖHLE, R., S. RAFII & M.A.S. MOORE. 1998. The role of endothelium in the regulation of hematopoietic stem cell migration. Stem Cells **16**(S1):159–165.

35. BISCHOFF, J., C. BRASEL, B. KRALING & K. VRANOVSKA. 1997. E-selectin is upregulated in proliferating endothelial cell *in vitro*. Microcirculation **4:** 279–287.

DISCUSSION

B. TOROK-STORB (*Fred Hutchinson Cancer Research Center*): In your experiments when you looked for induction of VEGF by different cytokines, you said c-kit ligand induced a little bit, but when you added a number of other factors, you got a lot. Did you look at G-CSF alone or GM-CSF alone?

MÖHLE: We did not look at G-CSF alone. We have always used a cytokine combination that had kit ligand as a basis for stimulation, but this would be an interesting question. We believe that G-CSF does not act directly, and we have done studies to see whether *in vitro* G-CSF has any effect on endothelium. We believe that G-CSF acts indirectly by increasing other cytokines, and so we think it is always a combination of cytokines that is involved in mobilization *in vivo*.

H.E. BROXMEYER (*Indiana University*): With regard to your VEGF production from CD34$^+$ cells, how pure were your CD34$^+$ cells, and what percent of those CD34$^+$ cells were endothelial cells?

MÖHLE: For these studies we used different CD34 cells including circulating and CD34+ bone marrow cells that were about 99% pure isolated by the magnetic-activated cell sorting (MACS) system. The production of VEGF was from CD34 cells isolated from peripheral blood, so there is virtually no contamination with endothelial cells. However, there are some indications that there may be some circulating endothelial progenitor cells. Since VEGF production increases during proliferation and we have replated the CD34 cells during culturing, it is clear that the VEGF is produced by the hematopoietic CD34$^+$ cells.

J.D. GRIFFIN (*Dana Farber Cancer Institute*): There are acute myeloid leukemia (AML) patients that have packed marrows and a high white count and others that have a packed marrow and a low white count. Was there any correlation between CXCR-4 expression and peripheral counts or any other phenotype?

MÖHLE: So far we are just doing those correlations. One interesting fact was that the greatest difference between bone marrow and peripheral blood and high overexpression of CXCR-4 in the bone marrow cells was observed in a patient who had skin infiltration and infiltration of other tissues. SDF-1 is also produced by stroma from other tissues, so we think this may play a role in the cell trafficking or tropism for other tissues.

Y. REISNER (*Weizmann Institute of Science*): In T cells we are seeing modulation of fusin upon activation. For example, if you follow phytohemagglutinin (PHA) stimulation, you can see some modulation in the expression. Do you find something similar in your endothelial cells?

MÖHLE: Are you asking about CXCR-4 expression on CD34 cells? We did a follow-up study doing culturing with cytokines. There was no clear picture. If the cells start to differentiate, and if the cell goes through megakarocytic differentiation, and also if the cells go into myeloid lineage, the CXCR-4 level goes up, but there is always a population similar to the starting population, which expresses CD34 and has a moderate level of CXCR-4. CXCR-4 expression seems to be related to differentiation of the cells. There is clearly no effect of short incubation for one or two days, where we do not see a clear effect on CXCR-4 expression.

Hematopoietic Stem/Progenitor Cell Mobilization

A Continuing Quest for Etiologic Mechanisms

THALIA PAPAYANNOPOULOU[a]

Department of Medicine, Division of Hematology, Box 357710, University of Washington, Seattle, Washington 98195-7710, USA

ABSTRACT: The physiologic egress of mature hemopoietic cells and of hemopoietic stem/progenitor cells from bone marrow to the circulation are poorly understood processes. Likewise, the mechanism of their enforced emigration or mobilization through the use of several agents has not been unraveled. Although mobilization is suspected to be a multi-step process, involving sequential and/or overlapping changes in adhesion and migratory capacity, a model of molecular hierarchy, like the one governing the extravasation of mature leukocytes to tissues of inflammation, has not been worked out. Understanding the *in vivo* mechanism of mobilization has been a challenge. Signals emanating from both stromal cells and from hemopoietic cells are likely involved. However, dissecting out their roles, specificity, and interactions has been difficult. Nevertheless insightful information is rapidly emerging, especially with the current availability of many mouse models bearing targeted disruptions of cytoadhesion or signaling molecules.

INTRODUCTION

Although proliferating hemopoietic cells at various stages of differention are held within the bone marrow environment, terminally differentiated, mature cells of all lineages (myeloid, erythroid, megakaryocytic) have the ability to migrate out of the bone marrow to systemic circulation, a process called *egress*. How normal mature cells egress to the circulation is not defined. Specifically, what the molecular and anatomical requirements are for their exit through the bone marrow sinuses is not clear. In addition to mature cells, it has been known for several decades that hemopoietic stem/progenitor cells are also present in circulation.[1,2] The molecular basis of hemopoietic stem/progenitor cell emigration to the periphery, although likely distinct from that of the mature leukocytes, is also poorly understood. Nevertheless, several empiric treatments in the past[3–6] were found to enforce emigration of stem/progenitor cells to the periphery, a process referred to as *mobilization*. Mobilization in recent years has gained increased importance in clinical transplantation and sparked a flurry of relevant studies.[6,7] Mobilization has been achieved in several experimental animal models (mice, dogs, primates) by numerous agents (i.e., cytokines, chemokines, chemotherapeutic agents) and by the *in vivo* use of antibodies to certain cytoadhesion molecules.[8] The mechanism by which these agents induce mobilization

[a]Phone, 206/543-5756; fax, 206/543-3050; e-mail, thalp@u.washington.edu

remains to be defined. In this brief review, I would like to provide an interpretive account of the main features of mobilization, when it is achieved through the use of cytokines or chemokines, as well as the use of antibodies to cytoadhesion molecules *in vivo*.

MOBILIZATION INDUCED BY CYTOKINES AND CHEMOKINES

Kinetics of Mobilization

A large body of data is now available regarding mobilization induced by a variety of cytokines or chemokines.[6] Most of the studies have made use of mobilized peripheral blood cells after treatment with G-CSF with or without chemotherapy and have addressed the kinetics and the biological properties of mobilized cells, as well as issues of practical importance in clinical transplantation (i.e., optimal mobilizing schemes, collection practices, and validation of surrogate markers for predicting transplantation outcomes).[7]

One of the interesting features in the mobilization process is the characteristic kinetics through which mobilized stem/progenitor cells accumulate in peripheral blood following treatment with a mobilizing agent. Thus, when one compares mobilization induced by cytokines to that induced by chemokines, there is a striking difference in mobilization kinetics. For example, IL-8 has a peak mobilizing effect 15–20 minutes following a single injection of IL-8,[9] compared to 4–6 days for G-CSF and even longer for kit ligand (KL)[10] and FLT-3 ligand (FL).[11–13] Not only is IL-8–induced mobilization complete in a short time, but it is also short-lived. These kinetic differences between chemokines (i.e., IL-8, IL-1, MIP1α) and cytokines (i.e., G-CSF, KL, GM-CSF, IL-7, IL-3, FL, etc.) were interpreted to suggest that different mechanisms are involved in mobilization by chemokines as opposed to cytokines. It was not clear, however, what the kinetic differences were telling us. Did they indicate that different target cells are involved, or that one step versus multiple steps culminating into a common pathway are needed for mobilization by the one but not the other treatment? Also, it was possible that pre-existing pools of progenitors in different anatomic sites were mobilized with chemokines compared to cytokines.

Recent data with G-CSF receptor *null* mice seem to shed some light on these questions. IL-8 has been completely ineffective in these mice.[14] Although a reduced number of neutrophils is present in these mice, it is suspected that this is not the main reason for their failure to respond to IL-8. A functional defect in neutrophils, yet to be uncovered, is probably the most likely explanation. Nevertheless, these data do indicate that the target cells for IL-8 treatment, not unexpectedly, are the neutrophils, and that the existence of a normal functional pool of neutrophils may be important for the mobilizing effect of IL-8. In normal mice treated with IL-8 the peak of neutrophilia coincides with the peak of progenitor mobilization.[9] It is very likely the neutrophil pool that is immediately mobilized by IL-8 is the marginal pool present in and around the bone marrow sinuses, or diffusely in other tissues. Experimental evidence in support of this supposition was presented recently suggesting that at least 50% of mobilized neutrophils must originate from the bone marrow pool.[15] A similar pool of hemopoietic stem/progenitor cells could also be present within the bone marrow sinuses, and this pool is mobilized along with neutrophils. In this case, however, the implication is that the mobilization of progenitor cells by IL-8 is passive rather than selective. Mobilizations induced by endotoxin, IL-1, MIP1α, steroids, or lithium[16] may have a similar basis. Should mobilization of progenitors be expected every time neutrophilia is induced? I do not think that such an effect can be generalized and it may depend on what type of triggering event is imposed on neutrophils, or what indeed is the mechanism for neutrophilia. For example, antibodies to CD18 integrin (a β2 integrin) are able to cause a dramatic neutrophilia within the first day of administration without a concomitant increase in progenitor mobilization.[8] However, in this case, the neutrophilia is likely due to accumulation of neutrophils in peripheral blood, because of their inability to move to the tissues, rather than because of their increased release from the bone marrow. Also, G-CSF causes an early peak of neutrophils, but this peak is not reportedly accompanied by a significant mobilization of progenitor cells, although detailed studies addressing this specific issue hours after G-CSF administration are not available. Future studies with selective abrogation of neutrophils (i.e., by antibody treatment) may help clarify some of these issues. Recently it was also noted that the IL-8 effect was abrogated by a single injection of antibody to LFA-1 (CD11a integrin).[17] Although this was interpreted to indicate that the LFA-1 function may be needed for mobilization,[17] this may not be necessarily true (see below), and only highlights the complexity of interpreting *in vivo* data either through the use of function blocking antibodies or with cytokines which have pleiotropic effects on both hematopoietic cells and on their stroma.

Progenitor Proliferation/Cell Cycling and Mobilization

Early proliferation of progenitors in bone marrow, preceding mobilization, has been documented in the case of Cytoxan and G-CSF treatments,[18] or G-CSF alone,[19] but this effect is not sustained, and after 4 days or so the marrow progenitor pool is either at basal levels or reduced compared to steady state. Other cytokines, like IL-3[20] or KL[10] or FL,[11-13] have a more pronounced effect on proliferation for the first few days following their administration, but this effect is not accompanied by mobilization until several days later. Furthermore, Cytoxan treatment of G-CSF receptor null mice did not induce mobilization during the recovery period, although it did induce a significant proliferative effect within the bone marrow.[14] Thus, although proliferation *per se* may have a role in mobilization, particularly by expanding the pools of cells to be mobilized, the data indicate that it does not appear to be sufficient for mobilization and in many cases proliferation is not necessarily accompanied by mobilization. Nevertheless, the proliferative effects that cytokines other than G-CSF may display have been exploited in cytokine combination treatments with G-CSF to increase the yield of mobilized stem/progenitor cells. It is of interest that irrespective of the cytokine that G-CSF is combined with, the kinetics of peak mobilization are similar to the ones observed with G-CSF alone, i.e., 4–6 days from the beginning of G-CSF treatment. However, the bone marrow progenitor pool, in contrast to treatments with G-CSF alone, is now dramatically expanded and could largely underlie the synergistic effect in mobilization with the combination treatments.

One of the most intriguing findings with mobilized cells has been the fact that most of the mobilized progenitor cells in peripheral blood are in a state quiescent.[21-24] Both primitive and differentiated subsets found in the peripheral blood differ significantly from those present in steady state bone marrow (CFU-GM: 2–5% in S-phase in peripheral blood compared to about 25% in steady-state bone marrow; LTC-IC: 1% in peripheral blood versus 21% in bone marrow).[24] Other surrogate markers of proliferation are also in accord with the low cycling status, i.e., low Rhodamine staining and low expression of CD71 antigen. Of interest, many markers that have been considered to be associated with cycling cells, i.e., CD38 or CD13, are now present in these quiescent progenitor cells. The low cycling status has been confirmed by all investigators that have studied this issue, whether the cells are found to be held in G_0/G_1, or are in an extended G_1 phase.[25] It needs to be emphasized that low cycling has been mainly found with G-CSF-induced mobilization and that the extent to which low cycling is seen with other cytokines or with combinations of cytokines (i.e., G + KL or G + FL) is not clear. For example, IL-7 + G-CSF mobilizes more cells in cycle compared to G-CSF alone.[26] It is unlikely that circulating inhibitors in peripheral blood are important for this finding, or that the progenitors that are circulating are hyporesponsive to cytokines once they find themselves in peripheral blood.[21] Therefore, the low cycling status has been attributed to several other reasons. For example, some investigators suggest that low cycling represents loss of contact with a hemopoietic microenvironment or with the hemopoietic stroma cells.[24] Although this may seem reasonable, this proposition is at odds with other *in vitro* information suggesting inhibition of proliferation once cells are found in adherence state, either in long-term cultures or on immobilized extracellular matrices.[27] Others have suggested that quiescent cells may selectively leave the bone marrow because of their competence to transmigrate.[28] Alternatively one may suggest that the state of quiescence is imposed upon progenitor cells after their exposure to high levels of inhibitors of cell cycling, like TGFα, concentrated within bone marrow sinuses, as a result of cytokine or other mobilizing treatments. It is of note, however, that mobilized cells, in contrast to quiescent cells from bone marrow at steady state, readily enter cycling after stimulation with cytokines *in vitro* and readily migrate *in vitro*.[29] This property has been exploited in retroviral gene transduction using peripheral blood mobilized cells.

Properties of Mobilized Cells

The surface properties of stem/progenitor cells mobilized, especially the expression of several classes of cytoadhesion molecules, has become the focus of many studies, which have compared them to either steady state bone marrow cells, or to bone marrow concurrently retrieved from patients treated with a mobilizing agent. A decrease in the expression of some cytoadhesion molecules, especially of β1 integrins (α4 and α5),[6,30] has been hailed as being causally related to the movement of progenitors out of bone marrow spaces. Establishing, however, a direct causative relationship between the level of expression of these molecules after they have migrated out of the bone marrow and the treatment that caused their mobilization has not been straightforward, notwithstanding the disparity of findings among the different studies. β1 integrins are highly expressed in hemopoietic progenitors and their ligands are abundant in hemopoietic stroma.[31] Their influence on hemopoiesis is indisputable, not only by the *in vitro* data where α4 or α5 along with β2 integrins and CD44 play significant roles,[32–35] but also by studies on mice with ablation of β1 integrins showing markedly reduced colonization of fetal liver.[36] Whether, however, the decreased expression and/or function of β1 integrins found in the peripheral blood is a cause rather than a consequence of their transmigration through the marrow sinuses cannot be sorted out. Furthermore, whether low cycling status and low integrin expression are interrelated events has not been established. Similarly, a reduced expression of kit has been found in mobilized cells compared to the same subsets present in steady state bone marrow.[6,18,37,38] This reduced expression of kit in CD34[+] cells was irrespective of the mobilizing agent used and it was found not only in peripheral blood but also in cells from the bone marrow of treated patients. Although this finding could be interpreted to indicate a preceding activation of kit and subsequent downmodulation, its importance in the mobilization process has not been clearly defined. *In vitro* kit ligand influences neither the adhesiveness nor the migration of mobilized cells[29] in some studies, whereas in others kit ligand was found to be both a chemokinetic and chemotactic agent for hemopoietic progenitors.[39]

Another interesting property of mobilized cells (CD34[+] cells) has been their ability to produce, in contrast to their bone marrow counterparts, gelatinases A and B.[40] Whether the peripheral blood environment is conducive to this property, especially when circulating progenitor cells at steady state have the same property, or it is an indication of their ability to promote degradation of bone marrow extracellular matrices facilitating their exodus from bone marrow, remains to be seen.

MOBILIZATION BY FUNCTION BLOCKING ANTIBODIES TO CYTOADHESION MOLECULES

To test whether it was possible to perturb cytoadhesive interactions *in vivo* through the use of monoclonal antibodies, we treated primates with antibody to α4 integrin (CD49d). Short 3-day treatment with anti-α4 provoked a wave of hemopoietic progenitors in the blood of these primates.[8] These initial experiments established for the first time the feasibility of progenitor mobilization by antibodies to integrins, especially β1 integrins, and have continued to provide additional insights into the mobilization process. The functional properties of the anti-α4 antibody used were critical for its action, as a non-adhesion blocking antibody was ineffective in inducing mobilization *in vivo*.[41] A humanized monoclonal antibody with a long half-life had a prolonged effect, whereas F(ab)$_2$' fragments with short half-life, were much less effective. The salient features of the antibody treatments, which they extended in mice and later confirmed by other investigators,[42] are as follows: (*a*) In contrast to IL-8, mobilization was not immediate and it was not seen until after ~8 hours in primates or 4 hours in mice and was progressively increased until the first 24 hours. Although we have used three injections, the effect was clearly present after a single injection in both primates and mice, and a dose effect could be seen (unpublished data). (*b*) In addition to increase in progenitors in the peripheral blood, there is up to a two-fold increase in granulocytes and in lymphocytes. The small increase in these mature cells contrasts with the up-to-100-fold increment in circulating progenitors[8] and suggests that the egress of progenitors is probably not passive, along with a demarginating neutrophil pool, but rather selectively achieved. Similarly, although intermediate myeloid and erythroid precursors (i.e., myelocytes, erythroblasts) are expressing VLA-4 and greatly outnumber the clonogenic progenitors within bone marrow, they are not found in peripheral blood to accompany stem/progenitor cells. This would indicate either a different state of activation of their integrins, or a different regulatory control. Alternatively, if there is a sizable marginal pool of stem/progenitor cells within bone marrow sinuses, this does not seem to include morphologically recognizable precursor cells. (*c*) The spectrum of progenitors mobilized was wide, like in many other treatments. In addition to committed progenitors, detected by clonogenic assays *in vitro*, CFU-S and long-term repopulating cells were mobilized.[43] In primates, however, some preferential increase in BFUe was seen, although this was not evident with the antibody used in mice.

But how did anti-α4 achieve its mobilizing effect *in vivo*? Was it by inhibiting cytoadhesive interactions, preferentially loosely established ones, within the bone marrow, or by acting mostly on cells with unoccupied integrins (i.e., newly made progenitors), or by inhibiting the hypothetical return of circulating progenitors to the bone marrow? If de-adhesion was taking place, was it sufficient to increase motility and transmigration, or are additional steps involved? Also, what are the important ligands *in vivo* for α4 in this case?

A series of experiments was subsequently planned to approach, if possible, some of these questions *in vivo*. As VCAM-1 is the most important ligand of VLA4 *in vitro*, we tested whether antibodies to VCAM-1 had any mobilizing effect, like anti-α4. Indeed, treatment of mice (there was no good antibody that could be tested in primates) with rat anti-murine VCAM-1 caused mobilization of progenitors, similar to the one achieved by anti-VLA-4 antibodies.[44] These results indicated to us that antibodies directed at stromal cells were also capable of inducing progenitor egress. It is tempting to speculate once again that anti-VCAM-1, like anti-α4, interfered with established cytoadhesion interactions between hemopoietic cells and bone marrow stroma or endothelial cells, and that VCAM-1 was indeed a dominant *in vivo* ligand for VLA-4. This conclusion was strengthened by subsequent observations showing that competitive inhibition of CS-1 binding by VLA-4 (through the use of CS-1 inhibitory peptides) was not effective in mobilization.[44] The spectrum of mobilized progenitors and their kinetics following anti-VCAM-1 treatment were not unlike the ones with the anti-α4. As was the case with anti-VLA-4, however, the mode of action *in vivo* for both antibodies was obscure. We suspected that cooperation of other molecules is required for completion of the mobilization process. The participation of other molecules may be particularly necessary for cells to increase their motility and their migratory capacity, according to the paradigm of extravasation of mature leukocytes to tissues of inflammation, requiring a cascade of cytoadhesion reactions.

Therefore, to gain further insights into the anti-α4-induced mobilization, we carried out experiments aiming to test the cooperation and/or participation of other molecules, either in the form of growth factor receptors, or of cytoadhesion molecules present on hemopoietic cells, and/or their stroma. First we explored whether anti-α4 was capable of augmenting the mobilizing effect induced by several cytokines.[43] It was previously discussed that such treatments were downmodulating adhesion molecules, especially α4 integrin.[6,30] In this case, how much could the anti-α4 treatment add to this effect? We documented that single cytokine treatments by G-CSF, KL, and FL in mice or primates were indeed all augmented by co-treatments with anti-α4.[43] Combinations of G + KL or G + FL were also showing the same effect. There was no apparent correlation between magnitude of cytokine-induced mobilization and effect of antibody (although none of the combined treatments was carried out to a maximum effect). This result was surprising and its explanation was not *a priori* straightforward. Are we dealing with exaggeration of a single mechanism (i.e., further downregulation of $\alpha 4$ by antibody co-treatments) or were two independent mechanisms at play? Was the effect just additive, even if it appears to be synergistic, because of expansion, by cytokine treatment, of progenitor pools targeted by antibody treatments, or was a true synergy present due to integrin/cytokine interplay? To answer some of these questions we drafted for the anti-$\alpha 4$ studies mutant mice with defects in growth factor receptor function. We found that the presence of G-CSF, IL-7, or IL-3α receptors was dispensable for the mobilizing effect of anti-$\alpha 4$.[45] In contrast to these data, kit kinase activity on hemopoietic cells appeared to be important for an optimum mobilizing effect.[45] W/W^v mice responded suboptimally to anti-$\alpha 4$, in contrast to their littermate controls, and in contrast to Sl/Sl^d mice. This effect was not due to a decrease in progenitor pools in their marrow, or a low $\alpha 4$ expression in their hemopoietic cells. To consolidate this observation we also treated W/W^v and Sl/Sl^d mice with antibodies to VCAM-1. Both sets of mice did not respond to anti-VCAM-1 treatments, in contrast to their normal control littermates. This was surprising, especially for W/W^v mice in which bone marrow stromal composition and function is normal. To explain this result, we hypothesized that both hemopoietic cells with normal kit kinase activity and signaling may be required in the mobilization process by anti-VCAM-1 in W/W^v mice. To test the validity of this hypothesis, donor bone marrow cells from +/+ littermate controls or from W/W^v animals were transplanted into W/W^v recipients. Eight weeks post-transplantation hematopoietic parameters were normal in the recipients of +/+ cells but not in the recipients of W/W^v. Anti-VCAM-1 was then administered to both groups of transplanted animals. We found that the W/W^v recipients of normal (+/+) cells responded to anti-VCAM-1 treatment, in contrast to the recipients of W/W^v cells (only two such animals were available for testing). Although these results provided a good explanation for the failure of W/W^v to respond to VCAM-1, the failure of Sl/Sl^d mice to respond to VCAM-1 (although these mice do respond to anti-VLA-4) was not readily interpretable. Perhaps for the anti-VCAM-1–induced mobilization in the latter animals signaling and putative intercommunication between VCAM-1 and membrane-bound kit ligand are needed. Whatever the explanation, we believe that the data with W/W^v and Sl/Sl^d mice provided a novel example of interplay of integrins and kinase receptors. In this context it was also of interest that $\alpha 4$ integrins and kit are both down-modulated in blast-like cells within bone marrow 3 days after anti-VLA-4 treatment, perhaps as a consequence of this interaction.[45] Furthermore, extrapolation of the above data to the untreated animal would suggest that both $\beta 1$ integrins and the kit/membrane found kit ligand pair contribute to the sustained anchoring of progenitors in bone marrow stroma under basal conditions. It can be predicted that perturbations of either (integrin or kinase) pathway may have consequences for the establishment of hemopoietic cells within the bone marrow (i.e., their homing) and for the cells to migrate out of the bone marrow (i.e., their mobilization).

In addition to the VLA-4/VCAM-1 pathway, it is suspected that other adhesion pathways may play a role in the mobilization process, either alone or in combination. For this purpose we initiated studies in which antibodies to other cytoadhesion molecules were used. We found (detailed data are to be published elsewhere) that other $\beta 1$ or $\beta 2$ integrins ($\alpha 5 \ \beta 1$, 11a, CD18) appear to exert a cooperative effect when they are combined with anti-VLA-4. However, in contrast to these data, anti-CD31 co-treatment had an inhibiting influence, raising a series of new questions about its mechanism of action and whether this could be a common downstream pathway in mobilization. These questions will be explored in future experiments. Recently antibodies to CD44 were reported to induce a modest mobilization in mice, bringing into action additional classes of cytoadhesion families.[42]

In summary, although the VLA-4/VCAM-1 pathway appears to play a dominant role in trafficking of hemopoietic stem progenitor cells, other molecular pathways, possibly working downstream of VLA-4, are important and remain to be explored. Insightful information, especially through the use of mice with targeted mutations of cytoadhesion molecules (i.e., P and E selectin, Fuc-TVII transferases, thrombospondin I and II) or of signaling molecules (i.e., Shp-1, Ship-1, etc.) will be instrumental in unraveling mechanisms of mobilization.

ACKNOWLEDGMENTS

The expert technical assistance of Greg Priestley and Betty Nakamoto is gratefully acknowledged. I am also indebted to Roy Lobb (Biogen, Cambridge, MA) for the gift of antibodies, and to Margaret Oppenheimer for secretarial assistance.

REFERENCES

1. BRECHER, G. & CRONKITE, E.P. 1951. Postirradiation para-biosis and survival in rats. Proc. Soc. Exp. Biol. Med. **77:** 292–294.
2. GOODMAN, J.W. & G.S. HODGSON. 1962. Evidence of stem cells in the peripheral blood of mice. Blood **19:** 702–714.
3. RICHMAN, C.M., R.S. WEINER & R.A. YANKEE. 1976. Increase in circulating stem cells following chemotherapy in man. Blood **47:** 1031–1039.
4. JUTTNER, C.A., L.B. TO, D.N. HAYLOCK, A. BRANFORD & R.J. KIMBER. 1985. Circulating autologous stem cells collected in very early remission from acute nonlymphoblastic leukaemia produce prompt but incomplete haemopoietic reconstruction after high dose melphalan or supralethal chemoradiotherapy. Br. J. Haematol. **61:** 739–745.
5. DURSTEN, U., J.L. VILLEVAL, J. BOYD, G. KANNOURAKIS, G. MORSTYN & D. METCALF. 1988. Effects of G-CSF on haematopoietic progenitor cells in cancer patients. Blood **72:** 2074–2081.
6. TO, L.B., D.N. HAYLOCK, P.J. SIMMONS & C.A. JUTTNER. 1997. The biology and clinical uses of blood stem cells. Blood **89:** 2233–2258.
7. WATTS, M.J. & D.C. LINCH. 1997. Peripheral blood stem cell transplantation. Vox Sang. **73:**135–142.
8. PAPAYANNOPOULOU, T. & B. NAKAMOTO. 1993. Peripheralization of hemopoietic progenitors in primates treated with anti-VLA₄ integrin. Proc. Natl. Acad. Sci. USA **90:** 9374–9378.
9. LATERVEER, L., I.J.D. LINDLEY, D.P.M. HEEMSKERK, J.A.J. CAMPS, E.K.J. PAUWELS, R. WILLEMZE & W.E. FIBBE. 1996. Rapid mobilization of hematopoietic progenitor cells in Rhesus monkeys by a single intravenous injection of interleukin-8. Blood **87:** 781–788.
10. ANDREWS, R.G., R.A. BRIDELL, G.H. KNITTER, T. OPIE, M. BRONSDEN, D. MYERSON, F.R. APPLEBAUM & I.K. MCNIECE. 1994. *In vivo* synergy between recombinant human stem cell factor and recombinant human granulocyte colony-stimulating factor in baboons. Blood **84:** 800–810.

11. SUDO, Y., C. SHIMAZAKI, E. ASHIHARA, T. KIKUTA, H. HIRAI, T. SUMIKUMA, N. YAMAGATA, H. GOTO, T. INABA, N. FUJITA & M. NAKAGAWA. 1997. Synergistic effect of FLT-3 ligand on the granulocyte colony-stimulating factor-induced mobilization of hematopoietic stem cells and progenitor cells into blood in mice. Blood **89:** 3186–3191.

12. PAPAYANNOPOULOU, T., B. NAKAMOTO, R.G. ANDREWS, S.D. LYMAN & M.Y. LEE. 1997. In vivo effects of Flt3/Flk2 ligand on mobilization of hematopoietic progenitors in primates and potent synergistic enhancement with granulocyte colony-stimulating factor. Blood **90**(2): 620–629.

13. ASHIHARA, E., C. SHIMAZAKI, Y. SUDO et al. 1998. FLT-3 ligand mobilizes hematopoietic primitve and committed progenitor cells into blood in mice. Eur. J. Haematol. **60:** 86–92.

14. LIU, F., J. POURSINE-LAURENT & D.C. LINK. 1997. The granulocyte colony-stimulating factor receptor is required for the mobilization of murine hematopoietic progenitors into peripheral blood by cyclophosphamide or interleukine-8 but not Flt-3 ligand. Blood **90:** 2522–2528.

15. TERASHIMA, T., D. ENGLISH, J.C. HOGG & S.F. VAN EEDEN. 1998. Release of polymorphonuclear leukocytes from the bone marrow by interleukin-8. Blood **92:** 1062–1069.

16. BALLIN, A., D. LEHMAN, P. SIROTA, U. LITVINJUK & D. MEYTES. D. 1998. Increased number of peripheral blood CD34+ cells in lithium-treated patients. Br. J. Haematol. **100:** 219–221.

17. PRUIJT, J.F.M., Y. VAN KOOYK, C.G. FIGDOR, I.J.D. LINDLEY, R. WILLEMZE & W.E. FIBBE. 1998. Anti-LFA-1 blocking antibodies prevent mobilization of hematopoietic progenitor cells induced by interleukin-8. Blood **91:** 4099–4105.

18. MORRISON, S.J., D.E. WRIGHT & I.L. WEISSMAN. 1997. Cyclophosphamide/granulocyte colony-stimulating factor induces hematopoietic stem cells to proliferate prior to mobilization. Proc. Natl. Acad. Sci. USA **94:** 1908–1913.

19. DICKE, K.A., D.L. HOOD, M. ARNESON, L. FULBRIGHT, A. DISTEFANO, B. FIRSTENBERG, J. ADAMS & G.R. BLUMENSCHEIN. 1997. Effects of short-term in vivo administration of G-CSF on bone marrow prior to harvesting. **25:** 34–38.

20. OTTMANN, O.G., A. GANSER, G. SEIPELT, M. EDER, G. SCHULTZ & D. HOELZER. 1990. Effects of recombinant human interleukin-3 on human hematopoietic progenitor and precursor cells in vivo. Blood **76:** 1494–1502.

21. ROBERTS, A.W. & D. METCALF. 1995. Noncycling state of peripheral blood progenitor cells mobilized by granulocyte colony-stimulating factor and other cytokines. Blood **86:** 1600–1605.

22. LEITNER, A., H. STROBL, G. FISCHMEISTER, M. KURZ, K. ROMANAKIS, O.A. HAAS, D. PRINTZ, P. BUCHINGER, S. BAUER, H. GADNER & G. FRITSCH. 1996. Lack of DNA synthesis among CD34+ cells in cord blood and in cytokine-mobilized blood. Br. J. Haematol. **92:** 255–262.

23. CROOCKEWIT, A.J., R.A.P. RAYMAKERS, M.E.P. SMEETS, G. VD BOSCH, A.H.M. Pennings & T.J.M. DE WITTE. 1997. The low cycling status of mobilized peripheral blood CD34+ cells is not restricted to the more primitive subfraction. Leukemia **12:** 571–577.

24. YAMAGUCHI, M., K. IKEBUCHI, F. HIRAYAMA, N. SATO, Y. MOGI, J.-I. OHKAWARA, Y. YOSHIKAWA, K.-I. SAWADA, T. KOIKE & S. SEKIGUCHI. 1998. Different adhesive characteristics and VLA-4 expression of CD34+ progenitors in G_0/G_1 versus S + G_2/M phases of the cell cycle. Blood **92:** 842–848.

25. LEMOLI, R.M., A. TAFURI, A. FORTUNA, M.T. PETRUCCI, M.R. RICCARDI, L. CATANI, D. RONDELLI, M. FOGLI, G. LEOPARDI, C. ARIOLA & S. TURA. 1997. Cycling status of CD34+ cells mobilized into peripheral blood of healthy donors by recombinant human granulocyte colony-stimulated factor. Blood **89:** 1189–1196.

26. GRZEGORZEWSKI, K.J., K.L. KOMSCHLIES, J.L. FRANCO, F.W. RUSCETTI, J.R. KELLER, & R.H. WILTROUT. 1996. Quantitative and cell-cycle differences in progenitor cells mobilized by recombinant human interleukin-7 and recombinant human granulocyte colony-stimulating factor. Blood 88: 4139–4148.

27. HURLEY, R.W., J.B. MCCARTHY, E.A. WAYNER & C.M. VERFAILLIE. 1997. Monoclonal antibody crosslinking of the alpha 4 or beta 1 integrin inhibits committed clonogenic hematopoietic progenitor proliferation. Exp. Hematol. 25: 321–328.

28. WRIGHT, D.E., S.J. MORRISON, S.H. CHESHIER & I.L. WEISSMAN. 1998. Cyclophosphamide/granulocyte colony-stimulating factor induces proliferation of all bone marrow hematopoietic stem cells, followed by selective egress of stem cells after mitosis [abstr.]. Exp. Hematol. 26: 689.

29. YONG, K.L., M. WATTS, N.S. THOMAS, A. SULLIVAN, S. INGS & S.C. LINCH. 1998. Transmigration of CD34$^+$ cells across specialized and no endothelium requires prior activation by growth factors and is mediated by PECAM-1 (CD31). Blood 91: 1196–1205.

30. PROSPER, F., D. STRONCEK, J.B. MCCARTHY & C.M. VERFAILLIE. 1998. Mobilization and homing of peripheral blood progenitors is related to reversible downregulation of $\alpha 4\beta 1$ integrin expression and function. J.C.I. 101: 2456–2467.

31. COULOMBEL, L., I. AUFFRAY, M.H. GAUGLER & M. ROSEMBLATT. 1997. Expression and function of integrins on hematopoietic progenitor cells. Acta Haematol. 97:13–21.

32. MIYAKE, K., K.L. MEDINA, S.-I. HAYASHI, S. ONO, T. HAMAOKA & P.W. KINCADE. 1990. Monoclonal antibodies to Pgp-1/CD44 block lympho-hemopoiesis in long-term bone marrow cultures. J. Exp. Med. 171: 477–488.

33. MIYAKE, K., I.L. WEISSMAN, J.S. GREENBERGER & P.W. KINCADE. 1991. Evidence for a role of the integrin VLA$_4$ in lympho-hemopoiesis. J. Exp. Med. 173: 599–607.

34. TEIXIDO, J., M.E. HEMLER, J.S. GREENBERGER & P. ANKLESARIA. 1992. Role of $\beta 1$ and $\beta 2$ integrins in the adhesion of human CD34^{hi} stem cells to bone marrow stoma. J. Clin. Invest. 90: 358–367.

35. OOSTENDORP, R.A. & P. DORMER. 1997. VLA-4 mediated interactions between normal human hematopoietic progenitors and stromal cells. Leuk. Lymphoma 24: 423–435.

36. HIRSCH, E., A. IGLESIAS, A.J. POTOCNIK, U. HARTMANN & R. FÄSSLER. 1996. Impaired migration but not differentiation of haematopoietic stem cells in the absence of $\beta 1$ integrins. Nature 380: 171–175.

37. TO, L.B., D.N. HAYLOCK, T. DOWSE, P.J. SIMMONS, S. TRIMBOLI, L.K. ASHMAN & C.A. JUTTNER. 1994. A comparative study of the phenotype and proliferative capacity of peripheral blood (PB) CD34$^+$ cells mobilized by four different protocols and those of steady-phase PB and bone marrow CD34$^+$ cells. Blood 84: 2930–2939.

38. KATAYAMA, N., J.-P. SHIH, S.-I. NISHIKAWA, T. KINA, S.C. CLARK & M. OGAWA. 1993. Stage-specific expression of c-kit protein by murine hematopoietic progenitors. Blood 82: 2353–2360.

39. OKUMURA, N., K. TSUJI, Y. EBIHARA, I. TANAKA, N. SAWAI, K. KOIKE, A. KOMIYAMA & T. NAKAHATA. 1996. Chemotactic and chemokinetic activities of stem cell factor on murine hematopoietic progenitor cells. BLOOD 87: 4100–4108.

40. JANOWSKA-WIECZOREK, A., L.A. MARQUEZ, M.L. CABUHAT, MONTAÑO, J.-M. NABHOLTZ, J.A. RUSSELL, D.R. EDWARDS & A.R. TURNER. 1998. CD34$^+$ stem/progenitor cells derived from peripheral blood express gelatinases and transmigrate through the reconstituted basement membrane: Role of cytokines [abstr.] Exp. Hematol. 26: 814.

41. NAKAMOTO, B. & T. PAPAYANNOPOULOU. 1994. Further insights on the anti-VLA4 induced hemopoietic progenitor (HP) peripheralization in primates [abstr.]. Blood **84:** 22a (abstr. suppl.).
42. VERMEULEN, M., F. LE PESTEUR, M.C. GAGNERAULT *et al.* 1998. Role of adhesion molecules in the homing and mobilization of murine hematopoietic stem and progenitor cells. Blood. **92**(3): 894–900.
43. CRADDOCK, C.F., B. NAKAMOTO, R.G. ANDREWS, G.V. PRIESTLEY & TH. PAPAYANNOPOULOU. 1997. Antibodies to VLA4 integrin mobilize long-term repopulating cells and augment cytokine-induced mobilization in primates and mice. **90:** 4779–4788.
44. CRADDOCK, C.F., B. NAKAMOTO, M. ELICES & T. PAPAYANNOPOULOU. 1997. The role of CS1 moiety of fibronectin in VLA4-mediated haemopoietic progenitor trafficking. Br. J. Haematol. **97:** 15.
45. PAPAYANNOPOULOU, TH., G.V. PRIESTLEY & B. NAKAMOTO. 1998. Anti-VLA4/VCAM-1–induced mobilization requires cooperative signaling through the kit/mkit ligand pathway. Blood **91:** 2231–2239.

DISCUSSION

D.A. WILLIAMS (*Riley Hospital for Children*): I assume that when you looked for the combined effects of the G-CSF receptor with anti-VLA-4 in the growth factor knock-outs that you lost the combined effect even though VLA-4 still mobilized. Is that correct?

PAPAYANNOPOLOU: I have not yet had the opportunity to test that owing to the unavailability of mice.

WILLIAMS: Your data would suggest that there is cross-talk between VCAM and a cytoplasmic tail of SCF. Is there any evidence for that?

PAPAYANNOPOLOU: The only evidence that we have is that Steel mice do not respond to anti-VCAM-1, but do respond to anti-VLA-4. It could be that once you start with the hemopoietic cells somehow a message gets through, because they do respond to the alpha-4. But when you start with the stroma the message does not go.

L. KANZ (*Eberhard Karls University*): I would like to come back to what we have observed and Robert Möhle has presented here, and what has been presented by G. Spangrude and you. Independent of the way mobilization is induced (e.g., toxins, chemotherapy, hematopoietic growth factors), there is—whether it is cause or consequence—a decreased expression of cytoadhesive molecules. What do you think it means that homing to the bone marrow might be decreased.

PAPAYANNOPOLOU: This is not necessarily the case because the integrins are very versatile molecules. They can change in a short time. We have transplanted monkey cells that were treated with the anti-alpha-4. We had a little delay in disappearance of cells from the circulation after they were injected. However, engraftment of neutrophils and platelets was not delayed.

D. METCALF (*P.O. Royal Melbourne Hospital*): You did not say whether anti-PECAM-1 (or CD31) was able to suppress the action of G-CSF. Are you are suggesting it was acting late to regulate the egress of cells from the bone marrow?

PAPAYANNOPOLOU: We have not done that experiment yet. We plan to test this concept in several ways of mobilization. I don't know yet whether it is a common inhibitor or whether the inhibition is specific for anti-VLA-4–induced mobilization.

J.D. GRIFFIN (*Dana Farber Cancer Institute*): I have a question about kinetics. An antibody like anti-VLA-4 would block integrin function almost instantly and yet the mobilization of stem cells occurs 1 to 3 days later. Is it possible that the antibody is really blocking a re-entry event rather than making stem cells leave the marrow? Perhaps there is continuous traffic of stem cells between marrow and blood and what is happening is an accumulation of cells because they cannot get back in.

PAPAYANNOPOLOU: We have looked at the kinetics. You start seeing the effect by 8 hours and it peaks in 24 hours. The effect builds up so it does not behave like an immediate event. It is conceivable that there is an early effect on adhesion, but additional steps are needed for the cells to get out. If the theory that we affect the re-entry of cells to the BM is correct, then these cells would have to be turning over very fast and it would predict a continous accumulation of cells in blood, something that we do not see.

S.T. ILDSTAD (*Alleghany University of Health Sciences*): Your studies are very elegant and my question regards the marrow compartment. In some simple studies we have performed, if we treat mice with G-CSF alone, we see an increase in stem cells out in the periphery, but in very low numbers. If we treat with Flt-3 alone, the expansion is in the marrow compartment and not in the periphery. With G-CSF and Flt-3 the stem cells migrate out to the periphery. Have you looked at the marrow compartment after treatment with your various antibodies?

PAPAYANNOPOLOU: When you combine something with G-CSF, you invariably get G-CSF kinetics. With the Flt-3 alone, it takes 7 days to get the effect, but if you combine G-CSF, it takes only 3 days. The reason that it is fast and massive is that despite the fact that the Flt-3 ligand has a peak mobilization effect at 7 days, the proliferation in the marrow peaks at days 3 to 4. Now, with the antibodies only, we do not see significant changes in the bone marrow.

P.J. QUESENBERRY (*University of Massachusetts Medical Center*): Is there any difference in the endothelial coverage or the actual structure or marrow sinusoids when you give the antibody? Do you know the old studies of actually opening up spaces for migration of different cell types?

PAPAYANNOPOLOU: Do you mean changes similar to ones occurring with irradiation or endotoxin?

QUESENBERRY: With erythropoietin also?

PAPAYANNOPOLOU: I have not done any studies that address any structural changes in the marrow.

S.J. SHARKIS (*Johns Hopkins Oncology Center*): You mentioned chemotherapy only in passing. Do you think that the chemotherapy mechanisms relate specifically to induction of specific cytokines/chemokines or is it some other mechanism that might be clearly working with chemotherapy-induced mobilization?

PAPAYANNOPOLOU: We do not know. The only thing that is known is that Cytoxan-induced mobilization does not work in the G-CSF receptor knock-out. These mice do not show neutrophilia and mobilization after Cytoxan treatment.

W.E. FIBBE (*University Medical Center, Leiden*): Dr. Papayannopoulou, in your combination studies with the cytokines, I noticed that you used what I would say are suboptimal doses of the cytokines, that is, 3 days of G-CSF or 5 days of Flt-3 ligand. What happens if you use optimal doses, let us say 5 days or 7 days of G-CSF or 10 days of Flt-3 ligand? Can you still mobilize cells with anti-VLA-4 antibody that are not responsive to mobilization with G-CSF or Flt-3 ligand?

PAPAYANNOPOLOU: That is a good question. The studies with G-CSF were done with 100 mg/kg in mice. To approach this point we treated mice and primates with combinations of cytokines, that is, G-CSF and Flt-3-L or G-CSF and KL, and super-imposed anti-VLA-4. In all cases augmentation was seen. However, it is theoretically possible that with a very high mobilization efficiency, the difference might not be very significant.

Characterization of Purified and *Ex Vivo* Manipulated Human Hematopoietic Progenitor and Stem Cells in Xenograft Recipients

THOMAS A. BOCK,[a] BENEDIKT L. ZIEGLER, HANS-JÖRG BÜHRING, STEFAN SCHEDING, WOLFRAM BRUGGER, AND LOTHAR KANZ

Department of Hematology and Oncology, University of Tübingen, Otfried-Müller-Str. 10, D-72076 Tübingen, Germany

ABSTRACT: Research on the biology, regulation, and transplantation of human hematopoietic stem cells requires test systems for the detection, monitoring, and quantitation of these cells. Xenografted animal models provide suitable stem cell assays, since they allow long-term engraftment, multilineage differentiation, and serial transfer of human hematopoietic cells. Recent techniques for the separation of hematopoietic cells have provided highly purified cellular subsets selected on the basis of the surface marker phenotype. The stem cell content of these subsets, however, is still unclear. Also, innovative approaches for the induction of hematopoietic cell proliferation and differentiation have generated *ex vivo* manipulated cells whose biological properties and functions still remain to be assessed. This paper reports on the biological characterization of these cell populations by the use of xenograft models.

INTRODUCTION

One major challenge in hematopoiesis research is directed towards the biology, the external and intracellular control, and the transplantation capacities of human hematopoietic stem cells. In the murine system, multiple *in vivo* assays have been established which define the properties of the most primitive hematopoietic cells.[1] In most of these assays, surface phenotyping and serial transplantation approaches have been used for testing the input cells for self-renewal and pluripotent capacity, the defined properties of pluripotent hematopoietic stem cells (PHSC). In humans, these studies cannot be performed for ethical reasons. Therefore, xenografted recipient animals have been recruited to provide a permissive environment for the study of primitive human hematopoietic cells.[2]

THE FETAL SHEEP XENOGRAFT MODEL

Human hematopoietic cells that have been injected into the peritoneal cavity of preimmune fetal sheep or monkeys do engraft and can mediate multilineage, long-term hematopoiesis.[3–7] Since xenografted donor cells are in competition with

[a]Corresponding author. Phone, +49 7071 298-2767; fax, +49 7071 29-2767; e-mail, tsbock@med.uni-tuebingen.de

the endogenous pool of stem cells, the level of engraftment of human cells is relatively low. Nevertheless, engraftment was successful of even as few as several hundred progenitor-enriched human bone marrow cells.[8]

THE IMMUNODEFICIENT MOUSE XENOGRAFT MODEL

Immunodeficient mouse strains provide a small animal model with a permissive microenvironment for the engraftment of human hematopoietic cells. Most commonly used mouse strains include beige, nude and X-linked immunodeficient (bnx) mice, severe combined immunodeficient (SCID) mice, and (non-obese diabetic-) NOD-SCID mice.[9–11] Human hematopoietic cells engraft in all three mouse strains with highest quantitative levels being reported in NOD-SCID mice.[12–15] The detection of small numbers of transplanted cells and the quantitation of primitive progenitor cells are still limited, however feasible.[15] In order to increase the engraftment level, multiple strategies have been pursued to provide complementary support for the proliferation and differentiation of xenografted cells. These include the injection of recombinant human cytokines,[16, 17] the endogenous expression of human cytokine transgenes,[14] and the cotransplantation of human fetal tissues [18, 19] or stromal cells engineered to produce human interleukin-3 (IL-3).[12]

XENOGRAFT MODELS AS AN ASSAY FOR PHSC

In PHSC assays, demonstration of long-term, multilineage hematopoietic repopulation and serial transfer capacity are required as evidence for the self-renewal and pluripotence of the input test cells.[1, 2] These criteria are fulfilled by the xenograft fetal sheep and immunodeficient mouse models, as shown in TABLE 1. Long-term engraftment has been observed for several months in immunodeficient mice[12–14] and for several years in the sheep model.[4, 6] Occasionally, engraftment even persisted for more than a year in murine recipients and for more than a decade in sheep. Xenografted cells differentiated into the granulocytic, erythroid, monocytic, megakaryocytic, and lymphoid lineages (own observations (see FIG. 1) and Refs. 15, 19). Whereas in the sheep model, differentiation along both, B- and T-lymphoid lineages has been reported,[5, 6] human lymphopoiesis in immunodeficient mice is only B-cellular (Ref. 15 and own data). However, T-lymphocytes were also reconstituted when human fetal thymus had been cotransplanted with fetal donor cells.[18, 20] Xenografted hematopoiesis was clonal as demonstrated by retroviral marking.[12, 24] Donor cells recovered from primary immunodeficinent mouse recipients had the capacity to reconstitute myelolymphoid hematopoiesis in secondary recipients.[19, 22] Also, human hematopoietic cells from the marrows of adult sheep, previously injected in utero with human fetal liver cells, could be transferred and engrafted secondary sheep recipients.[6, 22, 25] These data confirm that PHSC properties are reflected in xenograft models. Xenograft repopulating cells thus can be considered PHSC, and xenograft models therefore represent suitable assays for human PHSC.

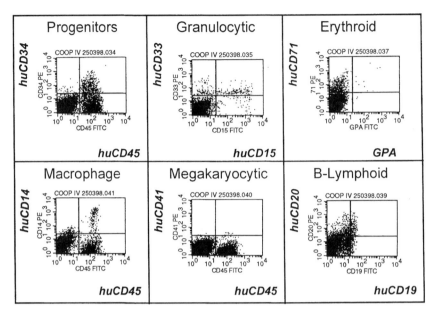

FIGURE 1. Human cell populations in NOD-SCID bone marrow.

STUDY OF PHENOTYPICALLY DEFINED HEMATOPOIETIC CELLULAR SUBSETS IN XENOGRAFT MODELS

Multiple surface markers have been positively or negatively correlated to early hematopoietic cells, such as CD34, CD38, c-kit, Thy-1, the AC133 antigen, or various tyrosine receptor kinases. A combination of these markers divides the pool of hematopoietic cells into multiple subsets. In order to test these fractions for the presence and concentration of PHSC, xenotransplantation approaches can be used and help to identify the PHSC phenotype.

CD34^{pos} Fraction

By magnetic immunoabsorption cell separation techniques (e.g., magnetic acivated cell sorting (MACS), AmCell Corp.) enrichment of CD34^{pos} cells up to a purity of greater than 99% has become feasible. Xenotransplantation of 1.5×10^5 of highly purified human CD34^{pos} cord blood engraftment in sublethally irradiated NOD/SCID mice was followed by long-term, multilineage for at least 3 months (FIG. 2). Also, mobilized human CD34^{pos} cells from the peripheral blood, CD34^{pos}lin^{neg} cells from fetal liver, or CD34^{pos}lin^{neg}Thy-1^{pos} bone marrow cells have engrafted immunodeficient mice long-term (own unpublished data, Refs. 21, 42).

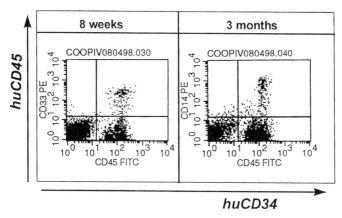

FIGURE 2. CD34$^+$ human cord blood engraftment in NOD-SCID bone marrow.

CD34$^+$38$^-$ fraction

SCID repopulating cells (SRC) have been contained in the CD34^{pos}CD38^{neg} but not in the CD34^{pos}CD38^{pos} fraction.[15,26,40] The frequency of SRC was determined at about 1 per 10^6 human cord blood and 1 per 3×10^6 bone marrow cells.[15] In these studies, the SRC appeared biologically distinct from long-term culture-initiating cells (LTC-IC) and ancestral to these progenitors. Similar results have been reported after transplantation of CD34$^+$CD38$^-$lin$^-$ cells.[27] Transplantation of CD34$^-$lin$^+$ cells as a control was not followed by successful engraftment. However, in one report SRC were contained in both, the CD34$^+$CD38 as well as the CD34$^+$CD38$^+$ fractions.[28]

CD34$^+$c-kit^{low} Fraction

In the murine system, PHSC have been characterized as FR25 (flow rate of 25 ml/min), Lin$^-$, c-kit bright cells. To test the c-kit expression on human repopulating stem cells, Kawashima *et al.* further separated CD34$^+$ enriched cells into c-kit^{bright}, c-kit^{low}, and c-kit^{negative} subsets. Engraftment was restricted to the c-kit^{low} as opposed to the c-kit^{bright} or c-kit^{negative} fractions.

CD34$^-$ Fraction

In spite of the studies above which identify xenograft repopulating cells within the CD34$^+$ fraction, there are murine data describing an apparently CD34^{negative} or CD34^{low} population of murine hematopoietic cells that can mediate long-term, multilineage engraftment even if transplanted as single cells.[31,32] In addition, Zanjani *et al.*[25]) transplanted both, CD34$^+$Lin$^-$ or CD34$^-$Lin$^-$ cells from the same human donors into preimmune fetal sheep, and reported long-term engraftment and multilineage hematopoietic cell expression from both fractions. Significant numbers of human CD34$^+$ cells were detected in sheep transplanted with CD34$^-$ grafts. The transplantation of human repopulating stem cells within the CD34$^-$ fraction was supported by secondary transplantation and limiting dilution studies.

In conclusion, murine and xenograft data on the CD34 surface marker phenotype of progenitor cells can suggest that various stem cell subsets exist which differ in their expression, splicing or glycosylation of the CD34 antigen. Explanations for reports of murine repopulating cells that were either CD34$^+$38) or CD34$^-$ also include genetic differences between murine strains with regard to CD34 expression in hematopoietic cells, as has been discussed for c-kit expression. Also, assay limitations have to be taken into account, since contamination by single cells is possible current separation techniques, and even a very small number of cells apparently can engraft xenograft recipients (particularly fetal sheep). This could generate false positive results.

AC133 Antigen$^+$ Fraction

AC133 is one of a new panel of murine hybridoma cell lines producing monoclonal antibodies to a novel glycoprotein antigen with a molecular weight of 120 kD. AC133 is selectively expressed on CD34$^+$ cells, and appears to be associated with early hematopoietic cells.[33,34] A first study has provided evidence for the long-term repopulation potential of AC133$^+$ cells:[33] AC133-selected cells successfully engrafted in the fetal sheep model, and human cells harvested from the bone marrow of primary recipients could be transferred to secondary sheep.

STUDY OF *EX VIVO* MANIPULATED HEMATOPOIETIC CELLS IN XENOGRAFT MODELS

Several studies have described culture conditions for the amplification of primitive human progenitor cells defined *in vitro* (e.g., long-term culture initiating cells, LTC-IC).[34,39] Xenograft studies, however, revealed that most of these protocols were unsuitable for the maintenance of long-term repopulating cells.[35–37]

Recently, culture conditions have been described that seemed to maintain and even to slightly expand the number of SRC. Human bone marrow cells that had been cultured in 6-day stroma-free medium supplemented with thrombopoietin, c-kit ligand, and flk2/flt3 ligand retained the capacity for *in vivo* marrow repopulation similar to freshly isolated CD34^{pos}lin^{neg}Thy-1^{pos} cells.[42] Incubation of purified CD34$^+$CD38$^-$ human cord blood cells in serum-free medium containing flt-3 ligand, stem cell factor, interleukin-3, interleukin-6, and granulocyte colony-stimulating factor for 5–8 days resulted in a 100-fold amplification of colony-forming cells, a 4-fold expansion of LTC-IC, and a 2-fold increase of SRC.[28] In another study,[27] maintenance or modest increase of SRC by a factor of 2–4 was described. However, maintenance of SRC was restricted to a maximum of 4 days in culture, and SRC were lost using extended culture periods.

SUMMARY

The study of early human hematopoiesis has been greatly enhanced by xenograft animal models which provide the feasibility to study human hematopoietic cells *in vivo* but outside the human body. It is generally suggested that human multipotent, long-term repopulating cells are contained in the $CD34^+$, the c-kit^{low} and the $CD38^-$ fractions. However, alternative data exist that may direct at different stem cell subsets or may be due to assay artefacts. Therefore, xenograftment by $CD34^{neg/low}$ or $CD34^+CD38^+$ cells has to be investigated further, and results cannot be evaluated at the present stage. Recent culture protocols for the *ex vivo* expansion of human hematopoietic progenitors are able to maintain PHSC, and early acting cytokines such as SCF, and Flt-3 ligand appear to be essential. As a prospect, it can be anticipated that the study of xenografted animal models will become increasingly valuable and will increase our knowledge about primitive human hematopoietic cells and the cellular phenotypes along the proliferation and differentiation processes.

REFERENCES

1. ORLIC, D. & D.M. BODINE. 1994. What defines a pluripotent hematopoietic stem cell (PHSC): Will the real PHSC please stand up! Blood **84:** 3991–3994.
2. BOCK, T.A. 1997. Assay systems for hematopoietic stem and progenitor cells. Stem cells **15**(Suppl. 1): 185–195.
3. FLAKE, A.W, *et al.* 1986. Transplantation of fetal hematopoietic stem cells in utero: the creation of hematopoietic chimeras. Science **233:** 776–778.
4. SROUR, E.F. *et al.* 1992. Sustained human hematopoiesis in sheep transplanted in utero during early gestation with fractionated adult human bone marrow cells. Blood **79:** 1404–1412.
5. ZANJANI, E.D. *et al.* 1992. *Ex vivo* incubation with growth factors enhances the engraftment of fetal hematopoietic cells transplanted in sheep fetuses. Blood **79:** 3045–3049.
6. ZANJANI, E.D. *et al.* 1994. Long-term repopulating ability of xenogeneic transplanted human fetal liver hematopoietic stem cells in sheep. J. Clin. Invest. **93:** 1051–1055.
7. ZANJANI, E. D. 1997. Transplantation of hematopoietic stem cells in utero. Stem Cells **15**(Suppl. 1): 79–93.
8. KAWASHIMA, I. *et al.* 1996. $CD34^+$ human marrow cells that express low levels of kit protein are enriched for long-term marrow-engrafting cells. Blood **87:** 4136–4142.
9. FLANAGAN, S. P. 1966. *Nude*, a new hairless gene with pleiotropic effects in the mouse. Genet. Res. **8:** 295–309.
10. BOSMA, G.C. *et al.* 1983. A severe combined immunodeficiency mutation in the mouse. Nature **301:** 527–530.
11. SHULTZ, L.D. *et al.* 1995. Multiple defects in innate and adaptive immunologic function in NOD-LtSz-SCID mice. J. Immunol. **154:** 180–191.
12. NOLTA, J.A. *et al.* 1994. Sustained human hematopoiesis in immunodeficient mice by cotransplantation of marrow stroma expressing human interleukin-3: analysis of gene transduction of long-lived progenitors. Blood **83:** 3041–3051.
13. VORMOOR, J. *et al.* Immature human cord blood progenitors engraft and proliferate to high levels in severe combined immunodeficient mice. Blood **83:** 2489–2497.
14. BOCK, T.A. *et al.* 1995. Improved engraftment of human hematopoietic cells in severe combined immunodeficient (SCID) mice carrying human cytokine transgenes. J. Exp. Med. **182:** 2037–2043.

15. LAROCHELLE, A. *et al.* 1996. Identification of primitive human hematopoietic cells capable of repopulating NOD/SCID mouse bone marrow: implications for gene therapy. Nat. Med. **2:** 1329–1337.
16. KAMEL-REID, S. & J.E. DICK. 1988. Engraftment of immune-deficient mice with human hematopoietic stem cells. Science **242:** 1706.
17. LAPIDOT, T. *et al.* 1992. Cytokine stimulation of multilineage hematopoiesis from immature human cells engrafted in SCID mice. Science **255:** 1137–1141.
18. MCCUNE, J.M. *et al.* 1988. The SCID-hu mouse: murine model for the analysis of human hematolymphoid differentiation and function. Science **241:** 1632.
19. CHEN, B.P. *et al.* 1994. Engraftment of human hematopoietic precursor cells with secondary transfer potential in SCID-hu mice. Blood **84:** 2497–2505.
20. PEAULT, B. *et al.* 1991. Lymphoid reconstitution of the human fetal thymus in SCID mice with CD34$^+$ precursor cells. J. Exp. Med. **174:** 1283–1286.
21. HUMEAU, L. *et al.* 1997. Successful reconstitution of human hematopoiesis in the SCID-hu mouse by genetically modified, highly enriched progenitors isolated from fetal liver. Blood **90:** 3496–3506.
22. CASHMAN, J. *et al.* 1997. Sustained proliferation, multi-lineage differentiation and maintenance of primitive human haematopoietic cells in NOD/SCID mice transplanted with human cord blood. Br. J. Haematol. **98:** 1026–1036.
23. SHIMIZU, Y. *et al.* 1998. Engraftment of cultured human hematopoietic cells in sheep. Blood **91:** 3688–3692.
24. NOLTA, J.A. *et al.* 1996. Transduction of pluripotent human hematopoietic stem cells demonstrated by clonal analysis after engraftment in immune-deficient mice. Proc. Natl. Acad. Sci. USA **93:** 2414–2419.
25. ZANJANI, E.D. *et al.* 1998. Human bone marrow CD34$^-$ cells engraft *in vivo* and undergo multilineage expression that includes giving rise to CD34$^+$ cells. Exp. Hematol.: 353–360.
26. VERSTEGEN, M.M. *et al.* 1998. Transplantation of human umbilical cord blood cells in macrophage-depleted SCID mice: evidence for accessory cell involvement in expansion of immature CD34$^+$ CD38$^-$ cells. Blood **91:** 1966–1976.
27. BHATIA, M. *et al.* 1997. Quantitative analysis reveals expansion of human hematopoietic repopulating cells after short-term *ex vivo* culture. J. Exp. Med. **186:** 619–624.
28. CONNEALLY, E. *et al.* 1997. Expansion *in vitro* of transplantable human cord blood stem cells demonstrated using a quantitative assay of their lympho-myeloid repopulation activity in nonobese diabetic-SCIS/SCID mice. Proc. Natl. Acad. Sci. USA **94:** 9836–9841.
29. ORLIC, D. *et al.* 1994. Biological properties of pluripotent hematopoietic stem cells enriched by elutriation and flow cytometry. Blood Cells **20:** 107–117.
30. KAWASHIMA, I. *et al.* CD34$^+$ human marrow cells that express low levels of kit protein are enriched for long-term marrow-engrafting cells. Blood **87:** 4136–4142.
31. OSAWA, M. *et al.* 1996. Long-term lymphohematopoietic reconstitution by a single CD34-low/negative hematopoietic stem cell. Science **271:** 242–245.
32. JONES, R.J. *et al.* 1996. Characterization of mouse lymphohematopoietic stem cells lacking spleen colony-forming activity. Blood **88:** 487–491.
33. YIN, A.H. *et al.* 1997. AC133, a novel marker for human hematopoietic stem and progenitor cells. Blood **90:** 5002–5012.
34. BÜHRING, H.J. *et al.* 1999. Expression of novel surface antigens on early hematopoietic cells. This volume.
35. PETZER, A.L. *et al.* 1996. Differential cytokine effects on primitive (CD34$^+$CD38$^-$) human hematopoietic cells: novel responses to Flt-3 ligand and thrombopoietin. J. Exp. Med. **183:** 2551–2558.

36. SHIMIZU, Y. *et al.* 1998. Engraftment of cultured human hematopoietic cells in sheep. Blood **91:** 3688–3692.
37. GAN, O.I. *et al.* 1997. Differential maintenance of primitive human SCID-repopulating cells, clonogenic progenitors, and long-term culture-initiating cells after incubation on human bone marrow stromal cells. Blood **90:** 641–650.
38. KRAUSE, D.S. *et al.* 1994. Characterization of murine CD34, a marker for hematopoietic progenitor and stem cells. Blood **84:** 691–701.
39. KANZ, L. & W. BRUGGER. 1998. obilization and *ex vivo* manipulation of peripheral blood progenitor cells for support of high-dose cancer therapy. *In* Stem Cell Transplanation. Blume, Ed.: 455–467.
40. BHATIA, M. *et al.* 1997. Purification of primitive human hematopoietic cells capable of repopulating immune-deficient mice. Proc. Natl. Acad. Sci. USA **94:** 5320–5325.
41. CIVIN, C.I. *et al.* 1996. Sustained, transplantable, multi-lineage engraftment of highly purified adult human bone marrow stem cells *in vivo*. Blood **88:** 4102–4109.
42. LUENS, K.M. *et al.* 1998. Thrombopoietin, kit-ligand, and flk2/flt3 ligand together induce increased numbers of primitive hematopoietic progenitors from human CD34+Thy-1Lin− cells with preserved ability to engraft SCID-hu bone. Blood **91:** 1206–1215.

DISCUSSION

P.J. QUESENBERRY (*University of Massachusetts Medical Center*): You mentioned that IL-6, IL-3, Flt-3, and steel factor treatment of cord blood maintained stem cells, but from your figure it looked like there was a major drop compared to your uncultured cell engraftment and you had much more engraftment from the uncultured cells.

BOCK: The engraftment level was low in both, but it was sustained at 8 weeks. You may infer from Dr. Eaves' data that 8-weeks' engraftment will continue, but this is part of ongoing projects. Our 3-month and 6-month data are not available yet.

QUESENBERRY: We have done a large number of this type of transplant in collaboration with Lenny Shultz (in the range of 20–25) using IL-3, IL-6, IL-11, and steel factor, and we find a chaotic variability between cord blood samples. A third of them are better, a third of them are much worse, and with markedly skewed differentiation. It is an interesting but very difficult system to interpret.

BOCK: This is true, and that is what I indicated in my introduction. In order to minimize variation, we used fresh cord blood, and we only used cord blood samples that contained sufficient cells for at least 3 mice (for every experiment group). At least we got the same cord blood samples in every group. However, there still is wide variation.

J.E. DICK (*University of Toronto*): I would not really agree with Dr. Quesenberry. We have looked at a lot of cord blood samples. Ninety-nine percent of them are fresh not frozen cells. We do not find a huge amount of variability from sample to sample, quantitatively, in terms of the level of engraftment we are getting, but particularly if you are putting in more than a few stem cells. I think it is a numbers issue more than anything and probably also the stability of the animals. That is where more variability does come in. You made the comment that you have maintenance of stem cells during culture, but until you really do it quantitatively, you cannot be sure. 1×10^5

or 1.5×10^5 CD34$^+$ Lin$^-$ cells contain quite a few stem cells, probably 10 or 15. So you are actually putting a lot of stem cells into your culture. You have some surviving to the end, but that may not be maintenance. It could just be a steady loss. Kinetically, that is what we tend to see.

BOCK: Experiments are running now for the 3-month and 6-month engraftment data.

DICK: I do not think that that is the issue. The readout is the readout whenever you do it, but quantitatively it is the number of stem cells you start with and the number you have at the end.

BOCK: Yes.

D.A. WILLIAMS (*Riley Hospital for Children*): I want to make a comment on variability. We have not done any studies with expanded cells. However, we have done a fair number of studies with G-CSF-mobilized peripheral blood cells, and we noted variability early on. When we checked our NOD-SCID colony, we found that there were occasional animals that had circulating mouse T cells. The presence of these T cells correlated very well with variability in engraftment. Now, in our colony we actually assay for mouse T cells before we do any transplants. We have not been able to determine any infectious agent in the colony after extensive testing, and we have not been able to determine at the genetic level a cause for these T cells. But they are consistent in some proportion of the animals. So people working with these animals probably need to be aware of that. Again, it correlates quite nicely with large differences in engraftment of human cells.

BOCK: The only thing to reduce variability is to use young mice that are not leaky. And in these experiments we have only used untreated allogeneic donors as opposed to pretreated cancer patients, whose variabilities are still higher.

EAVES: Since we are discussing technical issues, I would like to make two other comments. First, in our experience it is very difficult to do any meaningful experiments with human cells transplanted into sublethally irradiated NOD/SCID mice beyond about 4 months, because such a large proportion of the animals will begin to develop thymomas after that time and one would not want to be including such mice in a follow-up group. Given this problem, I am curious about your suggestion that you plan to look at animals 6 months posttransplant. Second, in our experience when more than 4 human competitive repopulating units (CRU) are transplanted per mouse, one loses linearity between the percent repopulation obtained and the number of CRU transplanted. Therefore, differences between suspensions can be misjudged just because of this.

BOCK: The real long-term may be a problem because the average survival of these mice is 8.5–9 months. So you are really limited, and you have to start at a young age.

QUESENBERRY: We were forced by a NIH Study Section to carry out our experiments to 6 months. A small number of animals got very good engraftment, and although we worried about the thymoma/lymphoma development, at least in the animals we get from Lenny, that has not been a major problem; just a small percentage develop thymomas.

BOCK: We had different sets of animals with different rates of thymoma. Lenny Shultz recently discovered that he had an endogenous virus, and he tried to back-cross them with the NOD-SCIDs to get it out. I do not know how far he has advanced in this, but that may help.

S.J. SHARKIS (*Johns Hopkins Oncology Center*): What we have done to avoid that problem is at about 4 months to retransplant these animals. Although there is concern that the transplant in itself may have an effect, you do avoid the thymoma issue, and these animals seem to continue to engraft over a long period of time.

BOCK: That is correct. If you want to say that you maintain pluripotent hematopoietic stem cells in your culture, you cannot do this without serial transfer experiments or even clonal proof of hematopoiesis. Cord blood might be suitable for this, but for engraftment of peripheral blood it is quite difficult to quantitatively do serial transplant experiments with NOD-SCIDs.

K. WELTE (*Hannover Medical School*): Do you get engraftment of all cell lineages? What does the peripheral blood look like in these mice?

BOCK: I get all the lineages that I showed except for the megakarocytes in all three groups and from both sources. I could not show you all the data, but we also get the progenitors, the early erythroid cells, granulocytes, and the B cells.

Y. REISNER (*Weizmann Institute of Science*): That brings us to my question. You, like many people, cannot get T cells to develop. Why, and have you tried to do something about it?

BOCK: You can get T cells in the SCID mouse system, but you have to cotransplant fetal thymus. There are five or six papers out about xenografted T cells and SCID mice. Some do not describe homing to the thymus. However, there are two papers that say that if you transplant human T cells, you can traffic them to the thymus. Then they rest there, and they do not develop or do not function. Others say they do not travel, they do not home to the thymus. The data are very inconsistent, and the interpretation is also very inconsistent. Most authors, including Dr. Dick in his large studies, found B cells but no T cells. There may be some trafficking to the thymus, but not differentiation to mature T cells.

G. KELLER (*Howard Hughes Medical Institute*): We have done some of these transplants, and in about one-third of the mice you certainly do see colonization of the thymus with human cells. They make it to the CD4$^+$CD8$^+$ stage of development.

REISNER: It is intriguing, because mouse thymus can support growth of T cells in culture. So you would expect it would be okay if they arrive in the thymus.

BOCK: In one of the two publications, the authors were looking at the T lymphocytes, and they saw a very limited rearrangement spectrum. So there are probably only a few clones, and whether they are really functional is debated and argued against.

WILLIAMS: I want to add to Dr. Keller's comment. We have a paper coming out (van der Loo *et al.*, Blood, 1998) with a large number of animals engrafted with peripheral blood CD34 cells. In those animals we did see T cell development at least to the CD4$^+$/CD8$^+$ double positive stage. Interestingly enough, from the same donor in multiple animals, we saw T cell development only in animals that were treated with G-CSF as part of a mobilization scheme. We could not tell if this was a pre-T cell that derived from the graft or was a legitimate SCID-repopulating cell derivative that moved from the marrow to the thymus with G-CSF mobilization. Clearly as Dr. Keller said, we see some human double positive cells in a percentage of the animals.

BOCK: In your graft, do you select against T cells?

WILLIAMS: No.

KELLER: Does the graft contain double positive cells?

BOCK: The only cell that we have with $CD4^+ CD3^-$ phenotype is a macrophage.

KELLER: If you have cells with an immature phenotype, it is unlikely due to contamination of the graft by mature cells.

Absence of CD34 on Some Human SCID-Repopulating Cells

JOHN E. DICK[a]

Programs in Cancer/Blood Research and Developmental Biology, Research Institute, Hospital for Sick Children , and Department of Molecular and Medical Genetics, University of Toronto, Toronto, Ontario, Canada

ABSTRACT: The availability of *in vivo* repopulation assays has greatly aided the study of human hematopoietic stem cells. Here, I shall review recent data that has identified a novel class of human repopulating cells that do not express classical stem cell markers including CD34 but still retain the ability to repopulate nonobese diabetic/severe combined immunodeficient (NOD/SCID) mice.

INTRODUCTION

The mammalian hematopoietic system consists of a heterogeneous array of cells ranging from large numbers of differentiated cells with defined function, to rare pluripotent stem cells with extensive developmental and proliferative potential that are able to repopulate conditioned recipients.[1–3] It is important to determine the composition and relationship of the cell types that comprise the human stem cell compartment both to identify the cellular and molecular factors that govern normal and leukemic stem cell development and to develop clinical applications such as transplantation, gene therapy, stem cell expansion and tumor cell purging. Significant progress has been made in purifying primitive cell populations by cell sorting based on the absence or presence of cell surface markers.[4] Determination of the developmental capacity of these putative primitive cells and their relationship to other cells within the hematopoietic hierarchy has depended, until recently, on detection of the purified cells by *in vitro* clonogenic or stromal-based long-term culture assays, on inference from transplantation experiments in other species (murine or primate), and on human clinical trials. The critical marker that all these studies have identified is the sialomucin, CD34, which is expressed on primitive cells and is downregulated as they differentiate into more abundant mature cells.[4] However, CD34 is not unique to stem cells, since it is also expressed on clonogenic progenitors and some lineage committed cells.[5] Nevertheless, all clinical and experimental protocols including *ex vivo* culture, gene therapy, and stem cell transplantation are designed for cell populations enriched for CD34[+] cells by a variety of selection methods.[4]

[a]Correspondence to: John E. Dick, Room 10-133, Programs in Cancer/Blood Research and Developmental Biology, Research Institute, Hospital for Sick Children and Department of Molecular and Medical Genetics, University of Toronto, 555 University Avenue, Toronto, Ontario M5G 1X8, Canada. Phone, 416/813-6354; fax, 416/813-4931; e-mail, dick@sickkids.on.ca

Recent evidence from the murine system indicates that some stem cells capable of long-term repopulation do not express detectable levels of cell surface CD34.[6–9] For example, cell populations selected by high efflux of Hoechst dye (side-population, SP),[7,9] or by aldehyde dehydrogenase (ALDH) expression.[6] are enriched for repopulating cells, and cell surface analysis demonstrated that the majority of the selected cells lack expression of lineage markers and CD34. The most definitive study demonstrated that single murine Lin⁻CD34⁻ cells transplanted into lethally irradiated mice could sustain long-term multilineage engraftment.[8] Recently, SP cells, similar to their murine counterpart, have been isolated from nonhuman primate and human hematopoietic tissue.[9] Interestingly, the nonhuman primate cells were able to expand in long-term culture systems generating CD34⁺ cells. By contrast the human SP were unable to initiate long-term stromal cultures or generate colonies in methylcellulose assays.[9] Therefore, the inability to detect hematopoietic activity from human SP cells makes it unclear whether the human stem cell compartment contains primitive Lin⁻CD34⁻ stem cells capable of repopulation or whether these novel cells do not read out in the assay systems that have been used to date. Together these data are provocative and suggest that further investigation is warranted to determine if such stem cells exist in the human.

The only conclusive assay for stem cells involves measuring repopulation capacity,[1–3] a requirement that confounds attempts to characterize the hematopoietic stem cell phenotype in humans. We have developed a system to assay primitive human repopulating cells, termed severe combined immunodeficient (SCID) repopulating cells (SRC), based on their ability to initiate multilineage engraftment in immune-deficient SCID and nonobese diabetic (NOD)/SCID mice.[10–12] Cell purification and gene marking studies have demonstrated that the SRC are more primitive than the majority of cells detected using clonogenic and long-term stromal assays.[13,14] The SRC, which we have re-termed CD34^pos-SRC, were found in the Lin⁻CD34⁺CD38⁻ cell fraction and not in the more mature Lin⁻CD34⁺CD38⁺ and Lin⁺CD34⁻ cells.[14] This knowledge of the cell surface phenotype, together with the ability to quantify SRC by limiting dilution analysis,[15] has enabled extensive purification[14] and identification of the signals that induce proliferation and differentiation during culture.[16]

Complementary to the NOD/SCID system, a second repopulation assay system has been developed based on the ability of human cells to be engrafted into fetal sheep.[17] To a large extent, the characteristics of the human fetal sheep repopulating cell are similar to the SRC. The sheep has two added features particularly attractive for stem cell studies. First, the adult sheep is a large animal, and the size of the human graft while modest in frequency terms (~5%) is huge in total engrafted human cells. Thus the engrafting stem cells are subjected to large proliferative stimuli. Second, the sheep have a long life span making long-term repopulation studies feasible. Again an important requirement for a stem cell assay. Details of this assay system have been reviewed here and elsewhere.[17]

Together, both these assays have been used to examine the question of whether human CD34⁻ stem cells exist. In the last 6 months, two reports have been published using these two assay systems that demonstrate that a Lin⁻CD34⁻ cell fraction exists in the human hematopoietic system and contains cells with repopulation activity.[18,19] In addition, a third report suggests the possibility that at least some SRC enriched by exposure to cytokines and *in vitro* cytotoxic agents may be derived from CD34[-] cells.[20] We have termed the CD34[-] human stem cell that repopulates NOD/SCID mice as CD34[neg]-SRC.[19] Analysis of the differentiation capacity of these cells, both *in vivo* and *in vitro*, indicates that they represent a novel class of human stem cells distinct from CD34[+] cells. Thus, these studies challenge the dogma that CD34 is expressed on the surface of all human hematopoietic stem cells and identify new complexity in the human stem cell compartment. This review will examine the data generated using the NOD/SCID model.

IDENTIFICATION OF A NOVEL CLASS OF HUMAN STEM CELLS

The hallmarks of the new class of human hematopoietic repopulating cells, termed CD34[neg]-SRC, are the absence of classical stem cell-associated cell surface markers and a distinct survival, proliferation, and differentiation response following *in vitro* cytokine stimulation. The distinguishing phenotypic feature of these cells is the absence of CD34, human leukocyte antigen (HLA)-DR, and Thy-1 markers on their cell surface. By contrast, the most primitive subfraction derived from the Lin[-]CD34[+] cell fraction expresses all three of these cell surface markers.[21–24] Consequently, our work challenges the long-standing dogma that CD34 is a marker for all human repopulating stem cells. In addition to phenotypic differences, four additional lines of evidence make a functional distinction between these two stem cell populations. 1) While the Lin[-]CD34[-]CD38[-] cells have limited hematopoietic activity in the colony-forming cell (CFC) and long-term culture-initiating cell (LTC-IC) assays, Lin[-]CD34[+]CD38[-] cells are highly clonogenic in these two assays; this surprising result explains why the Lin[-]CD34[-] cells had not been discovered earlier. Until the recent development of repopulation assays,[10] *in vitro* assays were the only methods that could be used to link cell surface phenotype with biological function. The absence of clonogenic activity in these directly sorted Lin[-]CD34[-]CD38[-] cells is identical to the result reported for SP cells collected based on Hoescht staining profiles.[9] 2) The differentiation and proliferation of Lin[-]CD34[-]CD38[-] cells in response to growth factor stimulation is clearly distinct from that of Lin[-]CD34[+]CD38[-] cells. The Lin[-]CD34[-]CD38[-] cells were unable to proliferate or increase their clonogenic capacity in culture conditions that induce large increases in cell number and clonogenic progenitors from Lin[-]CD34[+]CD38[-] cells. 3) The repopulating ability of Lin[-]CD34[-] and Lin[-]CD34[-]CD38[-] cells was increased by 5-fold during *ex vivo* culture in the presence of 5% fetal calf serum (FCS) or human umbilical vein endothelial cell-conditioned medium (HUVEC-CM), respectively. By contrast, Lin[-]CD34[+]CD38[-] cells rapidly lost their repopulating activity when cultured in the same conditions most likely due to a differentiation response.[14] The complete loss of repopulating cells after *ex vivo* culture of Lin[-]CD34[+]CD38[-] cells in 5% FCS or HUVEC-CM eliminates any possibility that the human cell engraftment is being initiated from CD34[pos]-SRC that may have been inadvertently copurified within the Lin[-]CD34[-]CD38[-] subfraction. 4) The Lin[-]CD34[-]CD38[-] cells can be induced to differentiate into cells that express CD34 following *in vivo* repopulation or *in vitro* cytokine stimulation. This differentiation result is concordant with the sheep xenograft studies where Lin[-]CD34[-] cells produced a full human graft including

CD34$^+$ cells[18] and with the nonhuman primate *in vitro* studies showing production of CD34$^+$ cells.[9] Together, these data indicate that the CD34^{neg}-SRC found within the Lin$^-$CD34$^-$CD38$^-$ cell fraction represent a novel stem cell within the human hematopoietic hierarchy.

COMPLEXITY OF THE HUMAN STEM CELL COMPARTMENT

The identification of CD34^{neg}-SRC within the Lin$^-$CD34$^-$CD38$^-$ subfraction establishes that the human hematopoietic stem cell compartment is more complex than previously recognized. The analysis we have made of the developmental capacity of CD34^{neg}-SRC *in vitro* and *in vivo* provides an understanding of their relationship to other cells that comprise the human stem cell compartment. Two lines of evidence suggest that the Lin$^-$CD34$^-$CD38$^-$ cells are developmentally earlier than at least some CD34$^+$ cells. First, the CD34^{neg}-SRC had extensive proliferation and differentiation capacity *in vivo* generating all hematopoietic lineages including primitive CD34$^+$ cells. Second, *in vitro* cytokine stimulation also resulted in the production, within 2 to 4 days, of CD34$^+$ cells. Since previously developed *in vitro* cultures for primary hematopoietic tissue have been shown to cause differentiation, especially in the presence of serum, the induction of CD34 expression is most likely due to a differentiation response. However, these newly generated CD34$^+$CD38$^-$ cells may still have unique growth requirements for their continued functional development. Lin$^-$CD34$^-$CD38$^-$ cultures with highest proportion of newly formed CD34$^+$CD38$^-$ cells (e.g., 5% FCS) only had a modest increase in clonogenic activity, and their repopulation capacity was still low. This result also highlights the caution that should be used in linking a particular cell surface phenotype with biological function. In support of this point, we have recently found that cytokine stimulation of Lin$^-$CD34$^+$ cells in the presence of low amounts of serum generates large numbers of CD34$^+$CD38$^-$ cells, but these cells have lost their repopulation capacity (Dorrell *et al.*, in preparation). Similar results have been obtained in murine transplant studies. Lin$^-$Ly6A/E$^+$Thy-1$^+$ cells isolated from primary recipients did not have the same reconstitution potential in secondary recipients compared to primary mice transplanted with cells of the same phenotype.[25] Taken together, the *in vitro* and *in vivo* data provide evidence that Lin$^-$CD34$^-$ cells can be positioned earlier than at least some CD34$^+$ cells in the hierarchy of human stem cells.

The *in vitro* cytokine stimulation studies also indicated that the stem cells within the Lin$^-$CD34$^-$CD38$^-$ cell population were heterogeneous. In the absence of *in vitro* stimulation, a low proportion (1 in 125,000) of these cells have CD34^{neg}-SRC activity, while after culture the total number of CD34^{neg}-SRC detected is increased (1 in 38,000). This increase in CD34^{neg}-SRC seems to occur while the total cell number in the culture is stable or declining, suggesting that the induction of repopulating activity is unrelated to self-renewal but instead is due to the stimulation of Lin$^-$CD34$^-$CD38$^-$ cells into a state that is required for their detection as CD34^{neg}-SRC. For example, the cells could acquire homing molecules necessary for their trafficking to the NOD/SCID bone marrow following intravenous injection. Those cells with the potential for repopulation could be termed "pre-SRC" and would not have been detected in the absence of *ex vivo* culture. The increase in CD34^{neg}-SRC from the Lin$^-$

CD34⁻CD38⁻ cell population was unrelated to the acquisition of the CD34 antigen, because cultures containing HUVEC-CM gave rise to similar increases in CD34^{neg}-SRC without differentiation into CD34⁺CD38⁻ cells. This enhanced repopulation in the absence of CD34 expression suggests that expression of CD34 is not a prerequisite to the acquisition of repopulating activity of Lin⁻CD34⁻CD38⁻ cells. This result is consistent with the finding that mice that are deleted for CD34 have normal hematopoiesis.[26, 27]

CLINICAL IMPLICATIONS

With the identification of CD34^{neg}-SRC, a new area of investigation will develop to examine the basic biology of these novel human hematopoietic stem cells, the cellular and molecular factors that regulate their developmental program, and the clinical applications of stem cell transplantation. Moreover, it will be important to determine if the CD34^{neg}-SRC might be a target for leukemic transformation. We have identified human acute myeloid leukemia (AML) stem cells and have shown recently that the initiating events occur in CD34⁺CD38⁻ cells.[28, 29] However, the Lin⁻CD34⁻ subfraction was not examined in this study. Thus it will be important to determine if the leukemogenic event could occur in the Lin⁻CD34⁻ cells.

It will be imperative to determine whether the findings that have come from the murine and xenograft studies have any bearing on human clinical work. At present, all manipulations of human stem cells are based on CD34⁺ stem cells, and the Lin⁻CD34⁻CD38⁻ cells are being discarded during the CD34 selection step, although most human transplants use CD34-enriched cells that are only 30–80% pure.[30] The data indicate that Lin⁻CD34⁻CD38⁻ cells are not only present in cord blood but can also be found in bone marrow and can be mobilized into the peripheral blood using granulocyte colony-stimulating factor (G-CSF). Therefore, all human stem cell transplants have included at least some Lin⁻CD34⁻CD38⁻ cells as a "contaminant," raising the possibility that it is these previously unidentified stem cells that sustain engraftment. Our data provide strong support for a new gene marking trial in humans addressing whether long-term repopulation can be derived from the Lin⁻CD34⁻CD38⁻ cells. However, the reduced ability to genetically modify repopulating stem cells represents a major barrier to directly address this question.[13] The NOD/SCID system will be ideal to optimize conditions for transduction of CD34^{neg}-SRC.

REFERENCES

1. PHILLIPS, R. 1991. Hematopoietic stem cells: concepts, assays, and controversies. Sem. Immunol. **3:** 337–347.
2. MORRISON, S., N. UCHIDA & I. WEISSMAN. 1995. The biology of hematopoietic stem cells. Annu. Rev. Cell Dev. Biol. **11:** 35–71.
3. ORLIC, D. & D. BODINE. 1994. What defines a pluripotent hematopoietic stem cell (PHSC): will the real PHSC please stand up. Blood **84:** 3991–3994.
4. KRAUSE, D.S. et al. 1996. CD34: structure, biology, and clinical utility [see comments]. Blood **87:** 1–13.
5. ANDREWS, R., J. SINGER & I. BERNSTEIN. 1989. Precursors of colony-forming cells in humans can be distinguished from colony-forming cells by expression of CD33 and CD34 antigen and light scatter. J. Exp. Med. **169:** 1721.

6. JONES, R.J. *et al.* 1996. Characterization of mouse lymphohematopoietic stem cells lacking spleen colony-forming activity. Blood **88:** 487–491.
7. GOODELL, M.A. *et al.* 1996. Isolation and functional properties of murine hematopoietic stem cells that are replicating *in vivo.* J. Exp. Med. **183:** 1797–1806.
8. OSAWA, M. *et al.* 1996. Long-term lymphohematopoietic reconstitution by a single CD34-low/negative hematopoietic stem cell. Science **273:** 242–245.
9. GOODELL, M. *et al.* 1997. Dye efflux studies suggest that hematopoietic stem cells expressing low or undetectable levels of CD34 antigen exist in multiple species. Nat. Med. **3:** 1337–1345.
10. DICK, J.E. 1996. Normal and leukemic human stem cells assayed in SCID mice. Semin. Immunol. **8:** 197–206.
11. LAPIDOT, T. *et al.* 1992. Cytokine stimulation of multilineage hematopoiesis from immature human cells engrafted in SCID mice. Science **255:** 1137–1141.
12. KAMEL-REID, S. & J.E. DICK. 1988. Engraftment of immune-deficient mice with human hematopoietic stem cells. Science **242:** 1706–1709.
13. LAROCHELLE, A. *et al.* 1996. Identification of primitive human hematopoietic cells capable of repopulating NOD/SCID mouse bone marrow: implications for gene therapy. Nat. Med. **2:** 1329–1337.
14. BHATIA, M. *et al.* 1997. Purification of primitive human hematopoietic cells capable of repopulating immune-deficient mice. Proc. Natl. Acad. Sci. USA **94:** 5320–5325.
15. WANG, J.C., M. DOEDENS & J.E. DICK. 1997. Primitive human hematopoietic cells are enriched in cord blood compared with adult bone marrow or mobilized peripheral blood as measured by the quantitative *in vivo* SCID-repopulating cell assay. Blood **89:** 3919–3924.
16. BHATIA, M. *et al.* 1997. Quantitative analysis reveals expansion of human hematopoietic repopulating cells after short-term *ex vivo* culture. J. Exp. Med. **186:** 619–624.
17. ZANJANI, E.D. 1997. The human/sheep xenograft model for assay of human HSC (discussion). Stem Cells **15:** 209.
18. ZANJANI, E.D. *et al.* 1998. Human bone marrow CD34⁻ cells engraft *in vivo* and undergo multilineage expression that includes giving rise to CD34⁺ cells. Exp. Hematol. **26:** 353–360.
19. BHATIA, M. *et al.* 1998. A newly discovered class of human hematopoietic cells with SCID- repopulating activity. Nat. Med. **4:** 1038–1045.
20. BERTOLINI, F. *et al.* 1997. Multilineage long-term engraftment potential of drug-resistant hematopoietic progenitors. Blood **90:** 3027–3036.
21. TERSTAPPEN, L.W.W.M. *et al.* 1991. Sequential generations of hematopoietic colonies derived from single nonlineage-committed CD34⁺CD38⁻ progenitor cells. Blood **77:** 1218–1227.
22. HUANG, S. & L.W. TERSTAPPEN. 1994. Lymphoid and myeloid differentiation of single human CD34⁺, HLA-DR⁺, CD38⁻ hematopoietic stem cells. Blood **83:** 1515–1526.
23. BAUM, C.M. *et al.* 1992. Isolation of a candidate human hematopoietic stem-cell population. Proc. Natl. Acad. Sci. USA **89:** 2804–2808.
24. CRAIG, W. *et al.* 1993. Expression of Thy-1 on human hematopoietic progenitor cells. J. Exp. Med. **177:** 1331–1342.
25. SPANGRUDE, G.J., D.M. BROOKS & D.B. TUMAS. 1995. Long-term repopulation of irradiated mice with limiting numbers of purified hematopoietic stem cells: *in vivo* expansion of stem cell phenotype but not function. Blood **85:** 1006–1016.
26. SUZUKI, A. *et al.* 1996. CD34-deficient mice have reduced eosinophil accumulation after allergen exposure and show a novel crossreactive 90-kD protein. Blood **87:** 3550–3562.

27. CHENG, J. *et al.* 1996. Hematopoietic defects in mice lacking the sialomucin CD34. Blood **87:** 479–490.
28. LAPIDOT, T. *et al.* 1994. A cell initiating human acute myeloid leukaemia after transplantation into SCID mice. Nature **367:** 645–648.
29. BONNET, D. & J.E. DICK. 1997. Human acute myeloid leukemia is organized as a hierarchy that originates from a primitive hematopoietic cell. Nat. Med. **3:** 730–737.
30. BENSINGER, W. *et al.* 1997. Transplantation of allogeneic CD34+ peripheral blood stem cells in patients with advanced hematologic malignancy. Blood **88:** 4132–4138.

DISCUSSION

G.J. SPANGRUDE (*University of Utah Medical Center*): Does your stromal culture system contain any added cytokines, or is it just what comes from the stromal cells?

DICK: No, it contains Flt-3 ligand, stem cell factor, interleukin-6 (IL-6) and granulocyte colony-stimulating facor (G-CSF), which is our standard cocktail when we look for plus/minus (CD34+CD38−) cells. We have not broken apart this combination to see what these cells respond to.

H.E. BROXMEYER (*Indiana University*): Your thought on the seeding efficiency was very important. We really do not know what the seeding efficiency is in the SCID mouse models. However, this seeding efficiency may be different for cord blood versus mobilized peripheral blood versus bone marrow. I am not sure how you would get the seeding efficiency like people used to do for the spleen colony-forming unit assay in mice. That is a lot of work, but I think this is very important and may be very important in the context of studying engraftment of ex vivo expanded cultured cells. You may not be changing a cell from one stage of maturity to another. You may just be activating or changing homing mechanisms, so in fact when you think you are going from one stage of maturity to another, actually you are not. You are just changing the homing characteristics of that cell. I know that this is a very difficult concept to experimentally evaluate. When you originally published that excellent paper in Nature Medicine where you suggested that the SCID repopulating cell (SRC) was more immature than the long-term culture-initiating cell (LTC-IC) or other cells we are assaying, that was based very heavily on the fact that you had few gene marked cells repopulating the SCID mice, whereas the LTC-IC were clearly very efficiently transduced. We have already seen some engrafted NOD-SCID mice from which you get reasonably good gene marked cells. So, if you get to the stage where you increase the ability to see gene marked cells in SCID mice, how are you going to say then that the SCID repopulating cell is more immature than other cells such as the LTC-IC.

DICK: We are very fortunate for those studies and that our gene transfer conditions did allow us to see the differential gene transfer into LTC-IC and SRC, which allows us to make this claim. It is important to remember that there is no one piece of evidence that conclusively supports that claim. We have a number of consistent pieces of evidence. These include differential support of the cells on stroma during ex vivo culture, purification, and gene marking. Obviously, if you find better ways of doing gene transfer and you hit 100% of the cells, it is going to be 100% of everything. So it does not address that question. You just have better gene transfer.

B.P. SORRENTINO (*St. Jude Children's Research Hospital*): As I looked at the data with the CD34$^-$ cells, it seemed to me that at limiting dilution, the number of human cells you get in the mouse were less than what you get with CD34$^+$CD38$^-$ cells. In some ways that surprised me. If, in fact, CD34$^-$ cells are more primitive cells, perhaps they should have a greater proliferative potential. But you are getting 0.1% reconstitution. Did I see the data correctly? What are your comments on that?

DICK: There are two points. First, if you look at the long bones, you are talking about 40 to 50 million mononuclear cells. So 0.1% of those cells is actually quite a large number of cells that would have derived from a few transplanted stem cells. We published this in Blood from work on limiting dilution experiments where we looked at the level of repopulation that you get at limiting dose in animals. The actual level of repopulation is not that dissimilar, ranging, as you would expect, between 0.5–1%. We are in the ball park with these cells if you believe that we are transplanting at limiting dilution. What we have not done is to transplant high numbers of CD34$^-$ stem cells, such as when we simply transplant whole cord blood or put in a large number of stem cells and you get 30/40/50% human repopulation in the animals. We have not been able to collect that many stem cells of this particular type to transplant them and to see whether we get those high levels. Second, if they are more primitive (and it appears from what Dr. Nakauchi says that they are), they do much better competing against the CD34$^+$ cells. We have not done the competition experiments, which would be important to do, to ask whether they have higher secondary repopulation. It is true, in our hands, you might expect a better graft from one of these cells being put into the animals. We do not see that. So this could be a limitation of the assay. We do not know. But certainly from that standpoint, these cells do not behave exactly the way the murine cells would.

D.A. WILLIAMS (*Riley Hospital for Children*): How are you going to address the question of whether acquisition of CD34 *in vitro* leads to the ability of repopulation of NOD-SCID, since you have to use serum? As you have noted, you have to use serum to acquire the phenotype, while you also say that for these cells you need stroma attachment or some sort of stroma interaction for engraftment. At least, that is what your hypothosis seems to suggest.

DICK: This topic came up at the Orcas Island meeting. If this is a unique cell type, we are working a black box. We have no idea what these cells respond to, so we are just taking our best guess based on what we know for other cells. Clearly, this is important. Our conditions are suboptimal, and we need to find out what these cells respond to. It reminds me of the embryonic stem cell (ES) work that has been going on for a long time, to try to get hematopoiesis out of these cells. We need to look at a whole different pattern of cells, potentially looking at mesoderm-inducing factors, fringes, and bone morphogenic proteins (BMPs). We just do not know. Until we really find out what those conditions are, we are not going to be able to do those kinds of experiments.

I. LEMISCHKA (*Princeton University*): It would be useful to have a positive selection marker on these cells. Clay Smith has suggested that CD7 may, in fact, be expressed on this compartment in cord blood. Have you looked at that?

DICK: We have. However, we do not have any functional data yet. We can agree that CD7 is on a proportion of these cells. We have sorted those, and they are in the mice. But we do not have any data back on that.

Engraftment and Multilineage Expression of Human Bone Marrow CD34− Cells In Vivo[a]

ESMAIL D. ZANJANI,[b,d] GRAÇA ALMEIDA-PORADA,[b] ANNE G. LIVINGSTON,[c] CHRISTOPHER D. PORADA,[b] AND MAKIO OGAWA[c]

[b]Department of Veterans Affairs Medical Center, University of Nevada Reno, Reno, Nevada 89520, USA
[c]Department of Veterans Affairs Medical Center, University of South Carolina, Charleston, South Carolina 29401, USA

ABSTRACT: The fetal sheep competitive engraftment model of human hematopoietic stem cells (HSC) was used to evaluate the in vivo engraftment potential of human bone marrow CD34− Lin− cells. Transplantation of CD34− Lin− cells into primary hosts resulted in the long-term (>1 year) engraftment and multilineage donor cell/progenitor expression with production of significant numbers of CD34+ cells. Secondary transplantation and limiting dilution studies confirmed the presence in human CD34− fraction of HSC with in vivo long-term engraftment and multilineage differentiation potentials.

INTRODUCTION

Hematopoiesis is characterized by the continuous, dynamic process of cell turnover. This cell renewal process is supported by a small number of hematopoietic stem cells (HSC) that are capable of self-renewal and differentiation into multiple hematopoietic lineages.[1] A great deal of progress has been made in the isolation and characterization of mouse and human HSC.[2–10] In the mouse, the ability to assay for HSC in vivo has allowed relatively extensive characterization of the physical properties and biology of HSC.[11,12] There is a large amount of evidence that murine HSCs lack lineage-specific surface marker expression, and express a number of other antigens, including Sca-1 and c-kit.[5,6] In contrast to murine studies, studies of human HSC have relied on a number of in vitro assays that identify cells with the capacity to generate hematopoietic progenitors in long-term culture, and to differentiate into multiple hematopoietic lineages.[13,14] More recently a number of immunodeficiency mouse engraftment models have been used as in vivo assay systems for human progenitors.[15,16] Studies in these in vitro and in vivo systems have generally supported the expression of the CD34 antigen as a requisite for long-term repopulating capacity.[7–10,17] These studies, as well as the successful reconstitution of baboons, using CD34 enriched cell populations,[18] has resulted in the current

[a]Supported by Grants HL40722, HL46566, HL39875, and DK51427 from National Institutes of Health, and by the Department of Veterans Affairs.

[d]Corresponding author: Esmail D. Zanjani, Ph.D., Professor of Medicine and Physiology, Department of Veterans Affairs Medical Center, 1000 Locust Street (151B), Reno, NV 89520. Phone, 702/328-1232; fax, 702/328-1745; e-mail, zanjani@scs.unr.edu

acceptance of experimental and clinical strategies for enrichment of human HSC based on positive selection for the CD34 antigen.[19,20]

Recent observations by a number of investigators, however, have supported the presence of a rodent CD34⁻ cell population that is markedly enriched for long-term reconstituting capacity and that may be a more primitive precursor to the CD34⁺ cell.[21–23] There is also evidence of a similar population of cells in other species.[24–27] To investigate this possibility for human HSC, we used the in utero human/sheep competitive HSC engraftment model in primary and secondary recipients to examine the *in vivo* engraftment and differentiative potential of human bone marrow CD34⁻ cells. In the preimmune sheep, human HSC from fetal liver, cord blood, mobilized peripheral blood, and bone marrow competitively engraft the bone marrow and undergo multilineage differentiation.[28] More importantly, as we reported recently,[9,29] the sheep model can distinguish between the different human HSC subsets. Unlike the immunodeficient mouse models that fail to engraft committed progenitors (e.g., CD34⁺, 38⁺ cells), but in agreement with allogeneic mouse transplants, in this model, committed human progenitors produce transient engraftment in primary recipients, but fail to engraft secondary hosts.[9,29] In contrast, primitive human HSC (e.g., CD34⁺, 38⁻ , or CD34⁺, c-kit^low) produce long-term engraftment in both primary and secondary sheep recipients.[9,29] The results presented here demonstrate that the CD34⁻ fraction of adult human bone marrow contains cells capable of engraftment and differentiation into CD34⁺ progenitors and multiple lymphohematopoietic lineages in primary and secondary hosts.

MATERIALS AND METHODS

Donor Cell Preparations

Bone marrow aspirates were obtained from the posterior iliac crest of healthy adult volunteers according to guidelines established by the Institutional Review Boards for Human Research at the University of Nevada, the Medical University of South Carolina, and the Department of Veterans Affairs Medical Centers, Reno, NV and Charleston, SC. Bone marrow low-density mononuclear cells (BMNC) were enriched for CD34⁺ cells ($73 \pm 14\%$ purity, $n = 9$) using an immunoaffinity column (CellPro, Bothel, WA) according to manufacturer's instructions. Populations of CD34⁻ and CD34⁺ cells were isolated from lineage-depleted CD34⁺-enriched fractions by sorting on a fluorescence-activated cell sorter (FACS) Vantage flow cytometer as reported.[29,30] The cells were suspended in α-medium containing 20% fetal calf serum (FCS) and 50 µg/ml each of recombinant human interleukin-3 (rHuIL-3) and granulocyte/macrophage colony-stimulating factor (GM-CSF)[31] at desired concentrations for transplantation into fetal sheep.

Transplantations into Primary and Secondary Fetal Sheep

The *in vivo* engraftment/differentiation potential of all cell preparations was evaluated in the human/sheep xenograft model. The amniotic bubble procedure was used to perform intraperitoneal injections of donor cell populations into both primary and secondary preimmune fetal sheep recipients (55–60 days old; term = 145 days) as previously described.[32] In the first series of studies involving CD34⁻ cells, each primary fetal sheep recipient was injected with either 6×10^4 CD34$^+$ cells or with 3.5 $\times 10^6$ CD34$^-$ cells. In the secondary transplant studies, each secondary fetal sheep recipient was transplanted with 1.5×10^5 CD45$^+$ cells obtained from bone marrow of primary recipients at 2 and 8 months posttransplant. Human CD45$^+$ cells were isolated by positive selection from bone marrow mononuclear cells of chimeric primary recipients as previously described,[33] pooled and suspended in Iscove's Modified Dulbecco's Medium (IMDM) (Gibco Laboratories, Grand Island, NY) containing 10% fetal sheep serum for injection into the fetus.

In subsequent experiments, engraftment efficacy of the CD34$^-$ cell population in primary recipients was compared to enriched CD34$^+$ or CD34$^+$, 38$^-$ cell populations by limiting dilution. Limiting dilution curves were generated in dose ranges of 1–64 $\times 10^3$ cells/fetus for enriched CD34$^+$ cells, 0.2–4.8×10^3 cells/fetus for more highly enriched CD34$^+$, 38$^-$ cells, and 3–15×10^4 cells/fetus for CD34$^-$ cell populations. All cell preparations were injected in 0.5 ml of volume/fetus and, except for the primary recipients, transplanted with 3.5×10^6 CD34$^-$ cells/fetus, each cell dose was suspended in 10^7 washed maternal red blood cells immediately before injection.

Monitoring of Engraftment

Primary and secondary recipients were examined for donor cell engraftment/expression either at 2 months posttransplant or soon after birth and at intervals thereafter as described.[9] Blood, bone marrow, liver, spleen and thymus of primary and secondary recipients sacrificed at 2 months posttransplant (i.e., 1 month before birth), and bone marrow aspirates from all recipients after birth, were analyzed for the presence of human cells by flow cytometry using a FACScan flow cytometer as previously described.[34] At sacrifice, peripheral blood was collected by cardiac puncture, and the liver, spleen, thymus, and bones harvested aseptically and placed in sterile saline. The eight long bones collected were then flushed with IMDM using an 18-gauge needle. Following washing and weighing, single cell suspensions were prepared from thymus, liver, and spleen using a glass tissue homogenizer followed by filtration through a 70-μm nylon strainer (Becton Dickinson, Franklin Lanes, NJ). Total mononuclear cell counts for each organ were determined and used to calculate the estimated total number of human cells of a given phenotype. Bone marrow from all recipients was also examined for the presence of human hematopoietic progenitors as reported.[33,34] Briefly, bone marrow mononuclear cells (BMNC; 0.4–2×10^5 cells/ml) were assayed for hematopoietic progenitor cells in methylcellulose assays as described.[33,34] All cultures were established with IMDM and erythropoietin (2 IU/ml). For optimal growth of sheep colony-forming unit-mix (CFU-Mix), granulocyte/macrophage colony-forming unit (CFU-GM) and erythroid burst-forming unit (BFU-E), the cultures were supplemented (5% vol./vol.) with a preparation of phytohemagglutinin (PHA)-stimulated leukocyte-conditioned medium[33,34] produced from a mixture of fetal sheep spleen, thymus, liver, and bone marrow cells in IMDM with 2% fetal sheep serum.[33,34] In these cultures maximal numbers of sheep colonies develop by day 9 of incubation. Optimal growth of human hematopoietic progenitors was achieved with the addition of 5 ng/ml each of human interleukin-3 and GM-CSF in the absence of sheep phytohemagglutinin-stimulated leukocyte-conditioned medium (PHA-LCM) with maximal colony growth at day 19. Colonies were enumerated by type on days 9 and 19 of incubation. On day 19 individual colonies were

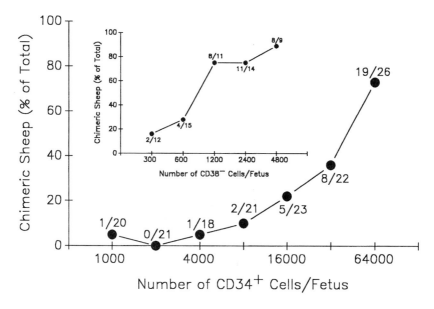

FIGURE 1. Limiting dilution studies with human bone marrow CD34⁺ and CD34⁺,38⁻ (*inset*) cells in sheep. The *first value* for each group indicates the number of animals found to be chimeric. The *second value* indicates the total number of animals transplanted in each group. Chimeric animals exhibited multilineage human cell/progenitor activity.

removed from the culture plates and processed for karyotyping as previously described.[33,34]

RESULTS

Results of limiting dilution assays established with CD34⁺ or CD34⁺, 38⁻ human BM cells were used to compare the relative engraftment efficacy of human CD34⁻ cells. FIGURE 1 summarizes the results of limiting dilution studies, conducted over the past 3 years, of transplantation of adult human BM CD34⁺ or CD34⁺, 38⁻ cells into preimmune fetal sheep. With very few exceptions, concentrations of $1-4 \times 10^3$ CD34⁺ cells/fetus failed to result in sustained chimerism. About 10% of recipients transplanted with 8×10^3 CD34⁺ cells exhibited human cell activity at 1 year of age (i.e., 15 months posttransplant). The percentage of chimeric animals increased with increasing doses of CD34⁺ cells with nearly 80% of sheep injected with 64×10^3 cells demonstrating human cell engraftment at 1 year of age (FIG. 1).

Two of 12 sheep transplanted with 300 CD34⁺, 38⁻ cells were chimeric at 1 year of age, while 4 of 15, and 8 of 11 recipients transplanted with 800 and 1200 CD34⁺, 38⁻ cells, respectively, exhibited chimerism (FIG. 1). Maximal percentage of chimeric recipients was obtained with 4800 CD34⁺, 38⁻ cells, which resulted in 8 of 9 animals being chimeric (FIG. 1).

Bone Marrow Mononuclear Cells

$\downarrow$

Lineage Depleted (MB) CD3, 14, 15, 16, 20, GlyA

$\downarrow$

FACS Sorted CD34 PE (HPCII) and CD3, 4, 8, 14, 15, 16, 20, GlyA FITC

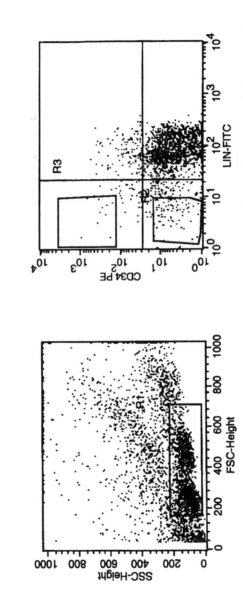
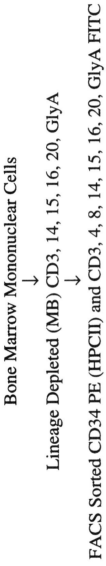

FIGURE 2. Sorting windows for donor CD34⁻ and CD34⁺ human bone marrow cells and the lineage depletion approaches used in this study. *Abbreviations:* MB, microbeads; Gly A, glycophorin A; FACS, fluorescence-activated cell sorter; PE, phycoerythrin; HPC, hematopoietic progenitor cells; FITC, fluorescein isothiocyanate; SSC, side scatter; FSC, forward scatter.

Table 1. Percentages and estimated total numbers of different human cells/progenitors in primary recipients at 60 days post-transplant[a]

Human Cells/ Progenitors	CD34$^+$ Group		CD34$^-$ Group	
	%	#	%	#
CD 3	0.52	7.7×10^7	0.24	1.2×10^9
CD 7	5.96	1.8×10^8	3.96	4.1%[b]
CD 13	0.36	1.1×10^8	0.00	0.00
CD 34	0.20	6.1×10^8	0.22	1.1×10^9
CD 45	1.02	7.9×10^{10}	2.49	1.4×10^{10}
HLA-DR	0.99	1.8×10^{10}	0.30	7.7×10^9
GLY-A	1.78	5.1×10^9	0.75	9.1×10^8
CFU-Mix[c]	7.10	1.3×10^5	7.10	2.5×10^5
CFU-GM[c]	13.70	2.2×10^5	4.30	4.3×10^5

[a]Each value represents mean of results from 2 animals/group and reflects the total numbers of each cell type detected in bone marrow, spleen, liver, and thymus.

[b]In CD34$^-$ group, CD7 was only detected in peripheral blood and is presented as % of total monnuclear cells only.

[c]The relative percentages of human CFU-Mix and CFU-GM were determined on day 19 of culture as described.[33] Because human progenitors were evaluated only in done marrow, the values reflect total numbers estimated to be present in the bone marrow from 8 long bones.

FIGURE 2 demonstrates the sorting windows for CD34$^-$ and CD34$^+$ cells used in studies in which the *in vivo* activities of these two cell populations from the same donor were directly compared. The results from primary recipients transplanted with either 6.4×10^4 CD34$^+$ or 3.5×10^6 CD34$^-$ cells/fetus are presented in TABLE 1.

Both groups presented with multilineage human cell expression including human myeloid (CD33$^+$), erythroid (glycophorin A (GlyA)) and lymphoid (CD3$^+$) cells, as well as human CFU-GM and CFU-Mix progenitors. TABLE 1 shows the relative percentages and the estimated total number of human cells/progenitors of different phenotypes in each primary recipient at 60 days posttransplant. It is of interest to note that there were about 10^9 CD34$^+$ cells in sheep transplanted with CD34$^-$ cells. This was nearly twice as many CD34$^+$ cells than were detected in the CD34$^+$ cell-transplanted recipient and supports the possibility that CD34$^-$ cells may serve as the precursor of CD34$^+$ cells.

Serial analysis of human cell/progenitor presence in bone marrow of primary recipients that were allowed to survive beyond term demonstrated the persistence of human cell expression for over 14 months after transplantation (FIG. 3). The long-term persistence of human cell activity in these primary recipients and the fact that bone marrow aspirated at 5 months posttransplant exhibited significant numbers of CD45$^+$, CD34$^+$ cells of donor origin[25] suggested that engraftment with long-term human HSC may have occurred. However, in our experience long-term activity of this duration in primary hosts can also occur with cells from the committed human progenitor pool.[9,29] In order to confirm the long-term engrafting nature of CD34$^-$ cells, human CD45$^+$ cells were isolated from bone marrow of primary recipients and

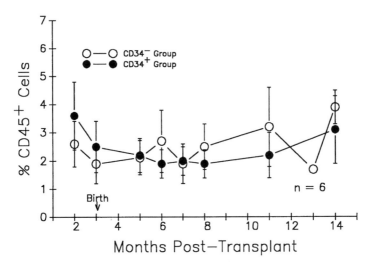

FIGURE 3. Human cell activity in primary sheep recipients transplanted with human bone marrow CD34$^+$ or CD34$^-$ cells. Each value represents the mean ± 1 SEM of results from 6 primary hosts. At all time points, the expression of human cells was multilineage.

transplanted into secondary preimmune fetal sheep. As shown in FIGURE 4, transplantation of CD45$^+$ cells obtained from bone marrow of primary animals transplanted with CD34$^-$ cells into secondary hosts resulted in human cell engraftment

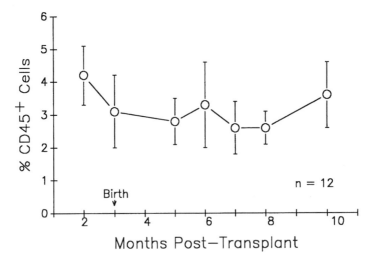

FIGURE 4. Human cell activity in secondary sheep recipients transplanted with human CD45$^+$ cells obtained from bone marrow of primary CD34$^-$ transplanted animals at 5 months posttransplant. Each value represents the mean ± 1 SEM of results from 12 animals.

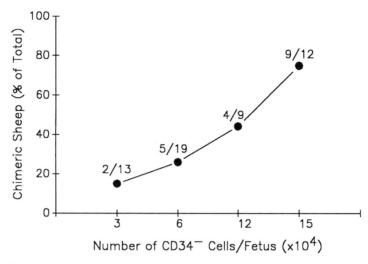

FIGURE 5. Limiting dilution studies with human bone marrow CD34⁻ cells in sheep. For details see legends to FIGURE 1.

that has persisted for at least 10 months. The ability to engraft secondary hosts has been associated only with stem/progenitor cell populations believed to represent the long-term repopulating HSC.[9,29,34]

The results of limiting dilution studies with CD34⁻ cells are presented in FIGURE 5. Overall, more CD34⁻ cells were required to achieve engraftment than CD34⁺ cells. However, the majority of sheep transplanted with 15×10^4 CD34⁻ cells were chimeric 60 days after transplantation.

DISCUSSION

The phenotype of the human pluripotent HSC remains to be defined. *In vitro*[1,13,14] and *in vivo*[15,16,28–33] studies designed to characterize repopulating capacity of human cell subpopulations have, in general, strongly supported expression of CD34 antigen as a requisite marker for long-term repopulating cells.[9,17,28,29,33] The majority of data supporting CD34 expression on human HSC is derived from *in vitro* assays, which phenotypically characterize cells capable of giving rise to committed hematopoietic progenitors after long-term culture. An example can be found in the long-term culture-initiating cell (LTC-IC) assay.[13] Although the relationship between LTC-IC and cells with *in vivo* reconstituting ability has recently been questioned,[38] the demonstration that CD34 enriched cells could provide rescue and long-term reconstitution in lethally irradiated baboons,[18] and that CD34⁺ cells could engraft in a variety of immunodeficient mouse and the preimmune fetal sheep models[15,16,26–29,31–35] has provided direct *in vivo* support for CD34 as a human stem cell marker. Because of these data, recent experimental and clinical strategies for enrichment of human HSC have been primarily based on positive selection for CD34 antigen and simultaneous lineage marker depletion.[19,20,36,37]

However, recent studies in the mouse have demonstrated the presence of CD34⁻ populations that contain progenitors capable of differentiation into CD34⁺ cells are highly enriched in HSC and have competitive long-term repopulating capacity *in vivo*.[21] Osawa *et al.*[21] reported that murine HSCs with long-term reconstitution capacity were present in the lin⁻c-kit⁺Sca-1⁺ CD34^{low}/⁻ cell population rather than CD34⁺ cells. Morel *et al.*[23] reported that the cells enriched in CD34⁺ fractions are largely short-term to mid-term engrafting cells, whereas the majority of the long-term engrafting cells are in the CD34⁻ cell population. In separate observations, Goodell *et al.*[22] have recently raised serious questions about CD34 expression on HSC. Their studies utilized dual-wavelength flow cytometric analysis of BM cells, stained with the fluorescent DNA-binding dye Hoechst 33342, to isolate a CD34⁻ population of murine HSC that is enriched over 3000 times in long-term repopulating capacity (side population or SP cells). They have subsequently applied the same methodology to porcine, rhesus monkey, and human BM cells, as well as umbilical cord blood cells, with findings of a remarkably similar population of SP cells.[22] SP cells derived from Rhesus BM are largely CD34⁻ and when cultured for 3 to 5 weeks on BM stromal cells, the CD34⁻ SP cells become largely CD34⁺,[24] consistent with a more primitive CD34⁻ HSC, which precedes the CD34⁺ progenitor. In this study, we used the human/sheep xenogeneic model as an assay to examine the *in vivo* long-term repopulating capacity of human CD34⁻ cell populations.

Our results demonstrate that transplantation of human CD34⁻, Lin⁻ populations results in long-term, multilineage human cell engraftment in the human/sheep model. In addition, harvest of human cells at various times after transplantation into primary hosts, with retransplantation into secondary recipients confirmed the presence of long-term engrafting cells in the CD34⁻, Lin⁻ population.[25] In our previous extensive experience with the sheep model, persistence of human cell engraftment for greater than 7 months after transplantation and the ability to engraft a secondary recipient 60 days after the primary transplant, reliably predicts long-term repopulating capacity, and chimeric sheep continue to express human cells for many years after transplantation.[28] In addition, in this study, animals transplanted with CD34⁻ cells demonstrated tremendous expansion of human hematopoiesis with the emergence of large numbers of CD34⁺ cells. This supports the existence of a CD34⁻ stem cell which can produce CD34⁺ progenitors. On comparison by limiting dilution, it was impressive that engraftment of the majority of animals could be achieved with as few as 2 to 3 times as many CD34⁻ cells as CD34⁺ cells, particularly since the CD34⁻ cell population used in this study is not highly defined.

We were concerned following our initial transplants that the human cell engraftment could be secondary to contaminating CD34⁺ cells in our CD34⁻ cell preparation which were below the threshold for detection by flow cytometry. We therefore performed limiting dilution studies to assess that possibility. If one assumes that the upper limit of undetectable CD34⁺ cells by flow cytometry is 3% (actual sensitivity is around 0.5%) then our primary recipients could have received as many as 1×10^5 contaminating CD34⁺ cells, which is enough to reliably engraft a fetal lamb. In the limiting dilution analysis, engraftment of recipient lambs was achieved in the majority of animals with 1.5×10^5 CD34⁻ cells. If one assumes 3% contamination by

CD34$^+$ cells (once again a gross overestimate), then a dose of 3600 to 4500 CD34$^+$ cells would have resulted in engraftment. This represents a dose in which only 2 of 59 sheep had evidence of human cell engraftment in the limiting dilution studies using CD34$^+$ cells, and represents approximately 1/15th the dose of CD34$^+$ cells required for consistent engraftment.

In the present study we cannot rule out a facilitating effect of cells in the CD34$^-$ population on engraftment of a minor contaminating population of CD34$^+$ cells, or the possibility that there were enough CD34$^+$, CD38$^-$ cells in the contaminating population to achieve engraftment. We feel a facilitating cell is unlikely, since the lineage depletion included CD8, which has been an associated marker in most identified "facilitating" populations.[39] In addition, CD38$^-$ cells represent a minor population of CD34$^+$ cells and therefore were unlikely to be present in adequate numbers for engraftment. Further studies using more defined CD34$^-$ cell populations will be required to definitively rule out these possibilities.

The results of this study provide further support for the existence of a primitive CD34$^-$ human cell population that contains in vivo long-term repopulating potential and is a precursor to the CD34$^+$ hematopoietic progenitors. The human/sheep xenogeneic model should prove invaluable in further characterization of this cell population.

REFERENCES

1. OGAWA, M. 1993. Differentiation and proliferation of hematopoietic stem cells. Blood **81:** 2844–2853.
2. SPANGRUDE, G.J., S. HEIMFELD & I.M. WEISSMAN. 1988. Purification and characterization of mouse hematopoietic stem cells. Science **241:** 58–62.
3. JONES, R.J., M.I. COLLECTOR, J.P. BARKER et al. 1996. Characterization of mouse lymphohematopoietic stem cells lacking spleen colony-forming activity. Blood **88:** 487–491.
4. JONES, R.J., J.E. WAGNER, P. CELANO et al. 1990. Separation of pluripotent haematopoietic stem cells from spleen colony-forming cells. Nature **347:** 188–189.
5. ORLIC D., R. FISCHER, S. NISHIKAWA et al. 1993. Purification and characterization of heterogeneous pluripotent hematopoietic stem cell populations expressing high levels of c-kit receptor. Blood **82:** 762–770.
6. VAN DE RIJN, M., S. HEIMFELD, G.J. SPANGRUDE et al. 1989. Mouse hematopoietic stem-cell antigen Sca-1 is a member of the Ly-6 antigen family. Proc. Natl. Acad. Sci. USA **86:** 4634–4638.
7. BRIDDELL, R.A., V.C. BROUDY, E. BRUNO et al. 1992. Further phenotypic characterization and isolation of human hematopoietic progenitor cells using a monoclonal antibody to the c-kit receptor. Blood **79:** 3159–3167.
8. BERARDI, A.C., A. WANG, J.D. LEVINE et al. 1995. Functional isolation and characterization of human hematopoietic stem cells. Science **267:** 104–108.
9. KAWASHIMA, I., E.D. ZANJANI, G. ALMEIDA-PORADA et al. 1996. CD34$^+$ human marrow cells that express low levels of Kit protein are enriched for long-term marrow-engrafting cells. Blood **87:** 4136–4142.
10. HUANG, S. & L.W. TERSTAPPEN. 1994. Lymphoid and myeloid differentiation of single human CD34$^+$, HLA-DR$^+$, CD38$^-$ hematopoietic stem cells. Blood **83:** 1515–1526.
11. SMITH L.G., I.L. WEISSMAN & S. HEIMFELD. 1991. Clonal analysis of hematopoietic stem-cell differentiation in vivo. Proc. Natl. Acad. Sci. USA **88:** 2788–2792.
12. OSAWA, M., K. NAKAMURA, N. NISHI et al. 1996. In vivo self renewal of c-Kit$^+$ Sca-1$^+$ Lin$^{low/-}$ hematopoietic stem cells. J. Immunol. **156:** 3207–3214.

13. EAVES, C., C. MILLER, J. CASHMAN et al. 1997. Hematopoietic stem cells: inferences from in vivo assays. Stem Cells 15 (Suppl. 1): 1–5.
14. LEARY, A.G. & M. OGAWA. 1987. Blast cell colony assay for umbilical cord blood and adult bone marrow progenitors. Blood 69: 953–956.
15. CASHMAN, J.D., T. LAPIDOT, J.D. WANG et al. 1997. Kinetic evidence of the regeneration of multilineage hematopoiesis from primitive cells in normal human bone marrow transplanted into immunodeficient mice. Blood 89: 4307–4316.
16. NOLTA, J.A., M.B. HANLEY & D.B. KOHN. 1994. Sustained human hematopoiesis in immunodeficient mice by cotransplantation of marrow stroma expressing human interleukin-3: analysis of gene transduction of long-lived progenitors. Blood 83: 3041–3051.
17. MOREL, F., S.J. SZILVASSY, M. TRAVIS et al. 1996. Primitive hematopoietic cells in murine bone marrow express the CD34 antigen. Blood 88: 3774–3784.
18. BERENSON, R.J., R.G. ANDREWS, W.I. BENSINGER et al. 1988. Antigen CD34+ marrow cells engraft lethally irradiated baboons. J. Clin. Invest. 81: 951–955.
19. BENSINGER, W.I., C.D. BUCKNER, K. SHANNON-DORCY et al. 1996. Transplantation of allogeneic CD34+ peripheral blood stem cells in patients with advanced hematologic malignancy. Blood 88: 4132–4138.
20. BERENSON, R.J., W.I. BENSINGER, R.S. HILL et al. 1991. Engraftment after infusion of CD34+ marrow cells in patients with breast cancer or neuroblastoma. Blood 77: 1717–1722.
21. OSAWA, M., K. HANADA, H. HAMADA et al. 1996. Long-term lymphohematopoietic reconstitution by a single CD34-low/negative hematopoietic stem cell. Science 273: 242–245.
22. GOODELL, M.A., K. BROSE, G. PARADIS et al. 1996. Isolation and functional properties of murine hematopoietic stem cells that are replicating in vivo. J. Exp. Med. 183: 1797–1806.
23. MOREL, F., A. GALY, B. CHEN et al. 1996. Characterization of CD34 negative hematopoietic stem cells in murine bone marrow [abstract]. Blood 88: 629.
24. JOHNSON, R.P., M. ROSENZWEIG, M.A. GODDELL et al. 1996. Isolation of a candidate hematopoietic stem cell population that lacks CD34 in rhesus macaques [abstract]. Blood 88: 629.
25. ZANJANI, E.D., G. ALMEIDA-PORADA, A.G. LIVINGSTON et al. 1998. Human bone marrow CD34− cells engraft in vivo and undergo multilineage expression including giving rise to CD34+ cells. Exp. Hematol. 26: 353–360.
26. GOODELL, M.A., M. ROSENWEIG, H. KIM et al. 1997. Dye efflux studies suggest that hematopoietic stem cells expressing low or undetectable levels of CD34 antigen exist in multiple species. Nat. Med. 3: 1337–1345.
27. BONNET, D., M. GHATIA & J.E. DICK. 1997. Development of conditions for the ex vivo culture of a novel CD34− population of primitive human hematopoietic repopulating cells [abstract]. Blood 90: 160.
28. ZANJANI, E.D., G. ALMEIDA-PORADA & A.W. FLAKE. 1996. The human/sheep xenograft model: a large animal model of human hematopoiesis. Int. J. Hematol. 63: 179–192.
29. CIVIN, C.I., G. ALMEIDA-PORADA, M-J. LEE, L.W.M.M. TERSTAPPEN et al. 1996. Sustained, retransplantable, multilineage engraftment of highly purified adult human bone marrow stem cells in vivo. Blood 88: 4102–4109.
30. KOBAYASHI, M., J.H. LAVER, T. KATO et al. 1996. Thrombopoietin supports proliferation of human primitive hematopoietic cells in synergy with steel factor and/or interleukin-3. Blood 88: 429–436.
31. ZANJANI, E.D., J.L. ASCENSAO, M.R. HARRISON et al. 1992. Ex vivo incubation with growth factors enhances the engraftment of fetal hematopoietic cells transplanted in sheep fetuses. Blood 79: 3045–3049.

32. FLAKE, A.W., M.R. HARRISON, N.S. ADZICK *et al.* 1986. Transplantation of fetal hematopoietic stem cells in utero: the creation of hematopoietic chimeras. Science **233:** 776–778.
33. ZANJANI, E.D., F.R. SROUR & R. HOFFMAN. 1995. Retention of long-term repopulating ability of xenogeneic transplanted purified adult human bone marrow hematopoietic stem cells in sheep. J. Lab. Clin. Med. **126:** 24–28.
34. ZANJANI, E.D., M.G. PALLAVICINI, A.W. FLAKE *et al.* 1992. Engraftment and long-term expression of human fetal hemopoietic stem cells in sheep following transplantation in utero. J. Clin. Invest. **89:** 1178–1180.
35. SUTHERLAND, D.R., E.L. YEO, A.K. STEWART *et al.* 1996. Identification of CD34⁺ subsets after glycoprotease selection: engraftment of CD34⁺Thy-1⁺Lin⁻ stem cells in fetal sheep. Exp. Hematol. **24:** 795–806.
36. CARELLA, A.M., I. CUNNINGHAM, E. LERMA *et al.* 1997. Mobilization and transplantation of Philadelphia-negative peripheral-blood progenitor cells early in chronic myelogenous leukemia. J. Clin. Oncol. **15:** 1575–1582.
37. MURRAY, L.J. *et al.* 1996. CD34⁺Thy-1⁺Lin⁻ stem cells from mobilized peripheral blood. Leuk. Lymphoma **22:** 37–42.
38. LAROCHELLE, A., J. VORMOOR, H. HANENBERG *et al.* 1996. Identification of primitive human hematopoietic cells capable of repopulating NOD/SCID mouse bone marrow: implications for gene therapy. Nat. Med. **2:** 1329–1337.
39. SHIZURU, J.A., L. JERABEK, C.T. EDWARDS *et al.* 1996. Transplantation of purified hematopoietic stem cells: requirements for overcoming the barriers of allogeneic engraftment. Biol. Blood Marrow Transplant **2:** 3–14.

DISCUSSION

R. HOFFMAN (*University of Illinois College of Medicine*): Does your last comment mean that for 11 years you have been transplanting CD34+ cells only?

ZANJANI: No. The animals that we reported in 1992 were already five years old. They were transplanted with human fetal liver cells, and we have been following these animals since then. Some have died, but others have been evaluated for about 10 years. We have never seen this type of increase in donor cell activity.

C.J. EAVES (*Terry Fox Laboratory*): Do you transplant an inbred line of sheep, and is that important for getting the consistency of data that you report?

ZANJANI: Our sheep are not truly inbred, but are inbred to some extent. Also we are getting much better technically, and this shows in the improved results. In general, at two months posttransplant, almost every animal is engrafted. At birth probably 80% show engraftment. At a year there is a slight decrease in percent chimeric lambs. Donor cell activity remains stable throughout.

B.P. SORRENTINO (*St. Jude Children's Research Hospital*): Have you tested to determine whether the CD34⁺ cells that develop in vitro from the CD34⁻ cells have repopulating activity?

ZANJANI: No. We get so few of them. We plan to do this in the future.

G.J. Spangrude (*University of Utah Medical Center*): I am a little puzzled by your statement that you have not seen this late increase in human cells, even in recipients of human fetal liver, because one would expect that these cells would have been present in that graft.

ZANJANI: I cannot explain it.

W.E. FIBBE (*University Medical Center Leiden*): I was surprised to see that almost 35–45% of your CD34⁻ cells express lymphocyte function-associated antigen

(LFA-1). Since most of the available data suggest that LFA-1–expressing cells are more primitive and since your CD34⁻ cell is obviously a very primitive cell, this is not what you would expect. Would you comment on that?

ZANJANI: That would fit with the idea of CD34⁻ cells serving as possible precursors of CD34⁺ cells.

Y. REISNER (*Weizmann Institute of Science*): I would like to ask two questions. First, I am puzzled by whether you are transplanting human to human or human to sheep. Human fetal transplants are being done now by some people. Also in primates people are doing primate-to-primate in utero transplants using many more CD34 cells than you used in this xenogeneic system. They too fail to get engraftment, probably because of the competition we hear about and the fact that they are not conditioned at all. No one wants to condition an embryo. This is a unique situation where human cells engraft a xenogeneic fetus.

ZANJANI: These transplants were in general done later in gestation in patients with functional marrow and with immune capabilities. In cases where there was immunodeficiency, there has been engraftment. In non-immunodeficient patients when transplants were performed early in gestation, there has been donor cell engraftment. The problem has been that donor cell levels have been low and not curative. Here we are transplanting very early in gestation. We are talking about a gestational age in sheep that is comparable to about 10–13 weeks in humans. However, human cases have been transplanted later.

REISNER: So obviously you have some advantage for donor cells in competing with the host cells.

ZANJANI: Not with a functioning host bone marrow. However, you can cotransplant autologous stroma, and donor cell engraftment will improve dramatically. You referred to monkeys; engraftment in monkeys has been reported. The levels are not in a curative range, but they are significant.

D.A. WILLIAMS (*Riley Hospital for Children*): In the cells that were put through "CD34 toxic laser treatment," it looked like the engraftment was diminished much more than the twofold reduction that you would predict from the loss of cells according to the number of cell input. It was at least a log less than what would be predicted.

ZANJANI: No, we have actually seen that in three cases. It does not make any difference though. Here we have a population of CD34⁻ cells that we believe have absolutely no significant low or high CD34⁺ cell contamination, and they are engrafting. At this point in our studies, the important thing is whether they engraft and undergo multilineage differentiation *in vivo*.

WILLIAMS: You can make that argument, but on the other hand, you did not show us any data on how efficient the kill is. I would argue that you do not know there is absolutely no contamination.

ZANJANI: By several criteria, we believe the killing was very efficient.

Ex Vivo Expansion and Genetic Marking of Primitive Human and Baboon Hematopoietic Cells

JEFFREY A. MEDIN,[a] JOHN E. BRANDT,[a] ELEN ROZLER,[a] MARY NELSON,[a] AMELIA BARTHOLOMEW,[a] CONGFEN LI,[a] JULIUS TURIAN,[b] JOHN CHUTE,[c] THEODORE CHUNG,[b] AND RONALD HOFFMAN[a,d]

[a]*Section of Hematology/Oncology and* [b]*the Department of Radiation Oncology, University of Illinois at Chicago, Chicago, Illinois, USA*
[c]*The Naval Medical Research Institute, Bethesda, Maryland, USA*

ABSTRACT: The achievement of positive outcomes in many clinical protocols involving hematopoietic stem cells (HSCs) has been handicapped by the limited numbers of marrow repopulating cells available to actually bring about therapy. This insufficiency has been especially problematic in stem cell transplantation and gene therapy. A number of studies have been initiated to attempt expansion of HSCs, mainly by manipulation of key cytokines in cell suspension cultures. Unfortunately, these expansion methods usually lead to altered properties in the amplified cells, mainly by reducing their self-renewal and multilineage differentiative potentials. Here we discuss our ongoing work, utilizing a unique endothelial cell line that supports primitive hematopoiesis, to attempt to generate expansion of primate HSCs that retain their elementary properties. Genetic marking of early hematopoietic cells to facilitate tracking will be mentioned as will the development and employment of assay systems designed to evaluate the long-term functional attributes of the expanded cells.

INTRODUCTION

True pluripotent hematopoietic stem cells (HSCs) by definition have the ability to self-replicate without changing their basal properties and yet also can program differentiation of their offspring into all lineages of blood cells. In practice, multiple outcomes potentially can occur when HSCs self-replicate after being transplanted into recipients (FIG. 1), ranging from engraftment and a total retention of functional stem cell activity to a complete alteration of the transplanted cells leading to the loss of proliferative potential or the ability to home to the marrow. The intra- and extracellular biochemical processes that govern these functions are not understood, although an interesting hypothesis concerning the importance of telomere length and stem cell transplantation has recently emerged.[1]

[d]Address correspondence to: Ronald Hoffman, MD, Section of Hematology/Oncology, Room 3150, MBRB, University of Illinois at Chicago, 900 South Ashland Avenue, Chicago, IL 60607-7173. Phone, 312/413-9308; fax, 312/413-7963; e-mail, ronhoff@uic.edu

F1 Generation in Host

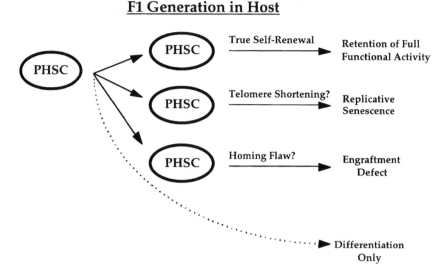

FIGURE 1. F1 generation in host: outcomes of transplantation of pluripotent hematopoietic stem cells.

Clinical therapeutic protocols involving HSC transplantation to ameliorate inherited and acquired disease would greatly benefit by the capability to synthetically produce large numbers of these cells that still retain their complete definitive functions. Efforts to expand HSCs towards this aim are currently being carried out by numerous research groups. Self-contained stromal cell coculture procedures as well as stromal-free suspension culture systems with added cytokines have been employed.[2] Most systems, to date, produce large increases in the numbers of more committed hematopoietic progenitor cells at the expense of the numbers of cells that retain true stem cell function.[2] Some data have been recently presented; however, these indicate that ex vivo expansion of actual HSCs may be possible.[3–5]

It seems reasonable to postulate that the most extensive HSC self-renewal occurs during the inauguration of the hematopoietic system during embryological development. Indeed, in the mouse the earliest identifiable HSCs are cells found in spatial contact with the vasculature.[6,7] Further, a common pluripotent precursor cell that leads to both HSCs and vascular endothelial cells upon progression has been recently identified.[8] In order to try to replicate this evolutionary 'nest,' which allows and even promotes HSC self-renewal, we sought to identify *ex vivo* cell culture conditions that could support or mimic this effect. An endothelial cell line from pig was identified that had been shown to demonstrate these supportive effects.[10] This PM-VEC (porcine microvascular endothelial cell) line allows expansion of cells that maintain some phenotypic functions of HSCs.[9–11] In fact, expansions in human CD34$^+$CD38$^-$ cells of over 100-fold have been described; a population of cells that have been shown to contain the earliest hematopoietic precursors.[10]

FUNCTIONAL EFFECTS OF EXPANSION OF PRIMITIVE HUMAN HEMATOPOIETIC CELLS IN SUSPENSION AND PMVEC COCULTURE

Experiments were initiated to test cell expansion products generated using this supportive PMVEC cell line and to compare the function of the outcome products with those resulting from incubations in suspension cultures containing exogenously added cytokines including stem cell factor (SCF), interleukin-3 (IL-3), interleukin-6 (IL-6), and granulocyte/macrophage colony-stimulating factor (GM-CSF).[9] Human bone marrow cells were isolated and CD34+Thy-1+Lin⁻ cell populations, enriched for HSCs, were sequestered and subjected to expansion under both conditions.[9] The total cell numbers, evaluated after three weeks, increased 1000-fold for the cells incubated on the PMVEC and 1500-fold for the suspension cultures. The numbers of cells expressing the CD34 stem cell surface antigen, measured by flow cytometrical analyses and again evaluated after 3 weeks, also increased 15- to 50-fold for both culture systems.[9] Large differences were seen after one week, however, in the expression pattern of the CD38 cell surface marker, for which a gain of cell surface expression is associated with differentiation, as a very high percentage of the cells in the suspension culture gained CD38 expression while a significant portion of the cells incubated in the PMVEC coculture system remained below the threshold of CD38 detection.

Comparative functional analyses of the PMVEC- and the suspension culture-expanded cells were performed on multiple levels. Expansion of hematopoietic progenitor colonies, measured by the number of granulocyte/macrophage colony-forming unit (CFU-GM) colonies formed after a 2-week incubation in a semisolid support media for various input cell number dilutions, was comparable between the two systems.[9] Cobblestone area-forming cells (CAFC), a measure of a more primitive hematopoietic cell, were enumerated after a 5-week incubation of input cells (which were previously expanded 2–3 weeks) on a permissive murine stromal cell line and found to be increased 4- to 30-fold for the PMVEC coculture and only 5- to 6-fold for the suspension cells.

However, it was on a more detailed *in vivo* engraftment study looking at the prevalence of even more primitive hematopoietic cells that the greatest differences in the constitution of the expanded cells became apparent. In this study the expanded cells from both systems (re-sorted for fidelity) were assayed for their ability to competitively engraft human fetal bone fragments implanted in severe combined immunodeficient (SCID) mice.[12] The results of these assays,[9] using various dilutions of the input cells and in comparison to freshly isolated cells, indicated large differences between the abilities of expanded cells from both systems to engraft (TABLE 1). Comparable engraftment was observed when similar numbers of the freshly isolated cells and those expanded on the supportive PMVEC cells, even at low dilutions, were engrafted in SCID-hu bone assays. In addition, input cells originating from the PMVEC coculture expanded cells or from freshly isolated cells produced multilineage progeny as the presence of cell surface markers including CD19 and CD33 could be observed on the offspring of input cells.[9] In marked contrast, the capacity for engraftment of the fetal human bone fragment was largely lost by the cells expanded in the suspension culture system (TABLE 1) even with much higher numbers of input cells and when the cytokine cocktail was varied.

TABLE 1. SCID-hu engraftment of adult marrow CD34[+] cells prior to and following expansion on the PMVEC coculture and expansion in suspension culture with added cytokines including: IL-3, IL-6, ±SCF, ±GM-CSF, ±leukemia inhibitory factor (LIF)[a]

Culture (sample #)	Day[1]	Cells/graft[1]	Positive grafts/bones[b]	Donor cells/graft[c]
Input				
(n = 6)	0	$1 \times 10^3 - 5 \times 10^4$	20/22	0–66%
PMVEC				
(n = 4)	12–15	$1 \times 10^3 - 1 \times 10^4$	8/10	0–89%
Suspension				
(n = 5)	14–23	$3 \times 10^3 - 5 \times 10^4$	1/8	ND[d]

[a] Note: Data from Brandt et al.[9]
[b] Eight weeks after injection, the bone implants were removed and analyzed for presence of donor human leukocyte antigen (HLA) by flow cytometric analyses.
[c] % Donor cells reflects the percent of donor to host marrow cells eight weeks postengraftment.
[d] Only CD19[+] cells were seen in the one positive graft.

Experiments were also performed to assess the proliferative status of the primitive cells expanded on the PMVEC and that of the cells expanded in the suspension culture with the added cytokine cocktail. For these studies, the dye PKH26 was used, which stably integrates into cell membranes of nondividing cells, is divided equally among daughter cells, and can be detected by flow cytometrical analysis.[13,14] For CD34[+] cells recovered from both culture systems, analysis of PKH26 intensity indicated that the primitive suspension/cytokine cells were largely quiescent as they maintained a bright staining pattern. This differs from the result seen with the primitive cells incubated with the PMVEC, as mainly PKH26[dim] cells were recovered indicating active proliferation.[9]

EXPANSION OF HUMAN CORD BLOOD STEM CELLS

The above experiments were performed on bone marrow-derived human HSCs. Another important clinical source of stem cells is those recovered from umbilical cord blood. This is especially true as a significant increase in public awareness of the potential future utility of these cells and the numbers of centers for banking human umbilical cord blood cells is occurring. Unfortunately, the total recovery of cord blood HSCs from the single isolation procedure is limited. Thus if the numbers of cord blood HSCs could also be increased, and as these cells may have engraftment or expansion properties that surpass HSCs obtained from mobilized peripheral blood or from adult bone marrow,[2] improved therapeutic outcomes for a number of disorders may occur.

Experiments were undertaken to examine the ability of human cord blood HSCs to be expanded by incubation with the PMVEC and in stromal-free suspension culture.[15] CD34[+] cells were isolated from numerous cryopreserved cord blood samples and incubated in coculture with PMVEC or in suspension culture with supplementary cytokines including GM-CSF, SCF, IL-6, and FLT-3. Additional cytokines that were added to some cultures included IL-3, thrombopoietin (TPO), and nerve growth factor (NGF). As was seen with the human bone marrow cells (above), total cell numbers again increased significantly in both culture systems to levels of 1000-fold higher than the input cell number by 3 weeks, although the kinetics of expansion differed as the cord blood cells had a longer lag period before the exponential increases occurred. Likewise, differential expansion of the more primitive human hematopoietic cells occurred over 1, 2, and 3 weeks with CD34$^+$CD38$^-$ cells expanding in number over 150-fold in the PMVEC coculture system but less than 10-fold in the stromal-free suspension culture after 21 days.[15] Little effect was observed with the addition of IL-3, TPO or NGF to the basic cytokine cocktail.

Functional analyses of the primitive cord blood cells expanded with both systems were also undertaken. No significant differences were observed in the numbers of CFU-GMs obtained from both culture systems, indicating that expansion of committed cells was unaffected by the culture conditions. Some slight differences were seen in the expansion of CAFC in that more cells capable of forming cobblestone areas were found in the PMVEC coculture than in the suspension culture after 7 days.[15] Engraftment analyses, *i.e.*, experiments testing the ability of expanded cord blood cells to competitively engraft SCID-hu bone, are currently underway. Preliminary results indicate that engraftment of expanded cells from both culture systems can occur, which highlights important ontogenetic differences of human HSCs from different tissue sources.

RETROVIRAL MARKING OF PRIMITIVE CELLS TO FACILITATE TRACKING

In order to facilitate tracking of expanded cells in SCID-hu engraftment assays and especially in the large animal model (see below), a recombinant retrovirus was developed that engineers expression of the enhanced yellow fluorescence protein.[16] This protein is a modified version of the *Aequorea victoria* green fluorescent protein (GFP) that is enhanced for high cytosolic expression in mammalian cells. The expressed enYFP protein (Clontech Labs) is excited at 488 nm and can be detected using a 530/30-nm bandpass filter, which is different than the green fluorescence protein, which is optimally detected using a 510/20-nm filter. Use of these fluorescence protein markers and flow cytometric analyses makes single cell detection and evaluation relatively simple for a variety of parameters including expression of cell surface antigens and the persistence or efficiency of retroviral-mediated cell transduction.[17] This gene transfer vector was constructed using the MFG vector backbone in plasmid pUMFG[18] and packaged in amphotropic GP+envAM12 cells.[19] A packaging cell line derived from a single cell clone was identified and was found to be of high titer and to produce only replication incompetent virus.[16] Test transductions of NIH3T3 cells demonstrated that a high percentage of cells could be transduced with even a single application of filtered viral supernatant and that the levels of expression of the enYFP protein were substantial and readily allowed distinction from untrans-

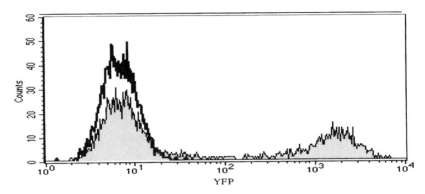

FIGURE 2. Flow cytometric histogram analysis of NIH3T3 cells transduced a single time with supernatant from the AM12pUMFGenYFP #6 producer cell line. The untransfected AM12 control cells are the *left-most peak* (*heavy black line*). The transduced cells are the *gray peaks.*

duced cells by flow cytometric analysis (FIG. 2). Indeed, fluorescence peak shifts into the third and fourth decade, on log-scale analyses, were seen for these and infected test hematologic cells (FIG. 2, and data not shown).

For initial experiments leading to the establishment of transduction procedures for human and nonhuman primate HSCs in our laboratories, cadaveric bone marrow CD34+ CD38− cells were isolated by flow cytometry to a high purity and infected with the filtered AM12enYFP retroviral supernatant in a 5-day infection course using fibronectin[20] and cytokines (including SCF, IL-3, IL-6, GM-CSF, and Flt-3 ligand). The cells were infected in suspension culture and in coculture with the PM-VEC supportive cells. The total percentages of functionally infected cells, as evidenced by the presence of measurable enYFP protein expression 7 days after the infection course, was over 11% in the suspension culture infections and about 2% in the PMVEC coculture infections.[16] The lower infection of the human HSCs in the coculture procedure could be due to sequestration of the virus on the PMVEC; an hypothesis that remains to be tested. Most important, however, was the fact that only the infection conditions with the PMVEC permitted a significant number of cells to be found after the infection course that were truly CD34+CD38− and also expressing the transgene. These data indicate that the infection, in conjunction with the PMVEC coculture, allows the maintenance of a very primitive human hematopoietic cell phenotype. Further functional analysis of these cells were performed including progenitor cell and CAFC assays. A high percentage of both CFU-GM colonies and cobble-stone areas were found to be positive for expression of enYFP for both infection systems.[16] Detailed SCID-hu bone assays to test the ability of transduced cells and to delineate possible differences in the ability of transduced cells from both culture systems to engraft are underway, along with further cell expansions of transduced cells. Nonetheless these preliminary data are encouraging and offer the possibility that we have actually transduced a true human stem cell with a recombinant retrovirus that is able to maintain its primitive phenotype.

DEVELOPMENT OF A LARGE ANIMAL STEM CELL TRANSPLANT MODEL

Since the above-mentioned surrogate assays for HSCs have critical limitations and shortcomings, a significant effort has been underway here at our facility to develop a large animal model for transplant studies.[21] This effort will allow us not only to improve expansion techniques of HSCs using the PMVEC and to study the biology of these clinically important cells *in vivo,* but also to refine conditions of gene transfer to later impact the efficacy of planned clinical gene therapy protocols. In this model system, bone marrow is harvested from juvenile baboons (*Papio anubis*) and mononuclear cells are isolated. A specific antibody has been identified that allows further segregation of baboon CD34[+] cells,[10] and detailed dose response optimizations have been performed with human cytokines. Animals undergoing either chemical or radiologic myeloablation are maintained on a tether assemblage and are given prophylactic antibiotics, antiviral agents and blood transfusions when needed.

In initial proof-of-principle studies, baboon bone marrow cells have been expanded to useful numbers using the PMVEC coculture system and infused into a lethally irradiated host.[21] Starting with a suboptimal graft size, total cell numbers were increased 14-fold with CD34[+] cells increasing 8-fold after a 10-day coculture on the PMVEC line.[21] These cells were then infused into an animal that had undergone a twice-daily total body irradiation regimen for 4 days resulting in a total of 1000 cGy. This level of irradiation has been shown to be lethal and myeloablative in control animals that did not receive a graft. Recovery of the animal receiving the expanded cells was established by an observed number of ANC at >500/ul at day 24 and a platelet count of >20,000 by day 27. This animal is now out approximately one year posttransplant and is considered to be hematologically normal. In addition, a second animal that received cells after expansion has also followed a similar course of recovery as the first animal (data not shown).

These studies clearly demonstrate the retention of marrow repopulating ability by *ex vivo* expanded cells. Further examination of stem cells that have undergone division will permit us to fully define the consequences of stem cell self-replication on marrow repopulating potential. Further experiments are also underway to begin to genetically mark baboon cells prior to transplantation using the recombinant retroviral construct that encodes the enhanced yellow fluorescence protein as mentioned above. Initial results have demonstrated that these baboon CD34[+] cells can also be infected with the transfer vector at some level of efficiency greater than or equal to the human HSCs, and these cells also express the marker transgene to a high level (data not shown).

REFERENCES

1. LANSDORP, P.M. 1995. Developmental changes in the function of hematopoietic stem cells. Exp. Hematol. **23:** 187–191.
2. EMERSON, S.G. 1996. *Ex vivo* expansion of hematopoietic precursors, progenitors and stem cells: the next generation of cellular therapeutics. Blood **87:** 3082–3088.
3. PETZER, A.L. *et al.* 1996. Self-renewal of primitive human hematopoietic cells (long-term-culture-initiating cells) *in vitro* and their expansion in defined medium. Proc. Natl. Acad. Sci. USA **93:** 1470–1474.

4. BHATIA, M. *et al.* 1997. Quantitative analysis reveals expansion of human hematopoietic repopulating cells after short-term *ex vivo* culture. J. Exp. Med. **186:** 619–624.
5. CONNEALLY, E. *et al.* 1997. Expansion *in vitro* of transplantable human cord blood stem cells demonstrated using a quantitative assay of their lympho-myeloid repopulating activity in nonobese diabetic-scid/scid mice. Proc. Natl. Acad. Sci. USA **94:** 9836–9841.
6. FENNIE, C. *et al.* 1995. CD34⁺ endothelial cell lines derived from murine yolk sac induce the proliferation and differentiation of yolk sac induce the proliferation and differentiation of yolk sac CD34⁺ hematopoietic progenitor. Blood **86:** 4454–4467.
7. SANCHEZ, M.J. *et al.* 1996. Characterization of the first definitive hematopoietic stem cells in the AGM and liver of mouse embryo. Immunity **5:** 513–525.
8. CHOI, K. *et al.* 1998. A common precursor for hematopoietic and endothelial cells. Development **125:** 725–732.
9. BRANDT, J.E. *et al.* 1998. Bone marrow repopulation by human marrow stem cells following long-term expansion culture on a porcine endothelial cell line. Exp. Hematol. In press.
10. DAVIS, T.A. *et al.* 1995. Porcine brain microvascular endothelial cells support the *in vitro* expansion of human primitive hematopoietic bone marrow progenitor cells with a high replating potential: required for cell-cell interactions and colony-stimulating factors. Blood **85:** 1751–1761.
11. DAVIS, T.A. *et al.* 1997. Conditioned medium from primary porcine endothelial cells alone promotes the growth of primitive human haematopoietic progenitor cells with a high replating potential: evidence for a novel early haematopoietic activity. Cytokine **9:** 263–275.
12. CHEN, S.P. *et al.* 1994. Engraftment of human precursor cells with secondary transfer potential in SCID-hu mice. Blood **84:** 2497–2505.
13. NORDIN, R.E., S.S. GINSBERG & C.J. EAVES. 1997. High-resolution cell division tracking demonstrates the Flt-3 ligand dependence of human marrow CD34⁺CD38⁻ cell production *in vitro.* Br. J. Haematol. **98:** 528–539.
14. TRAYCOFF, C.M. *et al.* 1995. Evaluation of *ex vivo* expansion potential of cord blood and bone marrow hematopoietic progenitor cells using cell tracking and limiting dilution analysis. Blood **85:** 2059–2068.
15. ROZLER, E. *et al.* 1997. Cocultivation with porcine endothelial cells leads to extensive amplification of cord blood CD34⁺CD38⁻ cell compartment [abstract]. Blood **90:** 394a.
16. MEDIN, J.A. *et al.* 1998. Genetic modification and expansion of human CD34⁺CD38⁻ cells. *In* collected abstracts of the 2nd Conference on Stem Cell Gene Therapy (Orcas Island, WA).
17. CHENG, L. *et al.* 1996. Use of green fluorescent protein variants to monitor gene transfer and expression in mammalian cells. Nat. Biotech. **14:** 606–609.
18. TAKENAKA, T. *et al.* 1998. Direct biochemical evidence for circulating α-galactoside A derived from transduced bone marrow cells. Submitted.
19. MARKOWITZ, D., S. GOFF & A. BANK. 1988. Construction and use of a safe and efficient amphotropic packaging cell line. Virology **167:** 400–406.
20. HANENBERG, H. *et al.* 1997. Optimization of fibronectin-assisted retroviral gene transfer into human CD34⁺ hematopoietic cells. Hum. Gene Ther. **8:** 2193–2206.
21. BRANDT, J. *et al.* 1997. *Ex vivo* stem cell expansion results in a graft capable of hematologically rescuing lethally irradiated nonhuman primates [abstract]. Blood **90:** 94a.

DISCUSSION

S.J. SHARKIS (*Johns Hopkins Oncology Center*): To my mind, in order to show that you have self-renewal you have to give back to the animal less than the number of cells, or the same number of cells that you have started with. Otherwise you are just showing maintenance of stem cells. I could not quite follow from the numbers seen whether you are actually giving stem cells that you have actually expanded versus just maintenance of stem cell population.

HOFFMAN: I think this is a difficult point to address. We started out prior to expansion with a graft that at least in several instances was incapable of repopulation; it contained inadequate numbers of stem cells in every instance. We have done several additional animals now. Following expansion, these grafts are now capable of hematological reconstitution. Therefore, by inference, we felt that that was evidence that we had actually increased the number of functional stem cells in these expanded grafts.

D.A. WILLIAMS (*Riley Hospital for Children*): Are the porcine endothelial cells CD34 positive?

HOFFMAN: We cannot detect $CD34^+$ expression using the monoclonal antibodies available to us.

WILLIAMS: Do you know whether in this system the PKH dye is transferred in the coculture to those cells?

HOFFMAN: We have not looked at that.

WILLIAMS: A third question is, in what way does this really differ from long-term marrow culture, that is, using autologous stroma in an expansion cocktail?

HOFFMAN: Using autologous stroma we do not get this degree of cell expansion, which favors the more primitive cells. In autologous stromal systems we get terminal differentiation.

J.E. DICK (*University of Toronto*): In the stromal-free conditions, did those contain serum?

HOFFMAN: Yes. All the culture systems included serum.

DICK: The level of expansion you were getting compared to the serum-free conditions for 10 days was a lot lower than you would get if it was serum-free.

L. KANZ (*Eberhard Karls University*): It is striking that it takes 10 days longer to get recovery with the expanded cells as compared to unmanipulated cells. We know from the clinical setting that there is a strong dose relationship between the number of cells transplanted and recovery time. Is it perhaps possible that you have recovery by a small number of stem cells surviving your culture and not losing stem cell properties and that leads to delayed recovery?

HOFFMAN: I think that is possible, although the number of stem cells in the original graft was inadequate for hematological reconstitution. By inference we believe we actually have increased the number of stem cells, and the time of engraftment surely was not related to the number of progenitor cells. The greatest degree of expansion was in the more primitive cells, the cobblestone area-forming cells. Whether those have any correlation to marrow repopulating ability is obviously open to debate.

B. TOROK-STORB (*Fred Hutchinson Cancer Research Center*): I am still confused by the very slow or failed engraftment observed with the unmanipulated marrow and then the very rapid engraftment with the enriched marrow, which was not expanded. I am wondering if there was a difference in the preparation of the marrow—specifically, the freeze-thaw and the quality of the product that was infused. Certainly an enriched product that is frozen and thawed is a better product than whole marrow that is frozen and thawed, in terms of cell quality.

HOFFMAN: Quality as assessed by what parameters?

TOROK-STORB: Assessed by viability after thaw. So were your determinations of cell number and phenotype made postthaw or prefreeze?

HOFFMAN: They were made postthaw.

TOROK-STORB: So there was no difference?

HOFFMAN: No. They were made postthaw.

C.J. EAVES (*Terry Fox Laboratory*): What was the procedure when you harvested your cocultures? Did you harvest the endothelial cells also, and were they part of what was infused?

HOFFMAN: There is a small contamination.

EAVES: How exactly were those harvests done?

HOFFMAN: These are very crude culture systems. The cells are in flasks, and essentially you aspirate out the cells and then hit the flasks against the side of the hood and get the rest of the cells off. So, there are likely some cells that are retained, but also some of the endothelial cells are present in the infusion.

EAVES: Have you tried to test the effect of infusing some endothelial cells in an uncultured graft?

HOFFMAN: Do you mean just directly infuse endothelial cells into the myeloablated animal?

EAVES: Yes. To test whether infusing some of these cells itself can contribute something to the engraftment obtained.

HOFFMAN: It was not done.

R. MÖHLE (*Eberhard Karls University*): Is direct contact with endothelium absolutely required, or do you get similar results with conditioned medium?

HOFFMAN: Those experiments are ongoing, because that is an important question. I did not get the chance to show the efficacy of gene transfer, which is impressive with this system. We are now getting conditioned media from our colleagues at the Naval Center in Bethesda, Maryland in order to determine if we can recapitulate this degree of marrow repopulation with the conditioned media.

Y. REISNER (*Weizmann Institute of Science*): How many CD34 cells were in the unexpanded population?

HOFFMAN: About 13.7×10^6.

REISNER: Was that suboptimal?

HOFFMAN: No, that is an optimal high dose

REISNER: What was the suboptimal dose?

HOFFMAN: It was about a tenth of that dose.

REISNER: In general, in the matched allogeneic transplants, a dose of 2 million CD34 cells per kg is sufficient to give a very nice engraftment. One expects that in the autologous setting, the suboptimal CD34 dose will be lower.

HOFFMAN: You have to understand that these antibodies are directed against human CD34, so when we isolate our cell populations, the CD34+ population contains all the progenitor cells and all the CAFCs, but there is a significant degree of nonspecific staining that probably leads to the higher percentages that do not accord with the human experience.

Isolation of Stem Cell-Specific cDNAs from Hematopoietic Stem Cell Populations

DONALD ORLIC, SHARI L. LAPRISE, AMANDA P. CLINE,
STACIE M. ANDERSON, AND DAVID M. BODINE[a]

Hematopoiesis Section, Genetics and Molecular Biology Branch,
National Human Genome Research Institute, National Institutes of Health,
Bethesda, Maryland 20892-4442, USA

ABSTRACT: We have begun to isolate gene sequences that are specifically expressed in hematopoietic stem cells (HSCs). There are at least three fundamental requirements for the isolation of HSC-specific transcripts. First, highly enriched populations of HSCs, and an HSC-depleted cell population for comparison must be isolated. Secondly, the gene isolation procedures must be adapted to accommodate the small amounts of RNA obtained from purified HSCs. Finally, a defined screening strategy must be developed to focus on sequences to be examined in more detail. In this report, we describe the characterization of populations of HSCs that are highly enriched (Lin⁻ c-kit^{HI}) or depleted (Lin⁻ c-kit^{NEG}) of HSCs. We compared two methods for gene isolation, differential display polymerase chain reaction (DD-PCR) and subtractive hybridization (SH), and found that the latter was more powerful and efficient in our hands. Lastly we describe the strategy that we have developed to screen clones for further study.

INTRODUCTION

Hematopoietic stem cells (HSCs) are a rare population of bone marrow cells that are capable of extensive proliferation and differentiation. This allows a limited number of HSCs to provide the millions of mature peripheral blood cells released into the circulation each day. At the same time, HSCs are also capable of self-renewal divisions, which allow a limited number of HSCs to repopulate the lymphohematopoietic system of a transplant recipient (for reviews, see Refs. 1,2). In the mouse, HSCs do not express lineage markers and are strongly positive for the markers Sca-1[3,4] and c-kit.[5] We and others have shown that Lin⁻ cells expressing the highest levels of c-kit are enriched for repopulating stem cells. As few as 10–30 cells will repopulated either genetically anemic *W/Wᵛ* mice and/or irradiated mice.[5–7] This same population is largely depleted of hematopoietic progenitor cells and spleen colony-forming units (CFU-S).[5]

[a]Corresponding author: David M. Bodine, Hematopoiesis Section, Genetics and Molecular Biology Branch, National Human Genome Research Institute, 49 Convent Drive, Rm. 3A14, MSC-4442, National Institutes of Health, Bethesda, MD 20892-4442. Phone, 301/402-0902; fax, 301/402-4929; e-mail: tedyaz@nhgri.nih.gov

The ability to isolate and enrich HSCs from populations of mature hematopoietic cells and hematopoioetic progenitor and precursor cells has allowed a detailed analysis of the cellular properties of HSCs. Elegant studies have shown repopulation of all lineages from single transplanted HSCs and demonstrated the extensive proliferative capacities of these cells.[5–8] Other studies have shown that the engraftment of HSCs is influenced by the cell cycle status of the transplanted cells.[9] Finally, HSCs have been shown to differ metabolically from more mature hematopoietic cells in their ability to export the Hoechst and Rhodamine dyes, presumably through the activity of the P-glycoprotein, MDR.[10–12]

In contrast to the rapidly expanding knowledge of HSC behavior at the cellular level, the genetic control of HSCs is not as well understood. Much of the problem is due to the rarity of HSCs among hematopoietic cells (1/10,000 to 1/100,000 cells).[1,5] The relatively few cells that can be isolated by these techniques do not provide enough cells for a molecular analysis of gene expression in HSCs by Northern blot or RNase protection assays, which require microgram quantities of RNA. Limited amounts of RNA have also complicated the construction of cDNA libraries.

The advent of polymerase chain reaction (PCR)-based analysis has allowed examination of mRNAs in populations of primitive hematopoietic cells. Using primers specific for individual genes reverse transcriptase PCR (RT-PCR), we and others have described the expression of a variety of genes in enriched populations of HSCs, embryoid bodies or mouse embryos.[5,14–21] Among our findings were that the c-kit, c-myb, and GATA-2 mRNAs are present at high levels in populations of Lin$^-$ c-kit^{HI} cells. In contrast, the c-fms, granulocyte colony-stimulating factor (G-CSF) receptor and interleukin-7 (IL-7) receptor mRNAs were not present at detectable levels in populations of Lin$^-$ c-kit^{HI} cells.[14,19]

PCR-based strategies can also be used to identify potentially novel gene sequences in HSCs.[22] We have explored two such methods: differential display PCR (DD-PCR)[23] and subtractive hybridization (SH).[24] Both techniques rely on cDNA generated from RNA extracted from enriched HSCs. In DD-PCR, the first strand of the cDNA reaction is primed using oligo dT linked to an adapter sequence, while the second strand is primed using degenerate oligonucleotides linked to a different adapter. After several rounds of low stringency amplification, adapter oligos are added and the annealing temperature raised to allow specific amplification of the population of cDNAs. The products of these reactions are compared to a population of cDNAs generated from a population of cells in which HSCs are rare (e.g., bone marrow). Bands of the same size from both reactions are taken to represent sequences common to both populations. Bands present in only one reaction are potentially expressed specifically in one population. These specific bands are excised from the gel for cloning and sequencing.[23]

There are many SH strategies, all based on the original model of Diatchenko et al.[24] In all cases, mRNA from cells with an activity of interest (tester) is transcribed into cDNA, and hybridized to an excess of cDNA from a population of cells that do not have the activity of interest (driver). Unhybridized cDNAs are either isolated or amplified for cloning and sequencing.[24] In this report, we present our approach to identifying novel sequences expressed in HSCs. The observations include the cell populations compared to identify novel sequences as well as a comparison of DD-PCR and the building of cDNA libraries by SH.

MATERIALS AND METHODS

Mice

All mice were purchased from the Jackson Laboratory, Bar Harbor, ME and housed under specific pathogen-free conditions. Young adult (6 to 8 weeks) female, C57BL/6J mice were used as donors of bone marrow in all experiments. Competitor marrow for the competitive repopulation assay was obtained from B6.C H-1b/ByJ (HW80) mice, which are congenic with C57BL/6J mice except for single allelic differences at the mouse β-globin locus.[25] Recipients for competitive repopulation assay experiments were genetically anemic WBB6F1-*W/W^v* mice[26] or lethally irradiated (1000 Gy ^{137}Cs source; 400 rad/min) WBB6F1-+/+ mice. No significant differences were observed between irradiated or genetically anemic recipients in the competitive repopulation assay.

Enrichment of HSCs

Mouse bone marrow HSCs were isolated as previously described.[5] Briefly, cells were incubated in a cocktail of rat anti-mouse monoclonal antibodies directed against lineage, and cells expressing lineage markers were removed using antibody-coated immunomagnetic beads. Lin⁻ cells were incubated with biotinylated anti-c-kit antibody (ACK-4; a gift of Dr. S.I. Nishikawa). Lin⁻ cells expressing high levels of c-kit (c-kit^HI), low levels of c-kit (c-kit^LO) and c-kit negative (c-kit^NEG) cells were collected.

Stem Cell Assays

For limiting dilution assays, the indicated numbers of cells were suspended in 0.4 ml of phosphate-buffered saline (PBS) supplemented with 1% fetal calf serum (Hyclone, Logan, Utah), and injected into the tail vein of WBB6F1-*W/W^v* mice. Repopulation with donor cells was demonstrated by conversion of the "single/diffuse" hemoglobin pattern of the recipient to the "single" hemoglobin pattern of the donor as described.[27] Repopulation of myeloid cells was demonstrated by Southern blot analysis of DNA extracted from the bone marrow, spleen, and thymus of transplanted mice. The restriction enzyme EcoRI defines a restriction enzyme polymorphism in the mouse β-globin gene that differs between the donor and recipient.[25] For competitive repopulation assays, the indicated number of C57Bl/6 sorted cells were mixed with 2×10^6 unfractionated bone marrow cells from congenic B6.C-H1b/By congenic mice and injected into the tail vein of irradiated WBB6F1-*W/W^v* mice or WBB6F1-+/+ mice.[28]

Isolation and Analysis of RNA

Total cellular RNA was isolated according to the manufacturer's instructions using RNAzol B. The relative amount of mRNA was estimated by limiting dilution RT-PCR analysis using primers specific for β-2 microglobulin (β-2 M) (primers and conditions shown below), with 0.1 ml α[32]PdCTP added per reaction. Phosphorimager analysis was used to identify the linear range of the β-2 M amplification curve. The signals from RNA extracted from fluorescence-activated cell sorter (FACS)-pu-

TABLE 1. Primers and PCR conditions

Gene	Primer Sequence	
	sense:	
Mouse β-2	5'TGC TAT CCA GAA AAC CCC TC3'	94°C-1 min
microglobulin	anti-sense:	55°C-1 min
	5'GTC ATG CTT AAC TCT GCA GG3'	72°C-2 min
	Fragment size: 258 bp	

rified cells were compared to known standards to estimate the amount of mRNA (TABLE 1).[14]

DD-PCR Conditions

DD-PCR was used to compare the transcript fingerprint of Lin⁻ c-kit^HI mRNA to the transcript finger print of unfractionated bone marrow DNA. The reactions were performed using the Clontech Delta Differential Display kit according to the manufacturer's instructions with the following exceptions. First, the amount of RNA used to start the reactions was scaled down to approximately 100 ng and 25 ng. Second, only three sets of "P" (arbitrary) and "T" (oligo dT) primers were used. Finally, multiple preps of both Lin⁻ c-kit^HI RNA (4–6) and unfractionated bone marrow RNA were compared simultaneously.

cDNA Subtraction Library Construction

The cDNA subtraction library was constructed using cDNA generated from 250 ng Lin⁻ c-kit^HI RNA using the Clontech CapFinder PCR cDNA Synthesis kit according to the manufacturer's instructions. This cDNA became the tester stock. The driver cDNA was generated from Lin⁻ c-kit^NEG RNA using the Clontech PCR-Select cDNA Subtraction kit. The tester stock was ligated to adapters and subtracted according to the manufacturer's instructions. Before plating control PCR experiments documented the amplification of c-kit cDNA and subtraction of β-2 M cDNA. Following ligation into plasmids and bacterial transformation, 1152 colonies were isolated, amplified by PCR, and spotted onto duplicate filters for screening. Filters were probed with ³²P-labeled unamplified tester cDNA and ³²P-labeled amplified tester cDNA. Clones showing the highest degree of amplification were selected for further analysis. A second screen was carried out using ³²P-labeled unamplified tester and ³²P-labeled driver cDNA. Clones with low signals in driver and strong hybridization to tester were selected for further analysis.

RESULTS

Over 90% of all bone marrow cells are identified and removed by our panel of lineage marker antibodies. Among Lin⁻ bone marrow cells three distinct populations of cells can be distinguished on the basis of c-kit expression (FIG. 1). Lin⁻ c-kit^NEG, Lin⁻ c-kit^LO, and Lin⁻ c-kit^HI cells account for ~90%, ~9.5%, and 0.5% of Lin⁻

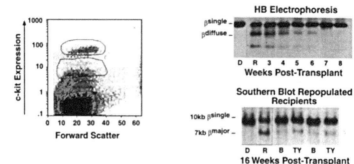

PHENOTYPE: Lin- c-kit^{HI}
ASSAY: Repopulation of irradiated or W/W^v mice

FIGURE 1. Characterization of mouse HSCs by FACS. *Left*, Lin⁻ bone marrow cells can be sorted into three distinct populations, c-kit^{HI}, c-kit^{LO}, and c-kit^{NEG}. Eighty-five percent (85%) or more of the repopulating ability is found in the c-kit^{HI} cells. *Right*, Limiting numbers of Lin⁻ c-kit^{HI} cells can repopulate the erythroid lineage, as demonstrated by hemoglobin (HB) electrophoresis, as well as the myeloid and lymphoid lineages, as demonstrated by Southern blot analysis. D = donor, R = recipient, B = bone marrow DNA (myeloid and lymphoid cells), TY = thymus DNA (lymphoid cells).

cells. Thus, the Lin⁻ c-kit^{HI} cells are enriched approximately 2000-fold compared to unfractionated bone marrow. As we have reported previously, the c-kit^{HI} population is highly enriched for long-term repopulating HSCs.[5] In limiting dilution assays performed in *W/W^v* mice, as few as 30 Lin⁻ c-kit^{HI} cells are sufficient to repopulate the erythroid, myeloid and lymphoid lineages of the recipient mouse (FIG. 1). Additional *W/W^v* mice were injected with up to 10^4 to 10^5 Lin⁻ c-kit^{LO} or Lin⁻ c-kit^{NEG} cells, respectively. This number of Lin⁻ c-kit^{LO} and Lin⁻ c-kit^{NEG} cells corresponds to approximately 10^6 unfractionated bone marrow cells, which is more than sufficient to repopulate *W/W^v* mice. No repopulation of *W/W^v* mice was observed after the injection of Lin⁻ c-kit^{LO} or Lin⁻ c-kit^{NEG} cells (Ref. 5 and TABLE 2).

The competitive repopulation assay provides a means to measure the relative repopulating ability of different populations of cells.[28] A mixture of 200 C57BL/6 Lin⁻ c-kit^{HI} cells (single Hb) and 2×10^6 HW80 unfractionated bone marrow cells was injected into cohorts of WBB6F1-*W/W^v* and WBB6F1-+/+ mice. The recipient animals had a mean of $11.25\% \pm 4.7\%$ C57BL/6 hemoglobin, indicating a 1274-fold enrichment of competitive repopulating ability in the Lin⁻ c-kit^{HI} cells (TABLE 2). A mixture of 2×10^6 C57BL/6 Lin⁻ c-kit^{HI} cells (single Hb) and 2×10^6 HW80 unfractionated bone marrow cells was injected into cohorts of WBB6F1-*W/W^v* and WBB6F1-+/+ mice. The recipient animals had a mean of $33.35\% \pm 1.1\%$ C57BL/6 hemoglobin, indicating a 6.6-fold depletion of competitive repopulating ability in the Lin⁻ c-kit^{NEG} cells (TABLE 2). From these data we estimate that as many as 15% of the competitive repopulating units in mouse marrow have a Lin⁻ c-kit^{NEG} phenotype.

TABLE 2. Repopulation of mice with purified populations of hematopoietic cells

A. Limiting Dilution Assays

Cells Injected	Strain	Number	Recipient	#Injected/ Repopulated
Lin⁻ c-kit^{HI}	C57BL/6	30 – 200	WBB6F1-WW^v	60–100%
Lin⁻ c-kit^{LO}	C57BL/6	1000 – 2.5 × 10⁴	WBB6F1-WW^v	0/14
Lin⁻ c-kit^{NEG}	C57BL/6	9 × 10⁴ – 4 × 10⁵	WBB6F1-WW^v	0/13

B. Competitive Repopulation Assays

Cells Injected	Strain	Number	Recipient	% B6 Hb	RRA[a]	fold enrichment
Lin⁻ c-kit^{HI}	C57BL/6	200	WBB6F1-+/+	11.3 ± 4.7%	1274	1274
Bone marrow	HW80	2 × 10⁶			1.0	
Lin⁻ c-kit^{NEG}	C57BL/6	2 × 10⁶	WBB6F1-+/+	33.4 ± 1.1%	0.15[b]	−6.6
Bone marrow	HW80	2 × 10⁶			1.0	

[a]Relative repopulating ability.
[b]Lin⁻ cells accounted for 30% of bone marrow cells in these experiments.

The relative enrichment of repopulating activity between Lin⁻ c-kit^{HI} cells and unfractionated bone marrow is 1274, and between Lin⁻ c-kit^{HI} cells and Lin⁻ c-kit-^{NEG} cells is 8400 (TABLE 2).

Isolation of HSC-Specific cDNAs by DD-PCR

A schematic representation of DD-PCR is shown in FIGURE 2. The "fingerprint" of transcripts between Lin⁻ c-kit^{HI} cells and unfractionated bone marrow cells was compared. To minimize artifacts caused by prep to prep variation of RNA, multiple samples of both RNAs were analyzed simultaneously. To minimize artifacts caused by the concentration of mRNA in the reaction, the amount of RNA was determined prior to the reactions using the β-2 M limiting dilution assay, and the reactions were performed at two different mRNA concentrations.

Multiple bands were present in RNA from both Lin⁻ c-kit^{HI} and unfractionated bone marrow cells. We established the following criteria for selection of bands to excise from the gel for cloning. First, the band must be present in all samples of Lin⁻ c-kit^{HI} RNA, and absent in all bone marrow RNA preps. Second, the band must be present at both concentrations of Lin⁻ c-kit^{HI} RNA. Using these criteria, we identified and cloned 25 bands. The size of the inserts ranged from ~100 to 400 base pairs. Sequence analysis of these 25 clones revealed that 5/25 (20%) represented ribosomal RNA sequences. Among the 20 other clones, a BLAST search identified sequences >95% homologous to the murine cbf-α[29] and the transcription factor CP2[30] (TABLE 3). PCR primers were generated from the sequence data for RT-PCR analysis. A total of 15/20 sequences were expressed at higher levels in HSCs than in unfractionated bone marrow. A similar result was observed when Lin⁻ c-kit^{HI} RNA and bone

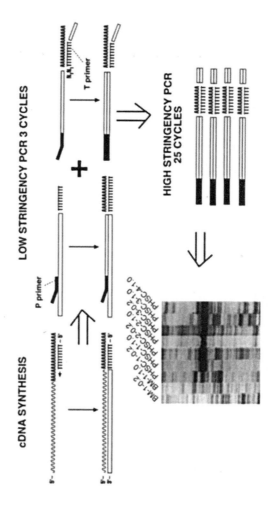

FIGURE 2. Identification of HSC-specific transcripts by DD-PCR. (Adapted from Liang and Pardee.[23]) A representative autoradiograph appears at the *left*.

249

TABLE 3. Isolation of sequences expressed in HSCs by DD-PCR

No. of clones sequenced	Average insert size	No. of rRNA/vector (%)	Known genes (%)	Novel genes/ESTs (%)
25	250 bp	5 (20%)	cbf-α2 CP2 transcription factor (10%)	18 (90%)

marrow RNA were ^{32}P-labeled and hybridized to identical slot blots of the 20 non-ribosomal RNA clones with an actin cDNA and empty vector as positive and negative controls.

The remainder of the clones did not show significant homology to known genes (TABLE 3). This analysis was complicated by the fact that the average insert was 250 bases in length, and that the sequence was mainly derived from the extreme 3' end of the mRNA, preventing a more detailed analysis of sequence homology.

Isolation of HSC-Specific cDNAs by Subtractive Hybridization

We have used sequence homology to known genes as a crucial aspect of the process of deciding which gene sequences to study in greater detail (see Discussion). Therefore, to obtain longer clones and increase the probability that the sequence we isolated represented coding (as opposed to 3' untranslated) sequence, we generated a library of cDNAs using subtractive hybridization (SH). A schematic representation of SH is shown in FIGURE 3. For the "tester" RNA, we used Lin⁻ c-kit[HI] RNA. Because of the greater difference between the relative repopulating abilities, we chose to use Lin⁻ c-kit[NEG] RNA as the "driver" RNA. A total of 1152 clones were isolated, and 151 clones represented at high levels in the "tester" cDNA and/or highly amplified after subtraction were identified and sequenced.

The average insert size among the selected clones was 1.3 kb. A total of 21 of the 151 clones (14%) represented vector (18), and tRNA (3) sequences. Of the remaining 130 clones, 93 (71.5%) represented known gene sequences, and 37 (28.5%) represented sequences that were either novel or homologous to expressed sequence tags (ESTs; TABLE 4). There was great redundancy among both the known genes and the novel/EST group. The 93 known gene sequences included 18 genes represented once, and 20 represented multiple times. The c-kit and c-myb genes were represented 3 times each, as predicted from our previous results.[14] Similarly, the 37 novel/EST sequences, represented 22 transcripts, represented 4 (1 sequence), three (3), two (10), or one (4) time each (TABLE 4).

TABLE 4. Isolation of sequences expressed in HSCs by subtractive hybridization

No. of clones sequenced	Average insert size	No. of rRNA/vector (%)	Known genes (%)	Novel genes/ESTs (%)
151	1.3 kb	21 (14%)	93 (71.5%) including c-kit, c-myb	37 (28.5%)

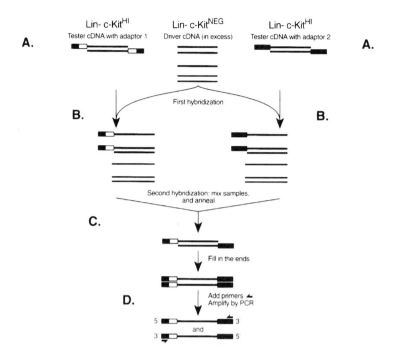

FIGURE 3. Identification of HSC-specific transcripts by SH. (Adapted from Diatchenko *et al.*[24])

DISCUSSION

The ideal comparison for isolating gene sequences specifically involved in hematopoietic repopulation would be RNA from pure repopulating HSCs versus the same population depleted of HSCs. The closest we can come to this ideal is a comparison of Lin⁻ c-kit[HI] cells to Lin⁻ c-kit[NEG] cells. We calculate that the relative enrichment in repopulating activity between these two cell populations is over 8000-fold (1274-fold enrichment × 6.6-fold depletion). While this enrichment is certainly favorable for molecular analysis of HSC-specific transcripts, there are two important caveats to a molecular analysis using these cell types. First, our Lin⁻ c-kit[HI] cell population is far from pure with regard to HSCs. As described above, an average of 30 cells is required to repopulate 100% of W/W^v mice, which compares favorably with the work of other groups. Estimates vary as to the "seeding efficiency" of transplanted hematopoietic cells. We calculate that if the seeding efficiency is 10%, that between 1/3 and 2/3 of the Lin⁻ c-kit[HI] cell population is not capable of repopulation. Secondly, despite the 8000-fold difference in repopulating ability between the Lin⁻ c-kit[HI] and Lin⁻ c-kit[NEG] cell populations, a small amount of repopulating activity is present in the Lin⁻ c-kit[NEG] cells. This cell population is phenotypically similar to the cell population identified by Jones *et al.* [31]. We are cautious about whether the

DD-PCR or SH procedures can absolutely prevent the subtraction of some HSC-related genes.

We hypothesize that mRNAs encoding gene products involved in maintaining stem cells in an undifferentiated state, and or mRNAs encoding gene products involved in promoting self renewal divisions will be present at high levels in HSCs and lower levels in either unfractionated bone marrow cells or Lin⁻ cells depleted of HSCs. In addition we predict that such genes would be expressed primarily in hematopoietic cells. In attempting to identify novel genes expressed in HSCs, we have devised a strategy that involves an integration of sequencing, Northern blot and RT-PCR analysis of gene expression in HSCs. Our screening strategy begins with sequence data from the clones identified by either the DD-PCR or SH procedures. The sequence data is used for BLAST searches of DNA sequence data bases to a) identify the gene sequence, or b) for novel genes to identify homology to known genes that may suggest a function for the gene product. The sequence data are used to generate RT-PCR primers to verify expression in HSCs. We eliminate genes that do not show higher levels of expression in Lin⁻ c-kit^{HI} RNA than in Lin⁻ c-kit^{NEG} and unfractionated bone marrow RNA. We also examine the expression of clones in different mouse tissues by Northern blot analysis. Our focus is on genes that are expressed primarily in hematopoietic cells and cell lines and not in other organs or non-hematopoietic cell lines. This analysis also demonstrates the size of the mRNA, and identifies libraries from which full length cDNAs can be cloned.

We explored two different procedures for the isolation of HSC-specific genes, DD-PCR and SH. Both procedures produces a low but persistent level of artifacts (14–20%), which consisted mainly of ribosomal RNA (DD-PCR) or vector sequences (SH). Using both procedures, we isolated cDNAs from genes that we or others have shown to be expressed in HSCs such as cbf-α[29] and c-kit.[5,14] Despite these similarities, in our hands the SH procedure is superior to DD-PCR in several ways. SH is a more powerful procedure, and we have generated a library of over 1000 amplified clones to screen with approximately the same amount of effort needed to isolate and characterize 25 clones by DD-PCR. In addition, the average length of the sequences cloned by SH was 5.2-fold longer than the sequences cloned by DD-PCR. These longer clones greatly increased the probability of identifying genes or gene families. For example only 2/20 (10%) of the sequences isolated by DD-PCR could be definitively identified in BLAST searches as opposed to over 70% of the clones identified by SH. We conclude that the longer sequences include more coding sequence that facilitates homology searches. More practical advantages of longer cDNAs are that they allow the cloning of the full length cDNA by rapid amplification of cDNA ends (RACE), which can bypass cDNA cloning, and they make superior probes for Southern and Northern blots.

In summary, our initial attempts to clone novel gene sequences expressed in HSCs have shown that Lin⁻ c-kit^{HI} and Lin⁻ c-kit^{NEG} cells have the greatest difference in the relative repopulating ability, and represent the best populations to compare. In our hands SH appears to be the most powerful and efficient method of identifying novel cDNAs. The redundancy of clones identified by SH indicates that there are a limited number of sequences that are differentially expressed in Lin⁻ c-kit^{HI} RNA rather than in Lin⁻ c-kit^{NEG} RNA, and suggests that many of the sequences we are seeking may be in the libraries we and others have generated.[32] Despite the fact that the number of differentially expressed sequences may be small, a carefully defined screening process must be established to allow detailed analysis of interesting genes.

REFERENCES

1. ORLIC, D. & D.M. BODINE. 1994. What defines a pluripotent hematopoietic stem cell (PHSC)?: Will the real PHSC please stand up. Blood **84:** 3991–3994.
2. MORRISON, S., N. UCHIDA & I. WEISSMAN. 1995. The biology of hematopoietic stem cells. Annu. Rev. Cell. Dev. Biol. **11:** 35–71.
3. SPANGRUDE, G.J., S. HEIMFELD & I.L. WEISSMAN. 1988. Purification and characterization of mouse hematopoietic stem cell. Science **241:** 58–62.
4. UCHIDA, N. & I.L. WEISSMAN. 1992. Searching for hematopoietic stem cells: evidence that Thy-1.1^{Lo} Lin$^-$ Sca-1$^+$ cells are the only stem cells in C57BL/Ka-Thy-1.1 bone marrow. J. Exp. Med. **175:** 175–184.
5. ORLIC, D., R. FISCHER, S-I. NISHIKAWA, A.W. NEINHUIS & D.M. BODINE. 1993. Purification and characterization of heterogeneous pluripotent hematopoietic stem cell populations expressing high levels of c-kit receptor. Blood **82:** 762–770.
6. SMITH, L.G., I.L. WEISSMAN & S. HEIMFELD. 1991. Clonal analysis of hematopoietic stem cell differentiation *in vivo*. Proc. Natl. Acad. Sci. USA **88:** 2788–2792.
7. MORRISON, S.J. & I.L. WEISSMAN. 1994. The long-term repopulating subset of hematopoietic stem cells is deterministic and isolatable by phenotype. Immunity **8:** 661–673.
8. JORDAN, C.T. & I.R. LEMISCHKA. 1990. Clonal and systemic analysis of long-term hematopoiesis in the mouse. Genes Dev. **4:** 220–228.
9. REDDY, G.P., C.Y. TIARKS, L. PANG, J. WUU, C.C. HSIEH & P.J. QUESENBERRY. 1997. Call cycle analysis and synchronization of pluripotent hematopoietic progenitor stem cells. Blood **90:** 2293–2299.
10. LI, C.L. & G.R. JOHNSON. 1992. Rhodamine 123 reveals heterogeneity within murine Lin$^-$ Sca-1$^+$ hematopoietic stem cells. J. Exp. Med. **175:** 1443–1447.
11. VISSER, J.W. & P. DEVRIES. 1988. Isolation of spleen colony forming cells (CFU-s) using wheat germ agglutinin and Rhodamine 123 retention. Blood Cells **14:** 369–384.
12. UCHIDA, N., J. COMBS, S. CHEN, E. ZANJANI, R. HOFFMAN & A. TSUKAMOTO. 1996. Primitive human hematopoietic cells displaying differential eflux of the Rhodamine 123 dye have distinct biological activities. Blood **88:** 1297–1305.
13. GOODELL, M.A., K. BROSE, G. PARADIS, A.S. CONNER & R.C. MULLIGAN. 1996. Isolation and functional properties of murine hematopoietic stem cells that are replicating *in vivo*. J. Exp. Med. **183:** 1797–1806.
14. ORLIC, D., S. ANDERSON, L.G. BIESECKER, B.P. SORRENTINO & D.M. BODINE. 1995. Pluripotent hematopoietic stem cells contain high levels of mRNA for c-kit, GATA-2, p45NF-E2, and c-myb and low levels or no mRNA for c-fms and the receptors for granulocyte colony stimulating factor and interleukins 5 and 7. Proc. Natl. Acad. Sci. USA **92:** 4601–4605.
15. ORLIC, D., L.J. GIRARD, C.T. JORDAN, S.M. ANDERSON, A.P. CLINE & D.M. BODINE. 1996. The level of mRNA encoding the amphotropic retrovirus receptor in mouse and human hematopoietic stem cells is low and correlates with the efficiency of retrovirus transduction. Proc. Natl. Acad. Sci. USA **93:** 11097–11102.
16. ORLIC, D., L.J. GIRARD, S.M. ANDERSON, L.C. PYLE, M.C. YODER, H.E. BROXMEYER & D.M. BODINE. 1998. Identification of human and mouse hematopoietic stem cell populations expressing high levels of mRNA encoding retrovirus receptors. Blood **91:** 3247–3254.
17. YODER, M.C., K. HIATT, P. DUTT, P. MUKHERJEE, D.M. BODINE & D. ORLIC. 1998. Characterization of definitive lymphohematopoietic stem cells in the day 9 murine yolk sac. Immunity **7:** 335–344.

18. SORRENTINO, B.P., K.T. MCDONAGH, D. WOODS & D. ORLIC. 1995. Expression of retroviral vectors containing the human multidrug resistance 1 cDNA in hematopoietic cells of transplanted mice. Blood **86:** 491–501.

19. ORLIC, D., L.J. GIRARD, D. LEE, S.M. ANDERSON, J.M. PUCK & D.M. BODINE. 1997. Interleukin-7Rα mRNA expression increases as stem cells differentiate into T and B lymphocyte progenitors. Exp. Hematol. **25:** 217–222.

20. RICHARDSON, C. & A. BANK. 1996. Developmental-stage-specific expression and regulation of an amphotropic retroviral receptor in hematopoietic cells. Mol. Cell. Biol. **16:** 4240–4247.

21. MCCLANAHAN, T., S. DALRYMPLE, M. BARKETT & F. LEE. 1993. Hematopoietic growth factor receptor genes as markers of lineage commitment during *in vitro* development of hematopoietic cells. Blood **81:** 2903–2915.

22. MATTHEWS, W., C.T. JORDAN, G.W. WIEGAND, D. PARDOLL & I.R. LEMISCHKA. 1991. A receptor tyrosine kinase specific to stem and progenitor enriched populations. Cell **65:** 1143–1152.

23. LIANG, P. & A. PARDEE. 1992. Differential display of eukaryotic messenger RNA by means of the polymerase chain reaction. Science **257:** 967–970.

24. DIATCHENKO, L., Y.-F.C. LAU, A.P. CAMPBELL, A. CHENCHIK, F. MOQADAM, B. HUANG, S. LUKYANOV, K. LUKYANOV, N. GUSKAYA, E.D. SVERDLOV & P.D. SIEBERT. 1996. Suppressive subtractive hybridization: a method for generating differentially regulated or tissue specific cDNA probes and libraries. Proc. Natl. Acad. Sci. USA **93:** 6025–6030.

25. WEAVER, S., N.L. HAIGWOOD, C.A. HUTCHISON III & M.H. Edgell. 1979. DNA fragments of the Mus musculus β globin haplotypes. Proc. Natl. Acad. Sci. USA **76:** 1385–1389.

26. RUSSELL, E.S. 1979. Hereditary anemias of the mouse: a review for geneticists. Adv. Genet. **20:** 357–459.

27. WHITNEY, J.B. III. 1978. Simplified typing of mouse hemoglobin (Hbb) phenotypes using cystamine. Biochem. Genet. **16:** 667–672.

28. HARRISON, D.E. 1980. Competitive repopulation: a new assay for long-term stem cell capacity. Blood **55:** 77–86.

29. WANG, Q., T. STACY, M. BINDER, M. MARIN-PADILLA, A.H. SHARPE & N.A. SPECK. 1996. Disruption of the Cbfa2 gene causes necrosis and hemmoraging in the central nervous system and blocks definitive hematopoiesis. Proc. Natl. Acad. Sci. USA **93:** 3444–3449.

30. JANE, S.M., A.W. NIENHUIS & J.M. CUNNINGHAM. 1995. Hemoglobin switching in man and chicken is mediated by a heteromeric complex between the ubiquitous transcription factor CP2 and a developmentally specific protein. EMBO J. **14:** 97–105.

31. JONES, R.J., M.I. COLLECTOR, J.P. BARBER, M.S. VALA, M.J. FACKLER, W.S. MAY, C.A. GRIFFIN, A.L. HAWKINS, B.A. ZHENBAUER, J. HILTON, O.M. COLVIN & S.J. SHARKIS. 1996. Characterization of mouse lymphohematopoietic stem cells lacking spleen colony-forming activity. Blood **88:** 487–491.

32. DOSIL, M., N. LEIBMAN & I.R. LEMISCHKA. 1996. Cloning and characterization of fetal liver phosphatase 1, a nuclear protein tyrosine phosphatase isolated from hematopoietic stem cells. Blood **88:** 4510–4525.

DISCUSSION

E. DZIERZAK (*Erasmus University*): I have a question related to expression of the tyrosine kinase gene and the HMG gene. Given that during development hematopoietic cells are developing in a number of different places within the embryo, perhaps *in situ* hybridization would be a nice technique to look further at the expression of these genes.

BODINE: Those studies are underway now in collaboration with Bill Paven, who studies mouse development. At this point what we can say from looking at tissue RNA by Northern blot is that the HMG gene is expressed almost exclusively in the yolk sac. You can see a little RNA in fetal liver by Northern blot. I agree that *in situ* hybridization would be important. The tyrosine kinase is expressed in a lot of tissues in the embryo, so I think that it will be important to look at specific cell types with *in situ* hybridization.

Embryonic Beginnings of Definitive Hematopoietic Stem Cells

ELAINE DZIERZAK[a]

Department of Cell Biology and Genetics, Medical Faculty, Erasmus University, P.O. Box 1738, 3000 DR Rotterdam, The Netherlands

ABSTRACT: The ability of the many cell types within the adult blood system to be constantly replenished and renewed from hematopoietic stem cells is an interesting problem in development and differentiation and has led to questions concerning how, when and where these stem cells for the adult hematopoietic system are generated within the embryo. During embryonic development many mature hematopoietic cells appear before adult-type hematopoietic stem cells thus the notion of a conventional hematopoietic hierarchy is challenged. Experiments probing the development of hematopoietic stem cells in the mouse embryo strongly suggest that at least two independent hematopoietic sites generate blood cells during development; the yolk sac, which produces the transient embryonic hematopoietic system, and the AGM (aorta-gonad-mesonephros) region, which initiates the long-lived adult hematopoietic system.

INTRODUCTION

The adult hematopoietic system is a complex series of pluripotent, multipotent and unipotent cellular intermediates which proliferate and differentiate into at least eight morphologically and functionally distinct mature blood cell types. Hematopoietic stem cells are at the foundation of this cellular hierarchy in the adult. The cells within this hierarchy have been defined by numerous *in vitro* and *in vivo* hematologic assays which measure proliferation and lineage differentiation. The most stringent of the assays, the radiation chimera assay, has been used to demonstrate the presence of pluripotential hematopoietic stem cells in bone marrow[1] and fetal liver.[14] *In vivo* transplantation of true adult-type hematopoietic stem cells into adult recipient mice depleted of endogenous hematopoietic stem cells by a lethal dose of irradiation leads to the complete, long-term engraftment of all blood lineages by donor-derived stem cells. Thus, pluripotential hematopoietic stem cells possess the following complex characteristics: 1) potential for all hematopoietic lineages as demonstrated by clonal markers; 2) high proliferative potential leading to 100% donor-derived engraftment; 3) long-term activity throughout the lifespan of the individual; and 4) self-renewal as demonstrated by *in vivo* serial transplantations. The clinical importance of stem cells with these characteristics is widely recognized in transplantation scenarios for blood-related genetic deficiencies and leukemias.

The developmental origins of adult-type hematopoietic stem cells in mammals are of current interest.[6,7] In developmentally early hematopoietic microenviron-

[a]Phone, +31-10-408-7172; fax, +31-10-436-0225; e-mail, dzierzak@ch1.fgg.eur.nl

ments, stem cells are induced and/or expanded from cells derived from the mesodermal germ layer. Subsequently, hematopoietic stem cells colonize the liver during fetal stages and the bone marrow of the adult where they remain throughout life.[13] Early hematopoietic development has been examined in both mammalian[19] and nonmammalian[4,5,24,25] vertebrate embryos. Mammalian vertebrates have the advantage of many *in vitro* and *in vivo* assays for defining the presence of an array of hematopoietic progenitors and stem cells within the embryo. Primitive erythroid cells, erythroid-myeloid progenitors, CFU-S and hematopoietic stem cells have been found in the yolk sac at E7, E8, E8.5, and E11, respectively.[19] These results led to the previously accepted notion that the yolk sac was the source of the adult hematopoietic system in mammals. However, orthotopic grafting experiments which can be performed with the large embryos of avian[4] or amphibian species[25] showed that while the yolk sac or ventral blood islands (yolk sac analogue) produced hematopoietic cells, these were transient blood cells present predominantly during embryonic stages. The long-lived adult hematopoietic system was generated instead by the cells in an intraembryonic site surrounding the dorsal aorta and pro/mesonephros. The dichotomy in these results of higher and lower vertebrates persisted for over twenty years leading to the assumption that mammalian hematopoietic development is different from that in nonmammalian vertebrate species. With the absence of previous studies examining this intraembryonic site in mammals, we set out to determine whether hematopoietic activity was present and could take its origins in the region comprising the dorsal aorta, gonads and mesonephros (AGM) of the early and mid-gestation mouse embryo.

THE AGM REGION CONTAINS HEMATOPOIETIC PROGENITORS AND STEM CELLS

To examine the hematopoietic potential of the intraembryonic AGM region we first performed the short-term *in vivo* spleen colony-forming unit (CFU-S) assay. We injected a single cell suspension of various tissues from E8, E9, E10, or E11 mouse embryos into lethally irradiated adult female recipient mice and examined their spleens at 9 and 11 days posttransplantation for the presence of macroscopic (erythroid-myeloid) colonies.[17] The donor injected cells were obtained from male embryos or transgenic embryos marked by either a Y chromosome or a human beta-globin gene locus (line 72), respectively. While E8 yolk sac, AGM, liver and blood contained no CFU-S, such progenitors are present in both E9 yolk sac and AGM. At E10 the number and frequency of CFU-S in the AGM region surpasses that in the yolk sac and peaks at late E10. Thereafter, CFU-S decrease rapidly in the AGM, with a concomitant increase in CFU-S in the liver. These results demonstrate the presence of potent multilineage progenitors in the AGM region, and their temporal and spatial distribution[16,17] suggest that CFU-S from the AGM region colonize the liver.

In addition to these data on the multipotent CFU-S progenitor, Godin and colleagues found the intraembryonic para-aortic splanchnopleura (PAS) at E8.5 to contain progenitors for the B1a subset of B lymphocytes by transplantation of this embryonic region under the kidney capsule of severe combined immunodeficiency (SCID) mice.[10] In a two step culture system multipotent progenitors for the B and T lymphoid lineages as well as erythroid-myeloid lineages were found in the PAS at E8.5.[9] These cells were found to be positive for the AA4.1 surface marker previously found to be on fetal liver hematopoietic progenitors and stem cells.

With these convincing data that multipotent hematopoietic progenitors could be found in the PAS/AGM region, long-term mouse radiation chimeras were generated to test whether the AGM region contains pluripotent adult-type hematopoietic stem cells.[21] Transplantations were performed as described for the CFU-S experiments, and mice were tested for engraftment at greater than 4 months posttransplantation. No donor-derived engraftment was observed for E8 or E9 yolk sac or AGM. However, transplanted E10 AGM region cells were able to fully engraft 3 out of 100 recipients, while E10 yolk sac resulted in no engraftment. Even at 8 months posttransplantation, E10 AGM region cells can repopulate the blood system of the recipients up to 100% in all hematopoietic tissues and lineages. Secondary and tertiary serial transplantations of bone marrow from these recipients indicated that the E10 AGM hematopoietic stem cells are self-renewing. Moreover, at E11 the AGM region contains a high frequency of such hematopoietic stem cells as demonstrated by the complete long-term engraftment of 11 out of 19 recipients. E11 yolk sac and liver also contained hematopoietic stem cells but at a lower frequency. Recently, Yoder and colleagues have shown that at E9 both the yolk sac and AGM region contain multipotent progenitors that can *in vivo* repopulate neonatal but not adult recipient mice.[26,27] These data suggest that the earlier progenitors in the yolk sac and AGM have some but not all the characteristics of adult hematopoietic stem cells. Thus, the AGM region appears to be the first site within the mouse conceptus to initiate fully competent adult-type hematopoietic stem cells.

THE AGM REGION AUTONOMOUSLY INITIATES HEMATOPOIETIC STEM CELL ACTIVITY

At E10 the AGM region contains the first hematopoietic stem cells at limiting numbers.[21] However, it is possible that these stem cells are generated at another site within the mouse conceptus and quickly migrate through the circulation or interstitially to localize in the AGM region. The circulation between the yolk sac and the embryo body is established at E8.5 in gestation.[3] Thus, to examine the site of initiation of the first hematopoietic stem cells, we instituted an organ explant culture step for AGM, yolk sac or liver before the *in vivo* transplantation assay.[15] Two to three days of organ culture of individual AGM, yolk sac or liver explants alleviates any cellular exchange between these tissues. When we examined E9 cultured tissues, no hematopoietic stem cells were found in AGM, yolk sac or liver. The first hematopoietic stem cells appeared in E10 cultured AGM explants. Quantitatively these stem cells outnumbered those found in uncultured AGMs by a factor of 15, strongly suggesting the induction and/or expansion of hematopoietic stem cells during the 3-day *in vitro* culture period. Interestingly, no hematopoietic stem cells were found in E10 yolk sac or liver but began to appear in E11 and late E11 cultured yolk sac and liver, respectively. These results show the autonomous and exclusive production of hematopoietic stem cells at E10 by the AGM region and suggest the colonization of liver by AGM-derived hematopoietic stem cells. The yolk sac may also be colonized by AGM-derived hematopoietic stem cells and/or endogenously generate its own hematopoietic stem cells beginning at E11.

A similar organ culture step was used to determine the site of generation of the first multipotent (lymphoid-myeloid-erythroid) progenitors.[2] At E7.5 and before the circulation is established between the embryo body and the yolk sac, these progenitors are found only in the para-aortic splanchnopleura. The yolk sac contains such progenitors only after E8.5. Thus, these definitive hematopoietic progenitors as well as the first fully competent adult-type hematopoietic stem cells are autonomously generated within the embryo body before they appear in the yolk sac.

THE FIRST HEMATOPOIETIC STEM CELLS ARE C-KIT⁺CD34⁺ AND LOCALIZE TO THE ANTERIOR AGM

The phenotypic characterization of the AGM hematopoietic stem cells was performed. Cell surface markers indicative of adult-type hematopoietic stem cells were found on AGM hematopoietic stem cells.[22] When transplanted in at various doses, E11 hematopoietic stem cells were always found in the c-kit⁺CD34⁺ double positive population. The E9 yolk sac and AGM cells that possess the ability to repopulate conditioned new born mice (but not adult recipients) to low levels are also c-kit⁺ and CD34⁺.[27] However, the Sca-1 hematopoietic stem cell marker, which is a marker of the hematopoietic stem cells of fetal liver[12] and adult bone marrow[23] but not yolk sac hematopoietc cells[11] is expressed on E11 AGM hematopoietic stem cells[8] suggesting this as a distinctive marker of only true definitive hematopoietic stem cells. Interestingly c-kit⁺CD34⁺ E11 AGM hematopoietic stem cells are negative for all mature lineage markers except Mac-1.[22] While fifty percent of the AGM stem cells were found to be Mac-1 negative, the other fifty percent were Mac-1 positive and have been suggested to be the subset of AGM stem cells ready to colonize the fetal liver (at E11, E12 and E13 all fetal liver hematopoietic stem cells are Mac-1 positive). These marker studies strongly suggest a direct lineage relationship between the hematopoietic stem cells of the AGM region and the fetal liver and together with the results of the organ culture studies suggest a colonization of the fetal liver with AGM-generated hematopoietic stem cells.

Using a transgenic mouse expressing the LacZ reporter gene in Sca-1-expressing cells, we examined the localization of Sca-1-LacZ-positive cells within intact AGM tissue.[18] When E10, E11, and E12 embryos were examined, beta-galactosidase-positive cells were found in the anterior portion of the AGM region. The cells lining the pronephric and mesonephric tubules stained brightly, while the cells in surrounding mesenchyme stained to an intermediate level. All yolk sac cells were negative. Moreover the kinetics of AGM beta-galactosidase staining coincided with the presence of hematopoietic stem cells in the AGM region, thus suggesting a localization for the first stem cells. By using the organ culture system we also tested whether we could further localize the first functional hematopoietic stem cells to the anterior and/or posterior portion of the AGM.[15] In two experiments we found all hematopoietic stem cell activity in the anterior portion of cultured E10 AGMs. Hence the beta-galactosidase-positive cells may provide a precise localization for the first hematopoietic stem cells in the AGM region, although at this time it is undetermined whether the beta-galactosidase positive-cells in the mesonephric tubules or the cells within the surrounding mesenchyme (which stain less intensely) are the functional stem cells. Further functional experiments are in progress to examine which positive population contains the hematopoietic stem cells.

CONCLUSIONS AND FUTURE DIRECTIONS

The results of our *in vivo* transplantation experiments using the mouse as a model for mammalian hematopoiesis, clearly demonstrate the potency of the AGM region in the initiation of adult-type hematopoietic stem cells. The AGM region autonomously and exclusively inititates the first adult-type hematopoietic stem cells at E10, one day earlier than these cells can be found in the yolk sac. Previously, in contrast to the intraembryonic source found in nonmammalian vertebrates, the yolk sac was thought to be the generating source of these stem cells in mammals. The discovery of the hematopoietic potential of the AGM region now yields a clear case for strong similarities in developmental hematopoiesis between all vertebrate species. It appears that the mouse yolk sac participates predominantly in the generation of the embryonic hematopoietic system, while the AGM region is dedicated to the initiation and production of the adult hematopoietic system.

Indeed this appears to be reflected in the genetic programming of cells destined to become embryonic or adult hematopoietic cells (reviewed in Ref. 7). Recent advances in targeted mutagenesis in mice have yielded results that demonstrate the differential requirement for some genes (AML-1, GATA-2, GATA-3, c-kit) in adult and fetal liver hematopoiesis but not embryonic hematopoiesis. In constrast the mutation of other genes (flk-1, tal-1/SCL) results in the impairment of hematopoiesis in both the yolk sac and fetal liver. Thus, the genetic programs of embryonic and adult hematopoietic cells appear to be initially overlapping during stages determining hematopoietic fate, but become unique as more complex programming is required in cells destined to become part of the adult hematopoietic system. It may be predicted that the primary cellular defects of the genes affecting fetal liver hematopoiesis occur in the induction, expansion or maintenance of hematopoietic stem cells and progenitors in the AGM region before they colonize the fetal liver. We are currently examining the roles of such genes in the AGM region and in the generation of the adult hematopoietic system by organ explant cultures and radiation chimera approaches.

Finally, the question remains how are the first fully competent adult-type hematopoietic stem cells generated in the AGM region? As the fetal thymic organ culture system has yielded great advances in knowledge concerning thymocyte differentiation and development, we hope to make use of chimeric AGM organ cultures to determine whether the precursors for the first hematopoietic stem cells are generated *in situ* within the AGM region or are recent emigrants from other embryonic sites such as the yolk sac. These cultures will also be used to test whether adult bone marrow hematopoietic stem cells can be increased in number in the AGM microenvironment. Recent findings of Mukouyama *et al.*[20] suggest that indeed hematopoietic progenitors from the AGM region can be increased *in vitro*. Hence, our future investigation will include differential cloning to address what are the unique signals within the AGM microenvironment that lead to the induction and/or proliferation of the first fully competent adult-type hematopoietic stem cells.

ACKNOWLEDGMENTS

The author would like to thank Drs. Alexander Medvinsky, Albrecht Muller, Maria-Jose Sanchez, Colin Miles, Angus Sinclair and Marella de Bruijn for their dedication and long hours spent in the laboratory to achieve the results presented here. My thanks also to all the members of my laboratory and the Department of Cell Biology, Erasmus University who contributed to this work. This research is supported in part by the Leukemia Society of America and The Netherlands Scientific Research Organization.

REFERENCES

1. ABRAMSON, S. *et al.* 1977. The identification in adult bone marrow of pluripotent and restricted stem cells of the myeloid and lymphoid systems. J. Exp. Med. **145:** 1567–1579.
2. CUMANO, A. *et al.* 1996. Lymphoid potential, probed before circulation in mouse, is restricted to caudal intraembryonic splanchnopleura. Cell **86:** 907–916.
3. DELASSUS, S. & A. CUMANO. 1996. Circulation of hematopoietic progenitors in the mouse embryo. Immunity **4:** 97–106.
4. DIETERLEN-LIEVRE, F. 1975. On the origin of haemopoietic stem cells in the avian embryo: an experimental approach. J. Embryol. Exp. Morphol. **33:** 607–619.
5. DIETERLEN-LIEVRE, F. & N.M. LE DOUARIN. 1993. Developmental rules in the hematopoietic and immune systems of birds: how general are they? Semin. Dev. Biol. **4:** 325–332.
6. DZIERZAK, E. & A. MEDVINSKY. 1995. Mouse embryonic hematopoiesis. Trends Genet. **11:** 359–366.
7. DZIERZAK, E. *et al.* 1998. Qualitative and quantitative aspects of haematopoietic cell development in the mammalian embryo. Immunol. Today **19:** 228–236.
8. DZIERZAK, E. *et al.* 1995. Hematopoietic stem cell development in the mouse embryo. *In* Molecular Biology of Hemoglobin Switching. G. Stamatoyannopoulos, Ed.: 109–121. Andover. Intercept.
9. GODIN, I. *et al.* 1995. Emergence of multipotent hemopoietic cells in the yolk sac and para-aortic splanchnopleura in mouse embryos, beginning at 8.5 days postcoitus. Proc. Natl. Acad. Sci. USA **92:** 773–777.
10. GODIN, I.E. *et al.* 1993. Para-aortic splanchnopleura from early mouse embryos contains B1a cell progenitors. Nature **364:** 67–70.
11. HUANG, H. & R. AUERBACH. 1993. Identification and characterization of hematopoietic stem cells from the yolk sac of the early mouse embryo. Proc. Natl. Acad. Sci. USA **90:** 10110–10114.
12. IKUTA, K. *et al.* 1990. A developmental switch in thymic lymphocyte maturation potential occurs at the level of hematopoietic stem cells. Cell **62:** 863–874.
13. JOHNSON, G. R. & M.A. MOORE. 1975. Role of stem cell migration in initiation of mouse foetal liver haemopoiesis. Nature **258:** 726–728.
14. JORDAN, C. T. *et al.* 1990. Cellular and developmental properties of fetal hematopoietic stem cells. Cell **61:** 953–963.
15. MEDVINSKY, A. & E. DZIERZAK. 1996. Definitive hematopoiesis is autonomously initiated by the AGM region. Cell **86:** 897–906.

16. MEDVINSKY, A.L. *et al.* 1996. Development of day-8 colony-forming unit-spleen hematpoietic progenitors during early murine embyrogenesis: spatial and temporal mapping. Blood **87:** 557–566.
17. MEDVINSKY, A. L. *et al.* 1993. An early pre-liver intraembryonic source of CFU-S in the developing mouse. Nature **364:** 64–67.
18. MILES, C. *et al.* 1997. Expression of the Ly-6E.1 (Sca-1) transgene in adult hematopoietic stem cells and the developing mouse embryo. Development **124:** 537–547.
19. MOORE, M. A. & D. METCALF. 1970. Ontogeny of the haemopoietic system: yolk sac origin of *in vivo* and *in vitro* colony forming cells in the developing mouse embryo. Br. J. Haematol. **18:** 279–296.
20. MUKOUYAMA, Y. *et al.* 1998. *In vitro* expansion of murine hematopoietic progenitors from the embryonic aorta-gonad-mesonephros region. Immunity **8:** 105–114.
21. MULLER, A. M. *et al.* 1994. Development of hematopoietic stem cell activity in the mouse embryo. Immunity **1:** 291–301.
22. SANCHEZ, M. J. *et al.* 1996. Characterization of the first definitive hematopoietic stem cells in the AGM and liver of the mouse embryo. Immunity **5:** 513–525.
23. SPANGRUDE, S.J. *et al.* 1988. Purificaiton and characterization of mouse heamtopoietic stem cells. Science **241:** 58–62.
24. TURPEN, J. B. *et al.* 1997. Bipotential primitive-definitive hematopoietic progenitors in the vertebrate embryo. Immunity **7:** 325–334.
25. TURPEN, J. B. *et al.* 1981. The early ontogeny of hematopoietic cells studied by grafting cytogenetically labeled tissue anlagen: localization of a prospective stem cell compartment. Dev. Biol. **85:** 99–112.
26. YODER, M.C. & K. HIATT. 1997. Engraftment of embryonic hematopoietic cells in conditioned newborn recipients. Blood **89:** 2176–2183.
27. YODER, M.C. *et al.* 1997. Characterization of definitive lymphohematopoietic stem cells in the day 9 murine yolk sac. Immunity **7:** 335–344.

DISCUSSION

G. KELLER (*Howard Hughes Medical Institute*): A technical question regarding your reaggregation experiments with the bone marrow stem cells. Were the reaggregated organs cultured?

DZIERZAK: The reaggregation culture is for 4 days.

KELLER: Could you speculate as to why cells with long-term repopulating potential would move from the AGM to the yolk sac?

DZIERZAK: In the avian system one finds movement of cells from the interbody region out to the yolk sac in the grafting experiments, so there is a precedent for it. Just by analogy I would think this probably does happen in the mouse, but we need to have direct evidence for these things. One really needs to *in situ* dye-mark those cells and see whether they actually go out. We would like to do these experiments. Time will tell.

S.J. SHARKIS (*Johns Hopkins Oncology Center*): If you take day 11 embryos and then put them in culture for only 1 day, so that it is at least equivalent in terms of time to your 10-day embryos that are in culture for two days, do you see an equivalent increase in progenitors that you would see otherwise?

DZIERZAK: We are trying to do some more quantitative experiments, and it requires a lot of competitive repopulation or limiting dilution transplantation analysis.

It is going to be difficult to be absolutely sure about how the *in vivo* data compare with this *in vitro* situation, because in the *in vitro* situation the cells do not move out. They can be generated there but not move out. So we have an accumulation of these cells, whereas in the embryo itself the cells are rapidly moving out as soon as they are produced to other places. So it is going to be very hard to be absolutely sure about how the cells are growing and their numbers in the culture versus *in vivo*.

SHARKIS: But *in vivo* you are actually seeing an increase at day 11 above day 10 *in vivo*.

DZIERZAK: Yes.

SHARKIS: So one would think that you could actually tell quantatively.

DZIERZAK: Yes, I think the production of these cells increases at day 11 in the AGM region, but we have to really measure that carefully.

T. PAPAYANNOPOULOU (*University of Washington*): In your reaggregation experiments, in which you mixed bone marrow cells with the AGM, you elected to use only the CD31$^+$/Ly-6$^+$/kit$^+$ cells. Why?

DZIERZAK: At Erasmus University the post doc M. de Bruijn has previously done sorting experiments for stem cells with Rob Ploemacher. They have developed these ERMP12/20 antibodies that they have used for many such sorting experiments. This was just the easiest way to get at an enriched population, because we did not want to use the whole bone marrow. There are too many cells, and the frequency of the stem cells is too limited. We wanted some fractionation procedure, so we just used the one that was close at hand.

G.J. SPANGRUDE (*University of Utah Medical Center*): One hypothesis that might explain the difference between your transplants into adult recipients compared to the transplants into perinatal or embryonic recipients is that you are actually following the emergence of what I am considering to be the "bank account" of stem cells that corresponds to the back-up source of reconstituting cells. So during the early course of embryogenesis, most of these cells are in an expanding phase, because they need to generate the hematopoietic system. But then you could say that around day 10 some of them start to go into a more quiescent compartment that eventually leads to the build-up of the back-up compartment. Along those lines I am wondering if you have looked at cell cycle analysis. Can you tell us whether these cells when you isolate them are actively cycling cells and if this correlates, as we see in adults, with engraftment by noncycling cells?

DZIERZAK: We are trying to look at this right now. It is very difficult for us to do it for numerous technical reasons. For the first look (and this is really preliminary, but you would expect this from embryonic cells), they are all cycling. But that is very preliminary, and we have to do a lot of engrafting experiments to be sure.

SPANGRUDE: So it does not really bother me if they are all cycling. Maybe the difference is time spent in G1 between cycles, and this is what allows these cells to engraft.

DZIERZAK: Yes, we do not know. We have to look very carefully at this question; it is very important.

D. METCALF (*P.O. Royal Melbourne Hospital*): There is a lot to be said for "seeing is believing." If one cultures a whole embryo with an intact yolk sac, it develops a heart that beats and that is pumping around blood cells. If one cultures the embryo alone, it develops a heart that pumps around cell free fluid. So I would like to know, in this sort of experiment what has happened to the function of the AGM, because the latter animal totally lacks hematopoietic cells? In relation to your organ culture experiments, can you be sure that the organ tissue survival and proliferation is equivalent in each case? I noticed, for example, that your liver cultures did not develop any repopulating cells. This is slightly odd, and liver is a difficult tissue to culture en masse. I think your chimeric organ cultures will approach this. I hope you use a combination of marked cells so that you can see whether with improved culture conditions, the yolk sac can generate repopulating cells.

DZIERZAK: Yes, we are using marked cells and, in combination in these chimeric organ cultures, we would like to use AGM region cells from knock-out embryos. We are testing to see whether they are deficient, say, in hematopoitic stem cells or stromal cells or whatever. The culture conditions for the liver certainly are not optimal. We would like to make them optimal. Late day-11 liver does give us hematopoietic stem cell activity.

As for the yolk sac culture experiment, we want to revisit that experiment, the one that you did long ago. It is a very provocative experiment and an interesting one. Yes, perhaps one needs a yolk sac not only very rapidly to produce red cells to oxygenate the tissues, but perhaps to help the heart in some form of development or setting up the liver to be accepting later-stage, developmentally more mature hematopoietic cells. I am curious whether the AGM region in such an animal is going to be functional with or without the AGM region. We would like now to do whole embryo cultures, and we are trying to establish that in the laboratory. It is a very good and interesting way to go about some of studies, and it may in fact give us many more answers than the individual organ explant culture will.

Asymmetric Cell Divisions in Hematopoietic Stem Cells

TIM H. BRÜMMENDORF,[a] WIESLAWA DRAGOWSKA,[a]
AND PETER M. LANSDORP[a,b,c]

[a]Terry Fox Laboratory, British Columbia Cancer Research Centre, Vancouver, British
Columbia V5Z 1L3, Canada
[b]Department of Medicine, University of British Columbia, Vancouver, British Columbia
V6T 2B5, Canada

ABSTRACT: In order to study cell kinetics involved in long-term hematopoiesis, we studied single sorted candidate hematopoietic stem cells (HSC) from fetal liver cultured in the presence of a mixture of stimulatory cytokines. After
8–10 days in culture, the number of cells varied from less than a hundred to
more than ten thousand cells. Single cells in slowly growing colonies were recloned upon reaching a 100–200-cell stage. Strikingly, the number of cells in
subclones varied widely again. These results are indicative of asymmetric divisions in primitive hematopoietic cells in which the proliferative potential and
cell cycle properties are unevenly distributed among daughter cells. The continuous generation of heterogeneity in cell cycle properties among the clonal
progeny of HSC appears a relevant mechanism to maintain long-term maintenance of hematopoiesis *in vitro* and *in vivo*.

INTRODUCTION

Blood formation originates in a small population of hematopoietic stem cells
(HSC) that have been defined as pluripotent cells with self-renewal capacity.[1,2] The
mechanisms underlying the proliferation and differentiation of HSC are incomplete-
ly understood.[3,4] Both extrinsic (e.g., growth factors and cell-matrix interactions)
and intrinsic factors (e.g., developmentally controlled transcription factors) are involved in the regulation of HSC. While hematopoietic growth factors and an adequate microenvironment are crucial for the survival and proliferation of HSC, self-
renewal/differentiation decisions in HSC seem to be determined intrinsically and
largely independent of cytokines.[4–8]

Studies aimed at dissecting the molecular mechanism involved in stem cell regulation have been hampered by difficulties in obtaining populations of HSC devoid of
more differentiated progenitor cells. Thus, despite intense efforts to establish deter-
minants by which primitive HSC can be defined prospectively, available *in vivo* and
in vitro stem cell assays only allow retrospective identification of HSC (reviewed in
Ref. 9). One prominent example of such an assay is the long-term culture initiating
cell (LTC-IC) assay.[10] LTC-IC are hematopoietic cells that are capable of generating

[c]Correspondence to: Dr. Peter Lansdorp, Terry Fox Laboratory, BC Cancer Research Centre,
601 West 10th Avenue, Vancouver, BC V5Z 1L3, Canada. Phone, 604/877-6070, Ext. 3026; fax,
604/877-0712; e-mail, peter@terryfox.ubc.ca

myeloid colony-forming cells after at least five weeks of culture in the presence of irradiated feeder cells. LTC-IC are highly enriched among cells with a CD34$^+$CD38$^-$ phenotype, and the yield of LTC-IC in such cells from adult human marrow and umbilical cord blood is around 20%[11] and 50%,[12] respectively. Based on these considerations, human CD34$^+$CD38$^-$cells are expected to be highly enriched for HSC. However, the frequency of CD34$^+$CD38$^-$cord blood cells capable of initiating hematopoiesis in immune deficient mice is only 0.1%.[13-15] In order to study the functional heterogeneity of CD34$^+$CD38$^-$candidate HSC, we followed the fate of single sorted fetal liver CD34$^+$CD38$^-$cells in cytokine-supplemented cultures. By combining observations on *in vitro* growth with a detailed characterization of individual cells produced in culture, we observed that functional heterogeneity is continuously generated among the clonal progeny of HSC. Details of this study are published elsewhere.[16]

MATERIALS AND METHODS

Purification of Fetal Liver Stem Cell Candidates (FL-SCC)

Cells with CD34$^+$CD38$^-$CD71$^-$CD45RA$^-$ phenotype were isolated from previously frozen samples of fetal liver obtained from elective, therapeutic abortions in the 10–16th week of gestation as described previously.[6,17] Populations of cells or single cells were sorted by flow cytometry and either collected in serum-free medium or individually sorted directly into round-bottom tissue culture plates (Nunc, Roskilde, Denmark) containing serum-free medium supplemented with hematopoietic growth factors (as indicated below) using an automatic cell deposition unit (Becton-Dickinson).

Culture of Cells

Single-cell Cultures

Single cells were sorted in 96-well round bottom plates (60 cells/plate) with each well containing 100 µl serum-free medium[17] containing steel factor (SF) or stem cell factor (SCF), Flt-3 ligand (each 100 ng/ml), interleukin-3 (IL-3), interleukin-6 (IL-6) and granulocyte colony-stimulating factor (G-CSF) (each 20 ng/ml). After 5–7 days of culture, another 100 µl growth factor-containing medium was added. After 6–9 days, the number of cells per well varied over a wide range from wells with more than ten thousand cells to wells with less than a hundred cells. Slowly growing colonies with 100–250 cells after 8–13 days in culture were recloned, and the number and morphology (shape, size and refractive index) of cells in each subclone were scored at various time intervals. Slowly growing colonies were recloned again at day 8–19. Such recloning of subclones was repeated until the sixth generation.

Expansion Culture

For the evaluation of the proliferative potential, slowly growing colonies that had reached a level of 5×10^4 cells were transferred in 1-ml cultures of 24-well plates. CD34$^+$CD38$^-$ cells were resorted every 5–10 days as described above if cultures be-

TABLE 1. Production of CD34$^+$CD38$^-$ cells by single cells in serum-free medium (SFM) supplemented with SF, Flt-3, Il-3, Il-6 and G-CSF

Category	Production of CD34$^+$CD38$^-$ Cells Up to Day	# of Clones ($n = 121$)	Proportion (%)	Maximum CD34$^+$CD38$^-$ Expansion[a]	Average Cell-cycle Time (in hours) Up to Day 9[b]
A	16	73	60	4.4 ± 10^3	20.8 ± 0.2
B	59	29	24	6.6 ± 10^7	24.8 ± 0.1
C	129	19	16	2.7 ± 10^{12}	32.0 ± 0.1

[a]Obtained by repeated sorting and reculture of CD34$^+$CD38$^-$ cells in 1-ml cultures until no more CD34$^+$CD38$^-$ cells were produced.

[b]Obtained by dividing the culture period in hours by the $\log_2$ of the estimated number of cells (n) at day 9.

came confluent ($>10^6$ cells/well) to initiate subcultures until the percentage of CD34$^+$CD38$^-$ cells per well dropped below 0.1% of viable cells.

RESULTS

Characterization of Primary Cultures Derived from Single CD34$^+$CD38$^-$ Fetal LiverCells

Single CD34$^+$CD38$^-$ FL-SCC were sorted in individual wells of microtiter plates containing serum-free medium supplemented with cytokines (see Methods section). The plating efficiency (number of wells containing visible single cells after sorting) was >90%, of which more than 80% appeared viable after 24 hr. After 6–9 days, the number of cells in the cultures varied over a wide range, indicating extensive heterogeneity among fetal liver CD34$^+$CD38$^-$ cells. Rapidly growing clones of more than a thousand cells as well as slowly growing clones of less than fifty cells were observed. All wells with growing cells ($n = 121$) were transferred to 1-ml cultures after 5×10^4 or more cells were present between 10 and 21 days of culture. Cells with a CD34$^+$CD38$^-$ phenotype were resorted from expanded 1-ml cultures when these cultures became confluent (0.5–2.0×10^6 cells) and used for continuation of cultures using identical culture conditions. This procedure was repeated until no more CD34$^+$ cells were produced. Three different categories (A–C) based on the ability to produce CD34$^+$CD38$^-$ cells in culture were defined. Clones producing CD34$^+$CD38$^-$ cells up to day 16 were named category A, whereas colonies producing CD34$^+$CD38$^-$ cells for up to day 59 or more were named category B and C, respectively.

Retrospective analysis revealed that colonies that gave rise to the highest number of CD34$^+$CD38$^-$ cells for the longest time period corresponded to primary clones with slow growth properties in the first 9 days of culture (TABLE 1). This fraction represented 16% of the clones analyzed, whereas the majority of clones (60%) were fast growing ($>10^3$ cells at day 9) with a relatively low expansion potential, indicative of functional heterogeneity within the CD34$^+$CD38$^-$ cell compartment of human fetal liver. The overall CD34$^+$CD38$^-$ expansion potential per clone varied over a wide range from 1.43×10^4 to 2.7×10^{12} with an average expansion of 8.65×10^8 CD34+CD38- cells in the 121 clones that were analyzed. The maximum continued production of CD34+CD38- cells was 129 days. Strikingly, a single clone produced 2.7×10^{12} CD34+CD38- cells over 106 days in culture (corresponding to at least 41 "self- renewal" population doublings).

Heterogeneity in Subclones Derived from Slowly Growing CD34+CD38- Fetal Liver Clones

To further analyze the functional heterogeneity within the most primitive, slowly growing CD34+CD38- fetal liver cells, we recloned cells recovered from slowly growing (category C) colonies at day 8–19, when cell numbers had reached between 100 and 250 cells. Individual subclones were analyzed with respect to cell number and morphology at different time intervals and, in some cases, also analyzed for total CD34+CD38- cell production as described above for primary clones. Surprisingly, the clonal heterogeneity observed in the primary single sorted CD34+CD38- fetal liver cells was preserved in the progeny of a single cell. This is shown for five consecutive generations of subclones of a single slowly growing colony of CD34+CD38- cells in FIGURE 1. Furthermore, as shown in FIGURE 2, the distribution

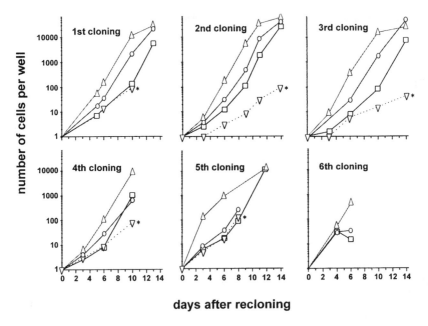

days after recloning

FIGURE 1. Clonal heterogeneity of subclones is preserved through at least five consecutive generations of recloning of slowly growing clones derived from single sorted CD34+CD38- fetal liver cells. The average number of cells in multiple clones of category A, B and C (see text) is plotted. A single "category C" clone (*dotted line and* *) was recloned when 100–200 cells were present and this was repeated for subsequent category C subclones that were produced from a single initial clone.

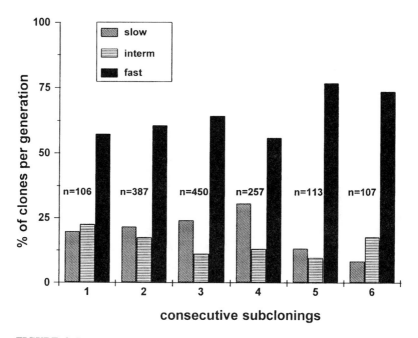

FIGURE 2. Percentage of slowly, intermediate and fast growing clones in the progeny of single sorted CD34⁺CD38⁻ fetal liver cells shown in FIGURE 1. (n = number of clones/generation; pooled data from 2 experiments).

pattern of the three categories remained more or less constant through multiple generations of recloning, with fast growing clones representing the majority. Slowly growing clones, which did not show morphological features of terminal (macrophage) differentiation, represented 20% of primary clones, rose to 20–30% of second to fourth generation subclones, and decreased to <10% at the sixth generation (FIG. 2). These result indicate that the number of CD34⁺CD38⁻ cells with extensive replating potential in slowly growing clones decreases upon multiple rounds of recloning.

DISCUSSION

The data presented in this paper provide novel information regarding three major aspects of stem cell biology. First, the data show that CD34⁺CD38⁻ candidate HSC from fetal liver display extensive functional heterogeneity when cultured as single cells in defined culture conditions. Secondly, this heterogeneity is most readily observed in the slowly growing progeny of single sorted fetal liver cells. Thirdly, cells with the highest overall proliferative potential could be recognized by their slow growth kinetics allowing relatively early (day 6–9) identification of colonies containing cells with a very high proliferative potential.

fetus

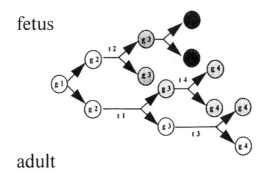

adult

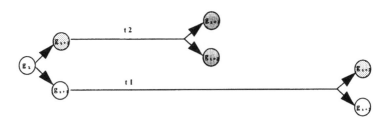

FIGURE 3. The Intrinsic Timetable (IT) model of stem cell biology. In this model, the functional properties of stem cells are 1) linked to the number of preceding cell divisions or generations (g) and 2) unevenly distributed among daughter cells upon each cell division. It is postulated that each stem cell division is asymmetric and results in daughter cells that differ in cell cycle properties. As a result, the time interval between successive generations (t1, t2, etc.) is variable between clones of the same generation, and the interval between divisions is subject to both intrinsic (developmental) and extrinsic (microenvironment and growth factors) control. Clonal variation in the time between cell divisions (t) results in an extreme hierarchy in the stem cell compartment with stem cells that differ in replicative history and related functional properties. Such a functional hierarchy is incompatible with the concept of stem cells as a homogeneous population of cells.

The majority of subclones derived from slowly growing $CD34^+CD38^-$ cells were fast growing clones with a low proliferative potential. However, a minority of subclones showed similar growth kinetics as the parental clone and this heterogeneity was preserved through four to six generations of recloning. Because in all these experiments, culture conditions were kept constant, our findings support the conclusion that differences in the fate of individual stem cells are continuously and intrinsically generated. What could be the mechanisms involved in the heritable functional heterogeneity within the clonal progeny of slowly growing candidate HSC? The simplest hypothesis is that daughter cells are endowed with different cell fates via asymmetric cell divisions (FIG. 3). Such asymmetric cell divisions would result in one daughter cell being similar to the mother cell and the other daughter cell being more committed to terminal differentiation. Alternatively, the observed differences in cell fate could be acquired postmitosis by unknown mechanisms. Data on ontogeny-related changes in the functional properties and telomere length of fetal liver compared to cord blood and adult bone marrow cells[18,19] have led to the speculation that the replicative life span of phenotypically identical HSC may decrease with age and could be limited to less than a hundred cell divisions.[4] Models of stem cell biology need to take asymmetric cell divisions as well as such ontogeny-related functional changes into account. In general, the data shown here provide further evidence that the fate of the most primitive HSC is primarily determined intrinsically and regulated only in a permissive way by extrinsic factors in agreement with previous studies in model systems[8] (reviewed in Ref. 20). The molecular mechanism(s) underlying the asymmetric divisions of HSC documented here appear to be a fruitful area for further studies.

ACKNOWLEDGMENTS

This work was supported by NIH grant AI29524 and by a grant from the National Cancer Institute of Canada with funds from the Terry Fox Run as well as a grant from the Deutsche Forschungsgemeinschaft (THB). The manuscript was typed by Colleen MacKinnon.

REFERENCES

1. TILL, J.E. & E.A. McCULLOCH. 1961. A direct measurement of the radiation sensitivity of normal mouse bone marrow cells. Radiat. Res. **14:** 213–222.
2. METCALF, D. 1977. Hemopoietic Colonies. *In Vitro* Cloning of Normal and Leukemic Cells. Springer-Verlag. Berlin and Heidelberg.
3. MORRISON, S.J., N.M. SHAH & D.J. ANDERSON. 1997. Regulatory mechanisms in stem cell biology. Cell **88:** 287–298.
4. LANSDORP, P.M. 1997. Self-renewal of stem cells. Biol. Blood Marrow Transplant. **3:** 171–178.
5. SUDA, T., J. SUDA & M. OGAWA. 1984. Disparate differentiation in mouse hemopoietic colonies derived from paired progenitors. Proc. Natl. Acad. Sci. USA **81:** 2520–2524.
6. MAYANI, H., W. DRAGOWSKA & P.M. LANSDORP. 1993. Lineage commitment in human hemopoiesis involves asymmetric cell division of multipotent progenitors and does not appear to be influenced by cytokines. J. Cell Physiol. **157:** 579–586.
7. STOFFEL, R., B. LEDERMANN, F.J. DE SAUVAGE & R.C. SKODA. 1997. Evidence for a selective-permissive role of cytokine receptors in hematopoietic cell fate decisions. Blood ed. 90th. **1:** (535)123a.
8. FAIRBAIRN, L.J., G.J. COWLING, B.M. REIPERT & T.M. DEXTER. 1993. Suppression of apoptosis allows differentiation and development of a multipotent hemopoietic cell line in the absence of added growth factors. Cell **74:** 823–832.
9. BOCK, T.A. 1997. Assay systems for hematopoietic stem and progenitor cells. Stem Cells **15:** 185–195.
10. SUTHERLAND, H.J., P.M. LANSDORP, D.H. HENKELMAN, A.C. EAVES & C.J. EAVES. 1990. Functional characterization of individual human hematopoietic stem cells cultured at limiting dilution on supportive marrow stromal layers. Proc. Natl. Acad. Sci. USA **87:** 3584–3588.
11. PETZER, A.L., D.E. HOGGE, P.M. LANSDORP, D.S. REID & C.J. EAVES. 1996. Self-renewal of primitive human hematopoietic cells (long-term-culture-initiating cells) *in vitro* and their expansion in defined medium. Proc. Natl. Acad. Sci. USA **93:** 1470–1474.

12. CONNEALLY, E., J. CASHMAN, A. PETZER & C. EAVES. 1997. Expansion *in vitro* of transplantable human cord blood stem cells demonstrated using a quantitative assay of their lympho-myeloid repopulating activity in nonobese diabetic-*scid/scid* mice. Proc. Natl. Acad. Sci. USA **94:** 9836–9841.
13. EAVES, C., C. MILLER, J. CASHMAN, E. CONNEALLY, A. PETZER, P. ZANDSTRA & A. EAVES. 1997. Hematopoietic stem cells—inferences from *in vivo* assays. Stem Cells **15:** 1–5.
14. BHATIA, M., D. BONNET, U. KAPP, J.C.Y. WANG, B. MURDOCH & J.E. DICK. 1997. Quantitative analysis reveals expansion of human hematopoietic repopulating cells after short-term *ex vivo* culture. J. Exp. Med. **186:** 619–624.
15. LAROCHELLE, A., J. VORMOOR, H. HANENBERG, J.C.Y. WANG, M. BHATIA, T. LAPIDOT, T. MORITZ, B. MURDOCH, X.L. XIAO, I. KATO, D.A. WILLIAMS & J.E. DICK. 1996. Identification of primitive human hematopoietic cells capable of repopulating NOD/SCID mouse bone marrow: implications for gene therapy. Nat. Med. **2:** 1329–1337.
16. BRUMMENDORF, T.H., W. DRAGOWSKA, J.M.J.M. ZIJLMANS, G. THORNBURY & P.M. LANSDORP. 1998. Asymmetric cell divisions sustain long-term hematopoiesis from single sorted human fetal liver cells. J. Exp. Med. **188:** 1117–1124.
17. LANSDORP, P.M. & W. DRAGOWSKA. 1992. Long-term erythropoiesis from constant numbers of CD34+ cells in serum-free cultures initiated with highly purified progenitor cells from human bone marrow. J. Exp. Med. **175:** 1501–1509.
18. LANSDORP, P.M., W. DRAGOWSKA & H. MAYANI. 1993. Ontogeny-related changes in proliferative potential of human hematopoietic cells. J. Exp. Med. **178:** 787–791.
19. VAZIRI, H., W. DRAGOWSKA, R.C. ALLSOPP, T.E. THOMAS, C.B. HARLEY & P.M. LANSDORP. 1994. Evidence for a mitotic clock in human hematopoietic stem cells: loss of telomeric DNA with age. Proc. Natl. Acad. Sci. USA **91:** 9857–9860.
20. CROSS, M.A. & T. ENVER. 1997. The lineage commitment of haemopoietic progenitor cells. Curr. Opin. Genet. Dev. **7:** 609–613.

DISCUSSION

S.T. ILDSTAD (*Allegheny University of Health Sciences*): Those are really nice studies. Have you examined which subpopulation of your asymetrically dividing cells has the most potent engraftmenmt potential for durable engraftment?

LANSDORP: No, we have not looked at *in vivo* engrafting potential. I would be surprised if there was any, because we have seen (as others have) that cells in culture in this particular serum-free medium with added cytokines in the absence of stromal cells very rapidly lose their grafting potential. These experiments document asymmetric cell divisions but may not be representative of what repopulating stem cells will do.

P. J. QUESENBERRY (*University of Massachusetts Medical Center*): On the recloning, you are sorting 200 cells. How difficult is that technically? We encounter difficulty when given 200 cells for single cell sorts.

LANSDORP: In reality, it is not that difficult. You have to set up the sorter to accept cells with other cell types and get the deposition units ready to go. Basically, you recover about 100 cells from the 200 that you counted visually in the wells. So it certainly is technically feasible.

B. TOROK-STORB (*Fred Hutchinson Cancer Research Center*): When you said that you had evidence that oogenesis required 25 divisions per generation and spermatogenesis 62, and that you could see the consequences of that in subsequent generations, is that because you looked at the karyotypes and you saw a complement of chromosomes with telomeres that were very short and a complement that were not so short?

LANSDORP: No, the differences in the length between parental telomeres are insufficient to be distinguished by fluorescence *in situ* hybridization (FISH). What I was referring to is that the average telomere length in each subsequent generation of telomerase knockout mice decreases by about 5 kb. Based on the observation that in normal somatic cells in the absence of telomerase there is a loss of about 50–200 bp, we speculated that that will translate into about 25–100 cell divisions between each subsequent generation of telomerase knockout mice.

H. NAKAUCHI (*University of Tsukuba*): Have you tried to see if it is possible to shorten the cell cycle, the type of asymmetry, or change the growth rate by adding cytokines or by any other method?

LANSDORP: Yes. There is some effect of thrombopoietin (TPO) in terms of the time it takes before the first cell division takes place. TPO seems to speed up this process, but it does not obliterate the type of asymmetry we observe.

Searching for Stem Cell Regulatory Molecules

Some General Thoughts and Possible Approaches

IHOR LEMISCHKA[A]

Department of Molecular Biology, Princeton University, Princeton,
New Jersey 08544, USA

ABSTRACT: Hematopoietic development in the mammal can be represented as a numerically expanding hierarchy of cell populations that are progressively restricted in their self-renewal and differentiation abilities. Classical functional studies have now been extended to provide exact physical descriptions of various stages in the hematopoietic hierarchy. In particular, much information is available that defines the properties of the most primitive stem cell compartment. In addition, a number of *in vitro* culture systems suggest the possibility of maintaining and expanding these cells in a defined context. In all developmental systems, unique profiles of expressed genes define distinct differentiation stages. Within these profiles are gene products that play crucial roles in the regulation of cell-fate decisions. Recent progress in hematopoietic biology provides the framework within which to define molecular phenotypes for hematopoietic stem cells and their immediate clonal progeny. Identifying novel gene products expressed predominantly in uncommitted stem cells together with functional loss and gain-of-function approaches should begin to unravel the molecular mechanisms that govern biological phenomena such as self-renewal, commitment, and proliferation in the hematopoietic system.

The mammalian hematopoietic system exists as a hierarchy of cells that collectively represent the sequential readouts of a developmental program. Traditionally, the elaboration of the hematopoietic hierarchy has been viewed as a unidirectional process involving: 1) progressive segregation of subsets of at least eight differentiation potentials, 2) an accompanying loss of self-renewal ability, 3) an increased tendency to reside in a cell cycle-activated state, and 4) ever larger populations of cells defining increasingly more mature hematopoietic cell compartments. Because of these features and because of the continuous nature of hematopoiesis during adult life, the blood system can be viewed as an experimentally attractive paradigm for general processes of mammalian development. The overall features of the hematopoietic hierarchy have emerged when data from a number of experimental approaches have been viewed together. For the most part, these have focused on the two ends of the hierarchy; 1) the most primitive, multipotent, self-renewing and generally quiescent or slowly cycling stem cell population and 2) progenitor cell populations, which may be uni- or multipotent, and which are endowed with limited self-renewal potential and are generally in active cell cycle. The rich tradition of clonal analysis

[a]Phone, 609/258-2838; fax, 609/258-2759; e-mail, ilemischka@molbio.princeton.edu

in hematopoiesis has resulted in a direct or indirect single cell level of resolution of the properties of stem/progenitor cells. Over the years studies originating at the two ends of the hematopoietic hierarchy have converged. Because the stem cell population is ultimately responsible for the formation of all blood cells, the global regulation of the hematopoietic system must have its mechanistic origins in the cellular and molecular regulatory pathways that govern the behavior of the most primitive stem cell. It is therefore crucial to understand the exact molecular circuitry that underlies the decisions to: 1) self-renew or commit to differentiation, 2) enter or exit the cell cycle, 3) home, localize and interact with the appropriate microenvironmental niches, and 4) respond to situations of stress, which may require the skewing of normal homeostatic behavior. It should also be pointed out that these decisions are likely to be interrelated. For example, because commitment events may occur as a function of asymmetric cell division, cell cycle regulation must be considered a fundamental facet of developmental decision-making pathways. Additionally, the basic features of the decisions that a stem cell must make can come in different flavors. For example, they can be stochastic or deterministic (or a combination of both). They can also be cell-autonomous or influenced by an instructive environment or other signals. In various hematopoietic and nonhematopoietic stem cell systems, one can encounter examples of all these.[1–4]

The only rigorous assay for the most primitive murine stem cell population has been *in vivo* transplantation into ablated hosts. A stem cell is defined as a long-term reconstituting activity (LTRA) that gives rise to permanent hematopoiesis in the engrafted host. Various transplantation assays have been devised, including radioprotection and quantitative competitive repopulation.[5] The existence of stem cells, their anatomical location, and estimates of their frequencies were first measured using donor vs. host marker combinations. Random karyotypic markers were used to demonstrate the multipotentiality of the stem cell.[6,7] More recently, studies using retroviral clonal markers have clearly shown that a single stem cell clone is both necessary and sufficient to sustain lifelong hematopoiesis in a recipient mouse.[8,9] These observations underscore the remarkable proliferative ability characteristic of a stem cell. Retransplantation of retrovirally marked marrow from a single primary recipient into numerous secondary mice demonstrated that the same stem cell clone could sustain multiple hematopoietic systems. This provided a minimal estimate for self-renewal capabilities. Sequential analysis of retroviral markers in mature hematopoietic cells also provided insight into stem cell dynamics and suggested that *in vivo* stem cell regulation may be governed at least in part by stochastic mechanisms. It is fair to say that most, if not all, of the biological properties of the hematopoietic stem cell were established prior to any knowledge of its physical properties. The physical characterization of stem cells and the resultant enrichment strategies constituted a major leap forward in hematopoietic studies.[10,11] A biological activity became a cellular entity, and this allowed the first direct approaches towards understanding stem cell regulation. It was shown that all purified stem/progenitor cell populations are still heterogeneous with respect to functional properties.[12,13] One example is the presence of other, more committed *in vitro* clonogenic progenitor cells in cell populations highly enriched for LTRA.[14,15] It is unclear if these *in vivo* and *in vitro* activities represent discrete cell subpopulations, or whether there is a continuum of functional potential. It is also not known if the specific assay systems influence the observed results; that is, if an *in vivo* transplantable cell can be "read out" as a progenitor *in vitro*. More recent studies have suggested that functionally different activities within the primitive population have distinct physical properties.[16–18] Other studies have suggested an inverse correlation between active bone marrow stem cell cycling and primitive, uncommitted developmental potential.[19] Based on these observations, it has been proposed that entry into active cell cycle may be intrinsically linked to stem cell commitment. Fetal liver derived stem cells have a much greater tendency to be actively cycling, and they are at least equal to, if not more potent than, their adult counterparts in transplantation.[20,21] These studies suggest that rapid stem cell cycling can be compatible with retention of primitive *in vivo* activity. Very recent studies suggest that the adult bone marrow stem cell compartment may be cycling at a very slow rate and therefore may not be truly quiescent.[22]

Although *in vivo* transplantation has provided invaluable insights into the properties of stem cells, whole animal studies are not amenable to precise definition of regulatory mechanisms. Novel, defined culture systems will need to be developed to stimulate and maintain cell cycling by purified stem cells and control the decision to self-renew or differentiate. Numerous stromal cell dependent and independent culture systems that facilitate cell cycle entry and proliferation of stem cells have been described. A general property of these systems is that almost invariably, *in vitro* proliferation is accompanied by differentiation.[23–26] Some recent studies have suggested that stem cells can be induced to proliferate *in vitro* without the loss of their uncommitted properties. It has been shown that colonies grown in cytokine-supplemented semisolid medium can retain erythroid, myeloid and B-lymphoid potentials.[27] It has also been possible to maintain LTRA in short-term suspension cultures supplemented with interleukin-6 (IL-6) and IL-11, together with ckit ligand or flk2/flt3 ligand.[28] A very recent report has shown that thrombopoietin (TPO) can support the short-term *in vitro* maintenance of LTRA as a single factor.[29] A most encouraging recent study has shown that LTRA can be detected in colonies grown in cytokine-supplemented semisolid conditions.[30] Our own studies have shown that a cloned stromal cell line can maintain quantitative and qualitative levels of LTRA for long-term *in vitro* periods of at least 4–7 weeks.[31] A precedent for the ability to achieve *in vitro* LTRA expansion or self-renewal also exists.[32,33] These important observations clearly suggest that stem cells can self-renew outside of an intact organism.

In the human stem cell system, where *in vivo* xenograft assays are costly and cumbersome, necessity has served as the mother of invention to yield even more sophisticated *in vitro* assay systems than those developed in the mouse. The long-term culture-initiating cell (LTCIC) assay measures the production of colony-forming progenitor cells from more primitive precursors.[34] These precursors overlap at least to some extent with the most primitive compartment. It has recently been possible to develop means with which to expand these precursors.[35] The extended LTCIC (ELTCIC) system has been suggested to measure even more primitive stem/progenitor cells.[36] It is likely that these will overlap to a large extent with the cells that "read-out" in xenograft transplantation systems.[37–39] Viewed collectively, the mouse and human *ex vivo* studies suggest optimism for the eventual development of defined culture systems supportive of both self-renewal and commitment decisions. These will serve as a crucial foundation for the unraveling of cell signaling and other molecular regulatory mechanisms.

In the simplest terms one can assume that the mechanisms that govern stem cell behavior must be composed of molecules that are expressed in the stem cell itself and/or in its supportive microenvironmental cell type. Such molecules may be expressed in each of these cells independently or as a function of their interaction. Because the biological properties of stem cells and mature blood cells are so distinct, it is reasonable to propose that the properties of stem cells will be governed at least in part by molecules whose expression is unique or preferential to the stem cell. In a sense, therefore, the unique biological phenotype of stem cells could be linked to a unique profile of expressed molecules. At least some of these molecules could be expected to play key roles in stem cell regulation. Very similar arguments can be made in comparisons of supportive and nonsupportive microenvironmental cell types. The overall challenge is to: 1) identify the gene expression profiles that uniquely or preferentially define the stem cell and its microenvironment, 2) devise rational ways to analyze the sequences of these genes and thus ascribe the predicted functions of their products, and 3) choose a limited number of genes with which to begin a full-scale functional analysis.

Before considering exact strategies to meet these challenges, it is worth summarizing previous and ongoing efforts to elucidate stem cell regulatory pathways. In general all of these are in their infancy, and most are based on the analysis of gene products identified in more mature cells or in situations leading to leukemic transformation. Additionally, many studies have extrapolated results obtained in transformed or factor-dependent cell lines to normal stem/progenitor cell populations. A particularly fruitful approach has been the use of gene targeting to analyze transcription factors and to demonstrate cell-intrinsic, global or cell type-specific roles in hematopoietic development.[40] Cell lineage-specific effects observed by gene targeting may reflect roles in a commitment process to "set up" a program of differentiation or in the completion of the program itself. This is a frequently encountered ambiguity, because in general the assays rely on the analysis of mature cell populations. In essence it is nearly impossible to directly measure effects on a committed "state" without simultaneously measuring effects in subsequent differentiation. Good examples of nonglobal lineage-specific regulatory roles are PU.1 and Ikaros.[41,42] Global regulatory effects revealed by gene targeting may be required for the actual specification of stem cells from mesodermal precursors, for their survival or for their self-renewal. Examples of such global regulatory transcription molecules are AML1 (CBF2), SCL (tal-1) and GATA-2.[40,43–46] Because it is experimentally difficult to define the developmental origin, survival, self-renewal and expansion of stem cells as separate processes, it is likewise difficult to ascribe the precise and earliest locus at which these factors act. Indeed, it appears likely that many such distinctions may be, at least in part, semantics. Global regulators such as AML1 (CBF2) or SCL (tal-1) may be necessary for the actual specification of stem cells during development. The exact origin of the stem cells responsible for definitive adult hematopoiesis is still controversial.[47,48] Therefore, the observed embryonic effects of mutations in such regulatory molecules can only be mechanistically extrapolated to general stem cell behaviors such as self-renewal with great caution. Other, gain-of-function experiments have suggested that the enforced expression of HOXB4 can expand the numbers of primitive stem/progenitor cells without abrogating their abilities to differentiate.[49] One interpretation of these data is that HOXB4 (and possibly other homeobox proteins) plays a role in regulating a quantitative balance between self-renewal and commitment decisions. It is of interest that AML1 (CBF2), SCL (tal-1) and HOXA9 have been implicated in leukemic transformation.[50] Other studies, also in transformed hematopoietic cell lines, have been informative; particularly by shedding light on processes such as lineage "programming." [51–54] Moreover, the constitutive expression of a dominant-negative mutant of retinoic acid receptor-alpha (RAR-α) in murine bone marrow stem/progenitor cells yields permanently growing ckit ligand-dependent cell lines that retain myeloid, erythroid, and B-lymphoid differentiation capacities.[55] These gain-of-function observations are intriguing; however, it remains to be determined if they reflect on actual regulatory pathways.

A most interesting set of observations initially made in an immortalized cell line suggest that the "ground state" of an uncommitted stem cell may be characterized by the low-level expression of many transcripts normally associated with individual mature cell lineages.[56] This has been extended to primary stem/progenitor cells and suggests that commitment processes may be based on choosing, reinforcing and amplifying a subset of the overall gene expression profile that preexists in an uncommitted cell. Such a model does not explain how these events would occur; however, it represents a novel viewpoint of a process normally considered to be based on the de novo "turning on" of gene expression programs. The existence of subtly fluctuating, baseline levels of gene expression in uncommitted stem cells also fits well with stochastic models of stem cell behavior.[2] An a priori prediction of such models is that stem cells "teeter on the edge" and, as a population, exist in a range of probabilistic "states." An intellectual challenge has always been to put such "states" on a firm molecular footing. In this regard, it is easily imaginable how one cell division could shift the balance of "titratable" regulatory molecules above or below the threshold levels required to initiate a cascade of subsequent events. Two somewhat sobering thoughts follow from the above observations: 1) A background of genes normally expressed in mature blood cells may exist in stem/progenitor cells, thus complicating efforts to identify unique gene expression profiles, and 2) If the key regulatory molecules responsible for self-renewal vs. commitment and other stem cell decisions exist in titratable amounts, then they will be difficult to identify. In spite of these complications it is possible to use such "ground state" models as a valuable framework to explain the suggested "balance-shifting" affects of HOXB4 and other molecules as phenoma mediated by quantitative up- or downregulation of key regulatory molecule levels.

All the above discussion is focused on transcriptional regulation. Two examples of other types of molecules that may be implicated in stem cell regulation are TPO and its receptor mpl as well as stromal derived factor-1 (SDF-1) and its receptor CXCR4. Gene targeting of either TPO or mpl reveals defects that extend to the level of primitive stem/progenitor cells.[58,59] The mpl receptor has been shown to be expressed on transplantable bone marrow stem cells, and mpl deficient mutant stem cells suffer a defect in competitive repopulation abilities.[60] In addition, as mentioned previously, TPO appears to be sufficient for the short-term *in vitro* maintenance of LTRA. Taken together these observations suggest an *in vivo* role for TPO as an extrinsic regulator of stem cell processes. The exact mechanism(s) of such regulation are still unclear. The SDF-1 and CXCR4 molecules appear to be required for bone marrow hematopoiesis as shown by gene targeting studies.[61,62] In these cases it has been suggested that this ligand and receptor combination may play a role in stem cell chemotaxis and homing to the bone marrow environment. It will be of interest to address the exact role of these molecules in the most primitive stem/progenitor cell compartment.

A common feature for all of the above suggested regulators of stem cell behavior is their prior identification in other systems. Therefore, the elucidation of their roles in stem cell biology can be viewed as somewhat fortuitous. It is very unlikely that most or all crucial stem cell regulatory molecules will be identified in this manner. An unbiased and comprehensive strategy to identify regulatory pathways can be based on saturation mutagenesis screens in genetically manipulable organisms. Such an approach has been very fruitful in identifying hematopoietically important genetic loci in the zebrafish.[63] At least some of these genes have been shown to act at the level of very primitive cells.[64] In a mammal this type of strategy is not feasible; however, it has been argued that a properly designed gene expression screen is, in many ways, formally equivalent.[65]

Several laboratories including our own have initiated attempts to identify novel molecules directly in purified stem cells.[66,67] Currently, the criteria employed to identify these molecules include predicted sequence homologies to known regulatory protein families as well as expression patterns. Using such criteria we have identified novel protein tyrosine kinases and phosphatases expressed in murine hematopoietic stem cells.[68–71] We have also initiated a global effort to identify molecules specifically expressed in stem/progenitor cells. Two issues arise in considering such an effort. The first is which stages or cell populations of the hematopoietic hierarchy are most suitable for gene expression comparisons. The basic properties of stem cells are likely to be similar regardless of fetal or adult origin. Moreover, these properties are likely to be similar in both mouse and human stem cell populations. As pointed out above, all purified stem cell populations are heterogeneous. Taken together, these observations suggest that the best approach may be to pursue parallel gene expression comparisons in several sources of stem cells obtained from both mouse and human. The gene products that are truly important for stem cell regulation should have similar expression patterns. The second issue is more technical; specifically, which exact molecular methodology is most feasible and reliable in gene expression comparisons?

To begin our studies we chose to use highly purified (AA4.1$^+$Lin$^{-/lo}$Sca$^+$c-kit$^+$) fetal liver cells that are 1,000–2,000-fold enriched for LTRA measured by competitive repopulation (Ly5.1/Ly5.2 congenic system).[20] Other primitive members of the stem/progenitor cell hierarchy are also present in this population. These include: 1) long-term culture-initiating cells (LTCIC),[34] 2) colony-forming unit (CFU)-blast progenitors,[2] 3) high proliferative potential colony-forming cell (HPP-CFC) progenitors,[72] and 4) stromal-dependent B-lymphoid progenitors.[73] The AA4.1$^+$Lin$^{-/lo}$Sca$^+$c-kit$^+$ subset is largely devoid of LTRA but contains significant numbers of *in vitro* progenitors. In contrast, the AA4.1– subset contains no stem/progenitor cell activity.[9] In order to generate progenitor populations at the expense of LTRA, short-term cultures of stem cells in differentiation-promoting cytokines (interleukin-3 (IL-3), IL-6, and c-kit ligand) were employed.[74] *In vivo* and *in vitro* assays confirmed a complete loss of LTRA and a significant retention of progenitor cells. In collaborative studies with Dr. G. Spangrude (University of Utah), Dr. Craig Jordan (University of Kentucky), and Dr. Clay Smith (Duke University) we have obtained biologically similar purified cell populations from murine adult bone marrow, human bone marrow, and human umbilical cord blood, respectively. In summary, we have several defined cell populations, which represent the beginning, the middle and the end points of the murine and human fetal and adult hematopoietic hierarchies.

There are many ways to compare profiles of expressed genes in defined cell populations. Exhaustive sequencing of representative cDNA collections obtained from stem cell and more mature cell sources followed by "electronic subtraction" would be the most direct approach. In an average cell there are 10–20,000 expressed genes. This number together with a statistical calculation suggest that approximately 50,000 sequences are required from a homogeneous cell population in order to insure a reliably complete representation. Clearly such an effort is beyond the economic (and other) means of an academic laboratory. Stem cell enrichment values can only be calculated in relation to an unenriched standard and cannot be converted into an absolute stem cell number. As discussed above, even the most highly purified stem cell population is functionally heterogeneous, and cell populations with the same cell surface phenotypes can differ in biological activity.[75] The unique properties of stem cells also suggest caution when extrapolating from expressed gene numbers estimated for other cells. Of particular relevance are the studies mentioned previously that suggest the low-level presence of mature blood cell gene products in uncommitted stem cells. Given all of these issues, it is not at present possible to reliably predict the extent of sequencing necessary to ensure complete coverage of gene expression in stem cells. Normalization procedures that "equalize" mRNA abundance classes are not appropriate, because they could obscure potentially important quantitative differences in levels of gene expression.[76] Additionally, a high-throughput sequencing effort is not applicable to numerous cell populations. As discussed above, a gene expression comparison among numerous sources of stem cell is likely to be invaluable. For these reasons, all of our studies begin with cDNA populations that are highly enriched in differentially expressed sequences. We have successfully employed three different gene expression comparison strategies: differential display (DD),[77] representational difference analysis (RDA),[78] and standard subtractive hybridization.[79] The latter underlies our whole approach. A key feature is that our differentially expressed cDNAs have a high probability of being full length, facilitating a rapid transition to functional studies. The DD and RDA approaches have certain advantages; however, both only yield fragments of gene products.

A series of high-quality, representative and directional cDNA libraries have been constructed from purified fetal liver stem cells. As a first approach, enough ($1–2 \times 10^6$) AA4.1$^+$Lin$^{-/lo}$Sca$^+$ c-kit$^+$ cells were purified to allow construction of a non-polymerase chain reaction (PCR)-based library using standard techniques. A second library was constructed using a new PCR-based technology called cap-finder (Clontech), designed to yield full-length cDNA copies. An aliquot of mRNA corresponding to approximately 20,000 cell equivalents was used for the synthesis of cDNA. For both libraries, the numbers of independent recombinants are on the order of several million. The quality of the libraries was verified by the detection of full-length cDNA copies corresponding to a number of known mRNAs. The average insert sizes are between one and two kilobase pairs. Further quality estimates are based on sequence analyses that suggest a high proportion of full-length cDNA clones.

Other fetal libraries constructed in similar ways include two libraries from AA4.1$^-$ cells, and two libraries from AA4.1$^+$Lin$^{-/lo}$Sca$^-$c-kit$^+$ cells. Finally, a library was constructed from AA4.1$^+$Lin$^{-/lo}$Sca$^+$c-kit$^+$ cells that were differentiated in culture. Using murine bone marrow stem cell enriched and depleted populations as well as human purified subsets, we are constructing very analogous libraries. When all these are completed, we shall have converted various stages of the murine and human hematopoietic hierarchies into large, well-defined panels of expressed genes. This will set the stage for the identification of gene expression profiles specific for different stem/progenitor subpopulations. In essence, it should be possible to obtain a molecular fingerprint for different stages of the hematopoietic hierarchy.

In order to initiate such efforts, we performed subtractive hybridization. Target libraries from AA4.1$^+$Lin$^{-/lo}$Sca$^+$c-kit$^+$ cells were subtracted with an AA4.1$^-$ driver cDNA library. These libraries should be enriched for all gene products expressed in the various stem/progenitor cells but not in terminally differentiated blood cells. Therefore, this panel of genes provides a molecular profile for the entire early portion of the hierarchy. The relative number of clones in a subtracted population is reduced by up to 200-fold. The effectiveness of the subtraction is directly verified by the depletion of "housekeeping" gene products such as ß-actin or glyceraldehyde-3-phosphate dehydrogenase (GAPDH) and by the concomitant enrichment of known, differentially expressed genes, such as flk2/flt3 and CD34. The absolute number of clones that "survive" the subtraction using AA4.1$^-$ driver material is 10–20,000. This does not necessarily imply that there are 10–20,000 differentially expressed genes. It is likely that individual clones are represented more than once. The exact number of unique sequences (complexity) in the subtracted library must still be determined. Two other subtracted libraries, potentially enriched for sequences expressed in the most primitive stem cell but not in clonogenic progenitors, were derived by subtracting the AA4.1$^+$Lin$^{-/lo}$Sca$^+$c-kit$^+$ libraries with material from the AA4.1$^+$Lin$^{-/lo}$Sca–c-kit$^+$ subpopulation.

We have embarked on a high-throughput sequencing effort with three subtracted libraries: two AA4.1$^+$Lin$^{-/lo}$Sca$^+$c-kit$^+$ cell libraries (standard and cap-finder) subtracted extensively with AA4.1– cell material and a standard AA4.1$^+$Lin$^{-/lo}$Sca$^+$c-kit$^+$ library subtracted with AA4.1$^+$Lin$^{-/lo}$Sca$^-$c-kit$^+$ material. To facilitate a rational handling of sequence information and to focus our attention on a small number of clones for functional analysis, we rely on bioinformatic analysis. This is central to our gene expression studies. It represents a major "filtering" device to focus on specific gene products, and it serves to integrate and analyze not only our own various sequence sets (local bioinformatics) but also other available sequence as well as functional databases (global bioinformatics). A good example of the former would be the sequence comparison of genes derived from subtracted fetal and adult stem cell sources or between mouse and human populations. Global bioinformatic analysis provides much information: 1) It can establish if a given nucleotide sequence is identical or closely related to an already identified murine, human, rat (or other mammalian species) gene. 2) Where the homologies are statistically significant but not identical, novel members of gene/protein families can be identified. 3) Conceptual translation of a nucleotide sequence can be used to expand the range of database comparisons. Examples are presented below where homologies to *Drosophila, C. elegans,* and even yeast proteins have been detected. "Virtual links" can thus be drawn between developmental regulation in invertebrates and in hematopoietic stem cells. An example is the Notch/Notch ligand pathway first defined in invertebrates and recently implicated in hematopoietic regulation.[80,81] It is also possible to categorize clones according to involvement in other mammalian stem cell systems such as the intestine. Bioinformatics can also facilitate the recognition of signature peptide motifs for epidermal growth factor (EGF) repeats, immunoglobulin (Ig)-like domains, various transcription factors and many other protein families. 4) Because the databases are annotated, predicted protein sequences can be assigned to cellular processes such as signal transduction pathways or apoptosis. 5) It is feasible to perform virtual expression studies and to construct overlapping expressed sequence tag contigs that can yield virtual full-length cDNAs.

To gain access to more sophisticated bioinformatics, we have established a collaboration with Dr. Christian Overton, the Director of the Bioinformatics Center at the University of Pennsylvania. A key feature of our collaboration is the automation of database searches, information cross-referencing, and annotation. One illustrative example is the potential for automated weekly database queries with our sequence set. New, previously unidentified homologies will be automatically noted and reported. A second example is the potential to query more sophisticated databases such as those based on protein family motifs or on empirically determined native protein structures. A World Wide Web site called Stem Cell Database (SCDB) is being constructed, which integrates sequence, expression and functional data.

To date we have analyzed a considerable number of sequences predominantly from the fetal liver AA4.1$^+$Lin$^{-/lo}$Sca$^+$c-kit$^+$ libraries subtracted with AA4.1$^-$ material. In addition, a similar number of sequences expressed in one stem cell-supportive stromal cell line have been analyzed. It is premature to present these data in detail, because our analyses are not yet sufficiently extensive; however, a number of interesting general points are beginning to emerge. Perhaps the most relevant of these is that the percentages of novel sequences in the subtracted clone population are quite high. This may indicate that focusing our efforts on rare cell populations and using subtraction techniques will uncover numerous molecules that have escaped detection in standard whole tissue gene expression studies. We are also beginning to detect numerous molecules whose predicted amino acid sequences are related to proteins identified in invertebrate organisms. Some of these have important roles in developmental processes such as oogenesis and neurogenesis. Taken together, validity of our overall strategies to search for novel hematopoietic regulatory molecules. The coming years should provide much work as well as much excitement.

ACKNOWLEDGMENTS

This article is not intended to be a comprehensive survey of the literature. I apologize for any omitted primary citations. I would like to thank the members of my laboratory who are involved in the actual experiments. The work was supported by grants from the NIH and ACS.

REFERENCES

1. MORRISON, S., N. UCHIDA & I. WEISSMAN. 1995. The biology of hematopoietic stem cells. Annu. Rev. Cell. Dev. Biol. **11:** 35–71.
2. OGAWA, M. 1993. Differentiation and proliferation of hemopoietic stem cells. Blood **81:** 2844–2853.
3. MORRISON, S.J., N.M. SHAH & D.J. ANDERSON. 1997. Regulatory mechanisms in stem cell biology. Cell **88:** 287–298.
4. LEMISCHKA, I.R. 1992. The haematopoietic stem cell and its clonal progeny: mechanisms regulating the hierarchy of primitive haematopoietic cells. Cancer Surv. **15:** 3–18.
5. HARRISON, D.E., C.T. JORDAN, R.K. ZHONG & C.M. ASTLE. 1993. Primitive hematopoietic stem cells: direct assay of most productive populations by competitive repopulation with simple binomial, correlation and covariance calculations. Exp. Hematol. **21:** 206–219.
6. BOGGS, D.R., S.S. BOGGS, D.F. SAXE, L.A. GRESS & D.R. CANFIELD. 1982. Hematopoietic stem cells with high proliferative potential; assay of their concentration in marrow by the frequency and duration of cure of W/W mice. J. Clin. Invest. **70:** 242–252.
7. ABRAMSON, S., R. MILLER & R. PHILLIPS. 1977. The identification in adult bone marrow of pluripotent and restricted stem cells of the myeloid and lymphoid systems. J. Exp. Med. **145:** 1567–1579.
8. JORDAN, C.T. & I.R. LEMISCHKA. 1990. Clonal and systemic analysis of long-term hematopoiesis in the mouse. Genes Dev. **4:** 220–232.
9. LEMISCHKA, I.R. 1992. What we have learned from retroviral marking of hematopoietic stem cells. Curr. Top. Microbiol. Immunol. **177:** 59–71.
10. BAUMAN, J., P. DE VRIES, B. PRONK & J. VISSER. 1988. Purification of murine hematopoietic stem cells and committed progenitors by fluorescence activated cell sorting using wheat germ agglutin and monoclonal antibodies. Acta Histochem. **36:** 241–253.
11. SPANGRUDE, G.J., S. HEIMFIELD & I.L. WEISSMAN. 1988. Purification and characterization of mouse hematopoietic stem cells. Science **241:** 58.
12. JONES, R., J. WAGNER, P. CELANO, M. ZICHA & S. SHARKIS. 1990. Separation of pluripotent hematopoietic stem cells from spleen colony-forming cells. Nature **347:** 188–189.
13. UCHIDA, N., W.H. FLEMING, E.J. ALPERN & I.L. WEISSMAN. 1993. Heterogeneity of hematopoietic stem cells. Curr. Opin. Immunol. **5:** 177–184.
14. 14.WEILBAECHER, K., I. WEISSMAN, K. BLUME & S. HEIMFELD. 1991. Culture of phenotypically defined hematopoietic stem cells and other progenitors at limiting-dilution on dexter monolayers. Blood **78:** 945–952.
15. TREVISAN, M. & N.N. ISCOVE. 1995. Phenotypic analysis of murine long-term hemopoietic reconstituting cells quantitated competitively *in vivo* and comparison with more advanced colony-forming progeny. J. Exp. Med. **181:** 93–103.
16. MORRISON, S. & I. WEISSMAN. 1994. The long-term repopulating subset of hematopoietic stem cells is deterministic and isolatable by phenotype. Immunity **1:** 661–673.
17. MORRISON, S., A. WANDYCZ, H. HEMMATI & I. WEISSMAN. 1997. Identification of a lineage of multipotent hematopoietic progenitors. Development **124:** 1929–1939.
18. JONES, R., M. COLLECTOR, J. BARBER, M. VALA, M. FACKLER, W. MAY, C. GRIFFIN, A. HAWKINS, B. ZEHNBAUER, J. HILTON, O. COLVIN & S. SHARKIS. 1996. Characterization of mouse lymphohematopoietic stem cells lacking spleen colony-forming activity. Blood **88:** 487–491.
19. FLEMING, W.H., E.J. ALPERN, N. UCHIDA, K. ITKUTA, G.J. SPANGRUDE & I.K. WEISSMAN. 1993. Functional heterogeneity is associated with the cell cycle status of murine hematopoietic stem cells. J. Cell Biol. **122:** 897–902.

20. JORDAN, C.T., C.M. ASTLE, J. ZAWADZKI, K. MACKAREHTSCHIAN, I.R. LEMISCHKA & D.E. HARRISON. 1995. Long-term repopulating abilities of enriched fetal liver stem cells measured by competitive repopulation. Exp. Hematol. **23:** 1011–1015.

21. PAWLIUK, R., C. EAVES & R.K. HUMPHRIES. 1996. Evidence of both ontogeny and transplant does-regulated expansion of hematopoietic stem cells *in vivo*. Blood **88:** 2852–2858.

22. BRADFORD, G., B. WILLIAMS, R. ROSSI & I. BERTONCELLO. 1997. Quiescence, cycling, and turnover in the primitive hematopoietic stem cell compartment. Exper. Hematol. **25:** 445–453.

23. VAN DER SLUIJS, J.P., C. VAN DEN BOS, M.R. BAERT, C.A. VAN BEURDEN & R.E. PLOEMACHER. 1993. Loss of long-term repopulating ability in long-term bone marrow culture. Leukemia : 725–732.

24. TRAYCOFF, C.M., K. CORNETTA, M.C. YODER, A. DAVIDSON & E.F. SROUR. 1996. *Ex vivo* expansion of murine hematopoietic progenitor cells generate classes of expanded cells possessing different levels of bone marrow repopulating potential. Exp. Hematol. **24:** 299–306.

25. PETERS, S.O., E.L.W. KITTLER, H.S. RAMSHAW & P.J. QUESENBERRY. 1995. Murine marrow cells expanded in culture with IL-3, Il-6, IL-11, and SCF acquire an engraftment defect in normal hosts. Exp. Hematol. **23:** 461–469.

26. KNOBEL, K.M., M.A. MCNALLY, A.E. BERSON, D. ROOD, K. CHEN, L. KILINSKI, K. TRAN, T.B. OKARMA & J.S. LEBKOWSKI. 1994. Long-term reconstitution of mice after *ex vivo* expansion of bone marrow cells: differential activity of cultured bone marrow and enriched stem cell populations. Exp. Hematol. **22:** 1227–1235.

27. BALL, T.C., F. HIRAYAMA & M. OGAWA. 1995. Lymphohematopoietic progenitors of normal mice. Blood **85:** 3086.

28. YONEMURA, Y., H. KU, S. LYMAN & M. OGAWA. 1997. *In vitro* expansion of hemato-poietic progenitors and maintenance of stem cells: comparison between Flt3/Flk2 ligand and Kit ligand. Blood **89:** 1915–1921.

29. MATSUNAGA, T., T. KATO, H. MIYAZAKI & M. OGAWA. 1998. Thrombopoietin pro-motes the survival of murine hematopoietic long-term reconstituting cells: compar-ison with the effects of FLT3/FLK-2 ligand and interleukin-6. Blood **92:** 452–461.

30. TREVISAN, M., X.-Q. YAN & N.N. ISCOVE. 1996. Cycle initiation and colony forma-tion in culture by murine marrow cells with long-term reconstituting potential *in vivo*. Blood **88:** 4149–4158.

31. MOORE, K.A., H. EMA & I.R. LEMISCHKA. 1997. *In vitro* maintenance of highly puri-fied, transplantable hematopoietic stem cells. Blood **89:** 4337–4347.

32. FRASER, C.C., C.J. EAVES, S.J. SZILVASSY & R.K. HUMPHRIES. 1990. Expansion *in vitro* of retrovirally marked totipotent hematopoietic stem cells. Blood **76:** 1071.

33. FRASER, C.C., S.J. SZILVASSY, C.J. EAVES & R.K. HUMPHRIES. 1992. Proliferation of totipotent hematopoietic stem cells *in vitro* with retention of long-term competitive *in vivo* reconstituting ability. Proc. Natl. Acad. Sci. USA **89:** 1968–1972.

34. SUTHERLAND, H.S., A.C. EAVES, W. DRAGOWSKA & P. LANSDORP. 1989. Character-ization and partial purification of human marrow cells capable of initiating long-term hematopoiesis *in vitro*. Blood **74:** 1563.

35. PETZER, A.L., D.E. HOGGE, P.M. LANSDORP, D.S. REID & C.J. EAVES. 1996. Self-renewal of primitive human hematopoietic cells (long-term-culture-initiating cells) *in vitro* and their expansion in defined medium. Proc. Natl. Acad. Sci. USA **93:** 1470–1474.

36. HAO, Q.-L., F.T. THIEMANN, D. PETERSEN, E.M. SMOGORZEWSKA & G.M. CROOKS. 1996. Extended long-term culture reveals a highly quiescent and primitive human hematopoietic progenitor population. Blood **88:** 3306–3313.

37. TRAYCOFF, C., R. HOFFMAN, E. ZANJANI, K. CORNETTA, P. LAW, A. GIANNI, M. BREGNI, S. SIENA, M. ABBOUD & J. LAVER. 1994. Measurement of marrow repopulating potential of human hematopoietic progenitor and stem cells using a fetal sheep model. Prog. Clin. Biol. Res. **389:** 281–291.

38. CASHMAN, J., L. WANG, M. DOEDDENS, L. SHULTZ, P. LANSDORP, J. DICK & C. EAVES. 1997. Kinetic evidence of the regeneration of multilineage hematopoiesis from primitive cells in normal bone marrow transplanted into immunodeficient mice. Blood **89:** 4307–4316.

39. BHATIA, M., J. WANG, U. KAPP, D. BONNET & J. DICK. 1997. Purification of primitive human hematopoietic cells capable of repopulating immune-deficient mice. Proc. Natl. Acad. Sci. USA **94:** 5320–5325.

40. SHIVDASANI, R.A. & S.H. ORKIN. 1996. The transcriptional control of hematopoiesis. Blood **87:** 4025–4039.

41. SIMON, M.C. 1998. PU.1 and hematopoiesis: lessons learned from gene targeting experiments. Semin. Immunol. **10:** 111–118.

42. NICHOGIANNOPOULOU, A., M. TREVISAN, C. FRIEDRICH & K. GEORGOPOULOS. 1998. Ikaros in hemopoietic lineage determination and homeostasis. Semin. Immunol. **10:** 119–125.

43. WANG, Q., T. STACY, M. BINDER, M. MARIN-PADILLA, A. SHARPE & N. SPECK. 1996. Disruption of the Cbfa2 gene causes necrosis and hemorrhaging in the central nervous system and blocks definitive hematopoiesis. Proc. Natl. Acad. Sci. USA **93:** 3444–3449.

44. OKUDA, T., J.W. DEURSEN, S.W. HIEBERT, G. GROSVELD & J.R. DOWNING. 1996. AML1, the target of multiple chromosomaltranslocations in human leukemia, is essential for normal fetal liver hematopoiesis. Cell **84:** 321–330.

45. PORCHER, C., W. SWAT, K. ROCKWELL, Y. FUJIWARA, F.W. ALT & S.H. ORKIN. 1996. The T-cell leukemia oncoprotein SCL/tal-1 is essential for development of all hematopoietic lineages. Cell **86:** 47–57.

46. ROBB, L., N. ELWOOD, A. ELEFANTY, F. KONTGEN, R. LI, L. BARNETT & C. BEGLEY. 1996. The scl gene is required for the generation of all hematopoietic lineages in the adult mouse. EMBO J. **15:** 4123–4129.

47. DZIERZAK, E., M. SANCHEZ, A. MULLER, C. MILES, A. HOLMES, H. TIDCOMBE & A. MEDVINSKY. 1997. Hematopoietic stem cells: embryonic beginnings. J. Cell. Physiol. **173:** 216–218.

48. YODER, M., K. HIATT, P. DUTT, P. MUKHERJEE, D. BODINE & D. ORLIC. 1997. Characterization of definitive lymphohematopoietic stem cells in the day nine murine yolk sac. Immunity **7:** 335–344.

49. SAUVAGEAU, G., U. THORSTEINSDOTTIR, C.J. EAVES, H.J. LAWRENCE, C. LARGMAN, P.M. LANSDORP & R.K. HUMPHRIES. 1995. Overexpression of HOXB4 in hematopoietic cells causes the selective expansion of more primitive populations *in vitro* and *in vivo*. Genes Dev. **9:** 1753–1765.

50. LOOK, A.T. 1997. Oncogenic transcription factors in the human acute leukemias. Science **278:** 1059–1064.

51. KULESSA, H., J. FRAMPTON & T. GRAF. 1995. GATA-1 reprograms avian myelomonocytic cells into eosinophils, thromboblasts and erythroblasts. Genes Dev. **9:** 1250–1262.

52. VISVADER, J., A. ELEFANTY, A. STRASSER & J. ADAMS. 1992. GATA-1 but not SCL induces megakaryocytic differentiation in an early myeloid line. EMBO J. **11:** 4557–4564.

53. MULLER, C., E. KOWENZ-LEUTZ, S. GRIESER-ADE, T. GRAF & A. LEUTZ. 1995. NF-M(chicken C/EBPb) induces eosinophilic differentiation and apoptosis in a hematopoietic progenitor cell line. EMBO J. **14:** 6127–6135.

54. FRAMPTON, J., K. MCNAGNY, M. SIEWEKE, A. PHILIP, G. SMITH & T. GRAF. 1995. v-Myb DNA binding is required to block thrombocytic differentiation of Myb-Ets-transformed multipotent haematopoietic progenitors. EMBO J. **14:** 2866–2875.

55. TSAI, S., S. BARTELMEZ, E. SITNICKA & S. COLLINS. 1994. Lymphohematopoietic progenitors immortalized by a retroviral vector harboring a dominant-negative retinoic acid receptor can recapitulate lymphoid, myeloid, and erythroid development. Genes Dev. **8:** 2831–2841.

56. HU, M., D. KRAUSE, M. GREAVES, S. SHARKIS, T. DEXTER, C. HEYWORTH & T. ENVER. 1997. Multilineage gene expression precedes commitment in the hemopoietic system. Genes Dev. **11:** 774–785.

57. ENVER, T. & M. GREAVES. 1998. Loops, lineage, and leukemia. Cell **94:** 9–12.

58. MURONE, M., D.A. CARPENTER & F.J. DE SAUVAGE. 1998. Hematopoietic deficiencies in c-mpl and TPO knockout mice. Stem Cells **16:** 1–6.

59. KIMURA, S., A.W. ROBERTS, D. METCALF & W.S. ALEXANDER. 1998. Hematopoietic stem cell deficiencies in mice lacking c-Mpl, the receptor for thrombopoietin. Proc. Natl. Acad. Sci. USA **95:** 1195–1200.

60. SOLAR, G.P., W.G. KERR, F.C. ZEIGLER, D. HESS, C. DONAHUE, F.J. DESAUVAGE & D.L. EATON. 1998. Role of c-mpl in early hematopoiesis. Blood **92:** 4–10.

61. NAGASAWA, T., S. HIROTA, K. TACHIBANA, N. TAKAKURA, S. NISHIKAWA, Y. KITAMURA, N. YOSHIDA, H. KIKUTANI & T. KISHIMOTO. 1996. Defects of B-cell lymphopoiesis and bone-marrow myelopoiesis in mice lacking the CXC chemokine PBSF/SDF-1. Nature **382:** 635–638.

62. ZOU, Y.R., A.H. KOTTMANN, M. KURODA, I. TANIUCHI & D.R. LITTMAN. 1998. Function of the chemokine receptor CXCR4 in haematopoiesis and in cerebellar development. Nature **393:** 595–599.

63. ORKIN, S.H. & L.I. ZON. 1997. Genetics of erythropoiesis: induced mutations in mice and zebrafish. Annu. Rev. Genet. **31:** 33–60.

64. LIAO, E.C., B.H. PAW, A.C. OATES, S.J. PRATT, J.H. POSTLETHWAIT & L.I. ZON. 1998. SCL/Tal-1 transcription factor acts downstream of cloche to specify hematopoietic and vascular progenitors in zebrafish. Genes Dev. **12:** 621–626.

65. WANG, Z. & D.D. BROWN. 1991. A gene expression screen. Proc. Natl. Acad. Sci. USA **88:** 11505–11509.

66. GRAF, L. & B. TOROK-STORB. 1995. Identification of a novel DNA sequence differentially expressed between normal human CD34+CD38hi and CD34+CD38lo marrow cells. Blood **86:** 548–556.

67. YANG, Y., K.R. PETERSON, G. STAMATOYANNOPOULOS & T. PAPYANNOPOULOU. 1996. Human CD34+ cell EST database: single-pass sequencing of 402 clones from a directional cDNA library. Exp. Hematol. **24:** 605–612.

68. MATTHEWS, W., C.T. JORDAN, G.W. WIEGAND, D. PARDOLL & I.R. LEMISCHKA. 1991. A receptor tyrosine kinase specific to hematopoietic stem and progenitor cell-enriched populations. Cell **65:** 1143–1152.

69. MATTHEWS, W., C.T. JORDAN, M. GAVIN, N.A. JENKINS, N.G. COPELAND & I.R. LEMISCHKA. 1991. A receptor tyrosine kinase cDNA isolated from a population of enriched primitive hematopoietic cells and exhibiting close genetic linkage to c-kit. Proc. Natl. Acad. Sci. USA **88:** 9026–9030.

70. MACKAREHTSCHIAN, K., J.D. HARDIN, K.A. MOORE, S. BOAST, S.P. GOFF & I.R. LEMISCHKA. 1995. Targeted disruption of the flk2/flt3 gene leads to deficiencies in primitive hematopoietic progenitors. Immunity **3:** 147–161.

71. DOSIL, M., N. LEIBMAN & I. LEMISCHKA. 1996. Cloning and characterization of fetal liver phosphatase 1, a nuclear protein tyrosine phosphatase isolated from hematopoietic stem cells. Blood **88:** 4510–4525.

72. LOWRY, P.A., D.M. DEACON, P. WHITEFIELD, S. RAO, M. QUESENBERRY & P.J. QUE-
    SENBERRY. 1995. The high-proliferative-potential megakaryocyte mixed
    (Hpp-Meg-Mix) cell: a trilineage murine hematopoietic progenitor with multiple
    growth factor responsiveness. Exp. Hematol. 23: 1135–1140.
73. WHITLOCK, C.A. & C.E. MÜLLER-SIEBURG. 1990. Long-term B lymphoid cultures
    from murine bone marrow. Methods Mol. Biol. 5: 303–322.
74. YONEMURA, Y., H. KU, F. HIRAYAMA, L.M. SOUZE & M. OGAWA. 1996. Interleukin 3
    or interleukin 1 abrogates the reconstituting ability of hematopoietic stem cells.
    Proc. Natl. Acad. Sci. USA 93: 4040–4044.
75. SPANGRUDE, G.J., D.M. BROOKS & D.B. TUMAS. 1995. Long-term repopulation of
    irradiated mice with limiting numbers of purified hematopoietic stem cells: in vivo
    expansion of stem cell phenotype but not function. Blood 85: 1006–1016.
76. SOARES, M.B., M.D.F. BONALDO, P. JELENE, L. SU, L. LAWTON & A. EFSTRATIADIS.
    1994. Construction and characterization of a normalized cDNA library. Proc. Natl.
    Acad. Sci. USA 91: 9228–9232.
77. Liang, P., L. Averboukh & A.B. Pardee. 1994. Method of differential display. In
    Methods in Molecular Genetics. : 3–16. Academic Press. New York.
78. HUBANK, M. & D.G. SCHATZ. 1994. Identifying differences in mRNA expression by
    representational difference analysis of cDNA. Nucleic Acids Res. 22: 5640–5648.
79. HARRISON, S.M., S.L. DUNWOODIE, R.M. ARKELL, H. LEHRACH & R.S.P. BEDDING-
    TON. 1995. Isolation of novel tissue-specific genes from cDNA libraries represent-
    ing the individual tissue constituents of the gastrulating mouse embryo. Dev. 121:
    2479–2489.
80. ARTAVANIS-TSAKONAS, D., K. MATSUNO & M.E. FORTINI. 1995. Notch signaling.
    Science 268: 225–232.
81. MILNER, L.A., A. BIGAS, R. KOPAN, C. BRASHEM-STEIN, I.D. BERNSTEIN & D.I.K.
    MARTIN. 1996. Inhibition of granulocytic differentiation by mNotch1. Proc. Natl.
    Acad. Sci. USA 93: 13014–13019.

DISCUSSION

D.M. BODINE (*National Human Genome Research Institute/NIH*): I agree with
the need for informatics. We have no informatics concerning stem cell gene expression, but the question is when you get down to doing these complicated Venn diagrams. Here you really are going to run up against the limit of technology. How deep
are your libraries? How will you represent everything in there?

LEMISCHKA: These are difficult questions. If, in fact, the estimates of the complexity of the genome are correct, and there are 80,000–100,000 expressed genes,
then given that we have screened 18,000 of them for expression and can come up
with a number that truly are differentially expressed (and, of course, these are early
days, so we have to confirm a lot of this), then we can extrapulate from these numbers and actually come up with a prediction that, when all is said and done, will be
within a factor of 2 or so of estimating the actual number of gene expression differences between these two cell populations. The real problem comes from the cell populations; that is, in every purification it is impossible to address the absolute degree
of purity. You can only address relative purity. When you take advantage of this, a
fetal stem cell population, no matter how it is purified, would likely have a different
set of contaminating cells than one from purified adult bone marrow. That is where
the power of the Venn diagram approach should be apparent. If you find something,

a subset of things, that are expressed in both fetal and adult purified stem cell populations, then these are likely to be interesting. There are differences between fetal and adult stem cells as well. One must keep in mind that there are going to be interesting gene products that are going to be overlooked.

Stem Cells, Pre-Progenitor Cells and Lineage-Committed Cells: Are Our Dogmas Correct?

D. METCALF[a]

The Walter and Eliza Hall Institute of Medical Research, P.O. Royal Melbourne Hospital, 3050 Victoria, Australia

ABSTRACT: Recent developments warrant careful reexamination of several of the central dogmas of hematopoiesis. The bioassays previously used may have predetermined which subsets of hematopoietic stem cells are regarded as having long-term repopulating activity and thus have produced misleading data. Lineage commitment in multipotential cells has been regarded as an immutable stochastic process but may be a process that can be modified by extrinsic signaling. Finally, loss of self-renewal activity has been regarded as progressive and irreversible but this response to signaling can be blocked by cytokine-inducible modulating proteins.

INTRODUCTION

Certain dogmas regarding hematopoiesis have become entrenched over the past thirty years which all of us pass on to our more junior colleagues or students as established truth. In brief, we describe the hematopoietic population as a three-tiered structure comprised of populations of increasing cell numbers, but with progressively decreasing capacity for self-renewal, proliferation and lineage potential. We describe traffic from one compartment to the next (stem cell → progenitor cell → immature differentiating cells) as being unidirectional and nonreversible for all of these defining parameters. Differentiation commitment is further described as being irreversible in terms of possible switching from one lineage to another. FIGURE 1 summarizes these familiar dogmas.

Without wishing to be gratuitously iconoclastic, questions need to be raised about how certain we are of the individual components of this dogma.

LINEAGE-COMMITTED PROGENITOR CELLS

Relatively few problems have arisen regarding the notion that there are such cells as irreversibly committed progenitor cells and, that their lineage commitment seems unchangeable. Moreover, these cells are numerous enough and have sufficient proliferative capacity to generate the required numbers of mature cells.

---

[a]Phone, +61 3-9345-2555; fax, +61 3-9347-0852.

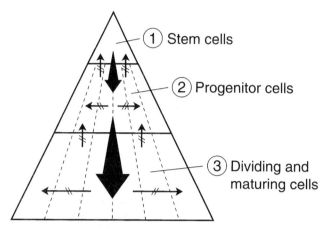

FIGURE 1. The conventional view of hematopoietic subpopulations. Cells in each compartment generate larger numbers of cells in succeeding compartments in a unidirectional process in which lineage-committed cells cannot switch their lineage commitment.

Committed progenitor cells can be enumerated with high detection efficiency as colony-forming cells in semisolid cultures and, when appropriately stimulated, can generate maturing progeny in the colonies they generate.[1,2] Within each lineage, there is a remarkable degree of heterogeneity evident between progenitor cells as indicated by the number of progeny generated or the responsiveness of different clones to proliferative stimulation. Some of this heterogeneity is certainly based on a parent-progeny relationship between different progenitor cells. In other instances, the heterogeneity *may* be based on derivation from differing stem cells with somewhat differing properties in a process of parallel, but independent, lineage development.

The cells of most colonies grown *in vitro* are of a single lineage and the cells do not exhibit aberrant morphological features, such as eosinophil granules in erythroid cells, even when the colonies are grown using a stimulating factor active on cells of multiple lineages. This argues strongly for the irreversibility of lineage-commitment and the consequent maturation events.

Some misinterpretation is possible with multipotential progenitor cells if adequate combinations of stimuli are not used to generate the colonies, in which case some lineages may not develop within particular colonies. Such clonogenic cells can then be misidentified as possibly being unilineage in nature. For example, in cultures of mouse fetal liver cells, stimulation by interleukin-3 (IL-3) can result in megakaryocyte colony development but, if erythropoietin (Epo) is also added, many mixed erythroid/megakaryocyte colonies develop. Has the added erythropoietin "committed" some megakaryocyte precursor cells to an erythroid maturation lineage? Most would not reach this conclusion and would interpret the observations either as the inability of IL-3 alone to stimulate a bipotential progenitor cell or as IL-3 being able only to stimulate the formation of megakaryocyte progeny by such cells, presenting the observer, by default, with what appears to be a unilineage megakaryocyte colony. More work needs to be done on such colony-forming cells, but it seems somewhat improbable that lateral lineage-switching is inducible by using combinations of stimulating factors.

The most compelling data on the reality of irreversible commitment in progenitor cells have come from the insertion of ectopic receptors into such progenitors. For example, when erythropoietin receptors are inserted into macrophage precursors or macrophage colony-stimulating factor (M-CSF) receptors are inserted into erythroid precursors. Under these conditions, erythropoietin will stimulate colony formation, but the colonies are macrophage in composition, not erythroid,[3] and conversely, M-CSF will stimulate erythroid colony formation.[4]

Certain major alterations in lineage maturation are inducible within populations of immature differentiating cells. The best documented example is the transformation of macrophage precursors to dendritic cells by the use of granulocyte/macrophage colony-stimulating factor (GM-CSF) plus tumor necrosis factor-α (TNF-α).[5,6] These are likely not to represent examples of lineage switching so much as phenotype modulation, a process by which immature macrophages can potentially be directed into the formation of mature cells of widely differing phenotypes such as Kupffer cells, alveolar macrophages, dendritic cells or osteoclasts. Such phenotypic modulation is dependent on the type of extrinsic stimulus used and possibly on subtle sublineage differences between cells of the broad macrophage-committed lineage. These phenomena are intriguing but do not constitute serious grounds for questioning this particular dogma of hematopoiesis.

STEM CELLS

Real grounds for concern have arisen in attempting to clarify the considerable confusion regarding the nature and possible heterogeneity of cells identified by surface marker criteria as likely to be members of the stem cell compartment. In the context of the present meeting, these uncertainties have one very practical aspect. Is it possible to define, isolate and amplify by selective *in vitro* culture, cells capable of sustained repopulation of a host with depleted hematopoietic tissue?

Present dogma identifies a small subset of such stem cells as being the genuine ancestral cells of hematopoietic populations and as being the only cells capable of long-term repopulation. A summation of stem cell data from the mouse, that most would be comfortable with, is set out in FIGURE 2. This indicates that three compartments of immature cells are segregatable by surface marker sorting.

The first, defined as $Lin^-Sca-1^+Rh^{lo}$, number 10 per 10^5 marrow cells. One in five of these cells is capable of long-term repopulation, but if the seeding efficiency of this assay is 20%, all such cells might be repopulating cells. This indicates a frequency for repopulating cells of 2 to 10 per 10^5 marrow cells. Other properties of these cells are less securely established. They probably are detected in assays for long-term culture-initiating cells (LTCICs) and cobblestone area-forming cells but do not respond in clonal culture to stimulation by single stimulating factors. With combinations of stimuli, 50% and possibly more can generate colonies. The colonies generated are usually characterized as being multipotential if scored late (2 weeks) and as blast colonies if scored earlier. A few (2%) of these cells can form day-12 spleen colonies but none day-7 colonies. With a seeding factor of 10%, this would have

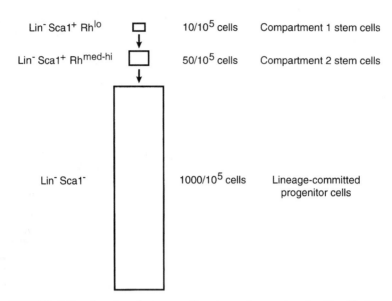

FIGURE 2. Fractionation of marrow cells using surface markers has identified two major subsets of multipotential cells with properties of stem cells and a larger population mainly composed of lineage-committed progenitor cells. The relative sizes of these populations are represented in scale by the areas of the *boxes*. Compartment 1 cells are regarded as the long-term repopulating cells, based on assays in irradiated recipients.

cells in this compartment contributing two day-12 colony-forming cells per 10^5 marrow cells.

Cells in the second compartment are defined as $Lin^-Sca-1^+Rh^{medhi}$ and number 50 per 10^5 bone marrow cells. Such cells have poor, but not zero, repopulating capacity. Presumably again these cells are detectible in LTCICs and cobblestone-forming assays. Ten percent can form day-12 spleen colonies but few day-7 colonies. With a seeding efficiency of 10%, this would indicate that essentially all cells in this compartment can form day-12 colonies, and they would then contribute 50 day-12 colony-forming cells per 10^5 bone marrow cells—the large majority of such cells in the bone marrow. Some colony formation in culture is possible using single stimuli like IL-3, but 50% to possibly 100% are clonogenic when stimulated by combinations of growth factors.

The third and largest compartment of immature cells is defined as Lin^-Sca-1^- and number 1000 per 10^5 bone marrow cells. Presumably this compartment contains the bulk of cells forming day-7 spleen colonies and most lineage-committed progenitor cells.

These data underpin the hematopoietic dogma of progressive population size increase in maturing compartments with concurrent progressive loss in proliferative and lineage potential. Compartments 1 and 2 could both be labeled stem cells with the smaller Compartment 1 being the "gold standard" repopulating stem cells and Compartment 2 a more mature and larger subset of cells, still clearly ancestral to the large Compartment 3 containing lineage-committed progenitor cells. Compartment 1 stem cells are those of likely clinical importance, because the ablated nature of the recipient patient parallels the defining repopulation assay for these cells, which uses irradiated recipient mice.

The model has some untidy features stemming from the limitations of the various assays and from differences between groups in the methodology of the various *in vitro* assays used to characterize the cells in the various compartments. It is still a little unclear what proportion of cells in the various compartments are LTCICs or cobblestone-area-forming cells of various types. Similarly, there is some uncertainty regarding the frequency of blast colony-forming cells in the various compartments and the responsiveness of these cells to growth factor stimulation.

It would be reasonable enough to anticipate that less mature cells would be detectable using assays for more mature cells, but this seems still a matter of dispute. If such detection is possible, the data using assays for more mature cells would not be seriously skewed by contributions from less mature cells because of their smaller numbers. However, some heterogeneity might be expected to result.

There are continuing problems regarding the efficiency of the various assays and/or the need to introduce seeding efficiency factors. Why do only 2% of Compartment 1 stem cells form day-12 spleen colonies? Is this only a question of seeding efficiency, or does it indicate further subset heterogeneity in this compartment? Is there a slight overlap with Compartment 2 stem cells arising from the limitations of cell sorting, or is there a certain variability in membrane marker expression by an otherwise uniform population of cells?

As is the case for committed progenitor cells, there is a danger that the assays used for Compartment 1 and 2 stem cells can lead to an artificial underestimation of the proliferative and lineage potential of the cells detected.

This introduces two key issues in need of resolution concerning stem cells: (a) the validity of the use of irradiated recipients to identify cells with long-term repopulating ability, and (b) the unidirectional movement of cells from stem cell Compartment 1 to Compartment 2.

While the irradiated recipient assay is clinically appropriate because it mimics a chemotherapy-pretreated patient, the assay may make unfair demands on repopulating cells and may fail to detect cells able to initiate long-term hematopoiesis under less demanding conditions of basal hematopoiesis.

The irradiated recipient is a very abnormal animal with major perturbations in regulatory systems and an overwhelming demand for the rapid generation of mature cells. Under these conditions, it is quite feasible that it detects a very special subset of repopulating cells or a repopulating cell that *at the time* expresses appropriate membrane proteins allowing it to function as a repopulating cell. There are alternative repopulation assays not demanding hematopoietic rescue of the animal, and it would not be surprising if Compartment 2 stem cells could then function as effective long-term generators of maturing progeny. This question needs reexamination using fluorescence-activated cell sorter (FACS)-sorted populations of Compartment 1 and 2 stem cells, paying particular attention to the possible ability of Compartment 2 cells, under some circumstances, to generate Compartment 1 cells.

This latter question of the possible plasticity of stem cells in response to differing environmental signals has become of importance from studies on developmental hematopoiesis. For years, a controversy has existed whether yolk sac hematopoiesis[7] and aorta-gonad-mesonephros (AGM) hematopoiesis[8] are independent processes and if so, whether the AGM is the only source of genuine adult-type repopulating cells. Assays using irradiated recipients indicated that yolk sac contains no long-term repopulating cells, and such cells appear merely to give rise to transient primitive hematopoietic cells.[9] However, embryological studies in *Xenopus* have shown that a common precursor population can generate the hematopoietic cells in the regions corresponding to both the mammalian yolk sac and AGM regions with the cells then generating their respective phenotypes.[10] The simple interpretation is that the particular host microenvironments can dictate by inductive stimuli the future behavior and properties of the migrating hematopoietic cells. This is supported by studies on murine embryonic stem cell clones that can generate both primitive and definitive erythropoietic cells, again indicating the existence of bipotential precursor cells.[11] The defect in these otherwise compelling *Xenopus* experiments is the inability so far to exclude the possibility that the original precursor population was in fact already heterogeneous and that the differing properties of the resulting stem cells were based merely on selective survival and proliferation in the recipient sites.

More intriguing is the observation that, while yolk sac cells fail to function as long-term repopulating cells in the standard adult irradiated recipient, they can do so if injected into pretreated neonatal recipients. Furthermore, cells from engrafted neonatal recipients can then repopulate irradiated adult recipients.[12] Is this an example of the assay system dictating the results observed or again merely a case of selective survival of heterogeneous populations of stem cells? Clearly the neonatal recipient represents a qualitatively different assay and one allowing the emergence of cells capable of repopulating conventional irradiated recipients. This system now needs to be used in a rigorous reappraisal of the properties of stem cell subpopulations currently excluded as having repopulating capacity, based on the rigid adult irradiated recipient assay. The ultimate key issue remains the possible plasticity of certain stem cells that appear to have irreversibly lost repopulating capacity in one assay but possibly being able to alter their behavior in another assay system to again exhibit long-term repopulating capacity.

Cells also worthy of reexamination using alternative repopulation assays are those in hematopoietic spleen colonies, either day-7 or day-12. In the earliest work on cells from such spleen colonies, an ability to repopulate an irradiated secondary recipient was documented.[13] However, cell separation studies in more recent times have reported that spleen colony-forming unit (CFU-S)-containing populations cannot reconstitute irradiated recipients on a long-term basis and thus that CFU-S are a more mature and partially committed population of stem cells. The two sets of data are incompatible, but only if it is assumed that cell movement from Compartment 1 to Compartment 2 is irreversible. No recent study seemed to have examined the surface markers or properties of the cells in day-7 or day-12 spleen hematopoietic colonies. CFU-S are accepted as being able to self-generate because spleen colonies contain CFU-S, but do they also contain repopulating cells of one or other type? In fact, can CFU-S function as long-term repopulating cells if tested under less demanding environmental conditions?

There are some early observations on the behavior of CFU-S that raise questions regarding the dogma of the progressive reduction in self-generative capacity during hematopoiesis and the irreversibility of this process. CFU-S can self-generate and also generate more mature progeny. It is logical to expect, in a situation where a large number of progeny cells needs to be generated quickly, that self-generation will be more evident early in clonal expansion to provide sufficient starting cells to generate the more mature progeny. This is also to be expected if progressive shutdown of self-generative capacity is irreversible and part of the maturation process—the central dogma of hematopoiesis. However, analysis of developing spleen colonies revealed the opposite situation. The total number of CFU-S detectable in developing spleen colonies was related inversely to the number of such colonies in any one spleen.[14] Furthermore, CFU-S in a developing spleen colony were more frequent at later stages of colony development than at earlier stages.[13] Since these progeny CFU-S are arising from a single CFU-S, this indicates that the bias between the formation of self-progeny and differentiative progeny may not be fixed and may be able to be changed as conditions change. Our early studies on the serial retransplantation of spleen colonies indicated that colonies generated by adult CFU-S could only be repassaged two or three times in irradiated recipients.[13] These experiments were criticized in that they may have placed unfair proliferative demands on the CFU-S and may have led us to underestimate the capacity of such cells for extended self-generation. This is probably valid criticism, but it applies equally to the current standard method for detecting repopulating cells. By using an extreme lethally-irradiated model are we preventing CFU-S from demonstrating their true capacity to self-generate and, under less demanding conditions, to generate progeny on a long-term basis? This may not be a relevant speculation for clinical work, where there is no option but to use such a heavily pretreated aplastic recipient, but it remains a valid speculation in the context of attempting to determine the true nature of hematopoiesis.

LINEAGE COMMITMENT AND SELF-RENEWAL

There are two further dogmas of hematopoiesis that need continuous reappraisal. The first is that the differentiation commitment seen during the formation of lineage-committed progenitor cells occurs by a random process and, the second, that cessation or restriction of self-renewal is an irreversible process. Both these questions require the use of clonal culture systems able to allow the progeny of individual cells to be analyzed.

LINEAGE COMMITMENT IN EARLY PRECURSOR CELLS

Current dogma regarding stem cells holds that lineage commitment in the progeny of stem cells occurs by a random process, a view that many equate with a nonregulatable event. This latter view is not in accord with embryological development or the process by which the original stem cells were generated. In both these situations there is clear evidence that extrinsic signaling is required to achieve the transcription of the appropriate nuclear transcription factors necessary to achieve the commitment event.[15] The actual murine data on this question in adult hematopoietic cells are

TABLE 1. Blast colony-forming cells in the bone marrow of C57BL mice with or without pretreatment with 5-fluorouracil[a]

Preinjected with	Mean Total Marrow Cells per Femur $\times 10^{-6}$	Blast Colony-Forming Cells per 10^5 Cells		
		SCF	SCF + IL6	SCF + IL3 + IL6
5FU	21.0	0.4 ± 0.4	12 ± 4	16 ± 4
Saline	46.5	22 ± 3	29 ± 9	$31 + 1$

[a]Mice were injected I.V. 2 days previously with 150 mg/kg 5fluorouracil or saline. Cultures of 50,000 normal marrow cells or 100,000 post5FU marrow cells were stimulated by 100 ng stem cell factor with or without 100 ng IL-6 or 10 ng IL-3. Colony formation was scored from stained whole mount cultures after 7 days of incubation.

from recloning studies on the daughter and granddaughter cells of blast colony-forming cells, most often those surviving initial treatment of the animal with 5-fluorouracil (5-FU). The data indicate that such progeny can have differentiation potentials in almost any combination.[16,17] This is certainly a random outcome, but the data do not provide any information on the actual processes responsible for the observed outcome.

For adult hematopoietic tissues, commitment in multipotential or stem cells is a difficult question to investigate experimentally, because such studies need to be undertaken using multipotential cells able to be cloned *in vitro*. Preprogenitor cells able to form blast colonies composed of committed progenitor cells can be detected either in normal marrow cells or in marrow cells surviving 5-FU pretreatment. As shown in TABLE 1, most blast colony-forming cells that survive pretreatment with 5-FU require stimulation by combinations of hematopoietic regulators, and few respond to stimulation by stem cell factor (SCF) alone. In contrast, blast colonies can be grown from normal marrow cells using SCF alone, and the numbers are only moderately increased by the use of combinations of regulators, although the size of such colonies can be enhanced by such combinations. Post-5-FU blast colony-forming cells can be presumed to have been out of cycle when 5-FU was administered and their noncycling status is supported by data on their resistance to subsequent tritiated thymidine treatment *in vitro*[18] and by the ability of comparable cells to survive for extended periods *in vitro* in the absence of added growth factors. In contrast, blast colony-forming cells in normal marrow are reduced in numbers by 30–40% by tritiated thymidine treatment and die *in vitro* with a half-life of less than 12 hours in the absence of added growth factors (D. Metcalf, unpublished data).

From consideration of the frequency data in TABLE 1, only 1% of the blast colony-forming cells in normal marrow, that are able to respond to SCF alone, survive 5-FU treatment, and only 25% of blast colony-forming cells responding to multifactor stimulation survive 5-FU treatment. Because of this, data on post-5-FU marrow monitors a highly selected population of blast colony-forming cells almost certainly of a less mature type than the majority of blast colony-forming cells present in normal marrow. Conversely, culture studies using normal marrow monitor blast colony-forming cells that, although the large majority in numerical terms, are cycling and of a more mature status than those monitored in post-5-FU marrow. The two types of starting populations may not, therefore, yield exactly comparable data when blast colonies are being analyzed.

In studies designed to explore the possible influence of extrinsic regulators on differentiation commitment in blast colony-forming cells, it is obviously of importance not to be forced to use combinations of multiple growth factors to elicit proliferation and, for this reason, we have focused our attention on blast colony-forming cells in normal marrow.

Approximately 30 per 10^5 normal marrow cells respond to stimulation by SCF alone to form blast colonies of one of three types—dispersed, multicentric or single center, compact.[20] These various blast colonies *may* be generated by distinct subsets of pre-progenitor cells. In the initial studies on SCF, inefficient rat SCF was used and, with this agent, it was evident that addition of G-CSF, GM-CSF, multi-CSF or IL-6 could enhance blast colony size.[21,22] Current studies use murine SCF which, acting alone, commonly stimulates the formation of blast colonies containing up to 6,000 cells.[20] Under these conditions, an enhancing action of additional factors is much less evident.

In analyses in this laboratory on the progenitor cell content of blast colonies, no special effort was made to detect erythroid progenitor cells, nor were studies undertaken to detect T- or B-lymphoid precursors. The studies were therefore artificially restricted to the detection of granulocytic, macrophage, eosinophil and megakaryocytic progenitors and specifically those responsive to stimulation by single stimulating factors. Even with such protocols, it was evident that all blast cell colonies contain lineage-committed progenitors and often in such high numbers that they constitute the majority of colony cells. This is particularly true of the smaller dispersed blast colonies where there is even a notable absence of cluster-forming cells, the immediate progeny of progenitor cells.

In the recloning protocols used, resuspended colony cells were stimulated in the secondary cultures by single stimulating factors. Possibly for this reason, multipotential progenitor cells were rarely detected. While SCF-stimulated blast colony forming cells (CFCs) exhibited some capacity for self-renewal, the frequency of colonies containing such cells was low (5%).[20] It has not been tested whether this frequency could be modified by addition of other stimulating factors and, because all analyses were restricted to day 7 colonies, the capacity of blast CFCs for self-renewal could have been underestimated.

Individual blast colonies stimulated by SCF vary widely in size after 7 days' stimulation, but this is not due to unusual asynchrony of onset of proliferation. There is a similar wide (up to 100-fold) variation in the content of lineage-committed progenitor cells between individual colonies.

Analysis in this laboratory of SCF-stimulated blast colonies has indicated that commitment is not a random process. Such colonies contained widely varying numbers of granulocyte, granulocyte-macrophage and macrophage committed progenitors and less often smaller numbers of eosinophil or megakaryocyte progenitors. If lineage commitment was random, a colony with high progenitor cell numbers should be more likely to contain one or other of these rarer-committed progenitor cells. However, the data indicated that there was no correlation between total progenitor cell numbers and whether or not these progenitors included eosinophil or megakaryocyte progenitors.[20] A similar lack of correlation between colony cell numbers and progenitor cell numbers was also noted in earlier studies.[23] Both sets of data are inconsistent with a random commitment process.

TABLE 2. Effect of thrombopoietin or IL-5 on lineage commitment in developing SCF-stimulated blast colonies[a]

		Percent Colonies Containing Lineage-Committed Progenitor Cells	
Stimulus	Blast Colony Type	Megakaryocytic	Eosinophil
SCF	Dispersed	16%	29%
	Multicentric	2%	30%
SCFplus TPO	Dispersed	47%	—
	Multicentric	33%	—
SCF plus IL5	Dispersed	—	27%
	Multicentric	—	71%

[a]Blast colonies analyzed were from 7 day cultures of normal C57BL bone marrow cells stimulated by 100 ng stem cell factor (SCF) with or without 50 ng thrombopoietin (TPO) or 10 ng interleukin5 (IL5). The presence of lineage-committed progenitor cells was established by secondary culture of individual resuspended blast colony populations.

Addition of thrombopoietin (TPO) to SCF increased the proportion of blast colonies containing megakaryocyte progenitor cells (TABLE 2) without increasing total progenitor cell numbers but, curiously, TPO acting alone was unable to stimulate the proliferation of the megakaryocyte progenitors present in such colonies.[20] Furthermore, combination of IL-5 with SCF increased the percentage of colonies containing eosinophil progenitors without increasing total blast progenitor cell numbers. However, this only occurred in multicentric blast colonies and not in dispersed colonies (TABLE 2), despite the fact that IL-5 was an effective proliferative stimulus for eosinophil progenitors present in either type of colony.[20]

These data cast doubt on the assumption that pre-progenitor (blast colony-forming) cells, when responding to stimulation by SCF, generate lineage-committed progeny on a random basis. By analogy, it could then be questioned whether the formation of pre-progenitor cells by stem cells is also unlikely to occur on a random basis.

The study of colony formation by SCF-stimulated pre-progenitor cells indicated that extrinsic growth factors can skew the commitment process in a situation where selective survival is not a satisfactory alternative explanation. However, the data also suggested that growth factor commitment effects of this type are relatively weak. Although the effects were quantitatively weak, their occurrence makes it reasonable to search for other extrinsic agents, not necessarily conventional hematopoietic regulators, that might have a stronger influence on these events.

This recent information on lineage commitment has merely indicated that the process is regulatable, but has not addressed the question of whether such commitment events can be reversed. At present, there are no data that compel a reappraisal of the current dogma of irreversibility of differentiation commitment.

SELF-GENERATION AND ITS REGULATION

Repopulation studies in irradiated recipients, whether analyzing long-term repopulation or merely spleen colony formation, indicate that the initiating stem cells

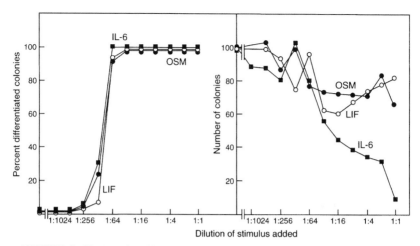

FIGURE 3. Clonogenic self-renewal by cells of the murine leukemic cell line, M1 can be suppressed by stimulation by leukemia inhibitory factor (LIF), interleukin-6 (IL-6) or oncostatin M (OSM). The parameters shown of reduction in colony numbers or the induction of differentiation in colonies reflect loss of clonogenic cells in the colonies if recloning analyses are performed on such colonies.

clearly have a capacity for self-generation. Conversely, examination of colonies formed *in vitro* by lineage-committed progenitor cells has equally clearly indicated that these cells do not exhibit significant self-generative capacity under the conditions used. These data are the basis for the dogma that, during hematopoiesis, there is a progressive and irreversible loss of self-renewal capacity.

No particular mechanisms have been proposed for this process in normal cells, nor has the process been claimed to occur on a stochastic basis. Little effort has been made using normal cells to determine whether the self-renewal characteristics of stem versus progenitor cells can be modulated by extrinsic signaling.

What has been studied extensively has been the capacity of hematopoietic regulators to suppress the high level of self-renewal exhibited by clonogenic cells within certain suitable leukemic cell lines such as HL60, U937, M1 or WEHI3B. Here the results are dramatic and readily reproducible. For example, stimulation of WEHI3B or U937 cells by G-CSF can irreversibly suppress self-renewal with those progeny that are generated either forming maturing cells or even failing to survive.[24,25] Similarly, IL-6, leukemia inhibitory factor (LIF) and oncostatin M (OSM) have dramatic effects on M1 leukemic cells leading to loss of clonogenic self-renewal as most readily observable by the reduction in colony numbers and the maturation induced in such colonies[25] (FIG. 3). Receptor insertion studies into the latter two cell lines have indicated that there is nothing special about the signals originating from the G-CSF receptor or the gp130 receptor chain. Similar results can be achieved by insertion of other receptors such as those for human GM-CSF[26] or thrombopoietin,[27] and then use of the appropriate ligand.

This regulator-induced suppression of self-renewal by clonogenic leukemic cells has been assumed to be a comparable process to that occurring when normal hemato-

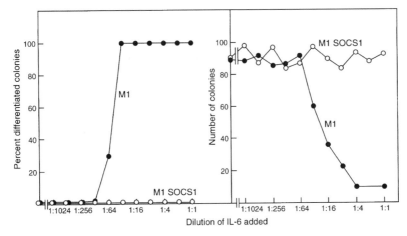

FIGURE 4. Overexpression of SOCS-1 in M1 leukemic cells renders them unresponsive to suppression or maturation induction when stimulated by IL-6. With IL-6 stimulation, colony cell numbers actually increase in developing colonies.

poietic stem cells generate progenitor cells, although this assumption is without formal proof. Furthermore, the apparent irreversibility of the suppression of self-renewal by clonogenic leukemic cells has supported the notion that the comparable changes in normal cells may equally be irreversible. While the leukemic cell line data indicate that suppression is the usual outcome of such signaling, parallel data from normal embryonic stem cell lines exposed to LIF equally clearly indicate that extrinsic signaling can *prevent* suppression of self-renewal.[28,29]

Although it remains to be established why the consequences for self-renewal can be opposite for leukemic cells versus normal embryonic stem (ES) cells, both sets of data raise the possibility that the process of self-renewal is able to be influenced by extrinsic signaling. If this is so, it can no longer be assumed that self-renewal and its suppression in normal hematopoietic stem cells are necessarily inevitable and immutable events. In the context of the present discussion, the progression of repopulating (Compartment 1) stem cells to nonrepopulating (Compartment 2) stem cells, which presumably involves questions of the level of expressed self-renewal, cannot be assumed to be unidirectional or irreversible.

Of potential relevance to these considerations has been the recent discovery of a family of cytokine-inducible proteins, the suppressor of cytokine signaling (SOCS) family, at least some members of which appear able to modulate responses to cytokine signaling that would otherwise result in suppression of self-generation, at least in leukemic cell lines.[30–33]

Overexpression of SOCS-1, -2, -3 and -5 in M1 leukemic cells can block the usual response of these cells to signaling by IL-6, LIF or OSM and prevent suppression of self-renewal (FIG. 4).[30] Indeed, with M1 cells overexpressing SOCS-1, stimulation by IL-6 actually results in an increase in colony size. Induction of transcription of SOCS-1 mRNA in leukemic and normal hematopoietic cells is observed following stimulation by IL-6 and other hematopoietic regulators.[30]

There is therefore a large family of proteins whose production is inducible by a wide range of cytokines. with at least some of these proteins being able to influence self-renewal decisions, at least in leukemic cell lines. Since these proteins are also inducible in normal bone marrow, a mechanism is potentially available for influencing self-renewal decisions made in normal hematopoietic stem cells. Because the induced transcription of SOCS proteins is transient, such decisions may potentially be reversible during subsequent cell divisions, a possibility of some interest if plasticity of the self-renewal behavior of normal stem cells is greater than at present assumed. This family of inducible proteins is clearly worthy of examination for their action on self-renewal by normal hematopoietic stem cells.

ACKNOWLEDGMENTS

The work from the author's laboratory was supported by the Carden Fellowship Fund of the Anti-Cancer Council of Victoria, the National Health and Medical Research Council, Canberra, the AMRAD Corporation, Melbourne, and the National Institutes of Health, Bethesda, MD, Grant No. CA22556.

REFERENCES

1. METCALF, D. 1984. The Hemopoietic Colony Stimulating Factors. Elsevier. Amsterdam.
2. METCALF, D. & N.A. NICOLA. 1995. The Hemopoietic Colony-Stimulating Factors. Cambridge University Press.
3. McARTHUR, G.A., G.L. LONGMORE, K. KLINGER & G.R. JOHNSON. 1995. Lineage-restricted recruitment of immature hematopoietic cells in response to erythropoietin after normal hematopoietic cell transfection with erythropoietin receptor. Exp. Hematol. 23: 645–654.
4. McARTHUR, G.A., L.R. ROHRSCHNEIDER & G.R. JOHNSON. 1994. Induced expression of cfms in normal hematopoietic cells shows evidence for both conservation and lineage restriction of signal transduction in response to macrophage colony-stimulating factor. Blood 83: 972–981.
5. INABA, K., M. INABA, N. ROMANI, H. AYA, M. DEGUCHI, S. IKEHARA, S. MURAMATSU & R.M. STEINMAN. 1992. Generation of large numbers of dendritic cells from mouse bone marrow cultures supplemented with granulocyte/macrophage colony-stimulating factor. J. Exp. Med. 176: 1693–1702.
6. YOUNG, J.W. & R.M. STEINMAN. 1996. The hematopoietic development of dendritic cells: a distinct pathway for myeloid differentiation. Stem Cells 14: 376–387.
7. MOORE, M.A.S. & D. METCALF. 1970. Ontogeny of the haemopoietic system: yolk sac origin of in vivo and in vitro colony forming cells in the developing mouse embryo. Br. J. Haematol. 18: 279–296.
8. MEDVINSKY, A. & E. DZIERZAK. 1996. Definitive hematopoiesis is autonomously initiated by the AGM region. Cell 81: 897–906.
9. MULLER, A., A. MEDVINSKY, J. STROUBOULIS, F. GROSVELD & E. DZIERZAK. 1994. Development of hematopoietic stem cell activity in the mouse embryo. Immunity 1: 291–301.
10. TURPEN, J.B., C.M. KELLEY, P.E. MEAD & L.I. ZON. 1997. Bipotential primitive-definitive hematopoietic progenitors in the vertebrate embryo. Immunity 7: 325–334.
11. KENNEDY, M., M. FIRPO, K. CHOL, C. WALL, S. ROBERTSON, N. KABRUN & G. KELLER. 1997. A common precursor for primitive erythropoiesis and definitive haematopoiesis. Nature 386: 488–492.

12. YODER, M. C. & K. HIATT. 1997. Engraftment of embryonic hematopoietic cells in conditioned newborn recipients. Blood **89:** 2176–2183.
13. METCALF, D. & M.A.S. MOORE. 1971. Haemopoietic Cells. North-Holland. Amsterdam.
14. SCHOFIELD, R. & L.G. LAJTHA. 1969 Mouse graft size considerations in the kinetics of spleen colony development. Cell Tissue Kinet. **2:** 147–155.
15. ZON, L. I. 1995. Developmental biology of hematopoiesis. Blood **86:** 2876–2891.
16. NAKAHATA, T., AJ. GROSS & M. OGAWA. 1982. A stochastic model of self-renewal and commitment to differentiation of the primitive hemopoietic stem cells in culture. J. Cell. Physiol. **113:** 455–458.
17. SUDA, T., J. SUDA. & M. OGAWA. 1984. Disparate differentiation in mouse hemopoietic colonies derived from paired progenitors. Proc. Natl. Acad. Sci. USA **81:** 2520–2524.
18. SUDA, T., J. SUDA & M. OGAWA. 1983. Proliferative kinetics and differentiation of murine blast cell colonies in culture: evidence for variable G_0 periods and constant doubling rates of early pluripotent hemopoietic progenitors. J. Cell. Physiol. **117:** 308–318.
19. LEARY, A.G., Y. HIRAI, T. KISHIMOTO, S.C. CLARK & M. OGAWA. 1989. Survival of hemopoietic progenitors in the G_0 period of the cell cycle does not require early hemopoietic regulators. Proc. Natl. Acad. Sci. USA **86:** 4535–4538.
20. METCALF, D. 1998. Lineage commitment in the progeny of murine hematopoietic preprogenitor cells: influence of thrombopoietin and interleukin 5. Proc. Natl. Acad. Sci. USA **95:** 6408–6412.
21. METCALF, D. & N.A. NICOLA. 1991. Direct proliferative actions of stem cell factor on murine bone marrow cells *in vitro*: effects of combination with colony-stimulating factors. Proc. Natl. Acad. Sci. USA **88:** 6239–6243.
22. METCALF, D. 1993. The cellular basis for enhancement interactions between stem cell factor and the colony stimulating factors. Stem Cells **11** (Suppl. 2)**:** 1–11.
23. HUMPHRIES, R.K., A.C. EAVES & C.J. EAVES. 1981. Self-renewal of hemopoietic stem cells during mixed colony formation *in vitro*. Proc. Natl. Acad. Sci. USA **78:** 3629–3633.
24. METCALF, D. 1982. Regulator-induced suppression of myelomonocytic leukemic cells: clonal analysis of early cellular events. Int. J. Cancer **30:** 203–210.
25. MAEKAWA, T., D. METCALF & D.P. GEARING. 1990. Enhanced suppression of human myeloid leukemic cell lines by combinations of Il6, LIF, GMCSF and GCSF. Int. J. Cancer **45:** 353–358.
26. SMITH, A., D. METCALF & N.A. NICOLA. 1997. Cytoplasmic domains of the common βchain of the GMCSF/IL3/IL5 receptors that are required for inducing differentiation or clonal suppression in myeloid leukaemic cell lines. EMBO J. **16:** 451–464.
27. ALEXANDER, W.S., A.B. MAURER, U. NOVAK & M. HARRISON-SMITH. 1996. Tyrosine-599 of the cMpl receptor is required for Shc phosphorylation and the induction of cellular differentiation. EMBO J. **15:** 6531–6540.
28. WILLIAMS, R.L., D.J. HILTON, S. PEASE, T.A. WILLSON, C.L. STEWART, D.P. GEARING, E.F. WAGNER, D. METCALF, N. A. NICOLA & N.M. GOUGH. 1988. Myeloid leukemia inhibitory factor (LIF) maintains the developmental potential of embryonic stem cells. Nature **336:** 684–687.
29. SMITH, A.G., J.K. HEATH, D.D. DONALDSON, G.G. WONG, J. MOREAU, M. STAHL & D. ROGERS. 1988. Inhibition of pluripotential embryonic stem cell differentiation by purified polypeptides. Nature **336:** 688–690.
30. STARR, R., T.A. WILLSON, E.M. VINEY, L. J.L. MURRAY, J.R. RAYNER, B.J. JENKINS, T.J. GONDA, W.S. ALEXANDER, D. METCALF, N.A. NICOLA & D.J. HILTON. 1997. A family of cytokine-inducible inhibitors of signalling. Nature **387:** 917–921.
31. ENDO, T.A., M. MASUHARA, M. YOKOUCHI, R. SUZUKI, K. MITSUI, T. MATSUMOTO, S. TANIMURA, M. OHTSUBO, H. MISAWA, T. MIYAZAKI, N. LEONOR, T. TANIGUCHI & T. FUJITA. 1997. A new protein containing an SH2 domain that inhibits JAK kinases. Nature **387:** 921–924.
32. NAKA, T., M. NARAZAKI, M. HIRATA, T. MATSUMOTO, S. MINAMOTO, A. AONO, N. NISHIMOTO, T. KAJITA, T. TAGA, K. YOSHIZAKI, S. AKIRA & T. KISHIMOTO. 1997.

Structure and function of a new STAT-induced STAT inhibitor. Nature **387**: 924–929.

33. HILTON, D.J., R.T. RICHARDSON, W.S. ALEXANDER, E.M. VINEY, T.A. WILLSON, N.S. SPRIGG, R. STARR, S.E. NICHOLSON, D. METCALF & N.A. NICOLA. 1998. Twenty proteins containing a C-terminal SOCS box form five structural classes. Proc. Natl. Acad. Sci. USA **95**: 114–119.

DISCUSSION

M. OGAWA (*Medical University of South Carolina*): You were concerned that the blast cell colonies from post-5-FU marrow cells may be unique. In 1981 or 1982 we published a paper in the *Journal of Cell Physiology* in which we compared the blast cell colonies from normal marrow and those from post-5-FU marrow. Late-developing small blast cell colonies, let us say those found on day-16 of culture, are quite comparable.

METCALF: That is correct but such cells are a small subset of blast colony-forming cells in normal bone marrow.

OGAWA: About your studies supporting the deterministic model, I think a critical experiment is to compare cultures containing steel factor and thrombopoietin with the cultures containing steel factor, thrombopoietin and IL-5. My predicition is that you do not see any negative effects of IL-5 on the megakaryocyte population. It is important to count the total number of cells rather than their ratios.

METCALF: This would be my prediction also, but it would be a hard experiment to do. The colonies are highly variable in their content of progenitor cells. You would probably need to do 1000 to be sure of any differences. I am too old to begin this experiment, but it would be a good experiment! If you believe certain authors, there is evidence that cytokines can compete for progenitor cell commitment.

S.J. SHARKIS (*Johns Hopkins Oncology Center*): Since you think that the SOCS proteins will ultimately inhibit self-renewal, do you think that they may be used to inhibit either engraftment or retransplant experiments with normal stem cells?

METCALF: That is an interesting possibility, and I would ask the people who have been looking at cDNAs from stem cells whether they did encounter cDNA for any of the SOCS proteins. That would be of great interest to us. I rather gather from the earlier papers that those have not yet been seen.

I. LEMISCHKA (*Princeton University*): We will certainly look. We have not analyzed all cDNAs, but it would be interesting.

METCALF: It would be great if some of these were present.

D.M. BODINE (*National Human Genome Research Institute/NIH*): The HMG protein that we talked about, the HMG cDNA that I showed, is a member of that same family.

METCALF: It was?

BODINE: Yes. The spelling I changed was my idea of a joke, but it is the same group of things, and I would predict that this is going to be more in the nucleus than anywhere else. It is probably not going to be in a signaling pathway, but it will be a recipient of a signal.

METCALF: So you are saying that in your stem cell preparation you have run into one of these cDNAs?

BODINE: We pulled the same one out twice . The question I was going to ask is have you looked at the ability of your SOCS-1, -2, and -3 in 32D or FDCP-1 cells to modulate responses to cytokines?

METCALF: No, we have not.

S.T. ILDSTAD (*Allegheny University of Health Sciences*): I wanted to follow up on your statement regarding 5-FU-treated marrow versus untreated. We rely heavily on an *in vivo* engraftment model for functional stem cell activity, and we have done a number of comparisons looking at the engraftment potential of stem cells after 5-FU treatment. It seems to be as good or better than unmodified marrow. Wouldn't it be the situation with 5-FU that you are enriching for more primitive cells rather than for committed, more mature cells?

METCALF: Yes, that is my interpretation. The type of cell in post-5-FU bone marrow that forms blast colonies is more ancestral to most blast colony forming-cells in normal marrow because the former cells are not in cycle; they are less dependent on cytokines for survival *in vitro*. We simply wanted to use a population that would respond to stimulation by a single cytokine. We could then add other ones to look for a clear change in generation of progenitor cells.

LEMISHKA: You mentioned that 5 of the SOCS proteins actually have this effect after transfection?

METCALF: We know that SOCS-1, SOCS-3, and SOCS-5 do.

LEMISHKA: I would suggest that because they seem to have other very different ankyrin, WD or SPRY domains appended, that perhaps what you are really seeing is a SOCS-Box/domain-mediated dominant-negative effect. I was wondering what would happen if you would transduce this domain alone?

METCALF: The SOCS-Box alone is functionally inactive. For SOCS-1 action, you need both the SH-2 domain and the N-terminal region.

Signaling Domains of the βc Chain of the GM-CSF/IL-3/IL-5 Receptor

KEIKO OKUDA, ROSEMARY FOSTER, AND JAMES D. GRIFFIN[a]

Department of Adult Oncology, Dana-Farber Cancer Institute, Boston, Massachusetts 02115, USA

ABSTRACT: The granulocyte/macrophage colony-stimulating factor (GM-CSF)/interleukin-3 (IL-3)/IL-5 receptors are a family of heterodimeric transmembrane proteins expressed by myeloid lineage cells. Each receptor has a unique ligand-binding α chain and they share a common β chain (βc chain). Binding of GM-CSF activates at least one receptor-associated tyrosine kinase, JAK2, and rapidly induces tyrosine phosphorylation of the GMR βc chain (GMRβ), but not the GMR α chain (GMRα). Mutation of each of the 8 tyrosine residues in the cytoplasmic domain of the human GMRβ to phenylalanine (GMRβ-F$_8$) reduced tyrosine phosphorylation of GMRβ, SHP2 and SHC, but not JAK2 or STAT5. Interestingly, GMRβ-F$_8$ was still capable of inducing at least short-term proliferation and enhancing viability. The role of each individual tyrosine residue was explored by replacing each mutated phenylalanine with the wild-type tyrosine residue. Tyrosine 577 was found to be sufficient to regenerate GM-CSF-dependent phosphorylation of SHC, and any of Y577, Y612, or Y695 were sufficient to regenerate GM-CSF-inducible phosphorylation of SHP2. Next, a series of four internal deletion mutants were generated, which deleted small sections from aa 518 to 626. One of these, deleting residues 566–589 was profoundly defective in signaling and supporting viability, and may identify an important viability signaling domain for this receptor family. Overall, these results indicate that GMRβ tyrosine residues are not necessary for activation of the JAK/STAT pathway, or for proliferation, viability, or adhesion signaling in Ba/F3 cells, although tyrosine residues significantly affect the magnitude of the response. However, internal deletion mutant studies identify critical domains for viability and proliferation.

INTRODUCTION

The granulocyte/macrophage colony-stimulating factor (GM-CSF) receptor consists of a ligand-binding α chain and a β chain, which is rapidly tyrosine phosphorylated in response to GM-CSF. The α chain may be preassociated with the β chain, but several studies, including our own, suggest that there is increased association in the presence of ligand. It is reasonable to expect that ligand may also increase oligomerization, creating clusters of 2 α chains with 2 β chains, or possibly higher order structures as well. The major tyrosine kinase activated by GM-CSF/interleukin-3 (IL-3)/IL-5 is JAK2, and the best available model suggests that the β chain constitutively or inducibly associates with JAK2 after ligand binding. This re-

[a]Corresponding author: James D. Griffin, M.D., Dana-Farber Cancer Institute, 44 Binney Street, Boston, MA 02115. Phone, 617/632-3360; fax: 617/632-4388; e-mail: james_griffin@dfci.harvard.edu

sults in rapid activation of JAK2 followed by tyrosine phosphorylation of JAK2 it-self, the β chain, and other JAK2 substrates, which include cytoplasmic components of transcription factor complexes termed STATs, particularly STAT 5a and 5b.[1] The autophosphorylation of JAK2 may attract signaling molecules via their SH2 do-mains and the phosphorylation of the β chain attracts signaling molecules through SH2 domains. The β chain is also phosphorylated on serine residues, but the function of this type of phosphorylation is unknown.

GM-CSF and GM-CSF βc chain knockout mice have no significant defects in he-matopoiesis, but develop a pulmonary lesion similar to pulmonary alveolar protei-nosis, possibly due to a macrophage defect in clearing surfactant-like material.[2-6] Importantly, the pulmonary lesion in GM-CSF βc chain (–/–) mice can be amelio-rated by transplantation of wild type marrow cells, but not by marrow from mutant mice. Similarly, there is no clear evidence from knockout mice that STAT 5 is re-quired for hematopoiesis, but Jak2 appears to be essential for signaling from many receptors.[7] IL-3 knockout mice have no significant hematopoietic defect, but are de-ficient in production of basophils and mast cells under stress conditions, and are also defective in certain types of hypersensitivity reactions.[8,9] IL-5 or IL-5 Rα-deficient mice have defects in production of eosinophils.

Previous studies have established that the βc chain is the source of signals for pro-liferation, viability, and adhesion from this receptor family.[10] Among the major con-sequences of this early signaling with regard to proliferation are activation of the p21ras pathway, induction of c-myc and other early response genes, induction of mo-tility, enhanced integrin-mediated adhesion, and inhibition of apoptosis. Preliminary studies using large deletion mutants of the βc chain from Sakamaki *et al.*,[11] followed by studies from our laboratory[12] and others, suggested that the membrane proximal and middle regions of the βc chain had quite distinct signaling functions (FIG. 1).

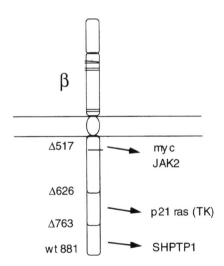

FIGURE 1. Common beta chain of the GM-CSF/IL-3/IL-5 receptor. Truncation mu-tants of the receptor are indicated, along with signaling pathways believed to originate in each segment.

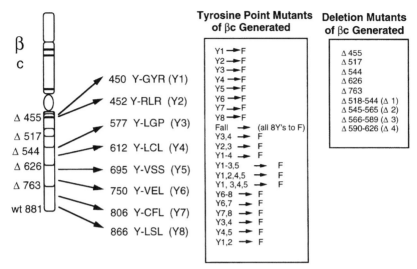

FIGURE 2. New mutants of the common beta chain prepared for this study.

The membrane proximal region, containing the box 1/box 2 domains, was responsible for JAK2 binding and activation, myc activation, and induction of piml; while the rnid-receptor segment was needed for viability signaling, optimal long-term proliferation, and activation of p21ras.

We have made a large number of mutants of the βc chain in an effort to link specific domains with signaling pathways and biological events. A summary of the mutants studied to date is shown in FIGURE 2.

SIGNALING FUNCTIONS OF THE βc TYROSINE RESIDUES

To examine the role of GMRβ tyrosine phosphorylation, each of the 8 tyrosine residues in the cytoplasmic domain of the human GMRβ was mutated to phenylalanine (GMRβ-F_8), and this mutant receptor was expressed with wild-type GMRα in the IL-3-dependent murine hematopoietic cell line, Ba/F3.[13] GM-CSF induced tyrosine phosphorylation of multiple cellular proteins in cells expressing GMRβ-F_8, including JAK2 and STAT5. However, GM-CSF-induced tyrosine phosphorylation of both SHP2 and SHC was reduced or absent compared to wild-type. Next, a series of eight receptors were generated, each containing only a single, restored, tyrosine residue. Tyrosine 577 was found to be sufficient to regenerate GM-CSF-dependent phosphorylation of SHC, and any of Y577, Y612, or Y695 were sufficient to regenerate GM-CSF-inducible phosphorylation of SHP2. Despite the signaling defect to SHC and SHP2, Ba/F3 cells expressing GMRβ-F_8 were still able to proliferate in response to 10 ng/ml human GM-CSF, although mitogenesis was impaired compared to wild-type GMRβ, and this effect was even more prominent at lower concentrations of GM-CSF (1 ng/ml). Overall, these results indicate that GMRβ tyrosine ressidues are not absolutely necessary for activation of the JAK/STAT pathway, or for

TABLE 1.

	Wild Type	βΔc1βc Mutant	Δ2βc Mutant	Δ3βc Mutant	Δ4βc Mutant
pTyr- βc chain	++	+	+	+	++
pTyr- JAK2	++	++	++	++	+
pTyr- STAT5	++	++	++	++	++
pTyr- Shc	++	+	++	—	++
pTyr- SHP2	+	+	+	+	++
Viability	Normal	Normal	Normal	Defective	Normal

proliferation, viability, or adhesion signaling in Ba/F3 cells, although tyrosine residues significantly affect the magnitude of the response. However, specific tyrosine residues are needed for activation of SHC and SHP2. A number of other mutants (shown in FIG. 2) are still under evaluation.

NOVEL VIABILITY DOMAINS OF THE βc CHAIN

Previous studies from our own and other laboratories have made large nested deletions of the βc chain in order to define biologically significant domains (FIG. 1). However, since the deletions are nested, it is impossible to define the contribution of a single, internal region, since previous mutants have always included all distal sequences also. Therefore, after showing that a Δ626 mutant retained most of the functions of the full length βc chain, but further truncation to Δ544 resulted in a profound viability defect, we constructed a series of βc mutants with internal deletions between aa 544 and 626 (shown in FIG. 2). The preliminary results are summarized in TABLE 1.

The results identify a segment of only 23 aa (aa 566–589; Δ3 βc deletion, see FIG. 2), which is absolutely required for viability, in contrast to all the other segments from 544 to 626. This segment contains Y577, which we have already shown to be required for tyrosine phosphorylation of Shc.[14] As would be predicted, Shc is not tyrosine phosphorylated by GM-CSF in the Δ3 βc deletion (FIG. 3), but this is not the sole important signaling effect, since a Y577F mutant also fails to phosphorylate SHC, but does not have a viability defect. Interestingly, this Δ3 βc mutant is not defective in activation of Raf, JAK2, PI3K, or Ras, and therefore there is another signaling pathway important for viability activated by aa 566–589. This deletion will be used in a 2-hybrid screen to identify potential signaling molecules responsible for this viability signal.

ACTIVATION OF P21 RAS

Several laboratories, including our own, have demonstrated that GM-CSF/IL-3 activate p21ras in myeloid cells in <5 min,[15,16] and that several signaling molecules generally thought to be downstream of ras are also activated, such as MAP kinase and Raf. Further, ras activation has been found to be critically important for viability

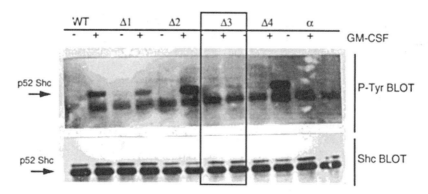

FIGURE 3. Reduced tyrosine phosphorylation of Shc by a GM-CSF beta chain receptor lacking amino acids 566–589.

signaling in many hematopoietic cell lines and also important for long-term proliferation of some lines. We found that the predominant form of ras is H-ras (> 90% of ras protein), and a focus of our efforts has been to define the links between the βc chain and the ras pathway. There are a number of insights as to how ras gets activated in other cell lineages, including well described links between tyrosine kinase receptors through GRB2, SOS, and Shc. Our studies support a key role for sequences between aa 544 and 626 of the βc chain. Using GRB2 as a probe, we have identified three distinct pathways to ras: GRB2 is linked to three different molecules, Shc, SHP2, and vav.[17–19]

ROLE OF Shc IN βc SIGNALING

Shc is a novel, SH2-containing, transforming protein, which has been previously implicated in the activation of p21ras. We prepared anti-Shc antibodies against a recombinant Shc SH2 GST fusion protein, which identified 2 Shc proteins in hematopoietic cells of approximate molecular weights 46 and 52 kDa, both of which were transiently tyrosine phosphorylated after stimulation with GM-CSF, IL-3, or SCF. We reported that Shc coprecipitated with a 140-kDa protein identified by Gerry Krystal's group as SHIP, an inositol 5-phosphatase involved in lipid signaling, and potentially involved in apoptosis. We also found that Shc was constitutively tyrosine phosphorylated in myeloid cell lines expressing p210[BCR/ABL] and at least a fraction of Shc was found to exist in a complex with p210[BCR/ABL].[18] We believe that Shc interacts indirectly with the βc chain, most likely through SHIP, which probably does interact directly with the βc chain at Y577.[14]

ROLE OF SHP2 IN βc SIGNALING

Multiple studies have demonstrated an important role for the Src homology SH2-containing tyrosine phosphatase 2 (SHP-2) in receptor tyrosine kinase-regulated cell proliferation and differentiation. SHP-2 (Syp/PTP-1D/PTP2C is a widely expressed SH2-containing protein tyrosine phosphatase, which is the homologue of the *Drosophila corkscrew* gene. In *Drosophila, corkscrew* transmits positive signals downstream from at least one tyrosine kinase receptor, *torso*. We found that: 1) SHP-2 coprecipitates with the βc chain after GM-CSF stimulation; 2) SHP-2 is tyrosine phosphorylated after GM-CSF, and 3) SHP-2 coprecipitates with GRB2 after GM-CSF stimulation; and 4) Tyrosines 577, 612, and 696 of the βc chain participate in binding to SHP2. We found two novel tyrosyl-phosphorylated proteins associated with SHP-2, in collaboration with Ben Neel.[17] The first, a 97-kDa cytosolic protein (p97), associates inducibly with SHP-2 upon cytokine stimulation and constitutively in Bcr-Abl-transformed cells. In contrast, p135, a 135-kDa transmembrane glycoprotein, forms a distinct complex with SHP-2, independent of cytokine stimulation or Bcr-Abl transformation. Far Western analysis reveals that SHP-2, via its Src homology 2 domains, interacts directly with both proteins. Thus, our results indicate that SHP-2 forms at least two separate complexes in hematopoietic cells, and the identification of these two new substrates is likely to provide significant advances in our understanding of the signaling of GM-CSF, IL-3, and IL-5.

CROSSTALK BETWEEN THE Shc AND SHP-2 PATHWAYS

We found that multiple cytokines, including IL-3, GM-CSF, thrombopoietin (TPO), and erythropoietin (EPO) induce transient formation of a complex composed of SHP-2 and SHIP.[20] Both phosphatases in the complex were tyrosine phosphorylated, and the amount of SHIP coprecipitating with SHP-2 was inversely related to the amount of SHIP coprecipitating with SHC. In hematopoietic cells transformed by the BCR/ABL oncogene, this phosphatase complex was found to be constitutively present with both components heavily tyrosine phosphorylated. Also, other proteins were detected in the complex, including BCR/ABL and c-CBL. However, transformation by BCR/ABL was associated with a reduced amount of SHIP protein, which could further affect the accumulation of various inositol polyphosphates in these leukemic cells. These data suggest that the function of SHIP and SHP-2 in normal cells are linked and that BCR/ABL alters the function of this signaling complex.

SUMMARY

Although GM-CSF, IL-3, and IL-5 are not absolutely required for hematopoiesis, each factor modulates functions of selected hernatopoietic cells, and at least one cytokine, GM-CSF has important clinical uses. While signaling for proliferation and viability are becoming better understood, the activities of GM-CSF and other cytokines in inducing mobilization of hernatopoietic progenitor cells is not understood at all. Further studies to link receptor signaling pathways to critical *in vivo* events, such as macrophage function and mobilization, are warranted.

REFERENCES

1. QUELLE, F.W., N. SATO, B.A. WITTHUHN, R.C. INHORN, M. EDER, A. MIYAJIMA, J.D. GRIFFIN & J.N. IHLE. 1994. JAK2 associates with the beta c chain of the receptor for granulocyte-macriphage colony-stimulating factor, and its activation requires the membrane-proximal region. Mol. Cell. Biol. **14:** 4335–4341.
2. IKEGANII, M., T. UEDA, W. HULL, J.A. WHITSETT, R.C. MULLIGAN, G. DRANOFF & A.H. JOBE. 1996. Surfactant metabolism in transgenic mice after granulocyte macrophage-colony stimulating factor ablation. Am. J. Physiol. **270:** L650–658.
3. HUFFMAN REED, J.A., W.R. RICE, Z.K. ZSENGELLER, S.E. WERT, G. DRANOFF & J.A. WHITSETT. 1997. GM-CSF enhances lung growth and causes alveolar type 11 epithelial cell hyperplasia in transgenic mice. Am. J. Physiol. **273:** L715–725.
4. NISHINAKAMURA, R., N. NAKAYAMA, Y. HIRABAYASHI, T. INOUE D. AUD, T. MCNEIL, S. AZUMA, S. YOSHIDA, Y. TOYODA, K. ARAI, A. MIYAJIMA & R. MURRAY. 1995. Mice deficient for the IL-3/GM-CSF/IL-5 beta-c receptor exhibit lung pathology and impaired immune response, while beta-IL-3 receptor-deficient mice are normal. Immunity **2:** 211–222.
5. NISHINAKAMURA, R., R. WILER, U. DIRKSEN, Y. MORIKAWA, K. ARAI, A. MIYAJIMA, S. BURDACH & R. MURRAY. 1996. The pulmonary alveolar proteinosis in granulocyte macrophage colony-stimulating factor/interleukins 3/5 beta-c receptor-deficient mice is reversed by bone marrow transplantation. J. Exp. Med. **183:** 2657–2662.
6. MUTO, A., S. WATANABE, A. MIYAJIMA, T. YOKOTA & K. ARAI. 1996. The beta subunit of human granulocyte-macrophage colony-stimulating factor receptor forms a homodimer and is activated via association with the alpha subunit. J. Exp. Med. **183:** 1911–1916.
7. PARGANAS, E., D. WANG, D. STRAVOPODIS, D.J. TOPHAM, J.C. MARINE, S. TEGLUND, E.F. VANIN, S. BODNER, O.R. COLAMONICI, J.M. VAN DEURSEN, G. GROSVELD & J.N. IHLE. 1998. Jak2 is essential for signaling through a variety of cytokine receptors. Cell **93:** 385–395.
8. MACH, N., C.S. LANTZ, S.J. GALLI, G. REZNIKOFF, M. MIHM, C. SMALL, R. GRANSTEIN, S. BEISSERT, M. SADELAIN, R.C. MULLIGAN & G. DRANOFF. 1998. Involvement of interleukin-3 in delayed type hypersensitivity. Blood **91:** 778–783.
9. LANTZ, C.S., J. BOESIGER, C.H. SONG, N. MACH, T. KOBAYASHI, R.C. MULLIGAN, Y. NAWA, G. DRANOFF & S.J. GALLI. 1998. Role for interleukin-3 in mast-cell and basophil development and in immunity to parasites. Nature **392:** 90–93.
10. EDER, M., T.J. ERNST, A. GANSER, P.T. JUBINSKY, R. INHORN, D. HOELZER & J.D. GRIFFIN. 1994. A low affinity chimeric human alpha/beta-granulocyte-macrophage colony-stimulating factor receptor induces ligand-dependent proliferation in a murine cell line. J. Biol. Chem. **269:** 30173–30180.
11. SAKAMAKI, K., I. MIYAJIMA, T. KITAMURA & A. MIYAJIMA. 1992. Critical cytoplasmic domains of the common beta subunit of the human GM-CSF, IL-3 and IL-5 receptors for growth signal transduction and tyrosine phosphorylation. Embo J. **11:** 3541–3549.
12. INHORN, R.C., N. CARLESSO, M. DURSTIN, D.A. FRANK & J.D. GRIFFIN. 1995. Identification of a viability domain in the granulocyte/macrophage colony-stimulating factor receptor beta chain involving tyirosine-750. Proc. Natl. Acad. Sci USA **92:** 8665–8669.
13. OKUDA, K., L. SMITH, J.D. GRIFFIN & R. FOSTER. 1997. Signaling functions of the tyrosine residues in the beta c chain of the granulocyte-macrophage colony-stimulating factor receptor. Blood **90:** 4759–4766.
14. DURSTIN, M., R.C. INHORN & J.D. GRIFFIN. 1996. Tyrosine phosphorylation of Shc is not required for proliferation or viability signaling by granulocyte-macrophage colony-stimulating factor in hematopoietic cell lines. J. Immunol. **157:** 534–540.
15. OKUDA, D., J. SANGHERA, S. PELECH, Y. KANAKURA, M. HALLEK, J. GRIFFIN & B. DRUKER. 1992. Granulocyte-macrophage colony-stimulating factor, interleukin-3, and steel factor induce rapid tyrosine phosphorylation of p42 and p44 MAP kinase. Blood **79:** 2880–2887.

16. OKUDA, K., T.J. ERNST & J.D. GRIFFIN. 1994. Inhibition of p2lras activation blocks proliferation but not differentiation of interleukin-3-dependent myeloid cells. J. Biol. Chem. **269:** 24602–24607.
17. GU, H., J.D. GRIFFIN & B.C. NEEL. 1997. Characterization of two SHP2-associated binding proteins and potential substrates in hernatopoietic cells. J. Biol. Chem. In press.
18. MATSUGUCHI, T., R. SALGIA, M. HALLEK, M. EDER, B. DRUKER, T. ERNST & J.D. GRIFFIN. 1994. Shc phosphorylation in myeloid cells is regulated by GM-CSF, IL-3, and steel factor, and is constitutively increased by p210[BCR/ABL]. J. Biol. Chem. **269:** 5016–5021.
19. MATSUGUCHI, T., R.C. INHORN, N. CARLESSO, G. XU, B. DRUKER & J.D. GRIFFIN. 1995. Tyrosine phosphorylation of p95Vav in myeloid cells is regulated by GM-CSF, IL-3 and steel factor and is constitutively increased by p210[BCR/ABL]. EMBO J. **14:** 257–265.
20. SATTLER, M., R. SALGIA, G. SHRIKHANDE, S. VERMA, J.L. CHOI, L.R. ROHRSCHNEIDER & J.D. GRIFFIN. 1997. The phosphatidylinositol polyphosphate 5-phosphatase SHIP and the protein tyrosine phosphatase SHP-2 form a complex in hematopoietic cells which can be regulated by BCR/ABL and growth factors. Oncogene **15:** 2379–2384.

DISCUSSION

J.E. DICK (*University of Toronto*): A few years ago when we put BCR/ABL into MO7E cells, we suggested that they are essentially setting up an autocrine loop secreting IL-3 and potentially stem cell factor as well. Is it possible that some of the effect that you are seeing is coming from secreted factor? For example, a molecule like SDF could block the receptor. This could cause increased effect on some of the nondirected migration, but you are not seeing the stimulatory effect if you had added exogenous molecule. For example, would neutralizing antibodies have some effect? I guess I am just wondering to what extent would the exogenous cytokine causes some of the effects you are seeing on adhesion and migration.

GRIFFIN: The issue of autocrine secretion of cytokines by BCR/ABL transformed cells continues to fascinate me, and there are a lot of new data here. I do not believe at this time that autocrine secretion of IL-3 will explain all the abnormalities of chronic myelogenous leukemia (CML). Let me just say that it is possible that the cell lines we use may at least secrete one or more cytokines in response to BCR/ABL. That said, BCR/ABL by itself has many aspects that make it look like an activated cytokine receptor. It activates many of the same pathways that the IL-3 receptor does, whether or not there is autocrine secretion of IL-3. It is more complicated, however, and I do not think (and I am willing to be shown to be wrong) that the entire phenotype of CML is going to be explained by autocrine secretion of IL-3. If it is, I would be delighted, but the kinds of adhesion assays I have shown you are not consistent with just an IL-3 effect.

H.E. BROXMEYER (*Indiana University*): I found those experiments really interesting. We have also been working with the Ba/F3 cells. A postdoctoral in our laboratory, Dr. Hiro Shibiyama, first shownend that IL-3 enhanced integrin-mediated adhesion of the Ba/F3 cells to fibronectin. Most recently he has overexpressed ras, Harvey ras in the cells, and found a tremendous amount of adhesion. You can enhance that a little bit with IL-3, but he has also taken the dominant negative form, put it into the cells and blocked the ability of the cells to adhere. So the whole system of ras, rac, rho is very intriguing.

GRIFFIN: There is large literature on the regulation of integrin function by ras. It is not Harvey ras, which is the major ras protein expressed by these cell lines. It is R-ras.

R. HOFFMAN (*University of Illinois College of Medicine*): Does interferon effect this pathway in any way?

GRIFFIN: Interferon is absolutely fascinating. It dramatically reduces the mortality of BCR/ABL-transformed cells to a fibronectin-coated surface, and it increases adhesion acutely. It does not effect the ruffling, the ability to make pseudopods and retract them, so the cells are stationary, but still trying to move. Those are acute effects. Interferon increases adhesive properties in many cells.

HOFFMAN: We have been working with Leon Platanias on the effects of interferon on CRKL in primary progenitor cells. Our data indicate that CRKL plays a major role in the effect of interferon on hematopoiesis.

GRIFFIN: I did not know that, but these results will be interesting.

D.A. WILLIAMS (*Riley Hospital for Children*): I just wonder if you have looked at using your retrovirus in primary cells and the effects on chemotaxis in primitive cells either human or mouse?

GRIFFIN: We will. For many reasons we prefer to work with cell lines. First, with primary cells you always have the problem of what the control is, and these are very tricky assays, and precise control cells are important. I believe there may even be differences between immature cells, of different lineages. I think that until we understand about the regulation of integrin signaling inside and out, it is going to be very difficult to start those kinds of studies and interpret them properly, unless you are absolutely sure you are comparing things with a good control. It does not mean that it should not be done. The viruses do work in primary cells and we are trying to get those studies going.

Thrombopoietin and Hematopoietic Stem Cell Development

KENNETH KAUSHANSKY[a]

Division of Hematology, Box 357710, University of Washington School of Medicine, Seattle, Washington 98195, USA

ABSTRACT: Thrombopoietin, the long sought primary regulator of thrombopoiesis, was cloned four years ago. In addition to its fulfilling most, if not all, of the expected biological activities relating to megakaryocyte and platelet development, the availability of the recombinant hormone and reagents to characterize its receptor have allowed detailed investigation of additional biological activities. In cultures of purified populations of candidate stem cells, thrombopoietin supports the survival, and augments the proliferation of hematopoietic stem cells when present together with interleukin-3 or steel factor. The progeny of such cultures are not skewed in their developmental potential; colony-forming cells of all lineages arise from thrombopoietin-stimulated stem cells. Evidence for an important effect of thrombopoietin on stem cell physiology *in vivo* are equally compelling. Genetic elimination of thrombopoietin or its receptor leads to a profound reduction not only of megakaryocytes and platelets, but also of committed myeloid progenitors of all types, primitive progenitors and hematopoietic stem cells. When administered to animals, thrombopoietin profoundly stimulates thrombopoiesis and enhances the number of hematopoietic progenitor cells of all lineages, and when used in most animal models of myelosuppressive therapy, accelerates the recovery of platelet, erythrocyte and leukocyte production. Thus, thrombopoietin appears to be more than a lineage-restricted growth factor.

The term thrombopoietin was first coined in 1958 to describe the primary regulator of thrombopoiesis,[1] although the concept of humoral control over platelet production dates somewhat earlier.[2] Over the several decades since these initial observations, multiple biological properties were predicted and reported, effects primarily restricted to megakaryocyte differentiation.[3,4] Whether the hormone also affects megakaryocytic progenitor cell proliferation was debated until recently, and effects on cells of other hematopoietic lineages were not seriously considered prior to the cloning of the molecule. All this uncertainty changed with the cloning of thrombopoietin in 1994.[5–8] It was immediately clear that thrombopoietin affected all aspects of megakaryocyte and platelet development, including stimulation of megakaryocyte progenitor cell proliferation, induction of platelet specific proteins and ultrastructural features, and augmentation of endomitosis (reviewed in Ref. 9). However, its effects on other aspects of hematopoiesis were not immediately clear. Nevertheless, two clues, one derived from the biologic effects of the murine myelo-

[a]Phone, 206/543-3360; fax, 206/543-3560; e-mail, kkaushan@u.washington.edu

proliferative virus (MPLV) on hematopoiesis,[10] the other from the cellular distribution of the thrombopoietin receptor,[11] suggested that the hormone may play a greater role in hematopoiesis than was initially anticipated. The present work will review our current understanding of the effects of thrombopoietin on hematopoietic stem cell biology.

Unfortunately, our current understanding of the factors that support the maintenance of hematopoietic stem cells and their commitment to various hematopoietic lineages is far from complete. Much evidence indicates that stem cell factor (SCF; also termed steel factor, c-kit ligand, or mast cell growth factor) is at least one of the proteins that helps to maintain normal numbers of hematopoietic stem cells. Naturally occurring SCF mutations in mice (Sl mutants), or that of its receptor *c-kit* (W mutants), lead to a profound reduction in the number of hematopoietic stem cells, assayed as marrow cells that can persistently repopulate all of hematopoiesis in a lethally irradiated recipient.[12,13] In addition, the administration of SCF to mice expands the number of transplantable hematopoietic stem cells.[14] Despite these results, SCF alone cannot even maintain the input numbers of stem cells in *ex vivo* "expansion cultures,"[15] suggesting that the *in vivo* effects of the cytokine are due to the interaction of SCF with other hematopoietic proteins. Candidate growth factors thought to fill such a role are Flt3 ligand (FL)[16] and interleukin-11 (IL-11).[17] Genetic elimination of the Flt3 receptor leads to a fivefold reduction in the number of long-term repopulating hematopoietic stem cells,[18] although in contrast to SCF, the administration of FL does not increase the number of stem cells. The argument for a role of IL-11 in stem cell biology is less convincing. Unlike the receptors for SCF and FL, genetic elimination of the IL-11 receptor does not affect hematopoietic stem cell numbers;[19] rather, the evidence that IL-11 affects stem cells derives almost entirely from *in vitro* expansion experiments. Neither SCF, FL, nor their combination is sufficient for maintaining the number of hematopoietic stem cells in serum-free culture.[20,21] However, the addition of IL-11 to either SCF or FL maintains, and the presence of all three cytokines modestly expands, the number of transplantable stem cells in serum-free cultures.[20] Finally, although several other cytokines (e.g., IL-1, IL-3, IL-6, and IL-12) have been tested for their capacity to maintain or expand hematopoietic stem cell populations, none has proved essential.

With the recent cloning of thrombopoietin much attention was focused on its role as the primary regulator of megakaryocyte and platelet development. Nevertheless, soon after the recombinant protein became available, evidence began to emerge that thrombopoietin can exert profound effects on primitive hematopoietic cells. A diverse range of studies have supported this concept, including studies of thrombopoietin receptor expression and function, the administration of the hormone to animals, genetic elimination of thrombopoietin or its receptor, and single cell *in vitro* tracking experiments.

The thrombopoietin receptor (c-mpl) was first recognized as the transforming oncogene (*v-mpl*) of MPLV, an acute transforming murine retrovirus,[11,22] and an agent that induces a pan-myeloid disorder.[10] Consistent with this effect, the normal receptor is expressed on a large fraction of CD34[+] cells[11] and acts to stimulate megakaryocyte formation.[23] Administration of thrombopoietin to normal animals expands the number of progenitor cells of all hematopoietic lineages, and if given following myelosuppressive therapy, accelerates their recovery to normal values.[24,25] Furthermore, in addition to a profound depression of thrombopoiesis, targeted disruption of the genes for thrombopoietin or its receptor greatly reduces the number of progenitor cells committed to both the erythroid and myeloid lineages.[26,27] This result, too, suggests that thrombopoietin might affect hematopoietic cells at an early stage of development.

While these *in vivo* experiments were being conducted, the direct effects of thrombopoietin on candidate populations of stem cells were also being tested. In a collaborative study with Makio Ogawa, we found that adding thrombopoietin to either IL-3 or SCF speeds entry of post-5-fluorouracil (5FU)/lin⁻/ly6⁺/kit⁺ murine cells into the cell cycle, and greatly increases the production of progenitor cells committed to multiple hematopoietic lineages.[28] Using an extremely enriched population of hematopoietic stem cells, containing virtually no *in vitro* colony-forming cells or CFU-S, we arrived at similar conclusions; thrombopoietin accelerates cellular entry into the cell cycle and induces a higher proportion of these cells to ultimately enter a proliferative phase and to increase the number of cell divisions per unit time compared to similar cultures lacking the hormone.[29] As these experiments were conducted in single cell cultures, thrombopoietin appeared to exert a direct effect on primitive hematopoietic cells.

Two recent studies were designed to directly assess the impact of thrombopoietin on hematopoietic stem cells. Kimura demonstrated that targeted disruption of the *mpl* gene greatly reduces the number of spleen colony-forming units (CFU-S$_{d12}$), and that marrow cells derived from the nullizygous mice were markedly inferior to those from wild type littermates in a competitive repopulation assay of stem cell activity.[30] And even more recently, Solar and his colleagues presented three lines of evidence that establish an important role for thrombopoietin in the maintenance of stem cell numbers.[31] These investigators found that compared to mpl- cells from normal mice, AA4⁺/Sca⁺/kit⁺/mpl⁺ fetal liver cells, or lin^lo^/Sca⁺/kit⁺/mpl⁺ adult marrow cell populations contain essentially all the hematopoietic repopulating activity when assessed at 24 weeks. Second, human marrow CD34⁺/CD38⁻/mpl⁺ cells were shown to engraft in a severe combined immunodeficient (SCID-hu) bone model of hematopoietic reconstitution far more efficiently than CD34⁺/CD38⁻/mpl⁻ cells. Finally, Solar and co-workers confirmed and extended the work of Kimura, quantifying the engraftment defect displayed by marrow cells from *mpl* nullizygous mice, a deficiency quite similar in magnitude (sevenfold reduction in repopulating units) to that found in Flt3- and SCF-deficient mice.

As thrombopoietin is the sole ligand for the mpl receptor, it is now firmly and directly established that the hormone affects hematopoietic stem cells. There are at least three immediate implications of these findings. First, the administration of thrombopoietin may evoke a far greater effect on hematopoietic recovery than initially anticipated. Proof of this principle has been provided by many preclinical trials of the agent,[32–34] and it would seem appropriate that clinical trials of thrombopoietin should be designed with this possibility in mind. Second, the hormone could provide an important adjunct in attempts to expand the numbers of hematopoietic stem cells for clinical use. The advantages of umbilical cord blood cells for transplantation and the use of stem cells in multiple gene therapy protocols have provided an important impetus to expand primitive hematopoietic cells. Evidence of the capacity of thrombopoietin to augment stem cell expansion is accumulating; the hormone is the most potent single agent at expanding long-term culture initiating cells (LTCIC) in serum-free culture,[35] a surrogate assay for the hematopoietic stem cell, and the combination of FL plus thrombopoietin greatly expands the output of these cells in long-term cultures of umbilical cord blood cells.[36] Moreover, an agent such as thrombopoietin, which accelerates stem cell entry into the cell cycle,[28,29] is particularly attractive for the expansion of stem cells destined for retroviral vector-based gene therapy. Third, the ability of thrombopoietin to support the survival and proliferation of hematopoietic stem cells may also herald adverse effects if the hormone is used in patients with myeloproliferative disorders. Similar warnings were sounded with the proposed use of granulocyte/macrophage (GM)- or granulocyte (G)-colony-stimulating factor (CSF) during therapy for acute myeloid leukemia, concerns that have not been realized.[37] However, G- and GM-CSF do not affect the hematopoietic stem cell, the likely cellular origin of most cases of myeloproliferative disease, making it once again incumbent upon us to carefully monitor the administration of thrombopoietin to such patients. Our understanding of hematopoiesis has advanced with the demonstration that thrombopoietin is one of the factors that support the survival and proliferation of pluripotent stem cells. However, many questions remain. The nature of the intracellular signals initiated by thrombopoietin and the other proteins that affect hematopoietic stem cell expansion and lineage determination are unknown, as are how these events interact with the developmental programs initiated by transcription factors such as SCL/TAL1, Rbtn-2 or GATA-2.[38] It is now up to basic scientists and clinical investigators to advance our understanding of this process and to exploit these effects for therapeutic benefit.

REFERENCES

1. KELEMEN, E., I. CSERHATI & B. TANOS. 1958. Demonstration and some properties of human thrombopoietin in thrombocythemic sera. Acta Haematol. (Basel) **20:** 350–355.

2. YAMAMOTO, S. 1957. Mechanism of the development of thrombocytosis due to bleeding. Acta Haematol. (Japan) **20:** 163–165.

3. McDONALD, T.P. 1988. Thrombopoietin: its biology, purification, and characterization. Exp. Hematol. **16:** 201–205.

4. HILL, R.J. & J. LEVIN. 1989. Regulators of thrombopoiesis: their biochemistry and physiology. Blood Cells **15:** 141–166.

5. DE SAUVAGE, F.J., P.E. HASS, S.D. SPENCER et al. 1994. Stimulation of megakaryocytopoiesis and thrombopoiesis by the c-Mpl ligand. Nature **369:** 533–538.

6. LOK, S., K. KAUSHANSKY, R.D. HOLLY et al. 1994. Cloning and expression of murine thrombopoietin cDNA and stimulation of platelet production in vivo. Nature **369:** 565–568.

7. BARTLEY, T.D., J. BOGENBERGER, P. HUNT et al. 1994. Identification and cloning of a megakaryocyte growth and development factor that is a ligand for the cytokine receptor Mpl. Cell **77:** 1117–1124.

8. SOHMA, Y., H. AKAHORI, N. SEKI et al. 1994 . Molecular cloning and chromosomal localization of the human thrombopoietin gene. FEBS Lett. **353:** 57–61.

9. KAUSHANSKY, K. 1995. Thrombopoietin: the primary regulator of platelet production. Blood **86:** 419–431.

10. WENDLING, F., P. VARLET, M. CHARON et al. 1986. A retrovirus complex inducing an acute myeloproliferative leukemia disorder in mice. Virology **149:** 242–246.

11. VIGON, I., J.-P. MORNON, L. COCAULT et al. 1992. Molecular cloning and characterization of *MPL*, the human homolog of the *v-mpl* oncogene: identification of a

member of the hematopoietic growth factor receptor superfamily. Proc. Natl. Acad. Sci. USA **89:** 5640–5644.

12. WITTE, O.N. 1990. Steel locus defines new multipotent growth factor. Cell **63:** 5–6.

13. BROUDY, V.C. 1997. Stem cell factor and hematopoiesis. Blood **90:** 1345–1364.

14. BODINE, D.M., N.E. SEIDEL, K.M. ZSEBO & D. ORLIC. 1993. *In vivo* administration of stem cell factor to mice increases the absolute number of pluripotent stem cells. Blood **82:** 445–455.

15. LI, C.L. & G.R. JOHNSON. 1994. Stem cell factor enhances the survival but not the self-renewal of murine hematopoietic long-term repopulating cells. Blood **84:** 408–414.

16. LYMAN, S.D. & S.E.W. JACOBSEN. 1998. c-Kit ligand and flt-3 ligand: stem/progenitor cell factors with overlapping yet distinct activity. Blood **91:** 1101–1134.

17. DU, X. & D.A. WILLIAMS. 1997. Interleukin-11: review of molecular, cell biology and clinical use. Blood **89:** 3897–3908.

18. YONEMURA, Y., H. KU, S.D. LYMAN & M. OGAWA. 1997. *In vitro* expansion of hematopoietic progenitors and maintenance of stem cells: comparison between flt3/flk2 ligand and kit ligand. Blood **89:** 1915–1921.

19. NANDURKAR, H.H., L. ROBB, D. TARLINTON *et al.* 1997. Adult mice with targeted mutation of the interleukin-11 receptor (IL11Ra) display normal hematopoiesis. Blood **90:** 2148–2159.

20. MILLER, C.L. & C.J. EAVES. 1997. Expansion *in vitro* of adult murine hematopoietic stem cells with transplantable lympho-myeloid reconstituting ability. Proc. Natl. Acad. Sci. USA **94:** 13648–13653.

21. MACKAREHTSCHIAN, K., J.D. HARDIN, K. A. MOORE *et al.* 1995. Targeted disruption of the flk2/flt3 gene leads to deficiencies in primitive hematopoietic progenitors. Immunity **3:** 147–161.

22. SOUYRI, M., I. VIGON, J.-F. PENCIOLELLI *et al.* 1990. A putative truncated cytokine receptor gene transduced by the myeloproliferative leukemia virus immortalizes hematopoietic progenitors. Cell **63:** 1137–1147.

23. ZEIGLER, F.C., F. DE SAUVAGE, H.R. WIDMER *et al.* 1994. *In vitro* megakaryocytopoietic and thrombopoietic activity of *c-mpl* ligand (TPO) on purified murine hematopoietic stem cells. Blood **84:** 4045–4052.

24. KAUSHANSKY, K., N. LIN, A. GROSSMANN *et al.* 1996. Thrombopoietin expands erythroid, granulocyte-macrophage and megakaryocytic progenitor cells in normal and myelosuppressed mice. Exp. Hematol. **23:** 265–269.

25. FARESE, A.M., P. HUNT, L.B. GRAB & T.J. MACVITTIE. 1996. Combined administration of recombinant human megakaryocyte growth and development factor and granulocyte colony-stimulating factor enhances multi-lineage hematopoietic reconstitution in nonhuman primates after radiation induced marrow aplasia. J. Clin. Invest. **97:** 2145–2151.

26. ALEXANDER, W.S., A.W. ROBERTS, N.A. NICOLA *et al.* 1996. Deficiencies in progenitor cells of multiple hematopoietic lineages and defective megakaryocytopoiesis in mice lacking the thrombopoietin receptor c-Mpl. Blood **87:** 2162–2170.

27. CARVER-MOORE, K., H.E. BROXMEYER, S.M. LUOH *et al.* 1996. Low levels of erythroid and myeloid progenitors in thrombopoietin and mpl-deficient mice. Blood **88:** 803–808.

28. KU, H., Y. YONEMURA, K. KAUSHANSKY & M. OGAWA. 1996. Thrombopoietin, the ligand for the Mpl receptor, synergizes with steel factor and other early-acting cytokines in supporting proliferation of primitive hematopoietic progenitors of mice. Blood **87:** 4544–4551.

29. SITNICKA, E., N. LIN, G.V. PRIESTLEY *et al.* 1996. The effect of thrombopoietin on the proliferation and differentiation of murine hematopoietic stem cells. Blood **87:** 4998–5005.

30. KIMURA, S., A.W. ROBERTS, D. METCALF & W.S. ALEXANDER. 1998. Hematopoietic stem cell deficiencies in mice lacking c-Mpl, the receptor for thrombopoietin. Proc. Natl. Acad. Sci. USA **95:** 1195–1200.
31. SOLAR, G.P., W.G. KERR, F.C. ZEIGLER *et al.* 1998. Role of c-Mpl in early hematopoiesis. Blood **92:** 4–10.
32. KAUSHANSKY, K., V.C. BROUDY, A. GROSSMANN *et al.* 1995. Thrombopoietin expands erythroid progenitors, increases red cell production, and enhances erythroid recovery after myelosuppressive therapy. J. Clin. Invest. **96:** 1683–1687.
33. NEELIS, K.J., L. QINGLIANG, G.R. THOMAS *et al.* 1997. Prevention of thrombocytopenia by thrombopoietin in myelosuppressed rhesus monkeys accompanied by prominent erythropoietic stimulation and iron depletion. Blood **90:** 58–63.
34. AKAHORI, H., K. SHIBUYA, M. OBUCHI *et al.* 1996. Effect of recombinant human thrombopoietin in nonhuman primates with chemotherapy-induced thrombocytopenia. Br. J. Haematol. **94:** 722–728.
35. PETZER, A.L., P.W. ZANDSTRA, J.M. PIRET & C.J. EAVES. 1996. Differential cytokine effects on primitive (CD34$^+$CD38$^-$) human hematopoietic cells: novel responses to Flt-3 ligand and thrombopoietin. J. Exp. Med. **183:** 2551–2558.
36. PIACIBELLO, W., F. SANAVIO, L. GARETTO *et al.* 1997. Extensive amplification and self-renewal of human primitive hematopoietic stem cells from cord blood. Blood **89:** 2644–2653.
37. ROWE, J.M. & J.L. LIESVELD. 1997. Hematopoietic growth factors in acute leukemia. Leukemia **11:** 328–341.
38. SHIVDASANI, R.A. & S.H. ORKIN. 1996. The transcriptional control of hematopoiesis. Blood **87:** 4025–4039.

DISCUSSION

D. METCALF (*P.O. Royal Melbourne Hospital*): With regard to your experiment with activated mpl receptors, a similar outcome is observed if murine fetal liver cells are infected with vmpl—also an activated mpl receptor. Cell lines emerge that are a mixture of megakaryocytic and erythroid cells. There seems to be a special mpl tropism for these two lineages.

J.W. ADAMSON (*New York Blood Center*): I would add to Dr. Metcalf's comment that whatever it was in culture seemed to have a large erythroid component as well. Was that a misinterpretation?

KAUSHANSKY: No. There were erythroid cells present, but there was a large number of megakaryocytes, much greater by day 40 than was present early on in the culture.

J.D. GRIFFIN (*Dana Farber Cancer Institute*): Truncation studies from a lot of other receptors suggest that the box 1/box 2 region by itself is not sufficient to activate ras. Have you tried to rescue your inactive truncation mutant receptors by putting in activated ras allele?

KAUSHANSKY: We have not done that experiment. It is a good experiment to do, and we have some other things that we are going to try to compliment these constructs with. We are also making mutants within the box 1/box 2 region. We believe that box 1 and box 2 is more than just binding of jak, and we hope to be able to find one or the other functional domains within that region.

G-CSF Receptor Mutations in Patients with Severe Congenital Neutropenia Do Not Abrogate Jak2 Activation and Stat1/Stat3 Translocation

A. HERBST,[a] M. KOESTER,[b] D. WIRTH,[b] H. HAUSER,[b] AND K. WELTE[a,c]

[a]Department of Pediatric Hematology and Oncology, Hannover Medical School, Hannover, Germany

[b]Department for Gene Regulation and Differentiation, GBF, Braunschweig, Germany

ABSTRACT: Severe congenital neutropenia (SCN) is an inherited disorder of myelopoiesis, characterized by a maturation arrest at the stage of promyelocytes and myelocytes in bone marrow, and absence or low levels of mature neutrophil granulocytes in peripheral blood. Recently, studies of patients with SCN who subsequently developed acute myeloid leukemia (AML) revealed nonsense mutations in the cytoplasmic domain of the granulocyte colony-stimulating factor (G-CSF) receptor messenger RNA. We focused our interest on the G-CSF-mediated signaling cascade to examine the consequences of the observed point mutations for the nuclear translocation of the transcription factors Stat1 and Stat3. Expression vectors encoding for truncated G-CSF receptors were transfected in the murine fibroblast cell line C243 expressing a fusion protein consisting of the transcription factor Stat1 and Stat3, respectively, and the green fluorescent protein (GFP). Nuclear translocation of the GFP fusion proteins was examined after G-CSF stimulation of the transfected cells.

INTRODUCTION

Before the era of growth factors, reports describing patients with congenital neutropenia who developed acute myeloid leukemia (AML) suggested that congenital neutropenia may be a premalignant condition.[4,8] Worldwide phase I–III clinical trials with recombinant human granulocyte colony-stimulating factor (G-CSF) and the International Register for patients with severe congenital neutropenia (SCNIR) have provided information on 506 chronic neutropenic patients: congenital neutropenia (249 patients), cyclic neutropenia (97 patients), and idiopathic neutropenia (160 patients). It was not unexpected that 23 cases of AML/myelodysplastic syndrome (MDS) were identified from the records of the 506 patients.[12] All 23 patients were originally found to have severe congenital neutropenia (Kostmann's syndrome) or Schwachmann-Diamond syndrome. None of the patients with cyclic or idiopathic neutropenia developed AML/MDS, suggesting that G-CSF was not involved in the development of leukemia. No relationship was found with amount or duration of G-

[c]Corresponding author: Prof. Dr. K. Welte, Pediatric Hematology and Oncology, OE 6781, Medical School Hannover, Carl-Neuberg-Strasse 1, D-30625 Hannover, Germany. Phone, +49 511 532 6711; fax, +49 511 532 9120; e-mail, Welte.Karl@MH-Hannover.de

CSF used. Leukemia conversion did not change significantly during G-CSF treatment over time. Patients with severe congenital neutropenia associated with progression towards MDS and AML have demonstrated a predictable pathway of transformation. In 8 out of 8 patients tested, point mutations in the G-CSF receptor gene were detected. Apart from these specific aberrations, more common abnormalities such as monosomy 7 or other chromosomal abnormalities and oncogene mutations (e.g., activating ras mutations) were found.[1] These data reveal that the only specific mutations were the G-CSF receptor mutations in patients with AML/MDS present in cells of the myeloid lineage. Retrospective studies demonstrated that these mutations were acquired mutations and present already months or even years prior to the overt AML.[11] These point mutations were nonsense mutations leading to the truncation of the C-terminal cytoplasmic region crucial for maturation signaling. In all patients both the mutated and the normal allels of the G-CSF receptor were expressed.[1] An additional 40 patients with severe congenital neutropenia who have no signs of AML/MDS were tested, and 7 patients were found to have G-CSF receptor mutations.[10] These findings support the notion that mutations in the G-CSF-R gene, resulting in the truncation of the membrane distal part of the cytoplasmic domain involved in differentiation signaling, are associated with progression from SCN to MDS/AML as mentioned above. The evolution from G-CSF-R mutation or monosomy 7 to overt AML has occurred over several months and years, suggesting a considerable variation in these patterns. To evaluate whether the G-CSF-R mutations are inherited or spontaneous somatic mutations, we evaluated six family members of two patients with severe congenital neutropenia who developed AML. All family members including the healthy parents, healthy sister, and one brother who has severe congenital neutropenia displayed both normal G-CSF-R gene and G-CSF-R messenger RNA.[11] From these data we concluded that the point mutations in the G-CSF-R gene occur spontaneously and are not inherited. It is important to emphasize that patients with either cyclic or idiopathic neutropenia and undergoing G-CSF treatment are not at risk for development of AML/MDS.

We were interested whether the G-CSF receptor mutations alter the signaling pathways and whether this altered signaling might be involved in leukemogenesis. To study the consequences of the truncation of the cytoplasmic domain for G-CSF receptor signaling, wildtype and mutated G-CSF receptor cDNA were transfected into the murine myeloid leukemic cell line L-GM.[2] This cell line proliferates interleukin-3 dependent and expresses no endogenous G-CSF receptor. After transfection of these cells with wildtype G-CSF receptors, they proliferate and differentiate in response to G-CSF stimulation. Compared to the wildtype G-CSF receptor transfected cells, cells transfected with a truncated G-CSF receptor protein showed an enhanced proliferation, but were defective in differentiation signaling.[2,9] Cytokine receptors like the erythropoietin (EPO) receptor or G-CSF receptor lack intrinsic tyrosine kinase activity, but activate cytoplasmic tyrosine kinases. Binding of the ligand G-CSF to its receptor results in rapid tyrosine phosphorylation of the Janus tyrosine kinases Jak1[5,9] and Jak2[3,9] and of the receptor protein itself.[5,6] The Jak kinases are thought to induce tyrosine phosphorylation of Stat molecules, resulting in their activation and translocation to the nucleus. Therefore, we focused our interest on the G-CSF-mediated signal transduction to examine the consequences of the observed point mutations in the G-CSF-R gene for the nuclear translocation of Stat1 and Stat3. To address this issue, we have generated deletion mutants of the G-CSF receptor protein by introducing stop codons in the receptor cDNA leading to the truncation of the expressed G-CSF receptor proteins. The expression vectors for the G-CSF deletion mutants were transfected in the murine fibroblast cell line C243, which overexpresses fusion proteins consisting of the transcription factors Stat1 and Stat3, respectively, and the green fluorescent protein (GFP), to study whether the nuclear translocation of these transcription factors is affected by point mutations found in patients with SCN and AML.

RESULTS

Activation of Jak2 in Neutrophil Granulocytes of Patients with Severe Congenital Neutropenia

The tyrosine kinase Jak2 is involved in the signaling pathway of the G-CSF receptor; therefore, we examined the expression and activity of Jak2 in neutrophils from SCN patients during G-CSF treatment. The immunoprecipitated Jak2 protein showed increased tyrosine phosphorylation in neutrophils from SCN patients as compared to the phosphorylation signal in neutrophils from healthy donors, suggesting that this kinase is activated. *In vitro* kinase assays of immunoprecipitated Jak2 confirmed that neutrophils from SCN patients show an increased autophosphorylation of Jak2 in comparison with that of neutrophils from healthy donors.[7]

Nuclear Translocation of Stat1 and Stat3 after Stimulation of the Wildtype G-CSF Receptor in C243 Cells

Using fusion proteins with the green fluorescent protein (GFP) fused to the C-terminal end of Stat1 and Stat3, we were able to monitor subcellular trafficking of these transcription factors. Wildtype G-CSF receptor-transfected C243 cells expressing either Stat1-GFP or Stat3-GFP were stimulated with G-CSF to study the kinetics of the nuclear translocation. Activation of these cells with G-CSF leads to the nuclear translocation of the fusion proteins as judged by the shift of the green fluorescence to the nucleus (TABLE 1).

Nuclear Translocation of Stat1 and Stat3 after Stimulation of the Truncated G-CSF Receptor

The nuclear translocation of Stat1 and Stat3 was studied after stimulation of a truncated G-CSF receptor S730 (nt 2429) containing a point mutation found in patients with SCN (FIG. 1). G-CSF stimulation of the transfected cells results in a translocation of the fusion proteins Stat1-GFP and Stat3-GFP from the cytoplasm to the nucleus as judged by the shift of the fluorescence signal. The kinetic and effiency of this nuclear translocation show no differences as compared to the nuclear translocation of Stat1 and Stat3 after stimulation of wildtype G-CSF receptor-transfected cells. Therefore, point mutations in the G-CSF receptor gene resulting in a truncated receptor protein do not abrogate the nuclear translocation of Stat1 and Stat3 (TABLE 1). The G-CSF receptor deletion mutant S649 containing only the Box 1

TABLE 1. Activity of the tyrosine kinase Jak2 and activation of the transcription factors Stat1 and Stat3[a]

G-CSF receptor	Jak2	Stat1	Stat3
wildtype	+	+	+
S730	++	+	+
S685	n.d.	+	+
S671	n.d.	+	+
S649	n.d.	−	−

[a]NOTE: The *in vitro* kinase activity of the tyrosine kinase Jak2 was studied in lysates of neutrophil granulocytes of healthy donors (wildtype) and of SCN patients (S730). To study the consequences of point mutations in the G-CSF receptor gene on the nuclear translocation of Stat1 and Stat3, different deletion mutants of the G-CSF receptor were generated and transfected into the murine fibroblast cell line C243 expressing fusion proteins consisting of the transcription factors Stat1 and Stat3, respectively, and the green fluorescent protein (GFP). Nuclear translocation of Stat1-GFP and Stat3-GFP was examined in the unstimulated state and after 1 hour of stimulation with 10^3 U G-CSF/ml in a fluorescence microscope. +, normal; ++, increased; −, no change; n.d., not determined. The number in the name of the G-CSF receptor mutants denotes the length of the protein in amino acids (wildtype = 813 amino acids (aa); S730 = truncated receptor with 730 aa; S685 = truncated receptor with 685 aa; S671 = truncated receptor with 671 aa; S649 = truncated receptor with 649 aa).

motif in the cytoplasmic domain is the longest mutant tested that is incapable of inducing the nuclear translocation of Stat1-GFP and Stat3-GFP.

DISCUSSION

Severe congenital neutropenia or Kostmann's syndrome is characterized by a maturation arrest of neutrophil granulocytes at the stage of promyelocytes or myelocytes in bone marrow, and absence or low levels of mature neutrophil granulocytes in peripheral blood.[12] Therefore, patients with SCN suffer from severe recurrent bacterial infections starting from birth. A subgroup of SCN patients (approximately 15%) developed a secondary acute myeloid leukemia, suggesting that severe congenital neutropenia might be a preleukemic condition.[12] Recently, point mutations

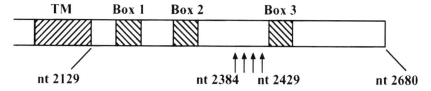

FIGURE 1. Schematic structure of the cytoplasmic domain of the G-CSF receptor protein. The cytoplasmic domain of the G-CSF receptor is shown including the critical region (nucleotides 2384–2429), where point mutations have been found in SCN patients. *Hatched boxes* indicate the conserved domains defined by homology to other members of the cytokine receptor family. TM, transmembrane domain; nt, nucleotide.

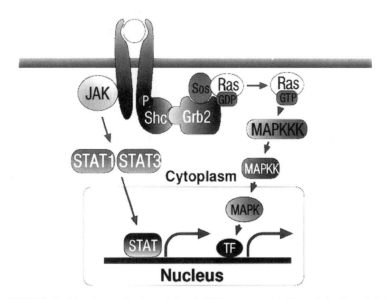

FIGURE 2. Signal transduction of the G-CSF receptor. Binding of the ligand G-CSF induces the homodimerization of G-CSF receptor molecules and the activation of tyrosine kinases of the Jak family. The Jak kinases are recruited to the membrane proximal part of the G-CSF receptor, become autophosphorylated, and can in turn phosphorylate tyrosine residues in the cytoplasmic domain of the G-CSF receptor. These phosphorylated tyrosine residues serve as potential docking sites for proteins with SH2- or phosphotyrosine binding sites (PTB), e.g., the adapter molecules Shc or Grb2, which are involved in the Ras-Raf-MAPK pathway, resulting in the phosphorylation of nuclear transcription factors and regulation of gene expression. Another important pathway is the activation of Stat proteins by Jak kinases. Upon activation of the G-CSF receptor, Stat1 and Stat3 are recruited to the receptor molecule, become phosphorylated by Jak kinases, and can dimerize in the phosphorylated form. The Stat homo- or heterodimers are transported to the nucleus, where they can bind to Stat recognition sites in the promotor regions of different genes resulting in regulation of gene expression.

were found in the G-CSF receptor gene of these patients, resulting in a nonsense mutation leading to the truncation of the cytoplasmic domain of the G-CSF receptor.[1–3,10,11] So far, two major signaling pathways are involved in the G-CSF receptor signal transduction. The Ras-Raf-MAPK-pathway and the Jak-Stat-pathway. Both pathways result in the activation of transcription factors and the regulation of gene expression (FIG. 2). To study the consequences of the observed point mutations in the G-CSF receptor gene on the G-CSF-related signal transduction, we focused our interest on the Jak-Stat-pathway. Using fusion proteins consisting of the transcription factors Stat1 and Stat3, respectively, and the green fluorescent protein, we were able to study the subcellular trafficking of these transcription factors. Stimulation of wildtype G-CSF receptor-transfected C243 cells expressing Stat1-GFP or Stat3-GFP leads to a nulear translocation of the fusion proteins, as judged by a shift of the green fluorescence from the cytosol to the nucleus. According to our experiments point mutations found in a subgroup of patients with SCN and AML should not abrogate nuclear translocation of Stat1-GFP and Stat3-GFP. These experiments do not rule out the possibility that mutations in the Stat molecules might interfere with the gene regulation, although the nuclear translocation and activation of the Stats is unaffected by point mutations in the G-CSF receptor gene.

In conclusion, we could demonstrate that the point mutations in one allele of the G-CSF receptor gene neither abrogate binding of Jak2 protein nor inhibit the translocation of the Stat proteins.

REFERENCES

1. DONG, F., R.K. BRYNES, N. TIDOW, K. WELTE, B. LOWENBERG & I.P. TOUW. 1995. Mutations in the gene for the granulocyte colony-stimulating-factor receptor in patients with acute myeloid leukemia preceded by severe congenital neutropenia [see comments]. N. Engl. J. Med. **333:** 487–493.
2. DONG, F., C. VAN BUITENEN, K. POUWELS, L.H. HOEFSLOOT, B. LOWENBERG & I.P. TOUW. 1993. Distinct cytoplasmic regions of the human granulocyte colony-stimulating factor receptor involved in induction of proliferation and maturation. Mol. Cell. Biol. **13:** 7774–7781.
3. DONG, F., M. VAN PAASSEN, C. VAN BUITENEN, L.H. HOEFSLOOT, B. LOWENBERG & I.P. TOUW. 1995. A point mutation in the granulocyte colony-stimulating factor receptor (G-CSF- R) gene in a case of acute myeloid leukemia results in the overexpression of a novel G-CSF-R isoform. Blood **85:** 902–911.
4. GILMAN, P.A., D.P. JACKSON & H.G. GUILD. 1970. Congenital agranulocytosis: prolonged survival and terminal acute leukemia. Blood **36:** 576–585.
5. NICHOLSON, S.E., A.C. OATES, A.G. HARPUR, A. ZIEMIECKI, A.F. WILKS & J.E. LAYTON. 1994. Tyrosine kinase JAK1 is associated with the granulocyte-colony-stimulating factor receptor and both become tyrosine-phosphorylated after receptor activation. Proc. Natl. Acad. Sci. USA **91:** 2985–2988.
6. PAN, C.X., R. FUKUNAGA, S. YONEHARA & S. NAGATA. 1993. Unidirectional cross-phosphorylation between the granulocyte colony-stimulating factor and interleukin 3 receptors. J. Biol. Chem. **268:** 25818–25823.
7. RAUPRICH, P., B. KASPER, N. TIDOW& K. WELTE. 1995. The protein tyrosine kinase JAK2 is activated in neutrophils from patients with severe congenital neutropenia. Blood **86:** 4500–4505.
8. ROSEN, R.B. & S.J. KANG. 1979. Congenital agranulocytosis terminating in acute myelomonocytic leukemia. J. Pediatr. **94:** 406–408.
9. TIAN, S.S., P. LAMB, H.M. SEIDEL, R.B. STEIN & J. ROSEN. 1 994. Rapid activation of the STAT3 transcription factor by granulocyte colony-stimulating factor. Blood **84:** 1760–1764.
10. TIDOW, N., C. PILZ, B. KASPER & K. WELTE. 1997. Frequency of point mutations in the gene for the G-CSF receptor in patients with chronic neutropenia undergoing G-CSF therapy. Stem Cells **1:** 113–119.
11. TIDOW, N., C. PILZ, B. TEICHMANN, A. MULLER-BRECHLIN, M. GERMESHAUSEN, B. KASPER, P. RAUPRICH, K.W. SYKORA & K. WELTE. 1997. Clinical relevance of point mutations in the cytoplasmic domain of the granulocyte colony-stimulating factor receptor gene in patients with severe congenital neutropenia. Blood **89:** 2369–2375.
12. WELTE, K. & L.A. BOXER. 1997. Severe chronic neutropenia: pathophysiology and therapy [61 refs]. Semin. Hematol. **34:** 267–278.

DISCUSSION

P.J. QUESENBERRY (*University of Massachusetts Medical Center*): I was informed by a New York physician about his seeing one case of cyclical neutropenia that evolved into leukemia. Do you know of any other cases outside the study group, or is that a very rare instance?

WELTE: I hope to learn about this case from David Dale. Until now I have not heard of any patient with cyclic neutropenia who developed leukemia. The problem from the clinical side is the definition of cyclic neutropenia. As you know, it is very hard to verify it at clinical levels. We have patients in our clinical registry who are diagnosed with cyclic neutropenia who really had congenital neutropenias (the Kostmann type) and the other way around. It is possible that if you have 100 cases or more during a period of time, one or another might develop leukemia.

QUESENBERRY: What was the average length of time that the patients were on G-CSF before you saw the mutations in the receptor?

WELTE: The patients I discussed today all started G-CSF treatment between 1988 and 1992. We have not seen any correlation with the age of the patient or with the time of treatment. If you do a dot plot analysis of age versus time of treatment, you see the leukemic patients distributed all over. There is no clear correlation. It may be that in the future there will be an increase in leukemia cases per year. So far we have 2 new AML cases per year. This number has not increased in the past 4 or 5 years.

R. HOFFMAN (*University of Illinois College of Medicine*): Do you have any archival data with cells from patients before the G-CSF era who transformed to acute leukemia? Did they have mutated receptors? And then, what is the receptor status after induction therapy for the leukemia? Does the mutated receptor persist?

WELTE: It is a good question. We tested three patients who developed leukemia. In one patient we saw that the mutation was not present anymore after induction therapy. I should say that the clinical outcome is very poor. Of the 24 patients, none survived, even with bone marrow transplantation. Having leukemia is very bad news for these patients. We should think about therapeutic approaches as soon as a patient develops a receptor mutation. We actually transplanted such a patient about 2 months ago from an HLA identical sibling.

HOFFMAN: Do the patients who do not get G-CSF also have the mutation?

WELTE: We have not had a chance to test it. We have no patient that is not on treatment. We know that prior to treatment with G-CSF, cases were reported in the US, e.g., by Rosen[8] and others who have shown that there is a higher risk for leukemic development.

D.A. WILLIAMS (*Riley Hospital for Children*): I think I am getting at the same thing Dr. Hoffman asked. The data on Kostmann's are strikingly similar to Fanconi anemia, where there is a high incidence of monosomy 7 as well as RAS mutations prior to or at the onset of AML. AML in these children is also fatal. At this point in time, that patient population has been treated, in many cases with G-CSF, because of severe neutropenia. In those children who develop AML, never having seen G-CSF, versus those who develop leukemia on G-CSF, do you see the mutation of the G-CSF receptor in either of those populations?

WELTE: In Germany we have a treatment protocol for patients with aplastic anemia, and there are patients who develop leukemia on G-CSF and not on G-CSF. There was no mutation seen in either group. I do not know about Fanconi's.

D. METCALF (*P.O. Royal Melbourne Hospital*): It seemed to me that most of your studies with truncated receptors were done using Ba/f3. Suppose the truncated mRNA acts in some way as a dominant inhibitor. In your experiments, you need a cell line that has no endogenous transcription of that receptor. Might this have influenced your failure to find an abnormal phenotype in your transfected cells?

WELTE: That is a good question. Since there is no endogenous G-CSF receptor expressed, there is no control mechanism for mutations of the G-CSF receptor protein or mRNA. These cells do not know the stop codon, and they do not know the truncated protein. The truncated protein may be expressed in opposite to the results from patients.

WILLIAMS: This is an interesting point, because we have looked at mutations of the c-kit receptor in cell lines, one of which should have kit expressed, but because the cell line is derived from a W mutant, it is not. The other is a cell line in which kit is a heterologous receptor. We see that the same mutation in these two cell lines leads to completely different phenotypes, even though the effect of the mutation on signaling is apparently similar. In one cell line you get differentiation, and in another cell line you get apoptosis on withdrawal of the supporting growth factor. It goes back to Dr. Kaushansky's talk, too. It makes you wonder whether you need to look at more than one cell line with the receptor mutations.

The Placental/Umbilical Cord Blood Program of the New York Blood Center

A Progress Report

PABLO RUBINSTEIN, JOHN W. ADAMSON,[a] AND CLADD STEVENS

The Lindsley F. Kimball Research Institute of the New York Blood Center, 310 East 67th Street, New York, New York 10021, USA

ABSTRACT: The transplantation of placental/umbilical cord blood (P/CB) has been used successfully to reconstitute bone marrow function in both related and unrelated recipients. We report here the experience of the New York Blood Center P/CB Program. Since its inception in 1992, over 400 unrelated transplants were supported between July 1993 and September 1997. Overall, event-free survival for all diagnoses and ages approached 0.45. Success and rapidity of engraftment correlated most strongly with the degree of human leukocyte antigen (HLA) disparity and cell dose/kg body weight recipient. Acute graft-versus-host disease (GVHD) was common in all patients but, surprisingly, did not differ between those patients who received grafts having one or more antigen mismatches. Chronic GVHD was uncommon and only rarely contributed to death. These results demonstrate the feasibility of large-scale P/CB banking for the provision of cryopreserved stem cell preparations for unrelated transplants. The degree of the program's success argues strongly for additional P/CB banks in order to increase the likelihood of finding a suitable stem cell preparation for patients for whom related matched donors do not exist.

INTRODUCTION

It has been recognized for a number of years that placental/umbilical cord blood (P/CB; neonatal blood) from a variety of mammals contains high concentrations of stem and progenitor cells. This led to the proposal that human P/CB might contain sufficient hematopoietic stem cells to successfully reconstitute bone marrow function if such cells were transplanted into an appropriately prepared recipient.[1–3]

Based on the early experimental evidence, the first P/CB transplant was carried out in a young man with Fanconi anemia in 1988, using a P/CB preparation obtained from the patient's sister at the time of her birth.[4] The patient successfully engrafted and remains alive and well, with no evidence of disease, 8 years after the transplant .

This "proof of principal" generated extreme interest in the possibility of collecting and cryopreserving P/CB stem cell preparations for transplantation into recipients who otherwise could not find a suitable human leukocyte antigen (HLA)-matched unrelated donor.[5,6]

[a]Corresponding author. Phone, 414/937-3803; fax, 414/937-6284; e-mail, jwadamson@bcsew.edu

With this as background, the New York Blood Center (NYBC) established a public P/CB collection, processing, cryopreservation and distribution effort to support patients in need of transplants who had no HLA-matched marrow donor (related or otherwise) available.[5] The program was initiated in 1992 with funding from the National Heart, Lung and Blood Institute of the National Institutes of Health. The first P/CB collection in support of the program was performed on February 1, 1993, and this was followed shortly by the first transplant at Duke University in July of the same year. A second transplant, also performed at Duke, was performed the next month, and that transplant recipient remains alive and well, having now passed the fifth anniversary of the transplant.

Since that time, the number of P/CB stem cell preparations released in support of unrelated patients has grown progressively. To date, the NYBC P/CB program has supported over 700 unrelated transplants world-wide. Currently, 20–30 P/CB stem cell preparations are released for transplantation per month, and the P/CB bank has nearly 8,000 usable units fully characterized, cryopreserved and readily available for those who might benefit. This report summarizes selected outcomes of the first 492 unrelated P/CB transplants.

RESULTS OF THE PROGRAM

As of December 31, 1997, search requests had been received for 5,559 patients from 272 transplant centers.

The level of transplant activity has increased steadily. As of September 1997, 493 patients in 93 transplant centers had undergone P/CB transplants using stem cell preparations from the NYBC bank. Two transplants were performed in 1993, 15 in 1994, 89 in 1995, 210 in 1996 and 225 in 1997.

As the program evolved, P/CB stem cell preparations were considered for transplantation if there were 0–1 HLA mismatches. P/CB stem cell preparations having greater than a 1-antigen mismatch were considered if requested by the transplant center.

Engraftment

Myeloid engraftment was defined as reaching and maintaining an absolute neutrophil count (ANC) of 500/µl on three consecutive days. Platelet engraftment was similarly defined as achieving a platelet count of 50,000/µl for 7 days without platelet transfusion support. In each case, the first day of ANC of 500 or platelet count of 50,000/µl was considered the day of engraftment.

Engraftment occurred in 71% of all patients. The median times to neutrophil and platelet engraftment were 25 and 71 days, respectively, for those who engrafted.

On multivariate analysis, engraftment rates were positively associated with nucleated cell dose and were negatively associated with specific diagnoses, being significantly lower in patients with severe aplastic anemia, Fanconi anemia and chronic myelogenous leukemia (CML), as shown in TABLE 1. The time to engraftment also correlated with nucleated cell dose, with disease category and with HLA disparity, as shown in TABLE 2. Platelet engraftment was also correlated with cell dose, post-transplant infection and graft-versus-host disease (GVHD).

TABLE 1. Incidence of myeloid engraftment by day 42 in recipients of unrelated P/CB transplants

Variable	No.	No.	Engrafted	
			% (Kaplan-Meier Estimates)	P
Diagnostic Group				
CML	40	19	62.6	
Fanconi anemia	34	18	65.5	
Sev. aplasic anemia	18	7	61.6	
All other	386	276	84.9	0.002
WBCs per Kg (pre-cryopreservation, $\times 10^6$):				
≥ 100	52	45	91.1	
75–99	40	32	87.4	
50–74	60	44	83.9	
25–49	179	116	80.3	
8–25	147	83	74.2	< 0.0001

Secondary graft failure occurred in only four patients, and all had posttransplant cytomegalovirus (CMV) infection; three of these four also had severe acute GVHD.

GVHD

Of the 347 patients who lived long enough to experience GVHD, 51% were graded as mild (grades 0–I) , 26% were graded as moderate (grade II) and another 23% were graded as severe (grades III–IV). Severity of acute GVHD correlated with age but only weakly with HLA incompatibility. The least degree of GVHD was seen in 6/6 matches but, after that, the severity and percent of individuals experiencing acute GVHD did not correlate with numbers of antigens mismatched (TABLE 3).

Chronic GVHD was unusual. It was seen in 40 patients and was listed as a contributor to death in only three. Among 145 patients surviving for 6 months or more, only 34 (23%) had chronic GVHD, which correlated with prior acute GVHD but not with HLA disparity. In most cases, acute GVHD was relatively easily managed.

Transplant-Related Events

Transplant-related events (TRE) were defined as death, autologous reconstitution or infusion of a second graft. Leukemic relapse was not included. By 100 days, 47% of patients had experienced a TRE.

Event-free survival (EFS) was defined as the time to the next transplant (of any kind) without autologous recovery or relapse. EFS correlated with diagnosis (worse with Fanconi anemia, severe aplastic anemia and CML), cell dose and HLA disparity. In examining the relationship with HLA disparity, it was found that there was no correlation with the class of mismatch or the level of resolution in Class II mismatches.

TABLE 2. Relative risk for (faster) time to ANC ≥ 500: all patients[a]

Variable	Number of Patients	Relative Risk for Time to ANC ≥ 500 (95% C1)	
		Univariate	Multivariate
Diagnosed with CML, Fanconi anemia, or severe aplastic anemia			
Yes	92	1.0	1.0
No	385	**2.0 (1.5–2.8)*****	**1.9 (1.3–2.6) P = 0.0003**
WBCs per Kg (pre-cryopreservation, $\times 10^6$):			
< 25	147	1.0	1.0
25–49	178	**1.3 (1.01–1.7)***	**1.4 (1.03–1.9) P = 0.033**
50–74	60	**1.7 (1.2–2.4)****	**1.9 (1.2–2.9) P = 0.0040**
75–99	40	**2.2 (1.5–3.4)*****	**2.4 (1.5–4.0) P = 0.0003**
≥ 100	52	**3.1 (2.2–4.5)*****	**3.4 (2.0–5.5) P < 0.0001**
Number of HLA-A, -B, -DR mismatches:			
≥ 2	267	1.0	1.0
1	177	**0.98 (0.8–1.2)**	**0.9 (0.7–1.1) P = 0.37**
None	30	**1.6 (1.05–2.4)***	**1.6 (1.06–2.5) P < 0.025**

[a]P (by univariate analysis): *< 0.05, **< 0.01, ***< 0.001.

The risk of viral infection correlated strongly with the patients' pretransplant CMV antibody status. Posttransplant CMV infection was reported in 24% of seropositive patients and only 3% of seronegative ($p < 0.001$) patients.

Of 316 leukemic patients for whom there are data, 14% experienced relapse. These included 17/151 with acute lymphocytic leukemia, 21/111 with acute myelogenous leukemia, 4/42 with CML, 2/11 with juvenile CML, and 2/10 with lymphoma.

The actuarial probability of leukemic relapse increased with disease stage. Thus, 18%, 25% and 38% of those characterized as having early stage, intermediate or advanced stage disease, respectively, had relapsed by one year.

DISCUSSION

P/CB is becoming more widely accepted as a source of stem cells for marrow reconstitution in both the related and unrelated settings.[7–10] The types of diseases that may benefit from CB transplantation are virtually identical to those for which unrelated bone marrow transplantation is performed.

In the results reported here, there are several insights to assist in guiding P/CB transplants in the future. First, there is a distinct cell dose effect in terms of failure to engraft. Thus, with nucleated cell doses below 5×10^7/kg, the likelihood of pri-

TABLE 3. Graft-versus-host disease among recipients of unrelated P/CB transplants[a]

Variable	No. Patients	Grade 0–I No. (%)	Grade II No. (%)	Grade III–IV No. (%)	P Value
Number of HLA-A, -B, -DR antigens mismatched:					
None	27	20 (74.1%)	5 (18.5%)	2 (7.4%)	
1	135	68 (50.4%)	36 (26.7%)	31 (23.0%)	
2	158	80 (50.6%)	39 (24.7%)	39 (24.7%)	
≥ 3	25	9 (36.0%)	9 (36.0%)	7 (28.0%)	NS

[a]Linear by linear association, $p = 0.027$; 0 vs. ≥1, $p = 0.01$.

mary graft failure increases. However, once engraftment has occurred, patient outcomes are similar above a cell dose of 2.5×10^7/kg.

Second, the cell dose also correlates with time to engraftment, although unpublished observations from this study indicate that a better correlation is between the dose of colony-forming cells/kg body weight than nucleated cell dose.

Third, while the expected degree of acute GVHD was observed, it was generally easily managed, infrequently progressed to chronic GVHD, and, beyond a full (6/6) HLA matched, was unrelated to HLA disparity.

In looking at the effectiveness of CB transplantation for specific disease categories, patients with severe aplastic anemia, Fanconi anemia or CML were less likely to have a successful outcome. The initial engraftment rates for these diseases were 61–64%, while the engraftment rate for all other disease categories was 84%. The EFS at 100 days was 29–32% for patients with diagnoses in the poor risk categories and 53% for those with diseases in the better risk categories.

In just a few short years, the New York Blood Center's Placental/Cord Blood Program has established the feasibility of a community-based P/CB collection, processing and cryopreservation effort and has defined a number of the clinical and laboratory parameters that predict successful engraftment in this setting. As was true in the early days of bone marrow transplantation, the types of patients and their overall clinical condition have improved with increasing experience using P/CB stem cell preparations. At its current level of activity, the Blood Center's P/CB Program is providing stem cell preparations at a rate that approximates 20–25% of the annual activity of the National Marrow Donor Program in the United States.

As the program has grown, and the value of P/CB as source of stem cells becomes better defined, a number of ethical and regulatory issues surrounding the activity have come to the fore.

Importantly, the United States Food and Drug Administration (FDA) has signaled that it plans to regulate P/CB collection, processing and cryopreservation.[11] While this will introduce a level of administrative and regulatory burden to the activity, we believe that it is critical to ensure that specimen handling and processing are carried out with the highest standards.[12,13] Failure to meet these standards could result in a defective P/CB stem cell preparation being released for transplantation, failure of the graft to take or other complication, and a loss of confidence in the reliability of P/CB stem cell preparations to support the transplantation process.

Other issues that will need to be dealt with involve some of the so-called ethical issues surrounding the activity.[14] These include the timing of obtaining consent from the mother/family, the content of the consent obtained, and the linkage of identifiers of the data to both the mother and the neonate. While these are all important considerations, it is critical to remember that the imposition of unwieldy or burdensome requirements, to the extent that they interfere with the efficient collection and banking of P/CB stem cell preparations, denies possible curative therapy for patients in need of transplantation.

REFERENCES

1. BROXMEYER, H.E., G.W. DOUGLAS, G. HANGOC, S. COOPER, J. BARD, D. ENGLISH, M. ARNY, L. THOMAS & E.A. BOYSE. 1989. Human umbilical cord blood as a potential source of transplantable hematopoietic stem/progenitor cells. Proc. Natl. Acad. Sci. USA **86:** 3828–3832.
2. BROXMEYER, H.E., E. GLUCKMAN, A.D. AUERBACH, G.W. DOUGLAS, H. FRIEDMAN, S. COOPER, G. HANGOC, J. KURTZBERG, J. BARD & E.A. BOYSE. 1990. Human umbilical cord blood: a clinically useful source of transplantable hematopoietic stem/progenitor cells. Int. J. Cell Cloning **8:** 76–89.
3. BROXMEYER, H.E., G. HANGOC, S. COOPER, R.C. RIBEIRO, V. GRAVES, M. YODER, J. WAGNER, S. VADHAN-RAJ, L. BENNINGER, P. RUBINSTEIN & E.R. BROUN. 1992. Growth characteristics and expansion of human umbilical cord blood and estimation of its potential for transplantation in adults. Proc. Natl. Acad. Sci. USA **89:** 4109–4113.
4. GLUCKMAN, E., H.E. BROXMEYER, A.D. AUERBACH, H.S. FRIEDMAN, G.W. DOUGLAS, A. DEVERGIE, H. ESPEROU, D. THIERRY, G. SOCIE, P. LEHN *et al.* 1989. Hematopoietic reconstitution in a patient with Fanconi's anemia by means of umbilical-cord blood from an HLA-identical sibling. N. Engl. J. Med. **321:** 1174–1178.
5. RUBINSTEIN, P., R.E. ROSENFIELD, J.W. ADAMSON & C.E. STEVENS. 1993. Stored placental blood for unrelated bone marrow reconstitution. Blood **81:** 679–690.
6. RUBINSTEIN, P. 1993. Placental blood-derived hematopoietic stem cells for unrelated bone marrow reconstitution. J. Hematother. **2:** 207–210.
7. WAGNER, J.E., N.A. KERNAN, M. STEINBUCH, H.E. BROXMEYER & E. GLUCKMAN. 1995. Allogeneic sibling umbilical-cord blood transplantation in children with malignant and non-malignant disease. Lancet **346:** 214–219.
8. KURTZBERG, J., M. LAUGHLIN, M.L. GRAHAM & C. SMITH. 1996. Placental blood as a source of hematopoietic stem cells for transplantation into unrelated recipients. N. Engl. J. Med .**335:** 157–166.
9. WAGNER, J.E., J. ROSENTHAL, R. SWEETMAN, X.O. SHU, S.M. DAVIES, N.K. RAMSAY, P.B. MCGLAVE, L. SENDER & M.S. CAIRO. 1996. Successful transplantation of HLA-matched and HLA-mismatched umbilical cord blood from unrelated donors: analysis of engraftment and acute graft-versus-host disease. Blood **88:** 795–802.
10. GLUCKMAN, E., V. ROCHA, A. BOYER-CHAMMARD, F. LOCATELLI, W. ARCESE, R. PASQUINI, J. ORTEGA, G. SOUILLET, E. FERREIRA, J.P. LAPORTE, M. FERNANDEZ & C. CHASTANG. 1997. Outcome of cord blood transplantation from related and unrelated donors. N. Engl. J. Med.**337:** 373–381.
11. 1998. Request for proposed standards for unrelated allogeneic peripheral and placental/umbilical cord blood hematopoietic stem/progenitor cell products. Federal Register **63**(12): 2985–2988.
12. WAGNER, J.E. 1997. Regulation of placental and umbilical cord blood stem cells. J. Hematother. **6:** 1–3.
13. SIRCHIA, G., P. REBULLA, L. LECCHI, F. MOZZI, R. CREPALDI & A. PARRAVICINI. 1998. Implementation of a quality system (ISO 9000 Series) for placental blood banking. J. Hematother. **7:** 19–35.

14. SUGARMAN, J., V. KAALUND, E. KODISH, M.F. MARSHALL, E.G. REISNER, B.S. WILFOND, P.R. WOLPE & THE WORKING GROUP ON ETHICAL ISSUES IN UMBILICAL CORD BLOOD BANKING. 1997. Ethical issues in umbilical cord banking. JAMA **278:** 938–943.

DISCUSSION

K. KAUSHANSKY (*University of Washington*): A question about a comment you made on platelet engraftment. John Wagner said he thought that platelet engraftment was no slower following cord blood transplants than those receiving matched adult unrelated transplants. Does that imply that many no longer believe there is an intrinsic defect in platelet engrafment using cord blood transplants, or do you think it is too early to be certain?

ADAMSON: I think it is too early to say, but that is a statement Wagner has made on more than one occasion. I am not that familiar with the platelet engraftment times in unrelated adult transplants. It is a little hard to tease out of the literature, but Wagner claims that they are very similar. I think that there probably is an opportunity to improve on platelet engraftment.

H.E. BROXMEYER (*Indiana University*): Two small questions and one small comment. With regard to what you said about the disparity in results of engraftment and GVHD between US centers and non-US centers, do you think it has anything to do with the type of disorders or recipients being treated or the severity of the disease prior to transplantation?

ADAMSON: It could be all of those. One of the things we have learned is that different centers have different ways of scoring GVHD. We have simply taken the reports as they have come to us.

BROXMEYER: Second question. What I gathered from the relationships you showed between matched transplants and mismatched transplants and GVHD is that you are seeing a significant difference between the complete match and the one antigen disparate and also between the complete match and the two antigens or the complete match and three-antigen mismatch. I was curious about your comments on this.

ADAMSON: That is true. If you look strictly at the percentage of individuals with the various grades 0–1, 2, and 3–4 acute GVHD, there is a relationship to HLA disparity, but the percent of individuals with GVHD does not change between 1 and 3 antigens mismatched. That was a surprise. Importantly, in terms of selecting a stem cell preparation for engraftment, this is an acute and relatively easily managed form of GVHD. There is very little chronic GVHD, and there is very little contribution to mortality from chronic GVHD. I would not use GVHD to argue against a one- or two-antigen mismatch. I think you have to look at graft failure and other parameters.

BROXMEYER: The quick comment is that I agree with what you said about John Wagner's comment made in Bormio, Italy about whether granulocyte colony-stimulating factor (G-CSF) is or is not enhancing engraftment. Even though he showed an enhanced effect when he combined the results of his work with those of Joanne Kurtzberg, he was very nervous about trying to make a statement that G-CSF was enhancing engraftment rates.

P.J. QUESENBERRY (*University of Massachusetts Medical Center*): You said that a key issue is whether there is graft-versus-tumor or graft-versus-leukemia. In the data on acute leukemias and unrelated marrow experience, is the relapse rate higher with acute leukemia compared to unrelated transplants?

ADAMSON: I would have to ask the transplant physicians that question, because we supported transplants, particularly early on, in patients that I would classify as high risk in terms of the state of their disease. Consequently, I am not sure that even if our relapse rates were higher than relapse rates observed in mature transplant centers, where you have a large single center experience, that it would count for much.

QUESENBERRY: Just one more question. What is the range of costs for cord bloods? I know some of them go for $15,000–$20,000. What is the cost for cord blood when you send it out?

ADAMSON: Currently, we are funding the activity through a cost recovery component that has been approved by the Food and Drug Administration. We are operating under an Investigational New Drug application (IND). This is something we worked out with the FDA. The cost recovery component means that we charge an amount of money that allows us to continue to collect the number of cord blood samples that matches, in some ratio, the number that are released for transplant purposes. That charge currently is $15,500 per cord blood sample that goes to a transplant center.

W.E. FIBBE (*University Medical Center Leiden*): I would like to go back to this graft failure issue. Cell dose determines the rate of reconstitution, and risk of graft failure is related to both cell dose and HLA disparity.

ADAMSON: There was a correlation. That is correct.

FIBBE: I would expect that in patients with HLA disparity, the risk of graft failure would be increased and that the risk can be reduced by giving more cells. Is that the case or not?

ADAMSON: I am not sure I understood the question.

FIBBE: I would expect that there is an increased risk of graft failure in patients with more mismatches and that you can reduce the risk by giving more cells.

ADAMSON: That could be, but by multivariate analysis, these were independent.

L. KANZ (*Eberhard Karls University*): Just to add to this, let me ask the question the other way around. If you have, for example, a 15-year-old patient with a one-mismatch situation and an intermediate cell dose transplanted, what is the mortality?

ADAMSON: I do not know.

KANZ: If we had a mortality rate of 70% in more than 18 years, I suspect the additional disparity in HLA would go higher.

ADAMSON: No, it is not a mortality of 70%.

FIBBE: In other settings, we know that the risk appears to relate to cell dose, so probably within the limits you are able to give here, you do not see such an effect.

C.J. EAVES (*Terry Fox Laboratory*): Is there any transplant center that has transplanted more than one cord blood sample into a single recipient, or is any center thinking of trying to do that, especially given the data that suggest that mismatches are not going to be as big a problem as one might have thought?

ADAMSON: To my knowledge, we certainly have not provided multiple cord blood stem cell preparations for use in a single patient at the same time. We have provided backup cord blood preparations if there was failure to engraft with the initial cord blood stem cell preparation. We have heard rumors that at least one transplant center in the United States has used multiple cord blood preparations. I have no knowledge of the outcomes.

The Role of Megadose CD34+ Progenitor Cells in the Treatment of Leukemia Patients without a Matched Donor and in Tolerance Induction for Organ Transplantation

YAIR REISNER,[a,c] ESTHER BACHAR-LUSTIG,[a] HONG-WEI LI,[a] FRANCO AVERSA,[b] ANDREA VELARDI,[b] AND MASSIMO F. MARTELLI[b]

[a]*Department of Immunology, The Weizmann Institute of Science, Rehovot, Israel*
[b]*Hematopoietic Stem Cell Transplant Program, Department of Internal and Experimental Medicine, University of Perugia, Perugia, Italy*

ABSTRACT: Throughout the 1980s, transplantation of unmodified (T cell-replete) bone marrow from full haplotype incompatible family donors was associated with an unsuccessful outcome because of graft failure and severe graft-versus-host disease (GVHD), at times affecting up to 90% of recipients. Although extensive T cell depletion of donor bone marrow was successful in preventing GVHD in children with severe combined immunodeficiency disease (SCID), results were disappointing in leukemic patients because the benefit of preventing GVHD was offset by graft failure. Resistance to engraftment appears to be mediated by host-derived cytotoxic T-lymphocyte precursors that survive supralethal conditioning. In the present paper, we review data that show that these genetic histocompatibility barriers can be overcome in stringent mouse models, employing lethally as well as sublethally irradiated recipients, by two major approaches that are synergistic to each other: escalation of hematopoietic progenitor cell dose and the use of nonalloreactive T cells. The former approach is already being successfully implemented in the treatment of leukemic patients.

BACKGROUND

Bone marrow transplantation presents a curative treatment of choice for many patients with leukemia or other hematolgical disorders.[1-5] Despite the world registry network, which includes more than 3 million human leukocyte antigen (HLA)-typed volunteers, about 40% of patients still fail to find a suitably matched donor. On the other hand, virtually every patient possesses a HLA full haplotype mismatched family member. However, the use of such donors has presented a major challenge during the past three decades due to major immunological problems, namely, graft-versus-host disease (GVHD) and graft rejection. During the early 1980s, we and others demonstrated that effective T cell depletion in man can completely prevent GVHD even when haploidentical 3-loci HLA mismatched bone marrow is used.[6] This approach was successfully implemented in the treatment of patients wih severe com-

[c]Corresponding author. Phone, +972 8-934-4023; fax, +972 8-934-4145; e-mail, bfrisner@weizmann.weizmann.ac.il

bined immune deficiency (SCID).[7] In leukemia patients, however, the clinical outcome was disappointing; the benefit of GVHD prevention was offset by a markedly increased rate of graft rejection.[8] This resistance to engraftment was shown to be mediated primarily by host-derived cytotoxic T lymphocytes, and therefore research with mouse models in the late 1980s was focused on the host immunity remaining after lethal total body irradiation (TBI), as well as on new approaches to overcome this barrier to bone marrow allografting. Attempts were made to eradicate the residual resistance by means of cytotoxic drugs or by use of specific monoclonal antibodies. While this approach was shown to effectively enhance engraftment, it has the disadvantage of being associated with an increased risk for infection and for nonspecific toxicity. Another line of investigation, which was more attractive since it avoids the use of additional cytoreduction, was based on manipulations of the donor bone marrow.

In the present paper, we describe two major approaches that led to impressive results in the mouse model: escalation of stem cell dose and the use of nonalloreactive T cells. These approaches are already being implemented in the treatment of leukemic patients.

ENHANCEMENT OF T CELL-DEPLETED BONE MARROW ALLOGRAFTS IN LETHALLY IRRADIATED MICE

Early studies by van Bekkum, Gengozian and others (for review, see Ref. 9) have shown that donor type chimerism can be achieved in lethally irradiated allogeneic as well as xenogeneic recipients upon escalation of bone marrow cell dose. However, engraftment was associated with lethal GVHD and therefore was short lived. The question, whether bone marrow cell escalation could still be effective in the absence of alloreactive T cells, was not trivial and it has been dealt with by several studies.[10–12] In 1989, we demonstrated the quantitative relationship that exists between residual host type immunity and the size of the T cell-depleted bone marrow inoculum by titering the cell dose in a fully allogeneic mouse model. We found that graft rejection could be a complex outcome of several mechanisms involving stem cell competition as well as immunological rejection.[10] We therefore designed a special stringent model that enabled us to evaluate the role of bone marrow cell escalation in dealing with T cell mediated immune rejection. As shown schematically in FIGURE 1, mice

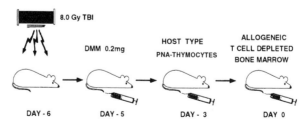

FIGURE 1. Schematic design of mouse model to evaluate the role of bone marrow cell escalation in dealing with T cell-mediated immune rejection. Mice were ablated by a supralethal radiochemotherapy, combining TBI with the myeloablative drug dimethyl myleran, and were reconstituted with different numbers of host type mature thymocytes.

were ablated by a supralethal radiochemotherapy, combining TBI with the myeloablative drug dimethyl myleran, so as to allow engraftment of T cell-depleted bone marrow allografts with minimal graft rejection, similar to that found in autologous transplants. These mice were then reconstituted with increasing numbers of purified host type T cells, as a result of which a marked incidence of graft rejection was documented. Interestingly, this T cell mediated rejection could be overcome by increasing the T cell-depleted bone marrow inoculum.[10] Similar conclusions were also obtained in another stringent mouse model employing recipients presensitized with host type spleen cells,[10] or even in xenogenic rat recipients when the bone marrow cells were from SCID mouse donors.[13]

MOBILIZED PERIPHERAL BLOOD PROGENITOR CELLS

The experiments in the mouse model described above led us to search in recent years for means to increase the availability of stem cells by an order of magnitude. Considering that bone marrow transplants already used the maximal dose that one can collect from the iliac crest by aspiration, we attempted for a while to increase the effective cell dose by expansion with cytokines *ex vivo*. However, with the advent of granulocyte colony-stimulating factor (G-CSF) mobilization, which was shown in the autologous setting to effectively mobilize human CD34 stem cells into the peripheral blood,[14,15] we began in 1993 to treat the donor rather than the recipient with G-CSF, aiming to collect 1 log more stem cells, in accordance with the prediction of the mouse model. The results of the first series of patients treated by this approach showed unequivocally that the problem of graft rejection was reduced to about 10%.[16, 17] These early results were performed in late-stage leukemia patients and therefore, although we showed the concept to be correct, the outcome of the transplants in this initial series was associated with high mortality.

This year we have concluded a study with a second series of patients who were high risk but were prereated with a less toxic conditioning protocol, employing fludarabine instead of cyclophosphamide as well as early posttransplant antiviral and antifungal prophilaxis.[18] Forty-three high-risk acute leukemia patients were conditioned with TBI, thiotepa, fludarabine and antithymocyte globulin. The graft consisted of recombinant human G-CSF-mobilized peripheral blood progenitor cells, and in 28 cases, also bone marrow. Bone marrows were depleted of T-lymphocytes by soybean agglutinin and E-rosetting. T cell depletion of peripheral blood mononuclear cells was achieved by E-rosetting followed by positive selection of CD34[+] cells. No posttransplant prophylaxis for GVHD was administered.

In all patients, full donor type engraftment was achieved (TABLE 1). None of the evaluable patients developed either acute or chronic GVHD. Regimen-related toxicity was minimal. Eleven of the twenty-three patients with acute lymphocytic leukemia (ALL) relapsed, but none of the twenty patients with acute myeloid leukemia (AML). Transplant-related mortality was 35%. With a median follow-up of 18 months (range 2.5–24), 12 of 43 patients are alive and free of disease. All surviving patients have a good quality of life. A major problem following T cell-depleted bone marrow transplantation is an increased risk of relapse.[19, 20] In the present study, relapses occurred in patients with ALL, particularly in those in relapse at the time of

TABLE 1. Hematological parameters and clinical outcome after haploidentical 3-loci HLA mismatched transplants in patients with acute leukemia[a]

		Perugia 2nd series	Tubingen	Vienna
Total number of patients		43	16	4
Median age (years)		22	9	8
Range (years)		4–53	1–18	4–18
Engraftment :	Primary	41/43	13/16	4/4
	Secondary	2/2	3/3	
GVHD (>1)		0/43	0/16	0/4
CD34+/kg × 10^6 (average)		12	15	15
CD3+/kg × 10^3 (average)		31	22	70
Days to ANC >500 (average)		10	12	13
Transplantation-related mortality		16/43	1/16	1/4
Relapse mortality:	ALL	11/23	4/8	0/3
	AML	0/20	3/5	0/1
	MDS	—	0/3	—
Months to CD4 T cells >100 (median)		8	3	n.d.
Disease-free survival		16/43	8/16	3/4
Median follow-up (months)		10	11	6.7
range (months)		2.5 to 24	1 to 29	3.5 to 21

[a]Additional data kindly provided by Dr. Rupert Handgretinger of Tübingen University and Dr. Christina Peters of St. Anna Kinderspital, Vienna (as at April, 1998).

transplant. This was not unexpected and mirrored the relapse rate in similar ALL patients after unmanipulated matched transplants.[19] To date, none of the twenty patients with AML has relapsed, even though all were at high risk. Although the present follow-up is short, in our previous pilot study the cumulative incidence of posttransplant relapse was 28 ± 17% at 4.5 years (minimum follow-up of 3 years) in twelve patients with advanced AML. These results suggest that T cell-depleted mismatched transplants trigger unique graft-versus-leukemia (GVL) effector mechanisms.

A major problem still remaining in our second series of patients is the high incidence of infectious complications, which was probably due to the delayed reconstitution of T cells. Because of this extended period of susceptibility to infection, we administered antiviral and antifungal prophylaxis, but bacterial and fungal infections still resulted in a large proportion of nonleukemic deaths. The slow T cell recovery appears to be due to the low T cell content of the graft. Immunological reconstitution was much faster in our previous series of patients who received one log more T lymphocytes. Unfortunately, this resulted in an 18% incidence of severe GVHD.[16] On the other hand, the growing experience with megadose stem cell transplants in mismatched children (TABLE 1) shows a significantly faster rate of T cell reconstituion. It seems that the slow T cell reconstitution in adults is associated in part with ineffective thymic differentiation.

The overall results, in terms of transplant-related mortality and disease-free survival, in our adult series as well as in the more recent pediatric series in Tübingen and in Vienna (TABLE 1), compare favorably with the expected outcome in patients at the same stage of disease receiving transplants from matched unrelated donors.[21] The high engraftment rate, the elimination of GVHD and the minimal nonhematological toxicity of the conditioning demonstrate that the main obstacles that limited the use of full haplotype mismatched transplantation have been overcome. Since virtually every patient with a hematological malignancy has a mismatched relative, further refinements of this strategy will increase the probability of a cure.

TOLERANCE INDUCTION BY HUMAN CD34+ HEMATOPOIETIC PROGENITOR CELLS

Our results in the first series of leukemia recipients of T cell-depleted megadose transplants could be attributed to several types of accessory cells, as previously shown in murine models employing lethaly irradiated recipients[22–29] or by in vitro studies measuring veto activity of different mouse[30] or monkey[31] bone marrow cell subpopulations.

In our second series of leukemia patients, we began to use megadoses of purified CD34 cells instead of the entire T cell-depleted megadose transplant, and found no reduction of engrafment rate or potency; it seemed that perhaps cells within the highly CD34-enriched cell fraction may possess marked tolerizing activity. We hypothesize that a possible explanation for the induction of tolerance by human CD34+ cells could be found in their unique phenotype, presenting both major hitocompatibility complex (MHC) class I and class II, in the absence of the appropriate B7 costimulatory molecule (FIG. 2) and thus rendering T cells anergic to both MHC class I and class II.

To further investigate the possibility that the CD34+ cells are endowed with veto activity, we purified CD34+ cells by the same procedure employed for transplantation into leukemia patients, and we demonstrated that indeed they are capable of specifically reducing the frequency of cytotoxic T lymphocyte precursors (CTL-p) directed against their antigens, but not against stimulator cells of a third party (TABLE 2).

This veto activity was not found in the unseparated peripheral blood stem cell fraction T cell-depleted by E-rosetting, or in the CD34-negative cell fraction.[32] This suggests that the observed veto activity exhibited by the CD34+ cell fraction could not be explained as an artifact due to cold target inhibition. Similarly to previous reports on other cells with veto properties,[31, 33] the specific reduction of CTL-p mediated by the CD34+-enriched cell fraction was completely ablated by 30 Gy gamma irradiation,[32] and it was also dependent on cell contact between the responder cells and the added CD34+ cells. Thus, when purified CD34+ cells were added to the primary mixed lymphocyte culture (MLC) in transwell flasks, and thereby were separated from the responder alloreactive cells by a membrane through which cytokines but not cells can pass, their veto activity was lost.

These results showed for the first time that the same CD34+ enriched fraction, which we used for transplantation in mismatched leukemia patients, possesses all the typical attributes of veto cells. This veto activity of CD34+ progenitor cells might be

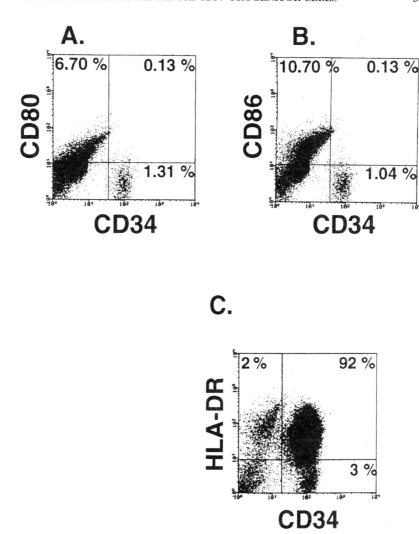

FIGURE 2. Phenotype of CD34⁺ cells. Donors received rhG-CSF (12 mg/kg/day, in two subcutaneous (s.c.) injections), and two leukaphereses were performed on days 4 and 5. The leukapheresis product was then washed and the cells were stained with the indicated fluorescently-labeled monoclonal antibodies and analyzed on a Becton-Dickinson FACScan analyzer (**A** and **B**). The CD34-positive cells were then purified and stained with anti-HLA-DR monoclonal antibody (**C**). (From Rachamim *et al.*[32] Reprinted by permission from *Transplantation*.)

mediated by cells other than the most primitive pluripotential hematopoietic stem cells and, therefore, while it is still very difficult to expand the latter cells *ex vivo*, it may be possible to expand the CD34⁺ veto cells *in vitro* and use them together with a small number of pluripotential cells for transplantation. Further fractionation of CD34⁺ cells might answer this possibility.

INDUCTION OF DONOR TYPE CHIMERISM ACROSS MAJOR HISTOCOMPATIBILITY BARRIERS IN SUBLETHALLY IRRADIATED MICE

A second major question raised by our finding that megadose stem cell transplants led to markedly stable and prompt engraftment in the leukemia patients, was whether it will be possible to reduce the toxicity of the preparatory protocol for patients whose treatment does not require exposure to supralethal radiochemotherapy. To address this question, we reinvestigated in the mouse model the quantitative relationship between cell dose and TBI dose in the sublethal range. Different groups of C3H/HeJ mice were conditioned by a single dose of TBI in the range of 5.5 to 8.5 Gy and then transplanted with increasing doses of T cell-depleted bone marrow from C57BL/6 donors. Donor type chimerism determination one month posttransplant revealed that while engraftment was, as expected, most effective in mice conditioned with lethal 8.5 Gy, requiring a transplant dose of only 10×10^6 cells, it could nevertheless also be generated following conditioning with a sublethal irradiation dose. When TBI was gradually decreased to 7.5 Gy, 6.5 Gy and 6.0 Gy, the bone marrow dose had to be increased by about 2-, 4- and 20-fold, respectively (FIG. 3) in order to obtain more than 50% donor type chimerism in the peripheral blood. Survival rate of control mice, receiving the same decreasing doses of TBI but without a transplant, was about 80% to 95%, whereas the control mice that received 8.5 Gy, without transplant, all died within the first 2 weeks post-TBI.[34]

Based on these initial results we chose to further evaluate the potential application of the minimal sublethal TBI dose (6.5 Gy) that can still be engrafted with donor

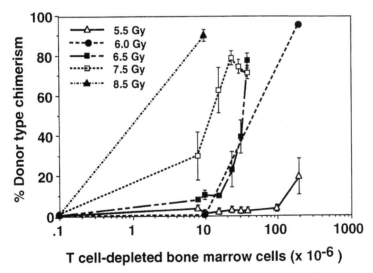

FIGURE 3. Induction of donor type chimerism in sublethally irradiated mice. Donor type chimera in different groups of C3H/HeJ mice conditioned with decreasing doses of TBI and transplanted with increasing numbers of T cell-depleted bone marrow from C57BL/6 donors. (From Bacher-Lustig *et al.*[34] Reprinted by permission from *Nature Medicine*.)

type cells upon transplantation of a relatively reasonable T cell-depleted bone marrow cell dose (40×10^6 cells). Thus, in six separate experiments, transplantation of 40×10^6 cells into recipients conditioned with 6.5 Gy TBI, led to donor type chimerism above 15% in 79 out of 99 recipients. The average donor type chimerism in the 79 engrafted mice was $77 \pm 3.8\%$, and the overall chimerism in the entire group of 99 transplanted mice was $67 \pm 3.7\%$.[34]

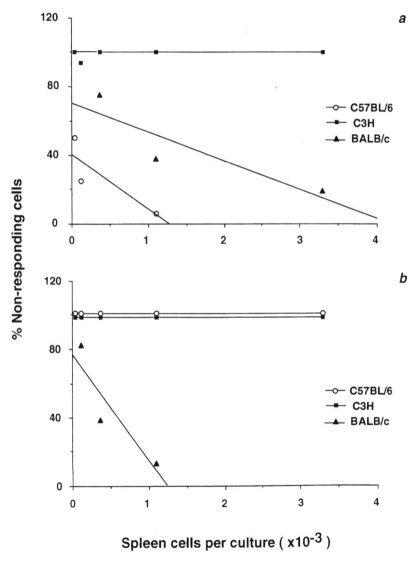

FIGURE 4. Analysis of CTL-p in spleen of sublethally irradiated mice following transplantation of a conventional dose and megadose of T cell-depleted bone marrow. (From Bacher-Lustig *et al.*[34] Reprinted by permission from *Nature Medicine.*)

The marked mixed chimerism found within the spleen T cell compartment of long-term chimera indicates that the substantial number of host type T cells present in these mice must be completely tolerized towards donor type antigens. To evaluate quantitatively the frequency of CTL-p against donor, host and third party cells, we performed limit-dilution analysis of CTL-p and we found that while in recipients of 10×10^6 T cell-depleted bone marrow cells the frequency of antidonor CTL-p was 1/333, no such cells could be detected in recipients of 40×10^6 T cell-depleted bone marrow cells (FIG. 4). Likewise, antihost CTL-p were undetectable, while anti-third party CTL-p were present at a level (1/167) comparable to that found in the recipients of 10×10^6 bone marrow cells (which rejected the graft) suggesting that the absence of antihost and antidonor CTL-p is due to specific tolerance induction and cannot be attributed to a general state of immune deficiency in the allogeneic chimera. The graft rejection in the recipients of the small bone marrow inoculum was found to be associated with antidonor CTL-p frequency (1/333) higher than that found against the third party target cells (1/500), demonstrating the relevance of the antidonor CTL-p to the rejection of the transplanted bone marrow.

In order to test the possible tolerizing activity of cells within the early hematopoietic stem cell fraction, we attempted to purify by magnetic beads Sca-1$^+$Lin$^-$ bone marrow cells from C57BL/6 donors, and we tested their capacity to induce tolerance in fully allogeneic C3H/HeJ recipients exposed to sublethal 7 Gy TBI.[35] The average frequency of these cells in the initial bone marrow fraction which was applied to the magnetic activating cell sorting (MACS) procedure (depleted of red cells and neutrophils by Ficoll separation) was $2.5 \pm 0.9\%$ (range = 1.8–2.7%) and after the two step fractionation it was enriched to an average of $65.0 \pm 7.5\%$ (range = 53.5–77.6%). Determination of donor type chimerism following infusion of different cell numbers from the Sca-1$^+$Lin$^-$ cell fraction revealed an exponential dose response curve similar to those described above for T cell-depleted transplants.[34] In the control group, in which the C3H/HeJ recipients of C57BL/6 Sca-1$^+$Lin$^-$ bone marrow cells were exposed to 10 Gy lethal TBI, about 50–100-fold less cells were capable of inducing donor type chimerism. It seems that in the sublethal model a large proportion of the cells are actually required in order to overcome the host immune cells remaining after 7 Gy TBI, which present a much larger barrier compared to the miniscule numbers surviving 10 Gy TBI.

In order to reduce the effective number of Sca-1$^+$Lin$^-$cells needed for tolerance induction, we were interested in studying the potential role of other facilitating or veto cells. Thus, very recently we found that the addition of nonalloreactive (donor $\times$ host)F_1 T cells, previously shown[11,12] to exhibit marked enhancement of engraftment of T cell-depleted transplants in mismatched lethally irradiated recipients, could also help to reduce the minimal number of stem cells required for chimerism induction in the sublethal model.

These experiments were not only useful for finding a novel approach to reduce the minimal number of Sca-1$^+$Lin$^-$ cells required for the induction of tolerance, but they also enabled us to address the possible duality of Sca-1$^+$Lin$^-$ stem cells that can affect chimerism induction, either by tolerizing the host immune system or by competing with host hematopoietic stem cells. Thus, by testing whether the engraftment of the latter cells is enhanced by Sca-1$^+$Lin$^-$ cells, we were able to separate *in vivo* the potent tolerizing activity associated with the purified Sca-1$^+$Lin$^-$ cells from their

TABLE 2. Specificity of CD34+ cells inhibitory activity

	Cell Origin		CTL Activity[a]	
	Stimulator and Target	CD34+	% Killing	% Inhibition
Experiment 1	A	—	42 ± 5.2	—
	A	A	6 ± 5.9	85.7
	B	—	55 ± 8.7	—
	B	A	43 ± 8.2	21.8
Experiment 2	A	—	25 ± 2.9	—
	A	A	4.4 ± 1.7	82.4
	B	—	45.4 ± 7.2	—
	B	A	30 ± 5.0	33.9
Experiment 3	A	—	63.0 ± 10.0	—
	A	A	32.3 ± 3.3	48.7
	B	—	43.3 ± 7.0	—
	B	A	41.8 ± 11.0	3.4

[a]CD34+ purified cells from donor A were added to a primary mixed lymphocyte culture (MLC), consisting of responder cells (from donor C) and irradiated allogeneic stimulator cells from either donor A or B. After 5 days, the responder cells were isolated, restimulated with allogeneic cells in a secondary MLC and 7 days later CTL activity against the appropriate target cells (having the same origin as the stimulators) was measured using a ^{51}Cr-release assay. The inhibition of CTL activity was calculated, taking as reference the killing activity in absence of stem cells. (Data from Rachamim *et al.*[32])

hematopoietic repopulating capacity, which might also contribute to donor type chimerism induction.

In man, nonalloreactive T cells can be generated by purging interleukin-2 receptor (CD25) mixed lymphocyte reaction (MLR)-reactive T cells[36] or by anergy induction upon incubation with CTLA-4.[20, 37]

CONCLUDING REMARKS

The conclusion that stem cell escalation can be used to induce transplantation tolerance in sublethally irradiated recipients has remarkable implications for many areas of clinical investigation as it might lead to the cure of diseases other than leukemia, for which the application of the lethal radiochemotherapy used in cancer patients is not ethical. For example, if we shall succeed in achieving hemopoietic chimerism in man under conditions that pose a minimal risk, we could think of curing sickle cell anemia, enzyme deficiencies, and autoimmunity, as well as use tolerance induction as a prelude for organ transplantation or for cell therapy with allogeneic cells in cancer patients.

As we have already achieved this goal in the mouse model, we have decided to embark on preclinical studies in a primate model. Preliminary results already show that, as can be expected, the challenge of overcoming rejection by stem cell escalation in the outbred setting is more difficult than in the mouse model. However, we hope that the application of nonalloreactive T cells in conjunction with megadose

CD34 cells, will pave the way for a successful induction of durable donor type chimerism in this sublethal preclinical primate model.

In addition, we shall attempt to identify the tolerizing cells within the CD34 cell fraction in the hope of expanding *ex vivo* these valuable cells. By achieving this goal, it may be possible to induce donor type chimerism in lethally irradiated primates upon infusion of regular doses of hematopoietic stem cells.

REFERENCES

1. THOMAS, E. 1983. Marrow transplantation for malignant disease. J. Clin. Oncol. **1:** 517–531.
2. KERNAN, N., G. BARTSCH, R. ASH, P.G. BEATTY, R. CHAMPLIN, A. FILIPOVICH, J. GAJEWSKY, J.A. HANSEN, J. HENSLEE-DOWNEY, J. MCCULLOUGH, P. MCGLAVE, H.A. PERKINS, G.L. PHILLIPS, J. SANDERS, D. STRONCEK, E.D. THOMAS & K.G. BLUME. 1993. Retrospective analysis of 462 unrelated marrow transplants facilitated by the National Marrow Donor Program (NMDP) for treatment of acquired and congenital disorders of the lymphohematopoietic system and congenital metabolic disorders. N. Engl. J. Med. **328:** 593–602.
3. CHAMPLIN, R. 1993. Bone marrow transplantation for leukemia utilizing HLA-matched unrelated donors. Bone Marrow Transplant. **11:** 74–77.
4. ANASETTI, C., R. ETZIONI, E. PETERSDORF, P. MARTIN & J. HANSEN. 1995. Marrow transplantation from unrelated volunteer donors. Annu. Rev. Med. **46:** 169–179.
5. BEATTY, P., M. MORI & E. MILFORD. 1995. Impact of racial genetic polymorphism on the probability of finding an HLA-matched donor. Transplantation **60:** 778–783.
6. REISNER, Y., N. KAPOOR, D. KIRKPATRICK, M.S. POLLACK, B. DUPONT, R.A. GOOD & R.J. O'REILLY. 1981. Transplantation for acute leukaemia with HLA-A and B non-identical parental marrow cells fractionated with soybean agglutinin and sheep red blood cells. Lancet **2:** 327–331.
7. REISNER, Y., N. KAPOOR, D. KIRKPATRICK, M.S. POLLACK, R.S. CUNNINGHAM, B. DUPONT, M.Z. HODES, R.A. GOOD & R.J. O'REILLY. 1983. Transplantation for severe combined immunodeficiency with HLA-A,B,D,DR incompatible parental marrow cells fractionated by soybean agglutinin and sheep red blood cells. Blood **61:** 341–348.
8. GALE, R.P. & Y. REISNER. 1986. Graft rejection and graft-versus-host disease: mirror images. Lancet **1:** 1468–1470.
9. VAN-BEKKUM, D.W. & B.E. LOWENBERG. 1985. Bone Marrow Transplantation: Biological Mechanisms and Clinical Practice. Marcel Dekker. New York.
10. LAPIDOT, T., A. TERENZI, T.S. SINGER, O. SALOMON & Y. REISNER. 1989. Enhancement by dimethyl myleran of donor type chimerism in murine recipients of bone marrow allografts. Blood **73:** 2025–2032.
11. LAPIDOT, T., I. LUBIN, A. TERENZI, Y. FAKTOROWICH, P. ERLICH & Y. REISNER. 1990. Enhancement of bone marrow allografts from nude mice into mismatched recipients by T cells void of graft-versus-host activity. Proc. Natl. Acad. Sci. USA **87:** 4595–4599.
12. LAPIDOT, T., Y. FAKTOROWICH, I. LUBIN & Y. REISNER. 1992. Enhancement of T-cell-depleted bone marrow allografts in the absence of graft-versus-host disease is mediated by $CD8^+ CD4^-$ and not by $CD8^- CD4^+$ thymocytes. Blood **80:** 2406–2411.
13. LUBIN, I., Y. FAKTOROWICH, T. LAPIDOT, Y. GAN, Z. ESHHAR, E. GAZIT, M. LEVITE & Y. REISNER. 1991. Engraftment and development of human T and B cells in mice after bone marrow transplantation. Science **252:** 427–431.
14. SHERIDAN, W.P., C. GLENN-BEGLEY, C.A. JUTTNER, J. SZER, T. BIK, D. MAHER, K.M. MCGRATH, G. MORSTYN & R.M. FOX. 1992. Effect of peripheral-blood progenitor cells mobilised by filgrastin (G-CSF) on platelet recovery after high-dose chemotherapy. Lancet **339:** 640–644.

15. BENSINGER, W., J. SINGER, F. APPELBAUM, K. LILLEB, K. LONGIN, S. ROWLEY, E. CLARKE, R. CLIFT, J. HANSEN, T. SHIELDS, R. STORB, C. WEAVER, P. WEIDEN & C.D. BUCKNER. 1993. Autologous transplantation with peripheral blood mononuclear cells collected after administrtion of recombinant granulocyte stimulating factor. Blood **81:** 3158–3165.

16. AVERSA, F., A. TABILIO, A. TERENZI, A. VELARDI, F. FALZETTI, C. GIANNONI, R. IACUCCI, T. ZEI, M.P. MARTELLI, C. GAMBELUNGHE, M. ROSSETTI, P. CAPUTO, P. LATINI, C. ARISTEI, C. RAYMONDI, Y. REISNER & M.F. MARTELLI. 1994. Successful engraftment of T-cell-depleted haploidentical "three-loci" incompatible transplants in leukemia patients by addition of recombinant human granulocyte colony-stimulating factor-mobilized peripheral blood progenitor cells to bone marrow inoculum. Blood **84:** 3948–3955.

17. REISNER, Y. & M.F. MARTELLI. 1995. Bone marrow transplantation across HLA barriers by increasing the number of transplanted cells. Immunol. Today **16:** 437–440.

18. AVERSA, F., A. TABILIO, A. VELARDI, I. CUNNINGHAM, A. TERENZI, F. FALZETTI, L. RUGGERI, G. BARBABIETOLA, C. ARISTEI, P. LATINI, Y. REISNER & M.F. MARTELLI. 1998. Transplantation for high-risk acute leukemia with high doses of T-cell-depleted hematopoietic stem cells from full-haplotype incompatible donors. N. Engl. J. Med. In press.

19. ALLISON, J.P. 1994. CD28-B7 interactions in T-cell activation. Curr. Opin. Immunol. **6:** 414–419.

20. BOUSSIOTIS, V.A., J.G. GRIBBEN, G.J. FREEMAN & L.M. NADLER. 1994. Blockade of the CD28 co-stimulatory pathway: a means to induce tolerance. Curr. Opin. Immunol. **6:** 797–807.

21. SIERRA, J., B. STORER, J.A. HANSEN, J. W. BJERKE, P.J. MARTIN, E.W. PETERSDORF, F.R. APPELBAUM, E. BRYANT, T.R. CHAUNCEY, G. SALE, J.E. SANDERS, R. STORB, K.M. SULLIVAN & C. ANASETTI. 1997. Transplantation of marrow cells from unrelated donors for treatment of high-risk leukemia: the effect of leukemic burden, donor HLA-matching and marrow cell dose. Blood **89:** 4226–4235.

22. COBBOLD, S.P., G. MARTIN, S. QIN & H. WALDMANN. 1986. Monoclonal antibodies to promote marrow engraftment and tissue graft tolerance. Nature **323:** 164–166.

23. STROBER, S., V. PALATHUMPAT, R. SCHWADRON & B. HERTEL-WULFF. 1987. Cloned natural suppressor cells prevent lethal graft-vs-host disease. J. Immunol. **138:** 699–703.

24. KIKUYA, S., M. INABA, H. OGATA, R. YASUMIZU & K. INABA. 1988. Wheat germ agglutinin-positive cells in a stem cell-enriched fraction of mouse bone marrow have potent natural suppressor activity. Proc. Natl. Acad. Sci. USA **85:** 4824–4826.

25. TSCHERNING, T. & M. CLAESSON. 1991. Veto-like down regulation of T helper cell reactivity *in vivo* by injection of semi-allogeneic spleen cells. Immunol. Lett. **29:** 223–228.

26. KIYOSHI, H., K. HIRUMA, H. NAKAMURA, P.A. HENKART & R.E. GRESS. 1992. Clonal deletion of postthymic T cells: veto cells kill precursor cytotoxic T lymphocytes. J. Exp. Med. **175:** 863–868.

27. PIERCE, G.E. & L.M. WATTS. 1993. Do donor cells function as veto cells in the induction and maintenance of tolerance across an MHC disparity in mixed lymphoid radiation chimeras? Transplantation **55:** 882–887.

28. PIERCE, G.E. & L.M. WATTS. 1993. Thy 1+ donor cells function as veto cells in the maintenance of tolerance across a major histocompatibility complex disparity in mixed-lymphoid radiation chimeras. Transplant. Proc. **25:** 331–333.

29. KAUFMAN, C.L., Y.L. COLSON, S.M. WREN, S. WATKINS, R.L. SIMMONS & S.T. ILDSTAD. 1994. Phenotypic characterization of a novel bone marrow-derived cell that facilitates engraftment of allogeneic bone marrow stem cells. Blood **84:** 2436–2446.

30. SAMBHARA, S.R. & R.G. MILLER. 1991. Programmed cell death of T cells signaled by the T cell receptor and the alpha 3 domain of class I MHC. Science **252:** 1424–1427.

31. THOMAS, J.M., F.M. CARVER, P.R. CUNNINGHAM, L.C. OLSON & F.T. THOMAS. 1991. Kidney allograft tolerance in primates without chronic immunosuppression—the role of veto cells. Transplantation **51:** 198–207.
32. RACHAMIM, N., J. GAN, H. SEGALL, R. KRAUTHGAMER, H. MARCUS, A. BERRREBI, M. MARTELLI & Y. REISNER. 1998. Tolerance induction by "megadose" hematopoietic transplants: donor-type human CD34 stem cells induce potent specific reduction of host anti-donor cytotoxic T lymphocyte precursors in mixed lymphocyte culture. Transplantation **65:** 1386–1393.
33. THOMAS, J.M., F.M. CARVER, J. KASTEN-JOLLY, C.E. HAISCH, L.M. REBELLATO, U. GROSS, S.J. VORE & F.T. THOMAS. 1994. Further studies of veto activity in rhesus monkey bone marrow in relation to allograft tolerance and chimerism. Transplantation **57:** 101–115.
34. BACHAR-LUSTIG, E., N. RACHAMIM, H.W. LI, F. LAN & Y. REISNER. 1995. Megadose of T cell-depleted bone marrow overcomes MHC barriers in sublethally irradiated mice. Nat. Med. **1:** 1268–1273.
35. REISNER, Y., E. BACHAR-LUSTIG, H.W. LI, N. RACHAMIM, H. SEGALL, H. MARCUS, A. BERREBI, M. F. MARTELLI & Y. GAN. 1997 Purified Sca-1$^+$Lin$^-$ stem cells can tolerize fully allogeneic host T cells remaining after sublethal TBI. (ASH meeting, San Diego, CA, Abst. 2507) Blood **90:** 2563a.
36. CAVAZZANA CALVO, M., J.L. STEPHAN, S. SARNACKI, S. CHEVRET, C. FROMONT, C. DE COENE, F. LE DEIST, D. GUY GRAND & A. FISCHER. 1994. Attenuation of graft-versus-host disease and graft rejection by *ex vivo* immunotoxin elimination of alloreactive T cells in an H-2 haplotype disparate mouse combination. Blood **83:** 288–298.
37. GRIBBEN, J.G., E.C. GUINAN, V.A. BOUSSIOTIS, X.Y. KE, L. LINSLEY, C. SIEFF, G.S. GRAY, G.J. FREEMAN & L.M. NADLER. 1996. Complete blockade of B7 family-mediated costimulation is necessary to induce human alloantigen-specific anergy: a method to ameliorate graft- versus-host disease and extend the donor pool. Blood **87:** 4887–4893.

DISCUSSION

L. KANZ (*Eberhard Karls University*): You indicate that the CD34$^+$ cells, per se, can induce anergy in the mismatched setting. So, in effect, it may be possible to expand those progenitor cells. You may not need to expand stem cells.

REISNER: Maybe. We do not know which cell is doing this within the CD34 compartment. It could be cells that are not pluripotential hematopoietic cells, and then we should be in good shape.

KANZ: Have you no data so far with your CTL assays?

REISNER: No, we are just beginning. Right now we are looking more at the mechanism of anergy. We are trying to establish this. It is not easy, because we need a large number of human CD34 cells from the same donor who is giving us his T cells.

KANZ: You imply that you do not need high-dose stem cells but high-dose CD34 cells.

REISNER: Perhaps. These are known in the literature as veto cells or tolerizing cells—many names. Maybe they are within this compartment.

B. TOROK-STORB (*Fred Hutchinson Cancer Research Center*): We have seen suppression of allograft reactions with the CD34-enriched product from peripheral blood mononuclear cells (PBMCs), but when you look at those cells, the vast majority of them are in fact CD33$^+$ and CD13$^+$. Very shortly upon culture they become CD14$^+$, and they make huge amounts of IL-10. We could neutralize their ability to inhibit an allograft reaction with antibodies against IL-10. So I would argue that it is not in fact the stem cell in that component that is responsible for this anergy-inducing effect, but more likely another cell type. So there would be a danger in trying to expand the product of possibly losing that cell type.

REISNER: Again, I do not know which cells within the CD34 population are responsible for the tolerizing effect, but I think we are talking about different cells. We try to remove CD14, CD13 cells. They are not there.

TOROK-STORB: I know they are not there to start, but they become that.

REISNER: CD13 or CD14 monocytes were shown in the literature to induce nonspecific tolerance. This is sort of nonspecific paralysis, so they will not be compatible with the control experiment, which is extremely important. In the control experiment, if you remember, the responder cells were reactive against a third party, in the presence of donor type CD34 cells. I know that monocytes and macrophages were described in the past to exhibit nonspecific immune suppression.

TOROK-STORB: I would still suggest it is not the stem cell.

REISNER: I think we still have to do some more work to identify, characterize and purify them. It may or may not be a pluripotential stem cell; it is a CD34 cell, but I do not know which yet. It is not a monocyte, or a T cell contaminant present in the initial CD34 cell fraction. It is not any of these, because we take great care to remove them, but it could be a cell derived from the CD34 cells within a very short time after the initiation of the culture. We know that if you add the CD34 cells 24 hours after initiation they cannot inhibit generation of CTLs.

KANZ: I would like to mention that the CD34⁺ fraction, expanded by stem cell factor (SCF), IL-3, IL-6, IL-1 and erythropoietin (Epo) is highly active in antigen presentation . So this goes in the same direction.

P.J. QUESENBERRY (*University of Massachusetts Medical Center*): To put it in a different context, it looks like you can come down to very low levels of radiation, say 100 cGy or maybe no radiation, if you get very high levels of stem cells and come in with a costimulator blockade in those settings. It has not been done with T cell depletion.

REISNER: It is my approach. The big challenge in my opinion is to achieve tolerance without T cells. The allograft reactive T cells that are in the unseparated transplants are a wild horse. It is very hard to control them. If we can do it without T cells, I think we have a nice open road for tolerance. I would take more time and maybe your approach of anti-CD40 ligand would synergize very nicely. Right now, in primates, we are up to 700 rads, which is still sublethal, fludarabine and antithymocyte globulin (ATG), together with a megadose of stem cells, and we are still seeing rejection. So I am very skeptical of going down to 100 rads. It may be possible with T cells in the bone marrow innoculum, but, again, you are limited to matched identical transplants and to GVHD prophylaxis, so as to reduce the likelihood of GVHD. However, it will not be acceptable for nonmalignant patients, because you do not want to take a sickle cell anemia patient and expose him to GVHD risk or infections. It may take another 2 years, but if we learn how to do it without T cells, with purified stem cells, we will really be in good shape. This is my more favorable approach.

B.P. SORRENTINO (*St. Jude Children's Research Hospital*): I have one comment. In terms of engraftment as a function of stem cell dose in unablated or minimally ablated patients, you really emphasize the immune effects. Is it not true that in SCID patients who receive haploidentical transplants, they very rarely engraft with myeloid cells or B cells when they receive no conditioning, suggesting that a really important effect is the stem cell dose? That is a naturally occurring experiment in a host that has no T cells.

REISNER: That is a very good point. It shows that you need some ablation. In SCID patients, megadose transplants were tested. Wilhelm Freidrich in Germany gave a megadose of stem cells to a SCID patient, and still he could only get engraftment within the T lineage, nothing in the myeloid. So maybe in humans, even in the absence of a significant immune system, such as in SCID, you may still need more than the large dose of $10–20 \times 10^6$ CD34 cells per kg that was given, in the absence of ablation. Clearly, those SCID patients are a very good test case, because they tell you it is very hard to compete with the existing stem cells for the myeloid lineage.

J.D. GRIFFIN (*Dana Farber Cancer Institute*): If you are really seeing induction of anergy in the CD34 cultures, you should see antigen-restricted suppression of IL-2 gene expression. Have you looked for IL-2 expression?

REISNER: We are looking at it now by RT-PCR as well as by intracellular staining, which is not the most sensitive method, but it shows you which cells are tolerized.

GRIFFIN: Could you not just measure IL-2 secretion in the culture?

REISNER: We could, and one way of doing it is by ELISPOT analysis, which is even more elegant. We are doing all these things. It will take time, about one experiment per month, because of the shortage of cells.

P.M. LANSDORP (*Terry Fox Laboratory*): In the clinical study that you were referring to, you had very encouraging results with AML in that there was little relapse, and you were relating that to a possible natural killer (NK) effect. However, you were using purified CD34 cells in the transplant. So where did the NK cells come from?

REISNER: It is very interesting, and I did not have time to cover this issue in detail. In all the haploidentical transplants, the first cells that come shooting up after the transplant are NK cells. Much later you see the T cells coming, and a large proportion of them bear the killer inhibitory receptor (KIR). And when you test those KIR-positive NK or T cells against blasts from patients, you always see very nice lysis by the NK cells of the AML blasts, but you hardly see killing of ALL blasts. This is something that Andrea Velardi from Perugia, Italy, is now doing and collecting all the data. He has already published some of it and has made very nice progress with this. Although it is very hard to prove the cause of relapse, which could involve several factors, there is a striking difference between AML and ALL. If we knew why ALL blasts are more resistant to KIR-positive alloreactive NK or T cells, we could get to new insight into GVL.

Transplantation of Megadoses of Purified Haploidentical Stem Cells

R. HANDGRETINGER,[a,d] M. SCHUMM,[a] P. LANG,[a] J. GREIL,[b] A. REITER,[c]
P. BADER,[a] D. NIETHAMMER,[a] AND T. KLINGEBIEL[a]

[a]Children's University Hospital, University of Tübingen, Germany
[b]Children's University Hospital, University of Erlangen-Nürnberg, Germany
[c]Children's University Hospital, Medical School, Hannover, Germany

ABSTRACT: Peripheral mobilized parental CD34+ progenitors were isolated and used for the hematopoietic reconstitution after a myeloablative therapy in 23 pediatric patients with various diseases. Fourteen donors were human leukocyte antigen (HLA) three-loci mismatches, 6 donors were two-loci and 3 donors were one-locus mismatches. For depletion of T-lymphocytes, a positive selection of the mobilized peripheral CD34+ progenitors using the method of magnetic-activated cell sorting (MACS) was used. The purity of the CD34+ cells after MACS-sorting was 98–99%, the average number of transplanted CD34+ cells was 14.2 × 10^6/kg (range 5.4–3 9 × I 0^6/kg) and the average number of infused T-lymphocytes was 1.4 × 10^4/kg. Due to this low T cell number, only a short-term or no prophylaxis of graft-versus-host disease (GVHD) was necessary and no GVHD was seen. A significant GVHD was only seen in patients after add-back of donor T-lymphocytes, which was performed in some patients for prevention of relapse or in patients who showed a transient mixed chimerism. Since the B lymphocyte contamination of the isolated CD34+ cells was low in the range of 0.2%, no Epstein-Barr virus (EBV)-associated lymphoproliferative syndrome was observed. A primary engraftment was seen in 18 patients. Nonengraftment and rejection occurred in three and two patients, respectively. In four of these 5 patients, a second transplant using purified CD34+ cells from the same donor after an *immunological* reconditioning regimen resulted in a complete and sustained hematopoietic reconstitution. The speed of the immunological recovery was dependent on the number of transplanted CD34+ cells and was more rapid if this number was >20 × 10^6/kg. Eleven of the 23 patients are alive and disease free with a median follow-up of 12 months (range 2–30). The main cause of death was relapse (7 patients), and only one fatal infection was seen. Our data suggest that the transplantation of megadoses of haploidentical CD34+ cells is a realistic therapeutic option for patients who otherwise have no suitable donor, and an alternative to the use of unrelated cord blood.

INTRODUCTION

Allogeneic transplantation is the only treatment modality for some malignant and nonmalignant diseases that might be able to offer a cure for these patients. Until re-

[d]Address for correspondence: Rupert Handgretinger, MD, Department of Pediatrics, Eberhard Karls University, Hoppe-Seyler-Str. 1, D-72076 Tübingen, Germany. Phone, +49 7071-2984744; fax, +49 7071-294713.

cently, only transplantations with matched related donors or matched unrelated donors were performed. For those patients for whom no suitable donors were identified, this treatment modality could not be used, and most of these patients waiting for a suitable stem cell donor died from the disease. Therefore, attempts have been made to transplant such patients with alternative stem cell sources such as related mismatch donors or parental donors.[1–3] However, these transplantations were at high risk for acute or chronic graft-versus-host disease (GVHD), rejection after T-cell depletion used for GVHD prophylaxis or severe infectious complications.[4–6]

In animal studies, it could be shown, however, that by increasing the number of transplantated stem cells completely depleted of T-cells, the human leukocyte antigen (HLA) barrier can be overcome and a sustained engraftment can be obtained in the absence of GVHD.[7] Therefore, we were interested whether the transplantion of highly purified granulocyte colony-stimulating factor (G-CSF)-mobilized peripheral CD34$^+$ stem cells from parental donors can reconstitute the hematopoiesis of children with malignant and nonmalignant diseases after myeloablative therapy. In order to deplete all contaminating cells including T- and B-lymphocytes, the CD34$^+$ cells were purified to a high degree using the method of magnetic-activated cell sorting (MACS).[8]

MATERIALS AND METHODS

Patient Characteristics

Twenty-three patients with various diseases (acute lymphocytic leukemia (ALL), 8; acute myeloid leukemia (AML), 3; myelodysplastic syndrome (MDS), 4; chronic myelogenous leukemia (CML), 3; immunodeficiency, 3; osteopetrosis, 1; and severe aplastic anemia, 1) were transplanted. The median age of the patients was 7 years (range 1–19 years).

Donors, Stem Cell Mobilization and Collection

For 21 patients, parental donors were used. In two patients, the stem cell donor was an adult brother. Fourteen donors had a three HLA-loci mismatch constellation, 6 donors were two-loci and 3 were one-locus mismatch. The peripheral blood progenitor cells (PBPCs) were mobilized with G-CSF (10 μg/kg/day) for 6 days and the stem cell collection was performed at day 5 and 6 using either a Fenwall CS3000 plus or a Cobe Spectra cell separator. In order to increase the stem cell dose or in the case of rejection, a second mobilization procedure identical to the first one had to be performed in 9 donors.

CD34$^+$ Positive Selection

CD34$^+$ selection was performed using a modified semiautomated method of magnetic-activated cell sorting (SuperMACS, Miltenyi Biotec, Bergisch-Gladbach, Germany) as described[9] or with the automated CliniMACS device (Miltenyi) as described.[10] The mean number of purified CD34$^+$ cells obtained from the 23 donors was 14.2×10^6/kg body weight of recipient (range $5.4–39 \times 10^6$/kg) and the number of contaminating T-lymphocytes was 1.4×10^4/kg body weight of the recipient

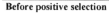

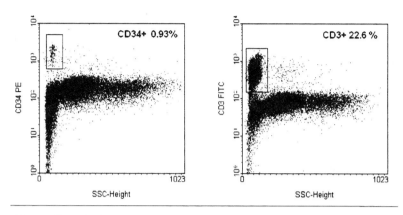

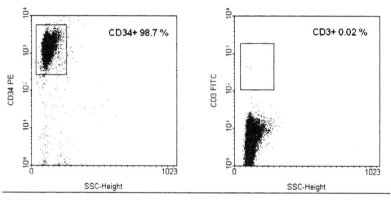

FIGURE 1. FACS analysis before and after positive selection of CD34$^+$ progenitors with the CliniMACS device.

(range $0.1–13 \times 10^4$/kg). The percentage of contaminating B-lymphocytes was in the range of 0.2.

In FIGURE 1, a representative example of CD34$^+$-positive selection and the resulting indirect T-cell depletion using the CliniMACS method is shown.

Engraftment Monitoring and T- Cell Add Back

The engraftment of the purified CD34$^+$ progenitors after the myeloablative therapy was monitored as described.[11] In 13 patients with mixed chimerism or patients who were considered to be at high risk of relapse, T-lymphocytes freshly obtained from the donor were added back at various numbers and time points after transplantation.

TABLE 1. Patients' characteristics, diagnosis, status of disease at transplantation, donors, HLA-disparity, conditioning regimen and GvHD prophylaxis

Patient	Weight (kg)/ Age (years)	Diagnosis	Status prior to transplantation	Donor	HLA-mismatch	Conditioning regimen	GvH Prophylaxis
1	13/4	CALL	early relapse	mother	A, B, DR	TBI,[a] TT, Cy, ALG	CsA 4 wks
2	15/4	MDS RAEB(T)	transformation	father	A, B, DR	Bu, TT, Cy, ATG	none
3	66/19	MDS	transformation	father	A, B, DR	Bu, Cy, ALG	CsA4 wks
4	20/9	AML	early relapse, PR	mother	A, B, DR	Bu, TT, Cy, ALG	none
5	6/1	Pre-B-ALL	poor responder	mother	A, B, DR	Bu, TT, Cy, ALG	none
6	10/2	AML	M7 early relapse	father	A, B, DR	Bu, TT, Cy, ALG	none
7	41/9	Pre-T-ALL	poor responder	father	A, B, DR	Bu, TT, Cy, ALG, OKT3, steroids	none
8	55/11	CML	Ph+, cP 1	father	A, B, DR	Bu, TT, Cy, ALG, OKT3, steroids	none
9	56/14	pro-B-ALL	early relapse	brother	A, B, DR	TBI, TT, Cy, ALG	CsA 4 wks
10	29/9	MDS RAEB(T)	relapse after MUD TP	father	A, DR	Bu, TT, Cy, ALG	none
11	46/18	TALL	relapse	brother	B, DR	TBI, TT, Cy, ALG	CSA 4 wks
12	15/3	Pre-B-ALL	early relapse, PR	father	B, DR	Bu, TT, Cy, ALG	none
13	16/3	CML	Ph+, cP 1	father	B, DR	Bu, TT, Cy, ALG	none
14	33/10	AML	M2, non-responder	father	A, B	Bu, TT, Cy, ALG	none
15	41/14	AML	early relapse	mother	B, DR	TBI, TT, Cy, ATG, OKT3, steroids	none
16	19/5	cALL	early relapse, PR	father	DR	Bu, TT, Cy, ALG	none
17	23/8	AML	non-responder	mother	B	Bu, TT, Cy, ALG OKT3, steroids	none
18	36/9	TALL	poor responder	father	A	Bu, TT, Cy, ALG	none
19	5/0.5	Osteopetrosis		father	A, B, DR	Bu, TT, Cy, ALG	none
20	30/12	SAA		father	A, B, DR	TBI, TT, Cy, ALG	none
21	5/0.5	SCID		father	A, B, DR	none	none
22	15/7	Immunodeficiency		mother	A, B	Bu, TT, Cy, ALG	none
23	9/1.6	Wiskoff-Aldrich		mother	A	Bu, TT, Cy, ALG	none

[a]TBI total body irradiation; TT Thiotepa; Cy cyclophosphamide; ALG Anti-lymphocyte immunoglobulin; Bu busulphan; OKT3 anti-CD3 antibody.

TABLE 2. Number of transplanted CD34+ progenitors and CD3+ T-lymphocytes, engraftment, GvHD before and after T-cell add-back and follow-up of the patients

Patient		CD34+/kg × 10^6	CD3+/kg × 10^3	days to ANC > 500	GvHD after Tx	T-cell add-back	GvHD after T-cell add-back	Overall survival (month)	Clinical outcome
1	1st	7.3	26	n.r.	I	none	—	11	non-engraftment
	2nd	8.7	47	9	none	none	—		dead of relapse
2		17.5	1.8	14	none	^{a}d28: 1 × 10^5/kg	I–II	9	not transplant-related death
3		8.3	11	10	none	dO: 5 × 10^4/kg d28: 5 × 10^4/kg	II–III resolved	> 21	alive and well
4	1st	18.4	9.3	10	none	d28: 2.5 × 10^4/kg	none	5	rejection
	2nd	14.2	1	11	none	d56: 5 × 10^4/kg	none		relapse
	3rd	6.7	9.1		none		none		dead of relapse
5	1st	25.5	2.7	12	none				relapse
	2nd	11	8.9		none	d28: 5 × 10^4/kg	none	6	dead of relapse
6		28.7	14.4	10	none	d19: 2.5 × 10^4/kg	11, skin	2	dead of relapse
7		17.4	6.1	9	none	d28: 2.5 × 10^4/kg	none	> 6	alive and well
8		16.7	13	11	I, skin	none	—	2	dead, VOD
9		9.8	30	12	none	none	—	2	dead of relapse and CMV infection
10	1st	6	6.1	n.r.	none	d3: 5 × 10^4/kg	chronic lung	> 18	non-engraftment
	2nd	13.6	17.1	13					alive and well
11		10.7	130	16	none	none	—	> 29	alive and well
12		8.6	5	15	I, skin	d28: 5 × 10^4/kg d56: 1 × 10^5/kg	II, skin, gut	9	dead of relapse

^{a}Indicate the days after transplant when a T-cell add back was performed; n.r., not reached; n.a., not applicable; VOD, venoocclusive disease.

TABLE 2. *Continued*

Patient		CD34+/kg ×10^6	CD3+/kg ×10^3	days to ANC >500	GvHD after Tx	T-cell add-back	GvHD after T-cell add-back	Overall survival (month)	Clinical outcome
13	1st	25	7	10	none	d56: 2.5 × 10^4/kg	none	>5	rejection
	2nd	26	7	10					alive and well
14		24.6	3.7	9	none	d14: 5 × 10^4/kg d28: 5 × 10^4/kg d56: 5 × 10^4/kg	none	5	dead of relapse
15		16.2	9.6	16	none	none	—	2	dead of adenovirus infection
16		39	14	9	none	d28: 5 × 10^4/kg d56: 5 × 10^4/kg	none	> 6	alive and well
17		11.6	13.6	12	none	d56: 5 × 10^4/kg	none	> 2	alive and well
18		5.4	26	10	none	d45: 5 × 10^4/kg d80: 5 × 10^4/kg d204: 1 × 10^5/kg	none	> 16	alive and well
19		29	2	11	I, skin	d180: 5 × 10^4/kg d210: 5 × 10^4/kg d240: 1 × 10^5/kg	none	> 24	alive and well
20	1st	12.3	8.3	n.r.	none	none	—		non-engraftment
	2nd	15.2	15.8	n.r.					non-engraftment
	3rd	3	5	n.r.				4	dead, sepsis
21		28	27.9	n.a.	I, skin	none	—	> 24	alive and well
22		37.5	18.7	9	none	none	—	6	dead due to preexisting lung disease
23		13.4	24	15	none	none	—	> 5	alive and well

RESULTS

In TABLE 1, the patients' characteristics, diagnosis, status of disease at transplantation, donors, HLA disparity, conditioning regimen and GVHD prophylaxis are shown. A short course of cyclosporin A (4 weeks) for prevention of GVHD was only used in the first 4 patients. In all other subsequent patients, the extensive indirect T-cell depletion obtained by the CD34$^+$-positive selection was the only GVHD prophylaxis. In TABLE 2, the number of transplanted CD34$^+$ cells, contaminating T-lymphocytes, engraftment, GVHD after transplantation and after T-cell add back and the clinical outcome is shown. In 13 patients, a nonengraftment was observed. Two of these patients could be regrafted from the same donor using a higher stem cell dose after an immunological reconditioning regimen consisting of an anti-CD3 antibody (Orthoclone OKT3, Janssen-Cilag, Germany) in combination with steroids for 4 weeks. The other patient with a long-lasting severe aplastic anemia showed no signs of engraftment despite the transplantation of high stem cell doses. In 2 patients, a rejection occurred. However, all patients engrafted after a second transplant using the same parental donor and the immunological reconditioning regime (anti-CD3 antibodies and steroids).

A significant GVHD was only seen in patients after T-cell add back. In the absence of this procedure, GVHD could completely be prevented even in the 3-loci mismatch transplants without any further pharmacological immunosuppression. The absence of any long-term pharmacological immunosuppression might be at least to some extent responsible for the relatively rapid immunological recovery. As is shown in FIGURE 2, there is a significant relationship of the number of transplanted CD34$^+$ cells and the speed of recovery of CD3$^+$ and CD4$^+$ T-lymphocytes. Among the 23 patients, 11 are alive and disease free with the longest follow-up of almost three years. The cause of death in the twelve patients was mainly relapse (7 patients), 1 adenoviral infection, 1 venoocclusive disease (VOD), 1 nonengraftment, 1 preexisting lung disease and 1 nontransplant-related death (TABLE 2).

DISCUSSION

The transplantation of T-cell-depleted, partially matched stem cells has been performed in the past in a number of patients for whom a stem cell transplantation was the only curative therapeutic option and for whom no suitable matched donor was available. However, these transplantations were associated with a high incidence of graft failures and severe infectious complications due to a delayed immunological recovery associated with T-cell depletion. However, with the possibility to use mobilized peripheral blood stem cells and the observation in animal models that the transplantation of megadoses of purified hematopoietic stem cells can overcome the HLA barrier, this transplantation procedure has become now a real therapeutic option. By using mobilized PBPCs the number of CD34$^+$ progenitors can be drastically increased compared to bone marrow. Since the number of contaminating T-lymphocytes increases with the number of collected stem cells, a T-cell depletion for prevention of GVHD must be performed in the mismatched situation. Therefore, we have focused on methods for the positive selection of CD34$^+$ progenitors for two

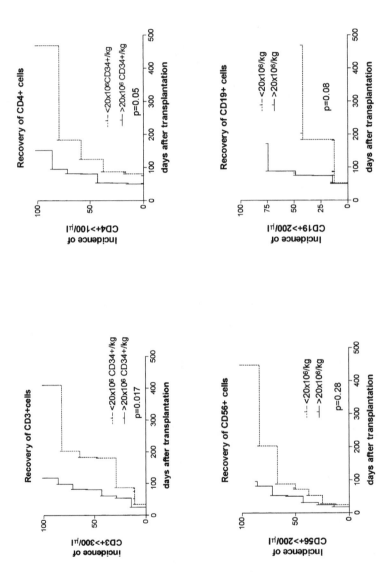

FIGURE 2. The speed of recovery of lymphocyte subsets after transplantation is dependent on the number of transplanted purified CD34[+] haploidentical stem cells.

reasons. First, positive selection of a target cell population is associated with less unspecific cell loss and second, positive selection of CD34$^+$ cells not only offers T-cell depletion for GVHD prevention, but also depletion of B-lymphocytes, which might prevent donor-derived Epstein-Barr virus (EBV)-associated lymphoproliferative diseases. And indeed, in none of our patients was an EBV-associated lymphoproliferative syndrome observed.

Since the method of magnetic-activated cell sorting (MACS) showed excellent results in the laboratory scale,[12] we optimized this method for clinical scale using the SuperMACS[9] and later the CliniMACS.[10] Since the purity of the CD34$^+$ cells with this method was in the range of 98–99%, the depletion of T- and B-lymphocytes was extremely effective, and the average number of transplanted T-lymphocytes was extremely low with 1.4×10^4/kg. Therefore, no further GVHD prophylaxis was necessary even in the three-loci mismatch situation. An additional advantage of the MACS method is the good recovery (between 70 and 90%) of the CD34$^+$ cells after positive selection, which is very important in order to augment the stem cell dose.[9] We have observed in our patients that the absence of any immunosuppression and the transplantation of high numbers of purified CD34$^+$ progenitors results in a rapid immunological recovery. When the number of transplanted CD34$^+$ cells was >20 $\times$ 10^6/kg, the time to reach subnormal or normal lymphocyte subsets was relatively short, which is associated with less severe infectious complications (FIG. 2).

Therefore, we conclude that the target cell dose of transplanted CD34$^+$ cells should be in the range of 20 $\times$ 10^6/kg.

In two patients, a rejection occurred despite the transplantation of high numbers of CD34$^+$ cells. The reason for these rejections was alloreactive residual host T-lymphocytes, which were not completely eliminated with the myeloablative therapy. However, the two patients were sucessfully retransplanted using the same stem cell donor, and a rapid and sustained three-lineage engraftment was seen after suppression of these residual T-lymphocytes using the immunological reconditioning regimen consisting of anti-CD3 antibodies and steroids. After this experience, we decided to combine the myeloablative therapy with this immunological conditioning by the application of anti-CD3 antibodies starting from day +1 until day +18. This preparative regimen is well tolerated, and up to now no rejection was seen in 4 patients (TABLE 2). However, more patients have to be transplanted with this preparative regimen in order to see whether the risk of rejection will be less. The transplant-related toxicities were acceptable, and the main cause of death in our patients was relapse of the malignant disease. This might be due to the T-cell depletion, since T-cell depletion and the absence of GVHD is associated with a higher risk of relapse.[13] Therefore, we have used T-cell add backs for some of the patients who were considered at high risk of relapse or who showed a transient autologous hematopoietic recovery. At this time, however, no clear conclusions can be drawn about whether the add back of T-cells in our setting has an antileukemic effect. However, we have noted that the T-cell number that can be safely added back without risk of severe GVHD is between 2.5×10^4/kg and 5×10^4/kg. The add back of other potential antileukemic lymphocyte subpopulations like natural killer (NK) cells as described in an animal model is currently under active investigation at our institution.[14,15] Another reason for the relapse might have been the status of disease at the time of transplant. Some of the patients were resistant to chemotherapy and not in remission at time of transplant. Such patients are at high risk of relapse, and additional posttransplant immunotherapeutic strategies have to be evaluated for such patients. Another aspect of our study is the existence of pluripotent long-term repopulating CD34-negative stem cells recently described.[16] Since the purity of our CD34+ cells is very high (98–99%), the possibility of transplanting this CD34-negative population is low. Our patients showed a complete donor engraftment and a complete hematopoietic recovery for almost up to three years. Therefore, we conclude, that the transplantation of highly purified CD34+ progenitors results in long-term repopulation in patients after myeloablative therapy. However, a longer follow-up of our patients will show the significance of long-term repopulating CD34-negative stem cells.

In summary, we have shown that the transplantation of megadoses of mismatched parental purified stem cells results in a complete and sustained engraftment. The incidence of transplant-related toxicities or severe infections is relatively low, and due to the permanent availability of the donor, a second transplant is possible in the case of nonengraftment or rejection. Moreover, posttransplant immunotherapy using defined antileukemic donor lymphocyte subpopulations can be systematically evaluated. Therefore, we conclude that this transplantation method is a real alternative to the use of unrelated umbilical cord blood,[17] where the stem cell number is low and the donor not available for further posttransplant immunotherapy.

ACKNOWLEDGMENTS

We thank A. Barbarin-Dorner, C. Faleyras, U. Krautter and R. Siedner for excellent technical assistance. This work is supported by a grant from the Deutsche Krebshilfe (W 44/93/Ni 6) and the German Jose Carreras Leukemia Foundation.

REFERENCES

1. HENSLEE-DOWNEY, P.J., R.S. PARRISH, J.S. MACDONALD *et al.* 1996. Combined *in vitro* and *in vivo* T lymphocyte depletion for the control of graft-versus-host disease following haploidentical marrow transplant. Transplantation **61:** 738–745.
2. AVERSA, F., A. TABILIO, A. TENEZA *et al.* 1994. Sucessful engraftment of T cell-depleted three loci incompatible transplant in leukemia patients by addition of recombinant human granulocytecolony-stimulating factor mobilized peripheral blood progenitor cells to bone marrow inoculum. Blood **84:** 3948–3955.
3. HENSLEE-DOWNEY, P.J., S.K. ABHYANKAR, R.S. PARRISH *et al.* 1997. Use of partially mismatched related donors extends access to allogeneic marrow transplant. Blood **89:** 3864–3872.
4. FERRARA, J.L. & H.J. DEEG. 1991. Graft-versus-host disease. N. Engl. J. Med. **324:** 667–674.
5. LAMB, L.S., F. SZAFER, P.J. HENSLEE DOWNEY *et al.* 1995. Characterization of acute bone marrow graft rejection in T cell depleted partially mismatched related donor bone marrow transplantation. Hematology **23:** 1595–1600.
6. FISCHER, A., P. LANDEIS, W. FRIEDRICH *et al.* 1990. European experience of bone marrow transplantaton for severe combined immunodeficiency. Lancet **336:** 850–852.
7. REISNER, Y. & M.F. MARTELLI. 1995. Bone marrow transplantation across HLA barriers by increasing the number of transplanted cells. Immunol. Today **16:** 437–438.
8. KATO, K. & A. RADBRUCH. 1993. Isolation and characterization of CD34+ hematopoietic stem cells from human peripheral blood by high-gradient magnetic activated cell sorting. Cytometry **14:** 384–392.

9. HANDGRETINGER, R., P. LANG, M. SCHUMM *et al.* 1998. Isolation and transplantation of autologous peripheral CD34$^+$ progenitor cells highly purified by magnetic-activated cell sorting. Bone Marrow Transplant. **21:** 987–993.
10. SCHUMM, M., P. LANG, G. TAYLOR et al. 1999. Isolation of highly purified autologous and allogeneic peripheral CD34$^+$ cells using the CliniMACS device. J. Hematother. In press.
11. BADER, P., W. HÖLLE, T. KLINBEBIEL *et al.* 1996. Quantitative assessment of mixed hematopoietic chimerism by polymerase chain reaction after allogeneic BMT. Anticancer Res. **16:** 1759–1764.
12. DE WYNTER, E.A., L.K. COUTINHO, X. PEI *et al.* 1995. Comparison of purity and enrichment of CD34$^+$ cells from bone marrow, umbilical cord blood and peripheral blood (primed for apheresis) using five separation systems. Stem Cells (Dayton) **13:** 524–532.
13. UHAREK, L., B. GLASS, M. ZEIS *et al.* 1998. Abrogation of graft-vs-leukemia activity after depletion of CD3$^+$ T cells in a murine model of MHC-matched peripheral blood progenitor cell transplantation (PBPCT). Exp. Hematol. **26:** 93–99.
14. ZEISS, M., L. UHAREK, B. GLASS *et al.* 1997. Allogeneic MHC-mismatched activated natural killer cells administered after bone marrow transplantation provide a strong graft-versus-leukemia effect in mice. Br. J. Haematol. **96:** 757–761.
15. GEISELHART, A., S. NEU, F. BUCHHOLZ *et al.* 1997. Positive selection of CD56$^+$ lymphocytes by magnetic-activated cell sorting (MACS). Nat. Immun. **15:** 227–233.
16. GOODELL, M.A., M. ROSENZWEIG, H. KIM *et al.* 1997. Dye efflux studies suggest that hematopoietic stem cells expressing low or undetectable levels of CD34 antigen exist in multiple species. Nat. Med. **12:** 1337–1345.
17. GLUCKMAN, E., R. VANDERSON, A. BOYER-CHAMMARD *et al.* 1997. Outcome of cord-blood transplantation from related and unrelated donors. N. Engl. J. Med. **337:** 373–381.

DISCUSSION

D. METCALF (*P. O. Royal Melbourne Hospital*): Can you give me an estimate of what percentage of candidates for transplantation still do not have a donor?

HANDGRETINGER: I think it is in the range that Dr. Reisner showed, 30–40%, and it depends upon the indication whether you are able to use this type of engraftment. This also changes your indications a little, because for such a patient who is not in remission it would be hard to find an unrelated donor for such a patient with such a poor prognosis. Probably you would not transplant such a patient with 50–60% blasts in the bone marrow. Using this setting with a related donor, the motivation is quite different than when you use an unrelated donor, where you would have problems to convince an unrelated donor to give bone marrow for such a poor prognosis patient. Some of these patients were high risk patients when we started this program. This also widens the indication for these patients, and the number of patients who profit from such kind of transplant is higher.

METCALF: What is the current percentage?

HANDGRETINGER: It is in the range of 30–40% still.

METCALF: If you use your approach, what percentage might remain?

HANDGRETINGER: It should be zero. If the patient is in the condition in which you can transplant him, then we do it. I misunderstood the question.

P.M. LANSDORP (*Terry Fox Laboratory*): The main role of the megadose CD34 cells seems to be to titrate out residual immunity in the recipient. Would you predict that if that particular problem could be addressed by improved immune suppression that you can in effect go down with your dose of CD34 cells?

HANDGRETINGER: We do not know yet. We have only this experience now with four patients with this immune-suppressive therapy with anti-CD3 antibodies from day +1 to day +18. These patients have a good engraftment at the moment. Probably, we will have to go down in the future, because not all donors mobilize the same stem cell numbers. But at the moment we are still in a position to collect as much as possible of CD34$^+$ cells, even if we have to work a second round of mobilization. I am not sure we can go down much further, because immunological recovery is another feature that reflects the number of stem cells that you give. We started this program with about 10 million/kg. We were happy to have this, but now we are focusing on 20 million/kg.

D.A. WILLIAMS (*Riley Hospital for Children*): I think in the United States a big advocate of this approach over the years has been Dr. Henslee-Downey. I just wonder what the difference in your preparative regimen and your approach is compared with hers.

HANDGRETINGER: I think that we tried all kinds of methods to get this and many combinations. With every additional step you lose quite a significant number of cells in an unspecific manner. The recovery of this method when we started (and we had to do it manually) was about 20%. It would not have been approved, but we came up with about 80% recovery of CD34 cells.

P.J. QUESENBERRY (*University of Massachusetts Medical Center*): It looks as though you can keep escalating your stem cell number; presumably you get progressively better results. Karl Dicke reported an interesting technique for outpatient harvest of marrow. He primed the marrow, used a little ativan, and even did a quality of life assessment. The patients tolerated this quite well. One of the things we have been discussing, and I would be interested in your comments, is combining the apheresis approaches with multiple outpatient marrow harvests, where you should be able to escalate your total number of CD34 cells tremendously.

HANDGRETINGER: I think you will have to have a highly motivated donor. In two of the patients we added bone marrow from the donors, but normally we want to avoid it. We would rather do several mobilization procedures. One other point that I did not make is the advantage of having the donor available after the transplant. We had one patient with MDS who relapsed after an unrelated transplant. Therefore, the patient got a second transplant with the haploidentical father as donor. However, the patient had very poor graft function for one year after the second transplant. Therefore, he got another graft from the father after one year without any conditioning regimen. He has a perfect graft now. It is really a big advantage to have the donor always available in constrast to the unrelated donor banks or the cord blood banks.

Approaches to Dendritic Cell-Based Immunotherapy after Peripheral Blood Stem Cell Transplantation

W. BRUGGER, P. BROSSART, S. SCHEDING, G. STUHLER, K. HEINRICH, V. REICHARDT, F. GRÜNEBACH, H.-J. BÜHRING, AND L. KANZ[a]

University of Tübingen, Medical Center II, Department of Hematology, Oncology, Immunology, and Rheumatology, Otfried-Müller Str. 10, 72076 Tübingen, Germany

ABSTRACT: High-dose chemotherapy with peripheral blood progenitor cell transplantation (PBPCT) is a potentially curative treatment option for patients with both hematological malignancies and solid tumors, including breast cancer. However, based on a number of clinical studies, there is strong evidence that minimal residual disease (MRD) persists after high-dose chemotherapy in a number of patients, which eventually results in disease recurrence. Therefore, several approaches to the treatment of MRD are currently being evaluated, including treatment with dendritic cell (DC)-based cancer vaccines. DCs, which play a crucial role with regard to the initiation of T-lymphocyte responses, can be generated *ex vivo* either from CD34+ hematopoietic progenitor cells or from blood monocytes. They can be pulsed *in vitro* with tumor-derived peptides or proteins, and then used as a professional antigen-presenting cell (APC) vaccine for the induction of antigen-specific T-lymphocytes *in vivo*. This paper summarizes our preclinical studies on the induction of primary HER-2/neu specific cytotoxic T-lymphocyte (CTL) responses using peptide-pulsed DC. As HER-2/neu is overexpressed on 30–40% of breast and ovarian cancer cells, this novel vaccination approach might be particularly applicable to advanced breast or ovarian cancer patients after high-dose chemotherapy and autologous PBPCT.

INTRODUCTION

Although the clinical outcome of cancer patients treated with high-dose chemotherapy is promising in various malignancies, a significant proportion of patients eventually relapse due to resistant disease. Therefore, it is important to provide effective strategies to treat minimal residual disease (MRD) after autologous peripheral blood progenitor cell transplantation (PBPCT) in order to potentially increase cure rates in otherwise incurable cancer patients. One possibility for treating MRD is the use of dendritic cell (DC)-based cancer vaccines.[1] DCs are professional antigen-presenting cells (APCs), which play a central role in the initiation of primary T-cell responses.[2,3] They express high levels of major histocompatibility complex (MHC) as well as costimulatory and adhesion molecules required for optimal T-cell activation. DCs can be generated *ex vivo* in the presence of various cytokine combina-

[a]Corresponding author: Phone, +49-7071-29-82726; fax, +49-7071-29-3671; e-mail, lothar.kanz@uni-tuebingen.de

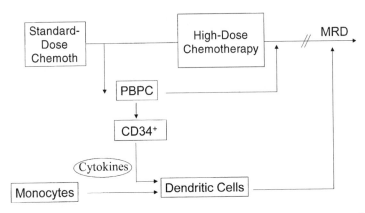

FIGURE 1. Approach to DC-based cancer vaccines after autologous PBPC transplantation.

tions either from CD34$^+$ progenitor cells[4–8] or from adherent blood monocytes[9–11] (FIG. 1). To study the functional capabilities of ex vivo- generated DCs in terms of induction of antigen-specific cytotoxic T-lymphocytes (CTLs), we used synthetic human leukocyte antigen (HLA)-A2 restricted peptides derived from the HER-2/neu protein as a model for tumor-associated antigens. The HER-2/neu oncogene encodes a transmembrane receptor tyrosine kinase that is overexpressed in approximately 30–40% of breast and ovarian cancer patients, and that has been shown to correlate with poor prognosis in these patients. Our results demonstrate that primary *in vitro* immunization using DCs pulsed with HER-2/neu-derived peptides can be efficiently used for the induction of primary CTL responses. These CTL lysed tumor cells that endogenously expressed HER-2/neu epitopes in an antigen and HLA-A2 specific fashion.[11] Similar approaches have now been performed by our group with DCs pulsed with synthetic peptides derived from the MUC-1 tumor antigen, and they have shown that MUC-1$^+$ targets can be recognized by MUC-1-specific CTLs *in vitro*, suggesting that epitopes derived from either HER-2/neu or MUC-1 proteins might be suitable candidates for broadly applicable cancer vaccines in patients with epithelial tumors.

MATERIALS AND METHODS

Purification of CD34$^+$ PBPC or Adherent Blood Monocytes

CD34$^+$ cells were positively selected from mobilized peripheral blood progenitor cells (PBPC) from cancer patients after chemotherapy plus granulocyte colony-stimulating factor (G-CSF) treatment[12] or from normal healthy volunteers after G-CSF priming for allogeneic transplantation. Cells were obtained after informed consent according to the guidelines of our local ethics committee. Cell selection was performed either using the Ceprate SC system (CellPro; Bothell, WA, USA), or by immunomagnetic enrichment using the MiniMACS cell selection system (Miltenyi, Bergisch Gladbach, Germany), according to the manufacturers' instructions.

Peripheral blood mononuclear cells (PBMNC) from healthy blood donors were obtained after Ficoll/Hypaque density gradient centrifugation, and monocytes were enriched by a 2-hour adherence step in RPMI 1640 medium supplemented with 10% heat-inactivated fetal calf serum (FCS) as described recently.[11] Purity of monocytes was >90%, as determined by flow cytometry.

Generation of DCs from CD34+ Cells

CD34+ cells were cultured in the presence of various cytokine combinations for up to 28 days in RPMI1640 medium supplemented with 10% FCS.[6] The following cytokines were used for DC generation: stem cell factor (SCF, 10–100 ng/ml), interleukin-1 (IL-1, 10 ng/ml), IL-3 (10 ng/ml), IL-6 (100 U/ml), erythropoietin (Epo, 1 U/ml), granulocyte/macrophage colony-stimulating factor (GM-CSF, 100 ng/ml), IL-4 (1,000 U/ml), transforming growth factor-β (TGF-β, 10 ng/ml), and FLT-3 ligand (FLT-3L, 10–100 ng/ml). Cells were analyzed by flow cytometry at various time points during culture.

Generation of DCs from Adherent PBMNC

Generation of DCs from blood monocytes was performed as described previously.[9–11] In brief, adherence purified monocytes were cultured for 7 days in serum (FCS) or in serum-free medium supplemented with GM-CSF (100 ng/ml; Leukomax, Novartis, Nürnberg, Germany) and IL-4 (1,000 U/ml; Genzyme, Rüsselsheim, Germany) with or without tumor necrosis factor-α (TNF-α, 10 ng/ml; Genzyme, Rüsselsheim, Germany). For additional experiments, DCs were generated in the absence of GM-CSF upon CD40 ligation using a CD40L transfected cell line (kindly provided by Dr. Banchereau, Dardilly, France).[13]

Induction of Peptide-Specific CTLs Using HLA-A2-Restricted Synthetic HIV Peptides

The pol HIV-1 reverse transcriptase peptide 476–484 was kindly provided by Dr. S. Stevanovic (Institute for Immunology, University of Tübingen). For CTL induction, 5×10^5 DCs generated under different culture conditions were pulsed with 25 μg/ml of the HIV peptide for 2 hours and incubated with autologous PBMNC, as described.[13] The cytolytic activity of induced CTLs was analyzed 5 days after the last stimulation in a ^{51}Cr-release assay.

^{51}Cr Release Assay

The CTL activity was measured in a standard ^{51}Cr-release assay, as described elsewhere.[11,13] In brief, target cells were pulsed with 50 μg/ml peptide for 2 hours and labeled with ^{51}Cr sodium chromate in RPMI1640 medium plus 10% FCS for 1 hour at 37°C. 10^4 cells were transferred into round-bottomed 96-well plates, and varying numbers of CTLs were added and incubated at a final volume of 200 μl for 4 hours at 37°C. Supernatants (50 μl/well) were harvested and counted in a β-plate counter.

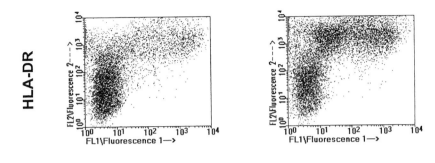

CD1a

FIGURE 2. Generation of DCs from purified CD34$^+$ cells. CD34$^+$ PBPCs were cultured for 21 days in the presence of SCF, IL-3, IL-6, IL-4, and GM-CSF with or without FLT-3L. Cells were analyzed by flow cytometry using anti-CD1a fluorescein isothiocyanate (FITC) and anti-CD80 phycoerythrin (PE) monoclonal antibodies (mAbs).

RESULTS AND DISCUSSION

Generation of DCs from Mobilized CD34$^+$ PBPCs

As shown by a number of investigators, DCs can be generated *in vitro* from purified CD34$^+$ cells using appropriate cytokine combinations (for review, see Ref. 3). We and others have convincingly shown that besides the well-known cytokines GM-CSF, IL-4, TNF-α and FLT-3L, TGF-β seems to be indispensible for the generation of DCs from CD34$^+$ cells under serum-free culture conditions.[14,15] By utilizing a SCF, IL-3 and IL-6-based growth factor combination, up to 40×10^6 CD1a$^+$ DCs can be generated starting from 1×10^6 CD34$^+$ cells (FIG. 2). These cells represent mature DCs with potent stimulatory capacity in an allogeneic mixed lymphocyte reaction (MLR, data not shown).

Generation of DCs from Adherence Purified Blood Monocytes

Monocytes were cultured for 7 days in the presence of GM-CSF and IL-4, and the resulting DCs were analyzed phenotypically by flow cytometry.[11,13] As expected, DCs expressed high levels of MHC class I and class II molecules as well as high levels of CD1a, CD80, CD86, CD40, and CD54. In addition, DCs generated in the presence of TNF-α or upon CD40 ligation strongly expressed CD1a and CD83, consistent with a mature DC phenotype (FIG. 3). The generation of monocyte-derived DCs in the absence of GM-CSF was particularly interesting and was shown by our group to occur solely upon CD40/CD40L interactions.[13] These data suggest that monocytes are a unique source of DCs, depending on external stimuli.[13] Indeed, CD40/CD40L interactions with antigen-presenting cells (APCs) and T-helper cells have been shown recently to be critical for cytotoxic T-cell activation.[16–18]

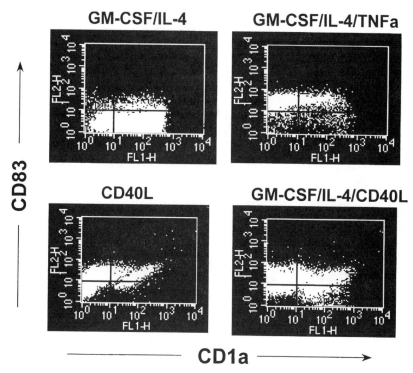

FIGURE 3. Generation of DCs from peripheral blood (PB) monocytes. Adherent PB monocytes from healthy volunteers were cultured for 7 days in the presence of various growth factor combinations. DCs were analyzed by flow cytometry at day 7, and data are shown in a dot-plot analysis.

Induction of Antigen-Specific CTLs Using Peptide-Pulsed DCs

The various DC populations, each of which was generated from blood monocytes under different growth factor combinations, were subsequently analyzed for their capacity to induce antigen-specific T-cell responses after pulsing with synthetic HIV peptides. As shown in FIGURE 4, DCs generated in the presence of GM-CSF, IL-4, and TNF-α were potent inducers of HIV peptide-specific CTL responses, while uncultured PBMNC did not prime CTLs after several rounds of restimulation. Consistent with the mature phenotype, DCs generated solely upon CD40/CD40L interactions were potent inducers of HIV-specific CTLs, similar to DCs generated with GM-CSF, IL-4, and TNF-α or DCs generated with GM-CSF, IL-4, and CD40 ligation (FIG. 4).[13]

Induction of HER-2/neu Peptide-Specific CTLs Using Peptide-Pulsed DCs and Lysis of HER-2/neu-Expressing Tumor Cells by HER-2/neu-Specific CTLs

For the potential clinical treatment of MRD after high-dose chemotherapy, we have chosen HER-2/neu-positive tumor cells as a model system. Therefore, we used

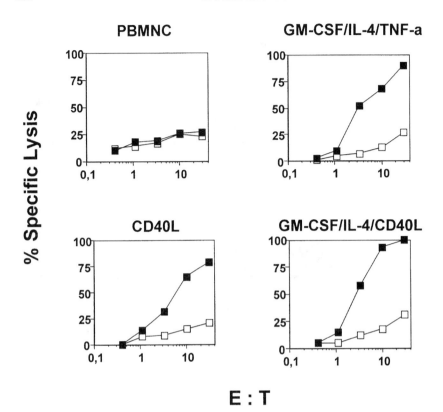

FIGURE 4. Induction of primary HIV peptide-specific CTLs by different populations of peptide-pulsed DCs. DCs were generated under different culture conditions from adherent HLA-A2[+] PBMNCs. The different DC populations were pulsed with the synthetic HLA-A2- restricted HIV peptide to induce a primary CTL response. The cytotoxic activity of induced CTLs was determined in a ^{51}Cr-release assay using T2 cells pulsed with the cognate HIV peptide (*closed symbols*) or an irrelevant peptide derived from the influenza matrix protein (IMP) (*open symbols*).

the previously published HLA-A2 restricted peptides E75 and GP2 derived from the HER-2/neu protein for the induction of CTLs by primary *in vitro* immunization of DCs.[11,19] We showed that the CTL lines obtained demonstrated peptide-specific and HLA-A2-restricted killing of targets coated with the cognate HER-2/neu-derived peptides E75 and GP2 (data not shown; see Ref. 11). More importantly, the induced CTL lines were able to lyse tumor cells naturally expressing the HER-2/neu protein. Among them, we found not only a peptide-specific and HLA-A2-restricted lysis of allogeneic HER-2/neu-positive breast and ovarian cancer cell lines, but also lysis of colon carcinoma cell lines and two renal cell carcinoma cell lines, suggesting that epitopes derived from the HER-2/neu protein might be candidates for broadly applicable cancer vaccines.[11]

CONCLUDING REMARKS

Our data show that DCs can be generated *ex vivo* by different growth factor cocktails, and that these DCs are functionally different, depending on the cytokines used. *Ex vivo*-generated DCs have a unique capacity to induce antigen-specific CTL responses, as demonstrated here for the induction of HIV- and HER-2/neu peptide-specific CTLs. These CTLs were able to lyse various allogeneic tumor cell lines naturally expressing HER-2/neu epitopes, providing the basis for clinical testing. Therefore, we have recently initiated a clinical phase I/II study in advanced breast and ovarian cancer patients using HER-2/neu peptide-pulsed DCs as a cancer vaccine. However, despite the fact that vaccination of follicular lymphoma, multiple myeloma or malignant melanoma patients with DCs showed some clinical responses in early clinical trials,[20–22] further comparative studies with DCs, each of which being generated in different ways and loaded under different conditions, are required to ultimately demonstrate effective antitumor immunity. Only if these requirements have been defined, DC-based cancer vaccines may prove useful for adoptive immunotherapy after high-dose chemotherapy in the setting of minimal residual disease.

ACKNOWLEDGMENTS

These studies were supported by the Deutsche Forschungsgemeinschaft (SFB 510, Project B2), by Deutsche Krebshilfe, and by grants from the *Fortüne* Research Program of the University of Tübingen. We thank S. Kurtz, A. Weber, and H. Becker for excellent technical assistance.

REFERENCES

1. PARDOLL, D.M. 1998. Cancer vaccines. Nat. Med. **4:** 525–531.
2. STEINMANN, A.M. 1991. The dendritic cell system and its role in immunogenicity. Annu. Rev. Immunol. **9:** 271–296.
3. CELLA, M., F. SALLUSTO & A. LANZAVECCHIA. 1997. Origin, maturation and antigen presenting function of dendritic cells. Curr. Opin. Immunol. **9:** 10–16.
4. CAUX, C., C. DEZUTTER-DEMBUYANT, D. SCHMITT & J. BANCHEREAU. 1992. GM-CSF and TNF-alpha cooperate in the generation of dendritic Langerhans cells. Nature **55:** 258–261.
5. YOUNG, J.W., P. SZABOLS & M.A.S. MOORE. 1995. Identification of dendritic cell colony forming units among normal human CD34+ bone marrow progenitors that are expanded by c-kit ligand and yield pure dendritic cell colonies in the presence of GM-CSF and TNFa. J. Exp. Med. **182:** 1111–1120.
6. FISCH, P., G. KÖHLER, H. E. SCHAEFER *et al.* 1996. Generation of antigen-presenting cells for soluble protein antigens *ex vivo* from peripheral blood CD34+ hematopoietic progenitor cells in cancer patients. Eur. J. Immunol. **26:** 595–560.
7. FLORES-ROMO, L., P. BJORCK, V. DUVERT *et al.* 1997. CD40 ligation on human cord blood CD34+ hematopoietic progenitors induces their proliferation and differentiation into functional dendritic cells. J. Exp. Med. **185:** 341–349.
8. KANZ, L. & W. BRUGGER. 1998. Mobilization and *ex vivo* manipulation of peripheral blood progenitor cells for support of high-dose cancer therapy. *In* Bone Marrow Transplantation. 2nd edit. E.D. Thomas, K.G. Blume & S.J. Forman, Eds.: 455–468. Blackwell Science, Inc. Boston, MA.

9. SALLUSTO, F. & A. LANZAVECCHIA. 1994. Efficient presentation of soluble antigen by cultured human dendritic cells is maintained by GM-CSF plus IL-4 and down regulated by TNFa. J. Exp. Med. **179:** 1109–1118.
10. ZHOU, L.J. & T.F. TEDDER. 1996. CD14$^+$ blood monocytes can differentiate into functionally mature CD83$^+$ dendritic cells. Proc. Natl. Acad. Sci. USA **93:** 2588–2592.
11. BROSSART, P., G. STUHLER, T. FLAD et al. 1998. HER-2/neu-derived peptides are tumor-associated antigens expressed by human renal cell and colon carcinoma lines and recognized by in vitro- induced specific cytotoxic T-lymphocytes. Cancer Res. **58:** 732–736.
12. BRUGGER, W., R. HENSCHLER, S. HEIMFELD et al. 1994. Positively selected autologous blood CD34$^+$ cells and unseparated peripheral blood progenitor cells mediate identical hematopoietic engraftment after high-dose VP16, ifosfamide, carboplatin, and epirubicine. Blood **84:** 1421–1426.
13. BROSSART, P., F. GRÜNEBACH, G. STUHLER et al. 1998. Generation of functional dendritic cells from adherent peripheral blood mononuclear cells by CD40 ligation in the absence of GM-CSF. Blood **92:** 4238–4247.
14. Strobl, H. et al. 1996. TGF-β1 promotes in vitro development of dendritic cells from CD34$^+$ hemopoietic progenitor cells. J. Immunol. **157:** 1499–1507.
15. SCHEDING, S., S. WIRTHS, H.-J. BÜHRING et al. 1997. FLT-3 ligand, TGF-β, and GM-CSF/IL-4 are critical growth factors for the induction of CD1a$^+$/CD14$^-$/CD80$^+$ dendritic cell (DC) development from CD34$^+$ PBPC in serum-free medium [abstract]. Blood **90:** 478a.
16. BENNETT, S.R.M., F. R. CARBONNE, F. KARAMALIS et al. 1998. Help from cytotxic T-cell responses is mediated by CD40 signalling. Nature **393:** 478–480.
17. SCHOENBERGER, S.P., R.E.M. TOES, E.J.H. VAN DER VOORT et al. 1998. T-cell help for cytotoxic T lymphocytes is mediated by CD40-CD40L interactions. Nature **393:** 480–483.
18. RIDGE, J.P., F. DI ROSA, P. MATZINGER et al. 1998. A conditioned dendritic cell can be a temporal bridge between a CD4$^+$ T-helper and a T-killer cell. Nature **393:** 474–478.
19. PIEPER, M., P.S. GOEDEBEBUURE, D.C. LINEHAN et al. 1997. The Her-2/neu derived peptide p654–662 is a tumor-associated antigen in human pancreatic cancer recognized by cytotoxic T lymphocytes. Eur. J. Immunol. **27:** 1115–1123.
20. HSU, F.J., C. BENIKE, F. FAGNONI et al. 1996. Vaccination of patients with B-cell lymphoma using autologous antigen-pulsed dendritic cells. Nat. Med. **2:** 52–58.
21. REICHARDT, V., C. OKADA, C. BENIKE et al. 1996. Idiotypic vaccination using dendritic cells for multiple myeloma patients after autologous peripheral blood stem cell transplantation [abstract]. Blood **88:** 481a.
22. NESTLE, F.O., S. ALIJAGIC, M. GILLIET et al. 1998. Vaccination of melanoma patients with peptide- or tumor lysate-pulsed dendritic cells. Nat. Med. **4:** 328–332.

DISCUSSION

S.T. ILDSTAD (*Allegheny University of Health Sciences*): Do you know which subpopulation of DCs you are generating? Are they more lymphoid or more myeloid?

BRUGGER: They are more myeloid.

P.M. LANSDORP (*Terry Fox Laboratory*): What would you recommend, to use CD34 cells or monocytes for the generation of dendritic cells?

BRUGGER: It is a good question. We have not done a direct comparison so far, but there is a paper from Gianni's group in Italy that directly compared them. They compared monocyte-derived DCs with CD34-derived DCs in terms of peptide-specific CTL induction. From this paper it is clear that the two populations are functionally different. I think it depends whether you would like to use peptide-pulsed DCs, or if you would like to use DCs that are highly efficient for uptake and presentation of exogenous soluble proteins. In the former case, it might be better to use monocyte-derived DCs, which have a mature phenotype expressing all the costimulatory molecules required for T-cell activation. But it is not totally clear at this stage.

L. KANZ (*Eberhard Karls University*): By preparing DCs from peripheral blood monocytes, you need a lower number of growth factors. That is a major point when thinking of a clinical application.

D. METCALF (*P.O. Royal Melbourne Hospital*): I am a little surprised that you are injecting the dendritic cells subcutaneously (s.c.). What do we know about the homing of intravenously (i.v.) injected dendritic cells? It seems to me that with your procedure you depend on recirculating T-cells just happening to come to the site of injection which would probably be rather inefficient if the antigen source was, for example, the breast. Do you know whether intravenously injected dendritic cells localize in lymph nodes?

BRUGGER: That is, of course, a relevant question. We finally decided to inject these cells s.c., because there are data from monkeys showing that dendritic cells given s.c. are able to migrate into the regional lymph nodes, where they come into contact with T-cells, of course. But you might be right about injecting these cells i.v. We have not done this clinically yet, but we have another trial in our institution with multiple myeloma patients, which is being done by Volker Reichert in our group. He injects these cells i.v., so we probably can get a comparison.

Y. REISNER (*Weizmann Institute of Science*): Do you find that G-CSF-mobilized stem cells are a reliable source for your dendritic cell generation, or do you have problems in repeating this experiment? We have tried, and we have some problems. I wonder if you find it less reproducible compared to using monocytes as a source.

BRUGGER: Yes, that is certainly true for cancer patients. Of course, if you do it in the cancer patient, you have a broad variability, and that is another reason why it is probably easier to use monocytes instead of CD34-derived DCs.

Mixed Hematopoietic Chimerism after Marrow Allografts

Transplantation in the Ambulatory Care Setting

RAINER STORB,[a] CONG YU, BRENDA M. SANDMAIER, PETER A. MCSWEENEY, GEORGE GEORGES, RICHARD A. NASH, AND ANN WOOLFREY

Clinical Research Division, Fred Hutchinson Cancer Research Center, Seattle, Washington 98109-1024, and the Department of Medicine, University of Washington, Seattle, Washington 98195, USA

ABSTRACT: This paper describes the development of nonmyeloablative marrow transplant programs that have little toxicity in a canine model and their translation to patients with malignant and nonmalignant hematological diseases.

Transplantation of allogeneic hematopoietic stem cells for the treatment of malignant and nonmalignant hematological diseases, as it is currently defined, includes three major components: 1) Intensive cytotoxic conditioning regimens to both eradicate the underlying disease and suppress the host's immune system in preparation for the allograft; 2) Infusion of the stem cell graft to both rescue the recipient from otherwise lethal marrow toxicity of the conditioning regimen and eliminate host resistance and residual leukemia via a graft-versus-host (GVH) reaction; and 3) Postgrafting immunosuppression to prevent graft-versus-host disease (GVHD) and to establish long-term graft host tolerance. A major limitation in the application of stem cell transplantation has been complications related to the conditioning regimens since, to accomplish their aims, regimens have been intensified to a point where organ toxicities are common, resulting in morbidity and mortality. Also, the pancytopenia caused by the regimens prepares the stage for serious and even lethal infections, in spite of the use of antibiotics. For these reasons, allogeneic grafts have been carried out in the setting of intensive care hospital wards. Given the severity of the complications, the use of transplantation has been restricted to relatively young patients at most transplant centers.

We have developed a radically different approach for major histocompatibility complex (MHC) matched allogeneic stem cell transplantation that has minimal toxicity and that is nonmarrow ablative and, thus, safe enough to administer in the ambulatory care setting, allowing inclusion of older patients currently ineligible for treatment with stem cell allografting (for more details, see Refs. 1 and 2). It is known

[a]Address all correspondence to: Rainer Storb, M.D., Fred Hutchinson Cancer Research Center, 1100 Fairview Avenue North, D1-100, P.O. Box 19024, Seattle, WA 98109-1024. Phone, 206/667-4407; fax, 206/667-6124; e-mail, rstorb@fhcrc.org

that both host-versus-graft (HVG) and GVH reactions are mediated by alloreactive T-lymphocytes in the MHC-identical setting. Accordingly, canine studies have been conducted that show that the intensive and toxic conditioning regimens can be rendered obsolete by employing nontoxic pretransplant immunosuppression combined with novel posttransplant immunosuppressive agents that control both HVG and GVH reactions and result in stable mixed donor-host hematopoietic chimerism. Specifically, mixed chimerism has been achieved by using a low and nonmarrow ablative dose of 200 cGy total body irradiation (TBI) before transplant and a combination of the antimetabolite mycophenolate mofetil (MMF) and the T-cell activation blocker cyclosporine for no more than 5 weeks after transplant. MMF blocks a key enzyme in the de novo purine pathway, inosine monophosphate dehydrogenase, and thereby inhibits replication of alloreactive host and donor T-lymphocytes. By substituting peripheral blood stem cells for marrow in this model, we have seen stable mixed chimerism after only 100 cGy TBI conditioning. It is likely that low-dose TBI given before transplant merely serves to provide host immunosuppression, as mixed chimerism, even including unirradiated marrow spaces, has now also been observed after conditioning with low-dose limited-field irradiation directed at cervical, thoracic, and abdominal lymph nodes. Current efforts are directed at replacing pretransplant TBI altogether by nontoxic anti-T-cell reagents. Studies include an antibody to the T-cell receptor $\alpha\beta$ and agents that block T-cell costimulatory pathways, such as CTLA4Ig and antibody to CD40 ligand. Blocking T-cell costimulation, while stimulating the T-cell receptor with stem cell donor antigen, may result in antigen-specific unresponsiveness, thereby facilitating engraftment.

The studies in healthy dogs have led to the development of the schema for using mixed donor-host hematopoietic chimerism in the treatment of hematological diseases as outlined in FIGURE 1. The hypothesis underlying the treatment schema postulates that creation of marrow space by cytotoxic agents is not obligatory for stable allogeneic hematopoietic engraftment to occur and that grafts can be established solely through immunosuppression. Given that, it follows that patients with various T-cell deficiencies, e.g., Wiskott-Aldrich syndrome, bare lymphocyte syndrome, adenosine deaminase deficiency, etc., will not need conditioning before stem cell transplantation. The only immunosuppression required will consist of MMF and cyclosporine given after transplantation. Indeed, two such patients have been transplanted, and early follow-up studies show evidence of donor engraftment consistent with our hypothesis. Patients with other genetic diseases and those with autoimmune diseases or malignant hematological diseases will need treatment with immunosuppression before transplantation. After transplant, these patients will also receive MMF/cyclosporine for further control of HVG reactions and for GVHD prevention. Due to the omission of cytotoxic and myeloablative therapy before transplant, host hematopoietic cells will survive along with grafted donor cells, and this will be manifested as stable mixed chimerism. The presence of donor cells in the mixture is anticipated to correct phenotypic expression of genetic hematological diseases, and this expectation is supported by sporadic observations that mixed chimerism after conventional high-dose conditioning regimens can result in control of sickle cell disease and thalassemia major. Early results in dogs with severe hereditary hemolytic anemia given marrow grafts using nonmyeloablative immunosuppression support the notion that mixed chimerism is sufficient for disease control. If these early data

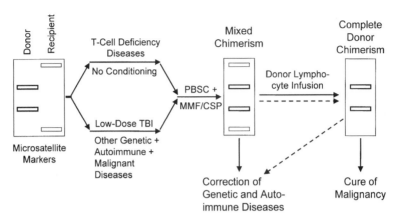

FIGURE 1. Conceptual basis for treatment of patients with nonmalignant and malignant hematological diseases by establishment of mixed chimerism. (From Storb *et al.*[2] Reprinted by permission from Springer-Verlag.)

can be confirmed, mixed chimerism transplants could be investigated as therapy in patients with sickle cell disease and thalassemia major. Conceivably, for some hereditary diseases complete chimerism might be required, and this could be accomplished through donor lymphocyte infusions (FIG. 1; broken arrow).

Perhaps mixed chimerism could also be used to treat patients with autoimmune diseases such as systemic sclerosis and lupus erythematosus in which pulmonary and renal complications would rule out a conventional transplant. Allotransplants have been reported to cure autoimmune diseases, and preclinical studies have suggested that mixed chimerism may suffice for this purpose.

In patients with malignant hematological diseases, mixed chimerism could serve as a platform for subsequent adoptive immunotherapy through donor lymphocyte infusions, and this would result in conversion to complete donor chimerism (FIG. 1; solid arrow). Perhaps those patients who developed GVHD despite postgrafting immunosuppression will not require lymphocyte infusions for conversion to complete donor chimerism to occur. The effectiveness of lymphocyte infusions in eradicating recurrent malignancy after a conventional transplant has been demonstrated for almost all hematological malignancies but appears most potent against chronic lymphocytic leukemia, chronic myelocytic leukemia, and multiple myeloma, and these diseases appear most suited to investigate mixed chimerism transplants. Four elderly human patients with hematological malignancies have now been successfully transplanted using exactly the same approach that has been developed in dogs. All transplants took place in the outpatient department without the need of posttransplant blood transfusions and without significant toxicities. For example, patients did not lose their hair or develop diarrhea or mucositis. The lead patient had chronic lymphocytic leukemia, and he is now 7 months after transplant with complete disappearance of his leukemic cells. Whether the novel transplant approach will be uniformly successful in such patients and whether it can be extended further to include patients with AIDS-related lymphoma or certain solid tumors is the subject of future investigations. Extending the outpatient transplant approach to include MHC-nonidentical transplants will be another future challenge.

REFERENCES

1. STORB, R., C. YU & P. MCSWEENEY. 1999. Mixed chimerism after transplantation of allogeneic hematopoietic cells. *In* Hematopoietic Cell Transplantation, 2nd edit. E.D. Thomas, K.G. Blume & S.J. Forman, Eds. Chap. 26: 287–295. Blackwell Science, Inc. Boston, MA.
2. STORB, R., C. YU, P. MCSWEENEY, R. NASH, B. SANDMAIER, J. WAGNER & A. WOOLFREY. New strategies for hematopoietic stem cell transplantation. *In* Proceedings of Transplantation in Hematology and Oncology Symposium, Münster, Germany, July 1–4, 1998. Springer-Verlag. Heidelberg. In press.

DISCUSSION

W.E. FIBBE (*University Medical Center Leiden*): Could you comment on the development of chimerism?

B. TOROK-STORB (*Fred Hutchinson Cancer Research Center*): If you want to treat sickle cell anemia or other genetic diseases, you are already there if you establish stable mixed hematopoietic chimerism. However, the first protocol dealt with malignant diseases in patients who were over 55 years of age, because they were ineligible for a standard conditioning regimen because of the toxicity. The first patient was a chronic lymphocytic leukemia (CLL) patient who was 54 years old. He is out 7 months now posttransplant and continues to receive cyclosporine. The GVH was controlled with some steroids, and because he had GVH, he never got the donor lymphocyte infusion. He is now about 210 days posttransplant, and he is 100% donor cells in all lineages. He was never hospitalized, he never had mucositis, he never had diarrhea, and he never lost his hair. Everything was done as an outpatient. There were two multiple myeloma patients and one patient with myelodysplastic syndrome (MDS)/acute myeloid leukemia (AML). All three of these patients are early posttransplant, about day 60 or 70. They all have mixed chimerism, and they have received their donor lymphocyte infusion because they did not get GVH. That was the experience in the dogs, also. They did not get GVH. Then there have been two patients with T-cell immune deficiencies who actually received no TBI. They just received the peripheral blood mononuclear cells and the MMF and the cyclosporine. The first T-cell deficiency patient is currently out 120 days; he is over 50% donor cells in all lineages. Interestingly, when he came to transplant he had a mycobacterium avian infection, and that responded very well to the transplant. This 30-year-old person says that he has never felt better in his 30 years of life and he received no TBI.

The adenosine deaminase (ADA) patient is out to day 30 and currently has 90% donor T-cells, 87% donor B-cells, but 5% donor granulocytes. The last patient, in fact, is a Basenji dog, Andy, that inherited a pyruvate kinase (PK) deficiency. He was 5 years old and had hemolytic anemia, so he looked very much like a sickle cell patient. He had iron overload. He was transplanted to look at the efficacy of this treatment in a disease where there is organ toxicity. Independently, he had also inherited inflammatory bowel disease. He was on a special diet. He had lots of diarrhea, and he had to be fed antibiotics. Now he is out about 4 months, and he is about 80% donor. He has normal hematocrit and reticulocyte counts, and his diarrhea has disappeared. And there is no GVH. This is a summary of our experience right now with this kind of conditioning. I remind you that these are all human leukocyte antigen (HLA)-identical matched siblings and that when you go into an unrelated donor it will be a different story. We know in the matched model that the GVH and the rejection are both mediated by T-cells, and introducing tolerance against that mechanism will be different from introducing tolerance against mechanisms mediating GVH or rejection in MHC-disparate grafts.

Clinical Applications of Mixed Chimerism

BEATE G. EXNER, MICHELE A. DOMENICK, MARIANNE BERGHEIM,
YVONNE M. MUELLER, AND SUZANNE T. ILDSTAD[a]

*Institute for Cellular Therapeutics, University of Louisville, 500 South Ridgeway Avenue,
Glenolden, Pennsylvania 19036, USA*

**ABSTRACT: Bone marrow transplantation (BMT) is currently a procedure
that is associated with high morbidity and mortality. Thus, the clinical application of this technique is limited to the treatment of life-threatening hematopoietic malignancies. The morbidity and mortality of BMT is mainly related to
graft-versus-host disease (GVHD), failure of engraftment, and toxicity related
to fully myeloablative conditioning. GVHD can be prevented by T-cell depletion. However, T-cell depletion increases the risk of failure of engraftment.
With the identification of a facilitating cell population that enables engraftment of hematopoietic stem cells across major histocompatibility barriers, the
dichotomy between GVHD and failure of engraftment has been resolved. If one
could overcome the toxicity of conditioning with the development of partially
ablative conditioning strategies, BMT could be used for the treatment of a variety of nonmalignant diseases, as well as in the induction of donor-specific
transplantation tolerance. This review outlines the development and advantages of partially ablative conditioning strategies and illustrates possible applications of the technique. Forty years ago E.D. Thomas discussed the potential of
BMT for treating immunodeficiencies and for the induction of transplantation
tolerance.[1] BMT can be viewed as a natural form of gene therapy to replace a
defective cell or enzyme with a functional and normally regulated one.**

INTRODUCTION

The clinical application of bone marrow transplantation is currently limited to the
treatment of hematological malignancy and other life-threatening diseases due to the
morbidity and mortality associated with the procedure. The complications are mainly caused by graft-versus-host disease (GVHD), failure of engraftment, and toxicity
associated with myeloablative conditioning. For a long time it seemed that engraftment could not be achieved without the risk of GVHD (FIG. 1). It has been shown
that GVHD can be successfully prevented by T-cell depletion of the bone marrow
graft.[2] However, when T-cell depletion was applied clinically, a dramatic increase
occurred in the incidence of graft failure.[3] This dichotomy seemed unresolvable until a cell population was identified in our laboratory that can prevent graft failure
without causing GVHD by facilitating engraftment through a mechanism that is yet
undefined.[4] Preliminary results from clinical trials using this cell to improve engraftment of T-cell-depleted bone marrow grafts are very encouraging. Rapid and reliable
engraftment has been achieved with heavily T-cell-depleted bone marrow grafts even
across major class I and II antigenic major histocompatibility complex (MHC) bar-

[a]Corresponding author. Phone, 610/237-7960; fax, 610/237-7773; e-mail, ildstads
@wpo.auhs.edu

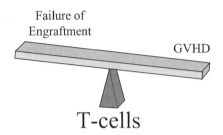

FIGURE 1. The dichotomy between GVHD mediated by T-cells and failure of engraftment with T-cell-depleted grafts.

riers.[5] Since the bone marrow grafts are T-cell depleted, the achieved engraftment is associated with only a limited degree of GVHD, which can usually be controlled with steroids. The dichotomy of GVHD and graft failure could be solved if this observation proved to be true. Thus, the major limitation in the widespread use of bone marrow transplantation (BMT) to treat nonmalignant diseases remains the toxicity associated with fully myeloablative conditioning.

DEVELOPMENT OF PARTIAL CONDITIONING STRATEGIES

Until the late 1970s it was believed that fully ablative conditioning was necessary to allow engraftment of bone marrow grafts. Now it has become clear that engraftment can be achieved with partial conditioning as well. The availability of novel nonspecific immunosuppressive agents to control rejection of solid organ transplants has ushered in a new era: the partial conditioning approach. Wood and Monaco were the first to achieve engraftment of MHC-identical bone marrow in mice conditioned with anti-lymphocyte serum in a mouse model.[6] McCarthy *et al.* achieved similar results using monoclonal antibodies (mAbs) against host MHC class I antigens in mice.[7] Transplantation of fully mismatched bone marrow grafts usually requires the use of low-dose total body irradiation (TBI) or another cytoreductive agent. The dose of TBI required to achieve engraftment across MHC barriers can be lowered by adding immunosuppressive agents to the conditioning protocol. Cobbold and Waldman were the first to use anti-CD4 and anti-CD8 mAbs in conditioning.[8] The use of these antibodies allowed engraftment across minor histocompatibility barriers with antibodies alone. However, for MHC-disparate recipients a low dose of TBI was essential. The combination of anti-CD4 and anti-CD8 mAbs was also successfully used by other investigators.[9,10] When recipient mice are pretreated with these antibodies plus thymic irradiation and a low dose of TBI, engraftment of MHC-disparate marrow can be achieved.[9] When very large doses of donor bone marrow are transplanted in this model, engraftment of MHC mismatched bone marrow cells even ocurs without requiring TBI.[11]

Other models to achieve engraftment in fully mismatched donor and recipient pairs are based on the use of cytoreductive and immunosuppressive agents. The combination of 1 mg anti-lymphocyte globulin (ALG) administrated intravenously three

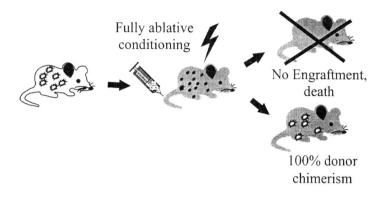

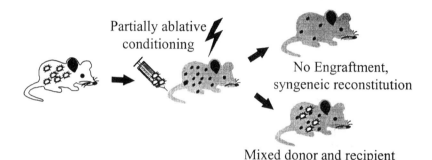

FIGURE 2. The difference between fully and partially ablative conditioning strategies. Fully ablative conditioning results in the death of the recipient when engraftment fails and in 100% donor chimerism when engraftment is achieved. In contrast, partially ablative conditioning allows syngeneic reconstitution in case of failure of engraftment, and mixed donor and host chimerism occur when engraftment is achieved.

days prior to BMT and 200 mg/kg cyclophosphamide intraperitoneally two days after BMT allows reliable engraftment with less than 300 cGy TBI in a fully MHC-mismatched mouse model.[12] By combining ALG plus cyclophosphamide and doubling the dose of donor bone marrow, the TBI dose can be reduced to 100 cGy.[12] In rats, a combination of ALG and tacrolimus is highly effective in conditioning for BMT with a minimum irradiation dose.[13] Partially ablative conditioning strategies have been developed not only in rat models, but also in large animal models. Storb *et al.* have developed an approach using mycophenolate mofetil and cyclosporin to achieve engraftment in dog leukocyte antigen matched littermate dogs with 200 cGy TBI.[14] These models show that fully ablative conditioning is not essential to achieve stable multilineage mixed chimerism, but that partially ablative conditioning regimens are sufficient.

ADVANTAGES OF PARTIAL ABLATIVE CONDITIONING STRATEGIES

With partially ablative conditioning strategies, the toxicity of conditioning can be minimized and partial conditioning has more advantages than just reducing transplantation-related toxicity. Individuals who receive a BMT after partial conditioning develop mixed multilineage chimerism in contrast to the 100% donor chimerism that develops in patients conditioned with fully ablative strategies (FIG. 2). Mixed chimeras show superior immunocompetence compared to fully allogeneic chimeras due to restriction.[15] Zinkernagel and Dougherty were awarded the Nobel Prize in 1996 for the discovery of this phenomenon. T-cells require "self" antigen-presenting cells (APCs) to be able to recognize antigen and initiate a primary immune response. T-cells must recognize the APCs as "self." T-cells that newly emerge from donor bone marrow are educated in the host thymus and thus are restricted to host MHC. With fully ablative conditioning, no APCs of host type are present in fully allogeneic chimeras, since all APCs are of donor-type. As a result, immunocompetence is impaired, the animals are susceptible to infections and exhibit impaired antibody production, and overall survival is inferior.[15,16] In contrast, in mixed chimeras donor and host-type APCs are present. Both host and donor T-cells that are restricted to host-derived APCs are therefore able to respond, since host-type APCs are present. As a result such chimeras are immunocompetent in B-cell and helper T-cell responses.[15,16] Colson *et al.* recently showed that lethally conditioned mice reconstituted with a mixture of xenogeneic rat and syngeneic mouse bone marrow have excellent survival when challenged with viruses. Moreover, the rat as well as mouse T-cells recognize mouse APCs as self and are restricted to them. In fact their survival is as good as in animals that were syngeneically reconstituted, while 100% of the fully xenogeneic chimeras die due to infection within 14 days.[17]

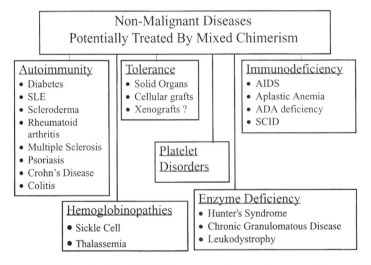

FIGURE 3. The potential of BMT. Many nonmalignant diseases could potentially be treated with the technique if the morbidity and mortality associated with GVHD, failure of engraftment, and toxicity of fully ablative conditioning could be solved.

NOVEL APPLICATIONS OF BONE MARROW TRANSPLANTATION

With an improved technique for BMT, including T-cell depletion, enrichment for facilitating cells, and partially ablative conditioning, many new possible applications for BMT can be considered (FIG. 3).

Induction of Allogeneic Tolerance to Solid Organ and Cellular Grafts

The association between chimerism and tolerance was first observed by Billingham, Brent, and Medawar.[18] They developed a technique of skin grafting and observed that skin grafts are accepted in genetically identical individuals, but rejected when transplanted across genetic disparities.[19] They were asked by the British agricultural system to apply this HLA-typing approach to cattle twins with a common placenta to differentiate monozygotic animals from dizygotic Freemartin cattle, since female Freemartin cattle are sterile and of lower market value for the farmers. To their surprise, although Freemartin cattle are dizygotic, they accepted the skin grafts from their genetically disparate siblings.[20] Reconciling an observation by Owen *et al.*[21] that cattle with a common placenta display red blood cell chimerism in the peripheral blood, they hypothesized that this was the reason for the unexpected graft acceptance. To prove their hypothesis, they performed a classical series of experiments in mice and chickens with inoculation of cell homogenates or blood into fetal recipients. The mice displayed donor-specific tolerance to skin grafts after birth. When the cells were inoculated into adult recipients, immunization with even more rapid rejection of consecutive skin grafts resulted.[18]

The significance of the association between chimerism and tolerance induction has been much discussed in the scientific community. In order to prevent confusion between different concepts in the induction of transplantation tolerance, two types of bone marrow chimerism must be differentiated: *microchimerism* and *macrochimerism*. Microchimerism occurs naturally with passenger leukocytes contained in solid organ and cellular grafts. It does not require conditioning to be induced, and it does not routinely include engraftment of the pluripotent hematopoietic stem cell. Most typing for microchimerism enumerates a single lineage: class II$^+$ dendritic cells.[22] Moreover, microchimerism has not been reliably associated with a drug-free state for solid organ acceptance. Some studies seem to indicate that microchimerism is more likely an epiphenomenon associated with tolerance to solid organ transplantation rather than the mechanism that induces tolerance. This is especially true in light of the fact that microchimerism has been reported in recipients of orthotopic liver transplantation during refractory rejection.[23,24]

Macrochimerism, in contrast, is the result of a BMT. BMT results in engraftment of the pluripotent hematopoietic stem cell, but also requires conditioning of the patient. Macrochimerism has been shown to induce donor-specific tolerance in the clinical setting. Patients are tolerant to donor-derived skin[25] or kidney grafts[26] of donor origin without immunosuppression after BMT for hematological malignancies. The difference in the effect of microchimerism and macrochimerism does not seem to be exclusively quantitative. Levels of chimerism as low as 1% achieved with 600 cGy of TBI and a single dose of cyclophosphamide two days after the transplantation of 80×10^6 xenogeneic bone marrow cells, are sufficient to induce donor-specific tolerance even across species barriers.[27] Perhaps a difference in the quality of the chimerism (like the presence of multiple lineages) accounts for the different effects in micro– and macrochimerism.

Re-Induction of Self-Tolerance in Autoimmune Diseases

Another potentially novel application of allogeneic BMT could be the treatment of autoimmune diseases. Data emerging from rodent work indicates that autoimmune diabetes can be prevented and to a certain degree even cured by BMT as indicated by reversed insulinitis in the nonobese diabetic mouse.[28] It has been shown that B27-associated spondyloarthropathies can be prevented by BMT in a rat model, and a lupus erythematosus-like syndrome can be cured by BMT in Fas-ligand-deficient mice.[30] Clinically evidence that patients with autoimmune diseases could benefit from BMT emerges from patients treated with BMT for a hematologic malignancy who suffer from an autoimmune disease. The autoimmunity did not recur after allogeneic BMT in patients suffering from psoriasis,[31] chronic inflammatory bowel disease,[32] rheumatoid arthritis,[33] autoimmune diabetes[34] and other autoimmune conditions[34] when transplanted with bone marrow from a healthy donor who is free of autoimmunity.

Nonmalignant Hematological Diseases

BMT is already performed in an attempt to treat hematological diseases that are classified as "nonmalignant" yet result in severe complications that impair the quality of life and the health of the patients. Unlike in malignant diseases where fully ablative conditioning is required to eliminate the tumor before BMT, most nonmalignant diseases could probably be cured with low levels of donor chimerism. One example is sickle cell anemia, which can be cured with allogeneic BMT as shown by Walters *et al.*[35] Donor chimerism of as low as 20% results in the production of 80% normal red blood cells (RBC) in the recipients' peripheral blood, suggesting a competitive advantage for hematopoietically normal RBC.[35] Another "nonmalignant" hematological disease that has been shown to profit from treatment with BMT is thalassemia.[36] BMT is already used in the treatment of patients with aplastic anemia (reviewed in Ref. 37). Even in conventional BMT, the advantages of the procedure far exceed the potential risks involved in select cases. The treatment of all these diseases could be significantly improved with improved techniques for BMT.

GENE THERAPY

As E.D. Thomas pointed out nearly 40 years ago, BMT has many potential applications and can be considered a natural form of gene therapy. With the successful engraftment of donor hematopoietic stem cells, normally regulated production of donor cells is established in the recipient. This could be used to provide cell types that are missing by an inherited immunodeficiency as well as produce enzymes and other substances deficient in the recipient. Many of these diseases have been reported to benefit from treatment with conventional BMT.[38,39] The majority of those diseases may not need 100% donor chimerism, but could be treated with mixed allogeneic chimerism that can be achieved with partially ablative conditioning.

SUMMARY

In summary, dramatic progress has been made in the development of techniques to improve BMT at the bench, and some of these developments are now in the process of being tested at the bedside. If we could optimize the graft composition by graft engineering for T-cell depletion and enrichment for engraftment-facilitating cells as well as define the most efficient yet least toxic conditioning strategies, BMT could potentially be used for the induction of donor-specific transplantation tolerance, the treatment of nonmalignant diseases, and gene therapy.

ACKNOWLEDGMENTS

This work was supported by NIH Grant R01DK43901-07 and by the German Society for Research (DFG; Grant Ex11/1-1).

REFERENCES

1. THOMAS, E.D., H.H. LOCHTE, W.C. LU & J.W. FERREBEE. 1957. Intravenous infusion of bone marrow in patients receiving radiation and chemotherapy. N. Engl. J. Med. **157:** 491–496.
2. KORNGOLD, B. & J. SPRENT. 1978. Lethal GvHD after transplantation across minor histocompatibility barriers in mice: prevention by removing mature T-cells from marrow. J. Exp. Med. **148:** 1687–1698.
3. MARTIN, P.J., J.A. HANSEN, C.D. BUCKNER *et al.* 1985. Effects of *in vitro* depletion of T cells in HLA-identical allogeneic marrow grafts. Blood **66:** 664–672.
4. KAUFMAN, C.L., Y.L. COLSON, S.M. WREN *et al.* 1994. Phenotypic characterization of a novel bone marrow-derived cell that facilitates engraftment of allogeneic bone marrow. Blood **84:** 2436–2446.
5. ILDSTAD, S.T., P.A. CRILLEY, R.A. SHADDUCK *et al.* 1997. Graft engineering: the facilitating cell (FC) protocol in HLA mismatched BMT for hematologic malignancy. Blood **90:** 484.
6. WOOD, M.L. A.P. MONACO, J.J. GOZZO & A. LIEGEOIS. 1971. Use of homozygous allogeneic bone marrow for induction of tolerance with antilymphocyte serum: dose and timing. Transplant. Proc. **3:** 676–679.
7. MCCARTHY, S.A., I.J. GRIFFITH, P. GAMBEL *et al.* 1985. Characterization of host lymphoid cells in antibody-facilitated bone marrow chimeras. Transplantation **40:** 12–17.
8. COBBOLD, S.P., G. MARTIN, S. QIN & H. WALDMANN. 1986. Monoclonal antibodies to promote marrow engraftment and tissue graft tolerance. Nature **323:** 164–166.
9. SHARABI, Y., M. SYKES & D.H. SACHS. 1992. Mixed allogeneic chimeras prepared by a non-myeloablative regimen: requirement for chimerism to maintain tolerance. Bone Marrow Transplant. **9:** 191–197.
10. EXNER, B.G., Y.L. COLSON, H. LI & S.T. ILDSTAD. 1997. *In vivo* depletion of host CD4+ and CD8+ cells permits engraftment of bone marrow stem cells and tolerance induction with minimal conditioning. Surgery **122:** 221–227.

11. SYKES, M., G.L. SZOT, K.A. SWENSON & D.A. PEARSON. 1997. Induction of high levels of allogeneic hematopoietic reconstitution and donor-specific tolerance without myelosuppressive conditioning. Nat. Med. **3:** 783–787.

12. COLSON, Y.L., H. LI, S.S. BOGGS et al. 1996. Durable mixed chimerism and tolerance by a non-lethal radiation-based cytoreductive approach. J. Immunol. **157:** 2820–2829.

13. GAMMIE, J.S., S. LI, N. KAWAHARADA et al. Mixed allogeneic chimerism prevents obstructive airway disease in a rat heterotopic tracheal transplantation model. J. Hematother. In press.

14. STORB, R., C. YU, J.L. WAGNER et al. 1997. Stable mixed hematopoietic chimerism in DLA-identical littermate dogs given sublethal total body irradiation before and pharmacological immunosuppression after marrow transplantation. Blood **89:** 3048–3054.

15. ILDSTAD, S.T., S.M. WREN, J.A. BLUESTONE et al. 1985. Characterization of mixed allogeneic chimeras. Immunocompetence, in vitro reactivity, and genetic specificity of tolerance. J. Exp. Med. **162:** 231–244.

16. RUEDI, E., M. SYKES, S.T. ILDSTAD et al. 1989. Antiviral T cell competence and restriction specificity of mixed allogeneic (P1 + P2øP1) irradiation chimeras. Cell. Immunol. **121:** 185–195.

17. COLSON, Y.L., R.A. TRIPP, P.C. DOHERTY et al. 1998. Antiviral cytotoxic activity across a species barrier in mixed xenogeneic chimeras: functional restriction to host MHC. J. Immunol. **160:** 3790–3796.

18. BILLINGHAM, R.E., L. BRENT & P.B. MEDAWAR. 1953. Actively acquired tolerance of foreign cells. Nature **172:** 603–606.

19. BILLINGHAM, R.E. & P.B. MEDAWAR. 1951. The technique of free skin grafting in mammals. J. Exp. Biol. **28:** 385–402.

20. BILLINGHAM, R.E., H.G. LAMPHIN, P.B. MEDAWAR & H.L. WILLIAMS. 1952. Tolerance of homografts, twin diagnosis and the freemartin conditions in cattle. Heredity **6:** 201.

21. OWEN, R.D. 1945. Immunogeneic consequences of vascular anastomoses between bovine twins. Science **102:** 400–401.

22. STARZL, T.E., A.J. DEMETRIS, N. MURASE et al. 1992. Cell migration, chimerism and graft acceptance. Lancet **339:** 1579–1582.

23. SCHLITT, H.J., J. HUNDRIESER, M. HISANAGA et al. 1994. Patterns of donor-type microchimerism after heart transplantation. Lancet **343:** 1469–1471.

24. SIVASAI, K.S., Y.G. ALEVY, B.F. DUFFY et al. 1997. Peripheral blood microchimerism in human liver and renal transplant recipients: rejection despite donor-specific chimerism. Transplantation **64:** 427–432.

25. KNOBLER, H.Y., U. SAGHER, I.J. PELED et al. 1985. Tolerance to donor-type skin in the recipient of a bone marrow allograft. Treatment of skin ulcers in chronic graft-versus-host disease with skin grafts from the bone marrow donor. Transplantation **40:** 223–225.

26. SAYEGH, M.H., N.A. FINE, J.L. SMITH et al. 1991. Immunologic tolerance to renal allografts after bone marrow transplants from the same donors. Ann. Intern. Med. **114:** 954–955.

27. NEIPP, M., B.G. EXNER & S.T. ILDSTAD. A nonlethal conditioning approach to achieve engraftment of xenogeneic rat bone marrow in mice and to induce donor-specific tolerance. Transplantation. In press.

28. LI, H., C.L. KAUFMAN, S.S. BOGGS et al. 1996. Mixed allogeneic chimerism induced by a sublethal approach prevents autoimmune diabetes and reverses insulinitis in nonobese diabetic (NOD) mice. J. Immunol. **156:** 380–388.

29. BREBAN, M., R.E. HAMMER, J.A. RICHARDSON & J.D. TAUROG. 1993. Transfer of the inflammatory disease of HLA-B27 transgenic rats by bone marrow engraftment. J. Exp. Med. **178:** 1607–1616.
30. SOBEL, E.S., V.N. KAKKANAIAH, P.L. COHEN & R.A. EISENBERG. 1993. Correction of gld autoimmunity by co-infusion of normal bone marrow suggests that gld is a mutation of the Fas ligand gene. Int. Immunol. **5:** 1275–1278.
31. EEDY, D.J., D. BURROWS, J.M. BRIDGES *et al.* 1990. Clearance of severe psoriasis after allogeneic bone marrow transplantation. Br. Med. J. **300:** 908–909.
32. LIU, Y.J. & S.N. JOWITT. 1992. Resolution of immune-mediated diseases following allogeneic bone marrow transplantation. Bone Marrow Transplant. **9:** 31–33.
33. LOWENTHAL, R.M., M.L. COHEN, K. ATKINSON *et al.* 1993. Apparent cure of rheumatoid arthritis by bone marrow transplantation for leukemia. J. Rheumatol. **20:** 137–140.
34. NELSON, J.L., R. TORREZ, F.M. LOUIE *et al.* 1997. Pre-existing autoimmune disease in patients with long-term survival after allogeneic bone marrow transplantation. J. Rheumatol. Suppl. **48:** 23–29.
35. WALTERS, M.C., M. PATIENCE, W. LEISENRING *et al.* 1996. Bone marrow transplantation for sickle cell disease. N. Engl. J. Med. **335:** 369–376.
36. LUCARELLI, G., M. GALIMBERTI, P POLCHI *et al.* 1990. New approach to bone marrow transplantation in thalassemia. Haematologica **75**(Suppl 5): 111–121.
37. BRODSKY, R.A. 1998. Biology and management of acquired severe aplastic anemia. Curr. Opin. Oncol. **10:** 95–99.
38. GOOD, R.A. 1987. Bone marrow transplantation for immunodeficiency diseases. Am. J. Med. Sci. **294:** 68–74.
39. RINGDEN, O., C.G. GROTH, A. ERIKSON *et al.* 1995. Ten years' experience of bone marrow transplantation for Gaucher disease. Transplantation **59:** 864–870.

DISCUSSION

E.D. ZANJANI (*Department of Veterans Affairs Medical Center*): The cells you get out of the vertebral column, what are they? Are they CD34$^+$ cells and facilitating cells? Are the cells given to the patient at the time of transplant?

ILDSTAD: It is embarassing, because it takes the surgeon much less time to transplant the heart or the kidney than it takes us to process the marrow. Thus, the patient was extubating 8 hours after the heart went in, and it was another 24 hours before we were done processing the marrow. We are working on ways to improve on that. We give the bone marrow transplant as soon as possible after the solid organ goes in.

ZANJANI: What cell populations do you give?

ILDSTAD: We give stem cells, progenitors, and facilitating cells. It is a heavily negatively selective process where we remove all of the mature types of cells that would mediate GVH reaction. My bias is that as you are processing major HLA disparities, if humans behave like mice, there are a lot of other cell types besides T-cells that mediate GVH including natural killer cells, B-cells, and APCs. What we do is graft engineering to keep what we think we need and take out all the rest.

Y. REISNER (*Weizmann Institute of Science*): Do you know how many CD34$^+$ cells per kilogram are being given?

ILDSTAD: I know what was given to this patient. Our formula is to give less than 1×10^4 T-cells and mature cells per kilo. We are not calculating a dose of CD34 we want to give, although we do want to give the maximum. Mr. Coombs received 0.3 $\times 10^6$ CD34$^+$ cells per kilo.

REISNER: You got that from just those few vertebrae?

ILDSTAD: Believe it or not a vertebral body has a billion bone marrow cells. It is an unbelievable source of marrow, and up until about the age of 60 donors are good. The military actually did those studies in the late 1970s. Our military had a plan in the event of a nuclear disaster to archive marrow and then transplant the President and then various other dignitaries. They found that the vertebral bodies were the best source of marrow, and they started archiving them. Then they realized that HLA matching was so important and the frequency of finding a donor was so difficult.

L. KANZ (*Eberhard Karls University*): What was the conditioning for the transplant?

ILDSTAD: He received a dose of 100 cGy TBI, which I think was too low.

KANZ: Immunosuppression?

ILDSTAD: Conventional. A lot of the drugs now being used for the partial conditioning strategies were drugs developed for solid organ transplantation, so he has been receiving conventional immunosuppression for 6 months, cyclosporine, mycophenolate mofetil (MFF) and prednisone, which is pretty much the standard. We do not know yet whether he has donor-specific tolerance, or whether he is chimeric at 6 months.

REISNER: We did monkeys at 700 cGy TBI (which is much more than 100 cGy) and infused approximately 2×10^6 CD34 cells/kg, and we have not seen any chimerism. None whatsoever. I doubt whether this treatment is ready for widespread use. I think we ought to do more with primates before we treat patients.

ILDSTAD: I think we will know, because if you look at the survival curve for cardiac transplants, within three years only 50% are surviving. Many people feel that the risk benefit ratio is justified.

Canine Lymphocyte Expression of Retrovirally Transferred Human Common Gamma Chain

TODD WHITWAM,[a] MARK E. HASKINS,[b] PAULA S. HENTHORN,[b]
DAVID M. BODINE,[a] AND JENNIFER M. PUCK[a,c]

[a]Genetics and Molecular Biology Branch, National Human Genome Research Institute,
National Institutes of Health, Bethesda, Maryland, USA
[b]Department of Genetics, University of Pennsylvania School of Veterinary Medicine,
Philadelphia, Pennsylvania, USA

X-linked severe combined immune deficiency (XSCID), the most common SCID in humans, is a profound immunodeficiency caused by mutations of *IL2RG*, encoding the interleukin-2 (IL-2) receptor common γ chain (γc).[1–4] Presently treatable only by bone marrow transplantation (BMT), XSCID is a favorable disease for treatment by gene transfer into hematopoietic stem cells (HSCs). Female carriers of *IL2RG* mutations show nonrandom X chromosome inactivation in their T, B and natural killer cells, reflecting *in vivo* positive selection of lymphoid progenitors with an active X chromosome bearing an intact copy of *IL2RG*.[5,6] The primary defect causes immunologic incompetence, rendering affected patients unlikely to reject transduced cells newly expressing γc protein. In addition, γc is expressed on immature and mature cells of all hematopoietic lineages,[7,8] suggesting that constituitive expression of γc from a retroviral long terminal repeat (LTR) would not be harmful. Animal models of XSCID include dogs with spontaneous mutations of *IL2RG*,[9] but the methods for transducing canine HSCs with amphotropic retroviruses required optimization in normal dogs. We have now achieved persistent lymphocyte expression of human γc in healthy dogs by transplanting cytokine mobilized, transduced canine bone marrow.

Previous mouse and primate studies demonstrated elevated numbers of HSCs and improved retroviral transduction efficiency in the bone marrow following priming *in vivo* with cytokines.[10,11] In this study, normal 8–10-week-old untreated donor dogs at the University of Pennsylvania School of Veterinary Medicine were compared to donors given 4 daily doses of recombinant canine stem cell factor (cSCF), 25 mg/kg/day, and canine granulocyte colony-stimulating factor (cG-CSF), 10 mg/kg/day (kindly provided by Fred Fletcher, Amgen, Thousand Oaks, CA). Bone marrow was harvested 10.5 days later for autologous BMT by multiple aspirations and for major histocompatibility complex (MHC)-matched allogeneic BMT by sacrificing the animal and flushing cells from the femur.

Between 3 and 4×10^8 nucleated cells were transduced with 4 successive daily exposures to amphotropic supernatants of a retrovirus called HGMDR (Harvey γc and multiple drug resistance gene-containing virus) with 2.0×10^7 cfu/ml.[12] This

[c]Address for correspondence: Jennifer M. Puck, NHGRI/NIH, Bldg. 49, Rm. 3A14, 49 Convent Drive, Bethesda, MD 20892-4442. Phone, 301/402-2194; fax, 301/402-4929; e-mail, jpuck@nhgri.nih.gov

virus contains the Harvey murine sarcoma virus LTR, human *IL2RG* cDNA and the human *MDR1* gene driven from an internal ribosome entry site.[13] One day prior to graft infusion, normal recipients received a low dose (200 cGy) of total body irradiation. The dogs experienced transient leukopenia and thrombocytopenia with no clinical complications. Peripheral blood and bone marrow samples were obtained at regular intervals for cell counts, semiquantitative polymerase chain reaction (PCR) measurement of total leukocyte proviral DNA, and determination of lymphocyte cell surface expression of γc by flow cytometry using the human-specific anti-γc TUGh4 (Pharmingen, San Diego, CA).

As in previous canine retroviral marking studies,[14,15] transduced proviral DNA and human γc expression were detected only transiently in recipients of non-cytokine-pretreated marrow. In contrast, bone marrow from cytokine-pretreated donors yielded up to 28% of peripheral blood leukocytes positive for provirus by PCR for 11–15 weeks in autologous recipients and for 23 weeks in allogeneic recipients. As illustrated in FIGURE 1A, 15–35% of lymphocytes expressed human γc by immunofluorescence, >5- to 50-fold higher than typical reported expression rates.[16,17] Long-term bone marrow expression of human γc was also found (not shown).

After 28 weeks, lymphocyte surface expression of human γc decreased to undetectable levels in all the dogs and did not spontaneously reappear during the following 10–20 weeks (FIG. 1B). However, provirus remained detectable by PCR. The

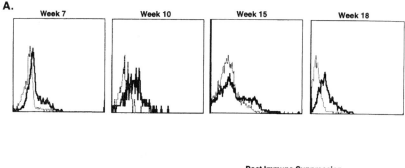

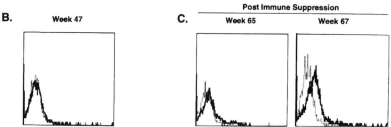

FIGURE 1. Immunofluorescence analysis of peripheral lymphocytes from a dog transplanted with autologous, cytokine-primed bone marrow transduced with HGMDR. Anti-γc rat monoclonal antibody, *solid tracings*; rat isotype control, *dotted tracings*. **(A)** Posttransplant 7–18 weeks, showing 15–35% of lymphocytes positive for human γc; **(B)** Nonexpression at week 47, prior to start of immune suppressive treatment; **(C)** Return of human γc-positive lymphocytes, 10–25%, following cyclosporin A and prednisone treatment.

loss of cells expressing human γc after strong expression was consistent with an immune reaction against either transduced human γc or the *MDR* gene product, P-glycoprotein. Therefore, two allogeneic recipients of cytokine-primed transduced marrow as well as one recipient of autologous cytokine-primed marrow were treated with cyclosporin A, 14–24 mg/kg, and prednisone acetate, 1–2 mg/kg, daily with doses adjusted to maintain peripheral absolute lymphocyte counts near 1×10^3 per μl. In all three dogs, lymphocytes bearing surface human γc reappeared, returning to nearly their original peak levels (FIG. 1C). After termination of immune suppression, expression again became undetectable 10 weeks later, consistent with the hypothesis that an immune response contributed to elimination of cells expressing foreign transduced protein.

Immune responses to transduced proteins have been noted before in the dog[18] and are a major issue in human gene transfer trials. Fortunately, for gene therapy of XSCID, the underlying primary immunodeficiency is predicted to render the host incapable of immune rejection of transduced cells. On the contrary, expression of normal γc on transduced lymphoid lineage progeny of long-term repopulating cells should confer a selective advantage over endogenous cells not expressing γc, as occurred in the related JAK3-deficient SCID in a knockout mouse model.[19] Our findings support previous studies with cytokine mobilization of stem cells in other species and indicate that pretreatment of canine donors with cSCF and cG-CSF improves transduction efficiency of canine long-term repopulating cells from bone marrow. This canine trial has demonstrated high levels and long duration of retrovirally transduced protein expression in lymphocytes. A similar approach in XSCID dogs and ultimately humans affected with XSCID may have therapeutic value.

ACKNOWLEDGMENTS

This work was supported by NIH Grants DK54481 and NS33526 to M. E. H. and AI3317 to P. S. H.

We thank Margie Weil and the University of Pennsylvania Veterinary Students for compassionate animal care; Fred Fletcher of Amgen for canine cytokines; Pat Miller-Wilson for canine irradiation; Stacie Anderson for flow cytometry and sorting; Ann Ferrero, Laurie Girard, Brian Hartnett and Jennifer Kraszewski for technical assistance; and Ian Dubé, Peter Felsburg and Michael Gottesman for helpful discussions.

REFERENCES

1. NOGUCHI, M., H. YI, H.M. ROSENBLATT, A.H. FILIPOVICH, S. ADELSTEIN, W.S. MODI, O.W. MCBRIDE & W.J. LEONARD. 1993. Interleukin-2 receptor gamma chain mutation results in X-linked severe combined immunodeficiency in humans. Cell **73:** 147–157.

2. PUCK, J.M., S.M. DESCHENES, J.C. PORTER, A.S. DUTRA, C.J. BROWN, H.F. WILLARD & P.S. HENTHORN. 1993. The interleukin-2 receptor gamma chain maps to Xq13.1 and is mutated in X-linked severe combined immunodeficiency, SCIDX1. Hum. Mol. Genet. **2:** 1099–1104.

3. PUCK, J.M, A.E. PEPPER, P.S. HENTHORN, F. CANDOTTI, J. ISAKOV, T. WHITWAM, M.E. CONLEY, R.E. FISCHER, H.M. ROSENBLATT, T.N. SMALL & R.H. BUCKLEY.

1997. Mutation analysis of IL2RG in human X-linked severe combined immunodeficiency. Blood **89:** 1968–1977.

4. LEONARD, W.J. 1996. The molecular basis of X-linked severe combined immunodeficiency: defective cytokine receptor signaling. Annu. Rev. Med. **47:** 229–239.

5. PUCK, J.M., R.L. NUSSBAUM & M.E. CONLEY. 1987. Carrier detection in X-linked severe combied immunodeficiency based on patterns of X-chromosome inactivation. J. Clin. Invest. **79:** 1395–1400.

6. WENGLER, G.S., R.C. ALLEN, O. PAROLINI, H. SMITH & M.E. CONLEY. 1993. Nonrandom X chromosome inactivation in natural killer cells from obligate carriers of X-linked severe combined immunodeficiency. J. Immunol. **15:** 700–704.

7. ISHII, N., T. TAKESHITA, Y. KIMURA, K. TADA, M. KONDO, M. NAKAMURA & K. SUGAMURA. 1994. Expression of the IL-2 receptor γ chain on various populations in human peripheral blood. Int. Immunol. **6:** 1273–1277.

8. ORLIC, D., L.J. GIRARD, D. LEE, S.M. ANDERSON, J.M. PUCK & D.M. BODINE. 1997. Interleukin-7R alpha mRNA expression increases as stem cells differentiate into T and B lymphocyte progenitors. Exp. Hematol. **25:**217–222.

9. HENTHORN, P.S., R.L. SOMBERG, V.M. FIMIANI, J.M. PUCK, D.F. PATTERSON & P.J. FELSBURG. 1994. IL2Rγ gene microdeletion demonstrates that canine X-linked severe combined immunodeficiency is a homologue of the human disease. Genomics **23:**69–74.

10. DUNBAR, C.E., N.E. SIEDEL, S. DOREN, S. SELLERS, A.P. CLINE, M.E. METZGER, B.A. AGRICOLA, R.E. DONAHUE & D.M. BODINE. 1996. Improved retroviral gene transfer into murine and rhesus peripheral blood or bone marrow repopulation cells *in vivo* with stem cell factor and granulocyte colony stimulating factor. Proc. Natl. Acad. Sci. USA **93:** 11871–11876.

11. ORLIC, D., L.J. GIRARD, S.M. ANDERSON, L.C. PYLE, M.C. YODER, H.E. BROXMEYER & D.M. BODINE. 1998. Identification of human and mouse hematopoietic stem cell (HSC) population expressing high levels of mRNA encoding retrovirus receptor. Blood **91:** 3247–3254.

12. WHITWAM, T., M.E. HASKINS, P.S. HENTHORN, J.N. KRASZEWSKI, S.E. KLEIMAN, N.E. SEIDEL, D.M. BODINE & J.M. PUCK. 1998. Retroviral marking of canine bone marrow: long term, high level expression of human IL-2 receptor common gamma chain in canine lymphocytes. Blood **92**. In press.

13. KLEIMAN, S.E., I. PATSAN, J.M. PUCK & M.M. GOTTESMAN. 1998. Characterization of an MDR1 retroviral bicistronic vector for correction of X-linked severe combined immunodeficiency. Gene Ther. **5:** 671–676.

14. STEAD, R.B., W.W. KWOK, R. STORB & A.D. MILLER. 1998. Canine model for gene therapy: inefficient gene expression in dogs reconstituted with autologous marrow infected with retroviral vectors. Blood **71:** 742–747.

15. BARQUINERO, J., H.-P. KIEM, C. VON KALLE, B. DAROVSKY, S. GOEHLE, T.C. GRAHAM, K. SEIDEL, R. STORB & F.G. SCHEUNING. 1995. Myelosuppressive conditioning improves autologus engraftment of genetically marked hematopoietic repopulating cells in dogs. Blood **85:** 1195–1201.

16. BIENZLE, D., A.C.G. ABRAMS-OGG, S.A. KRUTH, J. ACKLIND-SNOW, R.F. CARTER, J.E. DICK, R.M. JACOBS, S. KAMEL-REID & I.D. DUBÉ. 1994. Gene transfer into hematopoietic stem cells: long-term maintenance of *in vitro* activated progenitors without marrow ablation. Proc. Nat. Acad. Sci. USA **91:** 350–354.

17. KIEM, H.-P., B. DAROVSKY, C. VON KALLE, S. GOEHLE, T.C. GRAHAM, A.D. MILLER, R. STORB & F.G. SCHEUNING. 1996. Long term persistance of canine hematopoietic cells genetically marked by retrovirus vectors. Hum. Gene Ther. **7:** 89–96.

18. SHULL, R., X. LU, I.D. DUBÉ, C. LUTZKO, S.A. KRUTH, A.C.G. ABRAMS-OGG, H.-P. KIEM, S. GOEHLE, F.G. SCHUENING, C MILLAN & R.F. CARTER. 1996. Humoral immune response limits gene therapy in canine MPS I [letter]. Blood **88:** 377–379.

19. BUNTING, K.D., M.Y. SANGSTER, J,N, IHLE & B.P. SORRENTINO. 1998. Restoration of lymphocyte function in Janus kinase 3-deficient mice by retroviral-mediated gene transfer. Nat. Med. **4:** 58–64.

Effects of Several Cytokine Combinations on Retrovirus-Mediated Human MDR1 Gene Transfer into Bone Marrow Hematopoietic Cells

S. ZHOU,[a] Y. TONG, P.H. TANG, AND N. MAO

Department of Cell Biology, Institute of Basic Medical Sciences, Beijing, China

INTRODUCTION

Cytokine prestimulation of hematopoietic cells has been routine in gene transfer by retrovirus vectors. Kit ligand (KL), interleukin-3 (IL-3) and interleukin-6 (IL-6) are the most widely used cytokine combination.[1,2] Flt3 ligand (FL) and thrombopoietin (TPO) were reported to stimulate the expansion of primitive progenitor cells from cord blood and/or bone marrow.[3,4] Here we compare the effects of several cocktails of cytokines including KL, IL-3, IL-6, FL, and TPO on retrovirus-mediated mdr1 gene transfer into bone marrow hematopoietic cells.

MATERIALS AND METHODS

Retrovirus vector containing human mdr1 cDNA (SF-MDR) was kindly provided by C. Baum.[5] The vector was packaged in an amphotropic packaging cell line PA317. The titer of the virus was 2×10^5 cfu/ml and 2×10^4 cfu/ml when NIH3T3 cells and K562 cells were used as target cells of titering, respectively. Human bone marrow was obtained from individuals donating marrow for allogeneic transplantation with informed consent. Mononuclear cells were separated by centrifugation on a Ficoll-gradient. CD34$^+$ cells were enriched by a magnetic beads based magnetic-activated cell sorting (MACS) CD34 progenitor cell isolation kit (Myltenyi Biotech GmbH, Germany) according to the manufacturer's instructions. The purity of CD34$^+$ cells was more than 75% by fluorescence-activated cell sorting (FACS) analysis. The enriched CD34$^+$ cells were incubated in 1 ml Iscove's modified Dulbecco's medium (IMDM, Gibco-BRL) supplemented with 15% fetal calf serum (FCS), 1% bovine serum albumin (Stemcell Technologies Inc. Canada), 2 mM L-glutamine, 10^{-4} M 2-mecaptoethanol and cytokines at a concentration of 2×10^5 /ml in 24-well plates (Nunc, Denmark). Recombinant human KL(SCF) was from Amgen. FL, TPO, IL-3 and IL-6 were from Pepro Tech EC Ltd. KL and FL were used at 50 ng/ml; IL-3, IL-6 and TPO were used at 10 ng/ml. After 48 hours of incubation at 37°C, 1 ml fresh cell-free virus supernatant was added with 8 µg protamine (Sigma) and cytok-

[a]Corresponding author: S. Zhou, Department of Cell Biology, Institute of Basic Medical Sciences, 27 Taiping Road, Beijing 100850, P.R. China. Phone, (010)-66931320; fax, (010)-68213039; e-mail, s.zhou@cenpok.net

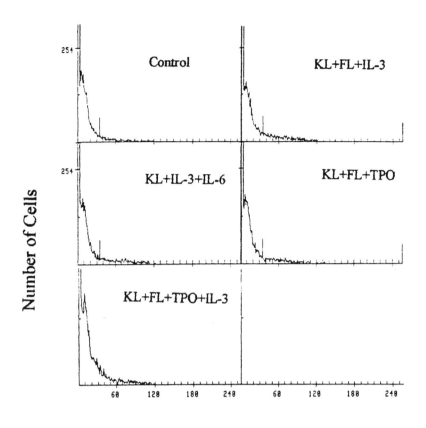

Fluorescence

FIGURE 1. Expression of P-glycoprotein on bone marrow hematopoietic cells after mdr1 gene transfer in the presence of various cytokine combinations. The cells were indirectly labeled with murine antihuman mdr1 monoclonal antibody (UIC2) and FITC-goat antimurine IgG and analyzed by a FACS440 machine. Four control groups had similar expression of P-glycoprotein and only one is included in the figure.

ines and incubated at 33°C. This process was repeated three times on three consecutive days except that 1 ml supernatant was removed from the culture before the second and third addition of virus. The cells were incubated for another four days at 37°C, collected and indirectly labeled with murine monoclonal antihuman P-glycoprotein antibody (UIC2) and fluorescein isothiocyanate (FITC)-goat antimurine immunoglobulin G (IgG, Immunotech S.A). The cells were analyzed by a FACS machine (FACS440, Becton Dickinson) for P-glycoprotein expression on the cell membrane.

RESULTS

Though KL + IL-3 + IL-6 was commonly used, other cocktails of cytokines may further increase the efficiency of retrovirus-mediated gene transfer into hematopoietic cells. In our experimental system here, the transduction efficiency of the KL + IL-3 + IL-6 group was 4.3% by analysis of cell membrane P-glycoprotein expression, while in the KL + FL + IL-3 group, the efficiency significantly increased to 8.4%. In the KL + FL + TPO and the KL + FL + TPO + IL-3 groups, the transduction efficiency was 2.1% and 4.0%, respectively (FIG. 1). Why addition of TPO to the KL + FL + IL-3 group decreased the transfer efficiency is unknown. The total number of cells after the nine days of culture increased 2.5-fold in the KL + FL + TPO group and 5-fold in the other groups.

DISCUSSION

The clinical results of mdr1 gene as well as other gene transfer into human hematopoietic cells as a gene therapy approach are disappointing. The main reason was supposed to be the low efficiency of gene transfer. Cytokine prestimulation of hematopoietic cells has been proved to increase gene transfer efficiency to some degree. Petzer *et al.* reported that KL + FL + IL-3 were necessary and sufficient to stimulate about 30-fold amplification of bone marow long-term culture-initiating cells (LTC-ICs) within 10 days.[3] Here we show that the same cytokine combination is superior to KL + IL-3 + IL-6 in enhancing retrovirus-mediated gene transfer into bone marrow hematopoietic cells and can be applied in future hematopoietic cell gene transfer experiments.

CONCLUSION

Increase of the efficiency of gene transfer into human hematopoietic cells may contribute to the clinical application of gene therapy. Several cytokine combinations including KL + IL-3 + IL-6, KL + FL + IL-3, KL + FL + TPO, and KL + FL + TPO + IL-3 were compared for their enhancing effect on retrovirus-mediated human mdr1 gene transfer into bone marrow hematopoietic cells. The mdr1 gene transfer efficiency in the presence of these cocktails of cytokines was 4.3%, 8.4%, 2.1%, and 4.0%, respectively, with the KL + FL + IL-3 group the most effective cytokine combination.

ACKNOWLEDGMENT

This work was supported by National High-Tech Grant BH-03.

REFERENCES

1. NOLTA, J.A., E.M. SMOGORZEWSKA & D.B. KHON. 1995. Analysis of optimal conditions for retroviral-mediated transduction of primitive human hematopoietic cells. Blood **86:** 101–110.

2. XU, L.C., S. KARLSSON, E.R. BYRNE, S. KLUEPFEL-STAHL, S.W. KESSLER, B.A. AGRI-
COLA, S. SELLERS, M. KIRBY, C.E. DUNBAR, R.O. BRADY, A.W. NIENHUIS & R.E.
DONAHUE. 1995. Long-term *in vivo* expression of the human glucocerebrosidase
gene in nonhuman primates after CD34+ hematopoietic cell transduction with
cell-free retroviral vector preparations. Proc. Natl. Acad. Sci. USA **92:** 4372–4376.
3. PETZER, A.L., P.W. ZANDSTRA, J.M. PIRET & C.J. EAVES. 1996. Differential cytokine
effects on primitive (CD34+CD38−) human hematopoietic cells: novel responses to
Flt3-ligand and thrombopoietin. J. Exp. Med. **183:** 2551–2558.
4. PIACIBELLO, W., F. SANAVIO, L. GARETTO, A. SEVERINO, D. BERGANDI, J. FERRARIO,
F. FAGIOLI, M. BERGER & M. AGLIETTA. 1997. Extensive amplification and
self-renewal of human primitive hematopoietic stem cells from cord blood. Blood
89: 2644–2653.
5. ECKERT, H.G., M. STOCKSCHLADER, U. JUST, S. HEGEWISCH-BECKER, M. GREZ, A.
UHDE, A. ZANDER, W. OSTERTAG & C. BAUM. 1996. High-dose multidrug resistance
in primary human hematopoietic progenitor cells transduced with optimized retroviral vectors. Blood **88:** 3407–3415.

Thrombopoietin and Interleukin-3 Are Chemotactic and Chemokinetic Chemoattractants for a Factor-Dependent Hematopoietic Progenitor Cell Line

CHANG H. KIM AND HAL E. BROXMEYER[a]

Departments of Microbiology/Immunology and Medicine and the Walther Oncology Center, Indiana University School of Medicine, Indianapolis, Indiana 46202, and the Walther Cancer Institute, Indianapolis, Indiana 46208, USA

Chemoattractants are possible regulatory signals for migration of hematopoietic progenitor cells (HPCs). Stromal cell-derived factor (SDF)-1 and steel factor are examples of HPC chemoattractants.[1] Thrombopoietin (TPO) induces megakaryocyte progenitor expansion and differentiation, and proliferation, survival and adhesion of diverse types of HPCs.[2–4] Interleukin-3 (IL-3) is an early-acting growth factor that induces adhesion of mature and immature hematopoietic cells to an extracellular matrix (ECM) component, fibronectin (FN),[5] and chemotaxis of eosinophils.[6] TPO induces mobilization of multipotent bone marrow (BM) HPCs to the periphery,[7] and IL-3 enhances granulocyte colony-stimulating factor (G-CSF)-induced mobilization of HPCs.[8] We examined whether TPO and IL-3 have chemotactic (directed movement) and/or chemokinetic (random movement) activity for the human factor-dependent cell line, MO7e cells. MO7e cells are ideal cells to study the chemotactic and chemokinetic effects of TPO and IL-3, because the proliferation/survival responsiveness of MO7e cells to both cytokines was previously established.[3] A chemotaxis chamber with two chambers (upper and lower), and a membrane (5 μm pore size) separating the two chambers was used.[1] MO7e cells were added to the upper chamber, and TPO, IL-3, and/or G-CSF were added to the upper and/or lower chambers in a combinatory manner to examine the chemoattractant effects of these cytokines. When TPO was added to the lower chamber, it induced a significant migration of MO7e cells, demonstrating the chemotactic activity of TPO (FIG. 1A). We also added TPO to both chambers to examine the possible chemokinetic effect of TPO. In this condition, TPO also induced significant migration of MO7e cells to the lower chamber (FIG. 1A). IL-3 in the lower chamber or both chambers induced MO7e cell migration to the lower chamber, an effect more potent than that of TPO (FIG. 1A). Thus TPO and IL-3 demonstrated both chemotactic and chemokinetic effects. However, G-CSF, another mobilizing cytokine for HPCs, did not show chemotactic or chemokinetic effects on MO7e cells (FIG. 1A). ECM proteins such as FN are important for HPCs to migrate by providing substratum for cells to attach

---

[a]Address correspondence to Dr. Hal E. Broxmeyer, Department of Microbiology/Immunology and the Walther Oncology Center, Indiana University School of Medicine, Building R4, Rm 302, 1044 West Walnut Street, Indianapolis, IN 46202. Phone, 317/ 274-7510; fax, 317/274-7592; e-mail, hbroxmey@iupui.edu

and move. Thus, we examined the chemotactic and chemokinetic effects of TPO and IL-3 using transwell membranes that had been coated with FN. In this adhesive condition, TPO and IL-3 again showed chemotactic and chemokinetic activity for MO7e cells, and the TPO- and IL-3-dependent chemotactic and chemokinetic activity were enhanced by at least six fold (FIG. 1B), when compared to the experiments using bare

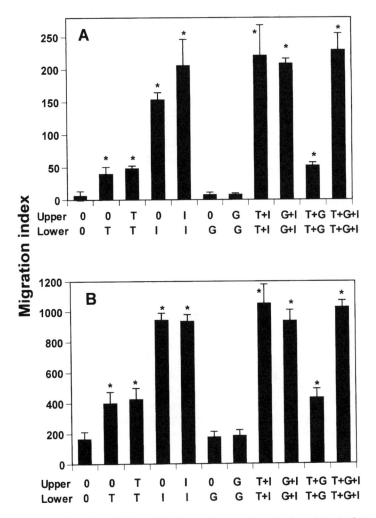

FIGURE 1. Thrombopoietin and IL-3 are chemotactic and chemokinetic factors for MO7e cells. 2.5×10^5 cells were used for input cells. Costar transwells were used without coating (**A**), or coated with 50 μg/ml FN (Collaborative Biomedical, Bedford, MA) (**B**), and chemotaxis was allowed to occur for 14 hr. Cells migrating into the lower chamber were counted by FACscan for 20 sec (migration index). TPO (T, final concentration of 20 ng/ml), IL-3 (I, final concentration of 400 U/ml), and G-CSF (G, final concentration of 400 U/ml) were added to the upper or lower chamber as indicated. *Significant migration ($p < 0.05$) compared to medium control.

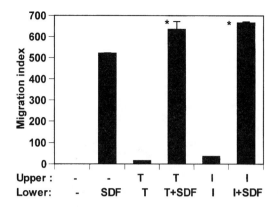

FIGURE 2. TPO and IL-3 enhance the chemotactic activity of SDF-1. Experiments were performed as in FIGURE 1 except that bare transwells were used, and chemotaxis was allowed to progress for 5 hr. *Significant enhancement ($p < 0.05$) compared to SDF-1 alone.

membranes (FIG. 1A). G-CSF, again, had no chemotactic or chemokinetic activity in this condition (FIG. 1B). We next examined the effect of TPO and IL-3 on SDF-1-dependent chemotaxis of MO7e cells. The chemotaxis chambers with cells were incubated for 5 hr, since SDF-1-induced chemotaxis is quicker and more efficacious than that of TPO and IL-3 (FIGS. 1 and 2). TPO and IL-3 were added to the both upper and lower chambers, and SDF-1 was added only to the lower chamber. In this situation, TPO and IL-3 significantly enhanced the chemotactic activity of SDF-1 (FIG. 2). This enhancing effect of TPO and IL-3 is not a simple additive effect, since it was greater than the sum of TPO- or IL-3-induced migration and SDF-1-dependent migration (FIG. 2). TPO and IL-3-dependent MO7e cell movement is better detected when the experiments were incubated for longer time (e.g., 14 hr), which suggests that TPO and IL-3 induce movement of cells slowly and consistently. This is different from that of SDF-1, because SDF-1-dependent cell movement occurs mainly within 5 hr when there is still an effective gradient of SDF-1.[1] This study demonstrates for the first time that TPO has chemoattractant activity for hematopoietic cells, and that IL-3 has chemotactic and chemokinetic activity for the factor-dependent cell line, MO7e.

ACKNOWLEDGMENTS

This work was supported by US Public Health Service Grants R01 DK 53674, R01 HL 56416, and R01 HL 54037, and by a project in National Institutes of Health Grant P01 HL 53586 to Hal. E. Broxmeyer.

REFERENCES

1. KIM, C.H. & H.E. BROXMEYER. 1998. *In vitro* behavior of hematopoietic progenitor cells under the influence of chemoattractants: SDF-1, steel factor and the bone marrow environment. Blood **91:** 100–110.
2. KAUSHANSKY, K. 1988. Thrombopoietin and the hematopoietic stem cell. Blood **92:** 1–3.
3. RITCHIE, A., S. VADHAN RAJ & H.E. BROXMEYER. 1996. Thrombopoietin suppresses apoptosis and behaves as a survival factor for the human growth factor-dependent cell line, M07e. Stem Cells **14:** 330–336.
4. GOTOH, A., A. RITCHIE, H. TAKAHIRA & H.E. BROXMEYER. 1997. Thrombopoietin and erythropoietin activate inside-out signaling of integrin and enhance adhesion to immobilized fibronectin in human growth-factor-dependent hematopoietic cells. Ann. Hematol. **75:** 207–213.
5. CONGET, P. & J.J. MINGUELL. 1995. IL-3 increases surface proteoglycan synthesis in haemopoietic progenitors and their adhesiveness to the heparin-binding domain of fibronectin. Br. J. Haematol. **89:** 1–7.
6. WARRINGA, R.A., L. KOENDERMAN, P.T. KOK, J. KREUKNIET & P.L. BRUIJNZEEL. 1991. Modulation and induction of eosinophil chemotaxis by granulocyte-macrophage colony-stimulating factor and interleukin-3. Blood **77:** 2694–2270.
7. CAVER-MOORE, K., H.E. BROXMEYER, S.-M. LUOH, S. COOPER, J. PENG, S. BURNSTEIN, M.W. MOORE & F.J. DESAUVAGE. 1996. Low levels of eryhtroid and myeloid progenitors in TPO and c-mpl deficient mice. Blood **88:** 803–808.
8. GEISSLER, K., C. PESCHEL, D. NIEDERWIESER, J. GOLDSCHMITT, F. HLADIK, A. FRITZ, L. OHLER, P. BETTELHEIM, C. HUBER, K. LECHNER *et al.* 1995. Effect of interleukin-3 pretreatment on granulocyte/macrophage colony-stimulating factor induced mobilization of circulating haemopoietic progenitor cells. Br. J. Haematol. **91:** 299–305.

A Human Factor-Dependent Cell Line Simulates Cobblestone Formation under Human Bone Marrow Stromal Cells *In Vitro*

CHARLIE R. MANTEL, ALESSANDRA BALDUINI, AND HAL E. BROXMEYER[a]

Departments of Microbiology/Immunology and Medicine and the Walther Oncology Center, Indiana University School of Medicine, Indianapolis, Indiana 46202, and the Walther Cancer Institute, Indianapolis, Indiana 46208, USA

Homing and local migration of hematopoietic progenitor and stem cells to stromal niches are critical to normal hematopoiesis and also to bone marrow and cord blood transplantation. Cells isolated from patients with acute and chronic myeloid and lymphoid leukemias are often defective in their stromal cell interactions. The mechanisms involved in these adhesion-dependent processes are poorly understood. *In vitro* studies using cell populations enriched for human hematopoietic progenitors and human stromal cell cultures have revealed that these primitive cells spontaneously migrate "under" a type of stromal cell sometimes referred to as a "blanket" cell.[1] As the progenitors multiply and differentiate, a characteristic structure called a "cobblestone" colony forms.[2] These cobblestone areas are most obvious when observed with a phase contrast microscope, which reveals cells that are under other cells as dark, flattened, and nonrefractive. Very little is known about the nature of the relationship between the progenitors and the blanket cell on a molecular level.

The study of hematopoietic progenitors has been hampered by their rarity, and many biochemical and genetic studies have relied on use of hematopoietic cell lines as models. One such cell line is MO7e. It is a human factor-dependent leukemic cell line that expresses various cytokine receptors on its surface and has been particularly useful in mechanistic studies of cytokine signal transduction.[3] In addition, model cell lines lend themselves well to genetic manipulation, allowing a wide range of other studies to be done.

We previously used MO7e cells as a model to study cytokine signal transduction,[4] cell cycle regulation,[5] growth factor responses,[6] and cell adhesion.[7] To begin to study molecules involved in the progenitor/blanket cell interactions, we have again turned to MO7e cells. We have now evaluated if MO7e cells will migrate under *in vitro* cultured human bone marrow-derived stromal cells similarly to primary human progenitors. We report here that MO7e cells behave in a similar fashion to primary human hematopoietic progenitor cells with respect to their migratory behavior *in vitro*, and thus may provide a convenient and useful model to study the migration/ interaction behavior of human progenitors on a molecular level. FIGURE 1 shows several examples of MO7e cells that have migrated under a stromal cell resembling

[a]Address correspondence to Dr. Hal E. Broxmeyer, Department of Microbiology/Immunology and the Walther Oncology Center, Indiana University School of Medicine, Building R4, Rm 302, 1044 West Walnut Street, Indianapolis, IN 46202. Phone, 317/ 274-7510; fax, 317/274-7592; e-mail, hbroxmey@iupui.edu

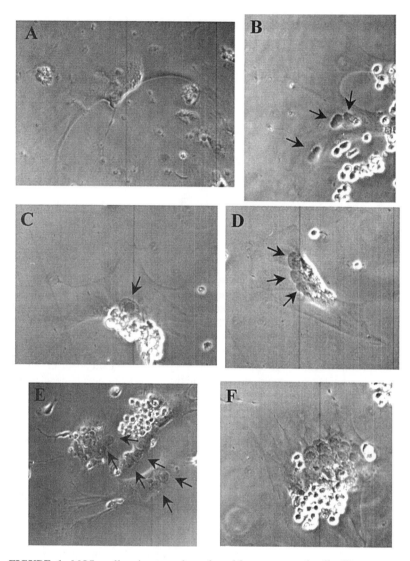

FIGURE 1. MO7e cells migrate under cultured human stromal cells. Phase-contrast photomicrographs of MO7e cells added to human bone marrow stromal cell cultures, which were established as previously described.[8] MO7e cells were added 48 hours after stromal culture setup so that individual stromal cells could be more easily visualized. (A) Blanket cell without MO7e cells. (B–F) Blanket cells with one or more MO7e cells under and adhered to the top surface. *Arrows* indicate phase-dark MO7e cells that are under the blanket cells. The original photomicrographs were digitally scanned, cropped, combined, and reproduced.

a blanket cell (MO7e cells under the blanket cells appear flat and dark; MO7e cells adhered to the top of the blanket cells are round and refractile). MO7e cells appear to begin migration at the lamellipods of the blanket cell (FIG. 1B) and are frequently found migrating toward the central region of the blanket cell (FIG. 1C–E). Other MO7e cells are seen to adhere to the surface of the blanket cell. This phenomenon begins within minutes of adding the MO7e cells to the stromal cultures and continues for at least three days. Once under, MO7e cells appear to remain there for the duration of the culture period. Sometimes so many MO7e cells crowd under the blanket cell that it appears to be "lifted" off the surface of the dish (FIG. 1F). We have not yet evaluated the growth kinetics of MO7e cells under the blanket cells.

We believe this behavior is similar to cobblestone formation by normal human progenitors. Further studies using this system as a model may help facilitate the identification of the molecules and processes that are important for stromal/progenitor cell interactions.

ACKNOWLEDGMENTS

This work was supported by US Public Health Service Grants R01 DK 53674, R01 HL 56416, and R01 HL 54037, and by a project in National Institutes of Health Grant P01 HL 53586 to Hal E. Broxmeyer.

REFERENCES

1. ALLEN, T.D. & T.M. DEXTER. 1984. The essential cells of the hematopoietic microenvironment. Exp. Hematol. **12:** 517–521.
2. ALLEN, T.D., T.M. DEXTER & P.J. SIMMONS. 1990. Colony Stimulating Factors: Molecules and Cellular Biology. Marcel Dekker. New York.
3. MIYAZAWA, K., P.C. HENDRIE, C. MANTEL, K. WOOD, L.K. ASHMAN & H.E. BROXMEYER. 1991. Comparative analysis of signaling pathways between mast cell growth factor (c-kit ligand) and granulocyte-macrophage colony-stimulating factor in a human factor-dependent myeloid cell line involves phosphorylation of Raf-1, GTP-ase activating protein and mitogen-activated protein kinase. Exp. Hematol. **19:** 1110–1123.
4. TAUCHI, T., G.S. FENG, M.S. MARSHALL, R. SHEN, C. MANTEL, T. PAWSON & H.E. BROXMEYER. 1994. The ubiquitously expressed syp phosphatase interacts with c-kit and grb-2 in hematopoietic cells. J. Biol. Chem. **269:** 25206–25211.
5. MANTEL, C., Z. LUO, J. CANFIELD, S. BRAUN, C. DENG & H.E. BROXMEYER. 1996. Involvement of p21cip-1 and p27kip-1 in the molecular mechanisms of steel factor induced proliferative synergy *in vitro* and of p21cip-1 in the maintenance of stem/progenitor cells *in vivo*. Blood **88:** 3710–3719.
6. MIYAZAWA, K., K. TOYAMA, A. GOTOH, P.C. HENDRIE, C. MANTEL & H.E. BROXMEYER. 1994. Ligand-dependent polyubiquitinization of c-kit gene product: a possible mechanism of receptor down modulation in MO7e cells. Blood **83:** 137–145.
7. GOTOH, A., A. RITCHIE, H. TAKAHIRA & H.E. BROXMEYER. 1997. Thrombopoietin and erythropoietin activate inside-out signaling of integrin and enhance adhesion to immobilized fibronectin in human growth-factor-dependent hematopoietic cells. Ann. Hematol. **75:** 207–213.
8. BALDUINI, A., S.E. BRAUN, K. CORNETTA, S. LYMAN & H.E. BROXMEYER. 1998. Comparative effects of retroviral-mediated gene transfer into primary human stromal cells of flt3-ligand, interleukin-3 and GM-CSF on production of cord blood progenitor cells in long-term culture. Stem Cells **16:** 37–49.

Index of Contributors